ALLE · ZEIT · WACH
1842

HLA Class II Antigens

A Comprehensive Review of Structure and Function

Edited by B. G. Solheim, E. Møller, S. Ferrone

With 128 Figures and 91 Tables

Springer-Verlag
Berlin Heidelberg New York Tokyo

Director Bjarte G. Solheim

Blood Bank and Immunohematological Laboratory
Rikshospitalet, National Hospital
Pilestredet 32
N-0027 Oslo 1/Norway

Professor Erna Møller

Karolinska Institute
Department of Clinical Immunology
Huddinge Hospital
S-141 86 Huddinge/Sweden

Professor Soldano Ferrone

Dept. of Microbiology and Immunology
New York Medical College
Valhalla, NY 10595/USA

ISBN-13:978-3-642-70369-0 e-ISBN-13:978-3-642-70367-6
DOI: 10.1007/978-3-642-70367-6

Library on Congress Cataloging in Publication Data. Main entry under title: HLA Class II Antigens. A Comprehensive Review of Structure and Function. 1. HLA Class II Antigens. I. Solheim, Bjarte G. II. Møller, Erna. III. Ferrone, Soldano, 1940– . IV. Title: HLA Class II Antigens. A Comprehensive Review of Structure and Function.
[DNLM: 1. HLA Antigens. WO 680 H918] QR184.32.H86 616.07'92 85-27945

Softcover reprint of the hardcover 1st edition 1986

Typesetting: Brühlsche Universitätsdruckerei, Giessen;

2123/3020-543210

Foreword

This volume deals with the structure and function of molecules that have, during the last decade, turned out to have a central role in immune responses. Transplantation antigens were discovered and characterized by Gorer about 50 years ago, and the biological basis for the unequalled complexity of their variability between individuals within a species, in spite of extreme conservation between species, was the subject of intense research and discussion for many years.

During the days of belief in "immune surveillance" against spontaneously developing tumors, it was suggested that histoincompatibility between members of one species would prevent cancer from being a contagious disease and thus a threat to the species.

Immunologists involved in human transplantation had to learn and care about the complexity, especially after 1967, when it was found that HLA antigens were the products of the human MHC. Rejection of HLA-identical sib kidney grafts was so rare, even in those days, that cases of rejection were described in scientific papers.

MLC reactivity correlated to transplant survival, whereas HLA "typing" for HLA-A and B antigens did not, as discussed by Terasaki at the Third Transplantation Society Congress in 1970. These findings came at a time when it was clarified that MLC activation is controlled by genes linked to, but separate from, the HLA-A and B antigens. Van Leeuwen et al. and Cone and Sachs described the class II antigens in man and mouse in 1973. They demonstrated that MLC activation could be inhibited by certain non-HLA-A,B antibodies and that the corresponding antigens were present on B but not on T lymphoid cells. These findings were subsequently confirmed by a number of investigators during the Fifth Histocompatibility Workshop in 1975. Data about the genetic organization of HLA class II antigens were one of the major topics at the Sixth Histocompatibility Workshop in 1977. These important discoveries formed the basis for the studies on the structure and function of HLA class II antigens, one of the most important research areas in immunogenetics and transplantation immunology today.

The first clear evidence of strong associations between HLA and disease was published in 1972. The knowledge of HLA genetics and the biological function of these molecules became of interest to an increasing scientific community. When Zinkernagel and Doherty, in 1973–1974, published data on the importance of MHC products as restriction elements, recognized in association with foreign antigenic determinants by T lymphocytes, the MHC molecules suddenly hit the front pages of all major immunology journals. Soon, it was also firmly established that the polymorphic class II antigens were, in fact, the true products of IR genes. Most probably class I antigens serve the same function for responses mediated by cytotoxic T cells. Thus class I and II antigens serve as markers for "self" in the ontogenetic development and selection of individual-specific T cell repertoires.

The fact that T cells can be either class I or class II restricted forms one of the bases for their subdivision into separate populations.

The MHC antigens are part of the "Ig super-gene" family, and share ancestral genes with immunoglobulins, T cell specific receptors, and certain other receptors involved in activation and regulation of T cells. The knowledge of the MHC antigens and their genes is basic in fundamental immunology and, in addition, has become increasingly important for the understanding of the pathogenesis of the long list of HLA-linked diseases. The new, refined, and rapid biochemical techniques, the use of monoclonal antibodies for purification and characterization, and the modern techniques of molecular biology and genetics have proven exceedingly fruitful for sulfit and clear evaluation of these genes and their products. A basic knowledge of structure is absolutely necessary for the understanding of evolution and the biological relevance of polymorphism of these molecules.

We believe that this is the optimal moment for the publication of a book on HLA class II antigens. Many questions are not yet resolved, but the knowledge has reached a level of sophistication that will form the basis for answers to some intriguing and relevant questions within the foreseeable future.

This volume gives a comprehensive up-to-date review of the HLA class II antigens. Many of the foremost scientists in the field contribute articles focused on their particular fields of interest and present updated and often unpublished information. The editors drew up the principal guidelines, and ensured that the volume covers both structure and function of HLA class II antigens, as well as their possible clinical relevance. Questions of major interest are, if possible, covered by contributions from more than one research group. The editors have also taken care that the chapters can be read as separate entities, although this inevitably results in some overlapping. We hope that the information presented in this way will be of interest to both nonexperts and experts in the HLA field.

We would like to thank all contributors for their cooperation and interest in preparing their chapters, and we are grateful to the publisher for the help during the various phases of preparation of this volume.

Bjarte G. Solheim
Erna Møller
Soldano Ferrone

List of Contributors

Accolla, R. S.
Ludwig Institute for Cancer Research, Lausanne Branch, Department of Biochemistry, University of Lausanne, 1066 Epalinges, Switzerland

Albrechtsen, D. H.
Kirurgisk avdeling B, Rikshospitalet, Pilestredet 32, 0027 Oslo 1, Norway

Ameglio, F.
Laboratorio di Biologia Cellulare, CNR, via Romagnosi 18A, and Regina Elena National Institute, viale Regina Elena 291, Roma, Italy

Ando, A.
Department of Transplantation, Tokai University, Isehara, Kanagawa, Japan 259-11

Anichini, A.
Immunobiology Research Center, Department of Lab. Med. and Pathol., Medical School, University of Minnesota, Box 724 Mayo Memorial Building, Minneapolis, MN 55455, USA

Bach, F.
Immunobiology Research Center, Department of Lab. Med. and Pathol., Medical School, University of Minnesota, Box 724 Mayo Memorial Building, Minneapolis, MN 55455, USA

Barnikol, H. U.
Max-Planck-Institut für Experimentelle Medizin, Abteilung Immunchemie, Hermann-Rein-Straße 3, 3400 Göttingen, FRG

Bell, J. I.
Dept. of Med. Microbiology, Stanford Univ. School of Medicine, Stanford, CA 94305, USA

Berg, K. J.
Medisinsk avdeling B, Rikshospitalet, Pilestredet 32, 0027 Oslo 1, Norway

Broudy, V. C.
Veterans Administration Medical Center, 3710 Southwest U.S. Veterans Hospital Road, P.O. Box 1034, Portland, OR 97207, USA

Bruserud, Ø.
Institute for Transplantation Immunology, Rikshospitalet, Pilestredet 32, 0027 Oslo 1, Norway

Carlsson, B.
Karolinska Institute, Department of Clinical Immunology and Center for Biotechnology, Huddinge Hospital, 141 86 Huddinge, Sweden

Carrel, S.
Ludwig Institute for Cancer Research, Lausanne Branch, Department of Biochemistry, University of Lausanne, 1066 Epalinges, Switzerland

Collins, T.
Dept. of Pathology, Brigham and Women's Hospital, Boston, MA 02115, USA

Colombani, J.
Inst. de Recherches sur les Maladies du Sang, Hôpital Saint Louis, 1, avenue Claude Vellefaux, 75010 Paris, France

Corredor, V.
Division of Immunogenetics, Dana-Farber Cancer Institute, 44 Binney Street, Boston, MA 02115, USA

Corte, G.
Universita degli Studi di Genova, Istituto Nationale per la Ricerca sul Cancro, Viale Benedetto XV, 16132 Genova, Italy

Curtoni, E. S.
Istituto di Genetica Medica dell'Università di Torino, Via Santena 19, 10126 Torino, Italy

Dolei, A.
Istituto di Virologia, Università di Roma, viale di Porta Tiburtina 28, Roma, Italy and Cattedra di Patologia Generale, Università di Camerino, Camerino, Italy

Duquesnoy, R.
University of Pittsburgh, Rm. 406, Scaife Hall, Pittsburgh, PA 15261, USA

Fainboim, L.
The London Hospital Medical College, Department of Immunology (Univ. of London), Turner Street, London E1 2AD, England

Ferremi, P.
Ludwig Institute for Cancer Research, Lausanne Branch, Department of Biochemistry, University of Lausanne, 1066 Epalinges, Switzerland

Ferrone, S.
Department of Microbiology and Immunology, New York Medical College, Valhalla, New York 10595, USA

Festenstein, H.
The London Hospital Medical College, Department of Immunology (Univ. of London), Turner Street, London E1 2AD, England

Fitchen, J.H.
Veterans Administration Medical Center, 3710 Southwest U.S. Veterans Hospital Road, P.O. Box 1034, Portland, OR 97207, USA

Flatmark, A.
Kirurgisk avdeling B, Rikshospitalet, Pilestredet 32, 0027 Oslo 1, Norway

Forsum, U.
Department Clinical Bacteriology, Box 552, 75122 Uppsala, Sweden

Giuffré, L.
Ludwig Institute for Cancer Research, Lausanne Branch, Department of Biochemistry, University of Lausanne, 1066 Epalinges, Switzerland

Götz, H.
Max-Planck-Institut für Experimentelle Medizin, Abteilung Immunchemie, Hermann-Rein-Straße 3, 3400 Göttingen, FRG

Goyert, S.M.
Cellular and Molecular Biology Unit, Dept. of Rheumatic Diseases, Hospital of Joint Diseases Orthopaedic Institute, 301 E 17th Street, New York, NY 10003, USA

Hilschmann, N.
Max-Planck-Institut für Experimentelle Medizin, Abteilung Immunchemie, Hermann-Rein-Straße 3, 3400 Göttingen, FRG

Igarashi, M.
Department of Microbiology and Immunology, New York Medical College, Valhalla, New York 10595, USA

Ikewaki, N.
Department of Transplantation, Tokai University, Isehara, Kanagawa, Japan 259-11

Imberti, L.
Department of Microbiology and Immunology, New York Medical College, Valhalla, New York 10595, USA

Inoko, H.
Department of Transplantation, Tokai University, Isehara, Kanagawa, Japan 259-11

Ivanyi, P.
Central Laboratory of the Netherlands Red Cross, Blood Transfusion Service, Plesmanlaan 125, P.O. Box 9190, 1006 AD Amsterdam, The Netherlands

Jaraquemada, D.
The London Hospital Medical College, Department of Immunology (Univ. of London), Turner Street, London E1 2AD, England

Jeannet, M.
Unité d'Immunologie de Transplantation, Hôpital Cantonal Universitaire, 1211 Genève 4, Switzerland

Klareskog, L.
Dept. of Medical and Physiological Chemistry, Box 575, 75123 Uppsala, Sweden

Kratzin, H.
Max-Planck-Institut für Experimentelle Medizin, Abteilung Immunchemie, Hermann-Rein-Straße 3, 3400 Göttingen, FRG

Kruse, T.
Max-Planck-Institut für Experimentelle Medizin, Abteilung Immunchemie, Hermann-Rein-Straße 3, 3400 Göttingen, FRG

Lepage, V.
Inst. de Recherches sur les Maladies du Sang, Hôpital Saint Louis, 1, avenue Claude Vellefaux, 75010 Paris, France

Mach, J. P.
Ludwig Institute for Cancer Research, Lausanne Branch, Department of Biochemistry, University of Lausanne, 1066 Epalinges, Switzerland

Maio, M.
Department of Microbiology and Immunology, New York Medical College, Valhalla, New York 10595, USA

Matsui, Y.
Division of Immunogenetics, Dana-Farber Cancer Institute, 44 Binney Street, Boston, MA 02115, USA

McDevitt, H. O.
Dept. of Med. Microbiology, Stanford Univ. School of Medicine, Stanford, CA 94305, USA

Møller, E.
Karolinska Institute, Department of Clinical Immunology, Huddinge Hospital, 141 86 Huddinge, Sweden

Moen, T.
Institute for Transplantation Immunology, Pilestredet 32, 0027 Oslo 1, Norway

Nakatsuji, T.
Department of Transplantation, Tokai University, Isehara, Kanagawa, Japan 259-11

Natali, P. G.
Laboratory of Immunology, Regina Elena Institute, 00161 Rome, Italy

Navarrete, C.
The London Hospital Medical College, Department of Immunology
(Univ. of London), Turner Street, London E1 2AD, England

Nose, Y.
Transplantation Immunology Center, Tokai University, Isehara, Kanagawa,
Japan 259-11

Nuñez, G.
Dept. of Internal Medicine, University of Texas, 5323 Harry Hines Boulevard,
Dallas, TX 75235, USA

Ohta, N.
Immunobiology Research Center, Department of Lab. Med. and Pathol.,
Medical School, University of Minnesota, Box 724 Mayo Memorial Building,
Minneapolis, MN 55455, USA

Pawelec, G.
Immunhaematologie, Medizinische Klinik, Abteilung Innere Medizin II,
Otfried-Müller-Straße, 7400 Tübingen, FRG

Perosa, F.
Department of Microbiology and Immunology, New York Medical College,
Valhalla, New York 10595, USA

Pescovitz, M. D.
Transplant. Biol. Section, Immunology Branch, National Cancer Institute,
Building 10, Room 4B17, Bethesda, MD 20205, USA

Peterson, P. A.
Dept. of Cell Research, The Wallenberg Laboratory, Box 562,
75122 Uppsala, Sweden

Pettaway, C.
Dept. of Internal Medicine, University of Texas, 5323 Harry Hines Boulevard,
Dallas, TX 75235, USA

Pla, M.
U 93 INSERM Hôpital Saint-Louis, 2 place du Dr A. Fournier,
75475 Paris Cedex 10, France

Pober, J. S.
Dept. of Pathology, Brigham and Women's Hospital, Boston,
MA 02115, USA

Qvigstad, E.
Institute for Transplantation Immunology, Rikshospitalet, Pilestredet 32,
0027 Oslo 1, Norway

Rask, L.
Dept. of Cell Research, The Wallenberg Laboratory, Box 562,
75122 Uppsala, Sweden

Reinsmoen, N. L.
Immunobiology Research Center, Department of Lab. Med. and Pathol.,
Medical School, University of Minnesota, Box 724 Mayo Memorial Building,
Minneapolis, MN 55455, USA

Richiardi, P.
Istituto di Genetica Medica dell' Universitá di Torino, Via Santena 19,
10126 Torino, Italy

Ruiter, D. J.
Pathologisch Laboratorium, Universitair Medisch Centrum Leiden,
Postbus 9603, 2300 RC Leiden, The Netherlands

Sachs, D. H.
Transplant. Biol. Section, Immunology Branch, National Cancer Institute,
Building 10, Room 4B17, Bethesda, MD 20205, USA

Sakaguchi, K.
Department of Microbiology and Immunology, New York Medical College,
Valhalla, New York 10595, USA

Sanchez-Perez, M.
Departamento de Microbiologia, Facultad de Farmacia, Universidad
Complutense de Madrid, Madrid, Spain

Sato, K.
Transplantation Immunology Center, Tokai University, Isehara, Kanagawa,
Japan 259-11

Schneider, E. M.
Immunhaematologie, Medizinische Klinik, Abteilung Innere Medizin II,
Otfried-Müller-Straße, 7400 Tübingen, FRG

Schreuder, G. M. T.
Department of Immunohematology and Bloodbank, University Hospital,
Leiden, Rijnsburgerweg 10,
2333 AA Leiden, The Netherlands

Shaw, S.
Immunology Branch, National Cancer Institute-NIH, Building 10, Room 4B17,
Bethesda MD 20892, USA

Silver, J.
Cellular and Molecular Biology Unit, Dept. of Rheumatic Diseases, Hospital of Joint Diseases Orthopaedic Institute, 301 E 17th Street, New York, NY 10003, USA

Sorrentino, R.
Dipartimento di Biologica Cellulare e dello Sviluppo, Università di Roma, Roma, Italy

Stastny, P.
Dept. of Internal Medicine, University of Texas, 5323 Harry Hines Boulevard, Dallas, TX 75235, USA

Steinmetz, M.
Basel Institute for Immunology, Grenzacherstraße 487, Postfach, 4005 Basel, Switzerland

Strominger, J. L.
Harvard University Med. School, Department of Biochemistry and Molecular Biology, 7 Divinity Ave., Cambridge, MA 02138, USA

Symington, F. W.
The Fred Hutchinson Cancer Research Center, Division of Oncology, Dept. of Medicine, University of Washington, 1124 Columbia Street, Seattle, 98104, USA

Tanigaki, N.
Department of Molecular Immunology, Roswell Memorial Park Institute, Buffalo, NY 14263, USA

Thinnes, F. P.
Max-Planck-Institut für Experimentelle Medizin, Abteilung Immunchemie, Hermann-Rein-Straße 3, 3400 Göttingen, FRG

Thorsby, E.
Institute for Transplantation Immunology, Rikshospitalet, Pilestredet 32, 0027 Oslo 1, Norway

Ting, A.
Nuffield Dept. of Surgery, University of Oxford, John Radcliffe Hospital, Oxford OX3 9DU, England

Torok-Storb, B.
The Fred Hutchinson Cancer Research Center, Division of Oncology, Dept. of Medicine, University of Washington, 1124 Columbia Street, Seattle, 98104, USA

Tosi, R.
Laboratorio di Biologia Cellulare, via G. Romagnosi 18 A, Roma, Italy

Tsuji, K.
Department of Transplantation and Transplantation Immunology Center, Tokai University, School of Medicine, Bhoseidai, Isehara, Kanagawa 259-11, Japan

Tsujisaki, M.
Department of Microbiology and Immunology, New York Medical College, Valhalla, New York 10595, USA

van Duinen, S.
Pathologisch Laboratorium, Universitair Medisch Centrum Leiden, Postbus 9603, 2300 RC Leiden, The Netherlands

van Leeuwen, A.
Department of Immunohematology and Bloodbank, University Hospital Leiden, Rijnsburgerweg 10, 2333 AA Leiden, The Netherlands

Wallin, J.
Karolinska Institute, Department of Clinical Immunology and Center for Biotechnology, Huddinge Hospital, 141 86 Huddinge, Sweden

Wernet, P.
Immunhaematologie, Medizinische Klinik, Abteilung Innere Medizin II, Otfried-Müller-Straße, 7400 Tübingen, FRG

Yunis, E. J.
Division of Immunogenetics, Dana-Farber Cancer Institute, 44 Binney Street, Boston, MA 02115, USA

Zeevi, A.
University of Pittsburgh, RM. 406, Scaife Hall, Pittsburgh, PA 15261, USA

Table of Contents

Cellular Detection

Regulation and Expression

Molecular Genetics

Biological Implications

Molecular Biology

Genes and Antigens of the HLA-D Region *

P. A. Peterson and L. Rask

Table of Contents

Introduction

The role of the major histocompatibility complex (MHC) in rejections of transplanted organs was recognized early. The combined efforts of immunologists and immunogeneticists demonstrated that the human MHC represents one of the most genetically polymorphic loci hitherto identified. The genetic polymorphism as such may have represented the greatest immunological obstacle to successful transplantations. However, it was soon realized that a surprisingly large number of cells of the immune system are committed to recognizing the products of the MHC. This made it clear that MHC molecules also have central roles in physiological immune responses. Thus, the obsession of the immune system with these polymorphic proteins sets them apart from other endogeneous molecules in initiating a graft rejection.

Population geneticists revealed the complexity of the human MHC by means of serological and cellular assays. A great number of alleles were identified, and could be arranged into several segregant series, which today are known as HLA-

* Work from the authors' laboratory was supported by grants from the Swedish Cancer Society and the King Gustav V 80th Birthday Fund

A, B, C, and D [1]. As a corollary to this work, it was observed that some alleles occurred in higher than expected frequencies in patients with certain diseases, mostly of autoimmune character [2]. These findings have generated much speculation as to the possible causal relationship between certain allelic products and the disease etiology, but so far our knowledge is limited.

The knowledge of the molecular biology of the MHC region has expanded rapidly. Due to its obvious importance in normal immune reactions as well as in clinical transplantations, this is particularly true for the HLA-D region. Most of the genes and antigens of this segment of the MHC have been isolated and examined in great detail. These analyses have also given some insight into the mechanisms generating the polymorphism. The biosynthesis of the class II antigens has been explored, and their expression under the control of γ-interferon has been documented.

This review gives some salient features of the molecular biology of the HLA-D genes and antigens. Since more detailed accounts of the subjects covered in this presentation are found elsewhere in this volume (J. Silver and S. M. Goyert; H. Kratzin et al.; M. Sanchez-Perez and S. Shaw, J. I. Bell and H. O. McDevitt; T. Collins et al.), the references are far from exhaustive.

Evolution of the HLA-D Region

Molecules derived from the HLA-D region are called class II antigens. They are heterodimeric glycoproteins [3, 4] expressed on the surface of B lymphocytes, macrophages, epidermal Langerhans cells, and, under certain circumstances, on activated T cells and some epithelial cells [5, 6]. Due to their genetic polymorphism, the number of different class II antigens expressed by a single cell varies depending on whether the cell is homozygous or heterozygous as regards the HLA-D region. All class II molecules are composed of one α and one β chain. The HLA-D region contains multiple genes encoding such polypeptide chains. The α and β chains have very similar structures and are obviously evolutionarily related. Even their gross configurations suggest that the ancestral class II molecule was a homodimer. Therefore, it seems reasonable to conclude that α and β chains diverged during evolution by processes involving gene duplication and specialization. Following the emergence of genes encoding heterodimers, further duplication events gave rise to an array of genes similar to those coding for the original α and β chains. By means of a number of techniques it has been possible to demonstrate that such genes occur to a large extent as clusters in the HLA-D region. Thus, most if not all class II genes appear to be localized to three well-defined loci called DP, DQ, and DR.

Structure of Class II Antigen α Chains

All α chains are composed of approximately 230 amino acid residues. About 80% of the structure is expressed on the cell surface, while the remainder of the chain is equally divided between an intramembranous and a cytoplasmic portion. The surface-exposed part of the α chain appears to be folded into two discrete domains of similar sizes. Each domain contains one asparagine-linked carbohydrate moiety. The structure of the domain in closest proximity to the membrane is stabilized by a single disulfide bridge. The membrane-spanning segment of the α chain comprises hydrophobic and neutral amino acid residues surrounded by negatively and positively charged residues, as is commonly found in other transmembrane proteins. The amino acid composition of the part of the α chain which resides on the cytoplasmic side of the membrane is hydrophilic [7].

Hitherto four different types of α chains have been shown to be expressed as protein or mature mRNA. Three of the chains have clearly been defined as products of the DP, DQ, and DR loci respectively [8], while the fourth chain may be derived from an as yet unidentified locus tentatively called DO [9]. The entire amino acid sequences of these chains have been elucidated from cDNA clones [9–15], and the correctness of the identification of the chains has been verified by partial amino acid sequencing.

Comparisons of the amino acid sequences of the different chains reveal a high degree of homology. Any two sequences compared display between 50% and 60% identity. The differences occur along the whole length of the chains, although the membrane-integrated portions may exhibit as much as 80% homology, while the short cytoplasmic tails vary considerably. The N-terminal domains are slightly less homologous than the C-terminal domains. On close inspection it is obvious that short stretches of amino acid residues in any pair of α chains may show an unusually high degree of homology. However, such stretches are not conserved between three or more chains, and are therefore not informative in revealing whether any two α chains are evolutionarily particularly closely related.

Several sequences of DP α chains reveal that this polypeptide displays a low degree of genetic polymorphism [15]; where only about 3% of the residues differ. The amino acid substitutions are scattered over the entire length of the α chain and no obvious clusters of replacements are discerned. The situation is dramatically different as regards the DQ α chains, which exhibit a high degree of amino acid sequence variability [13]. While the overall differences between any two DQ α chains comprise about 10% of the amino acid residues, the regional differences in the chain vary considerably. Thus, the domain in juxtaposition to the membrane, the membrane-spanning segment, and the cytoplasmic tail do not reveal any polymorphism greater than that recorded for DP α chains. Virtually all the differences between allelic DQ α chains are accordingly confined to the N-terminal domain, whose amino acid sequence varies to about 20%. This unusual distribution of the polymorphism is reminiscent of immunoglobulin variability, but is not as strictly confined to a few discrete regions of the domain, although one stretch of "hypervariability" has been identified in murine I-A α chains [16]. Do α chains are less polymorphic. Thus, the DQ α chains are unusual in terms of both magnitude and distribution of their polymorphism.

Structure of Class II Antigen β Chains

Despite the fact that four different types of α chains have been identified, only three types of β chains have been encountered. DP, DQ, and DR β chains have been structurally examined [17–22], but the reasonable assumption of the existence of a DO β chain has not yet been experimentally verified. However, a class II β chain gene has recently been isolated which may code for the elusive DO β chain (B. Servenius, in preparation).

The three types of β chains share structural features. They are all transmembrane polypeptides with a short cytoplasmic tail. Like the α chains, the predominant portion of the β chains is expressed on the surface of the cell. All human β chains seem to contain a single asparagine-linked carbohydrate moiety whose position appears invariable. The extracellular portion of the polypeptide is most likely folded into two about equally large domains. Each domain is stabilized by a single disulfide bond. Sequence determinations of cDNA clones and isolated β chains have unambiguously identified the products of the DP, DQ, and DR loci. These β chains display considerable homology, and the differences between any two polypeptides are no greater than 30%–40%. Thus, β chains of different loci appear to be somewhat more closely related than the corresponding α chains [19]. The distribution of amino acid residues which differ between chains of the three loci is not confined to any particular region of the polypeptide, although the N-terminal domains are slightly more divergent than the domains closest to the membrane. The greatest identity between the chains is displayed by the membrane-integrated portions, while the cytoplasmic tails vary considerably both in amino acid sequences and length [22].

β chains of all loci display extensive genetic polymorphism [23], which on the average engages approximately 10% of the polypeptide chain. The amino acid sequence variability is largely confined to the N-terminal domain [24], where 15%–20% of the residues may differ between nonallelic β chains, while available data suggest that it may be somewhat less pronounced for the DP β chains [22].

Class II Antigen α and β Chains Are Members of the Immunoglobulin Superfamily

Structural analyses of class II antigen α and β chains revealed their relatedness [10]. They are similarly organized in terms of extracellular domains, membrane-integrated segments, and cytoplasmic tails. In addition, both contain conspicuous disulfide bonds formed by cysteines separated from each other by approximately 60 amino acid residues. The similarities between the two types of polypeptides are strengthened by their amino acid sequences. Thus, the domains closest to the membrane display significant sequence homology, leaving little doubt that the predecessor α and β chains originated from the same ancestral gene. These portions of the polypeptides also display homology to the two subunits of class I MHC antigens. Likewise, significant homology to immunoglobulin light and heavy chains and to T cell antigen receptor α and β chains exist. Thus, the class II antigens obviously belong to the same superfamily of proteins as several other immunologically important recognition molecules [7].

The amino acid sequence homology between class II antigen α and β chains and the other members of the superfamily is confined to the domains located closest to the membrane. The N-terminal domains do not exhibit statistically significant homologies to other proteins, despite the fact that the β chain domain contains an immunoglobulin-like disulfide bridge. These observations do not, of course, rule out the possibility that the N-terminal domains of both α and β chains are related to immunoglobulin constant domains in their tertiary structures. This is the case for immunoglobulin variable domains which show the basic immunoglobulin fold although their primary structures are only poorly homologous to the constant domains. Since the tertiary structure of immunoglobulin variable domains can obviously accommodate a great number of amino acid variations without this causing gross structural alterations, it is conceivable that this basic structure has been fundamental in allowing β chains and DQ α chains to accumulate mutations to establish the genetic polymorphism.

Structure of Class II α and β Genes

Several class II α and β genes have been isolated and their structures elucidated. The genes are all very similar in their exon-intron organizations [25, 26]. The α genes are composed of five exons which encode the signal sequence; the N-terminal domain; the domain in juxtaposition to the membrane; the membrane-spanning segment; and the cytoplasmic tail and the 3′ untranslated region. This general outline applies to the DP [27], DQ [28], DX [14], DR [25], and DZ [15] α genes, all of which have been sequenced.

The organization of the β genes differ from that of the α genes only as regards the exons encoding the membrane-spanning segment and the cytoplasmic tail [22, 26, 29]. In contrast to the α chain genes, which encode these portions of the polypeptide chain in a single exon, the β genes use two or more exons for these regions. Alternate splicing also seems to occur, which may give rise to cytoplasmic tails of somewhat varying lengths [22]. It is conceivable that the heterogeneity in the C-terminal region, which arises by structural differences in the β genes of different loci, as well as by alternate splicing, signifies discrete functional differences between the different types of β chains [30]. However, evidence to this effect is hitherto lacking.

Enumeration of Class II α and β Chain Genes

In contrast to the genes for the class I MHC antigen subunits, which reside on separate chromosomes, all class II antigen α and β chain genes seem to occur in the HLA-D region. The numbers of α and β genes discovered so far are greater than the number of polypeptide chains. Thus, six HLA-D α genes have been structurally identified, and the corresponding number of β genes is between six and nine. The uncertainty over the number of β genes is due to the fact that the HLA-DR locus appears to contain a haplotype-specific number of β chain genes [31]. Thus, the DR8 haplotype may comprise only one DR β chain gene, while DR4 appears to contain no less than four such genes.

The number of genes in the DP region is firmly established, and a molecular map of this region has been drawn [27, 32, 33]. The region contains two pairs of alternating α and β genes which are clustered together within a chromosomal segment encompassing 60 kb. The two types of genes are transcribed in opposite directions. Since only one set of DP α and β chains has been observed [34], it is not surprising to find that one pair of α and β genes displays pseudogene characteristics [22, 27]. Therefore, they are unlikely to code for any polypeptides. From these observations it seems reasonable to conlude that most haplotypes will only express a single DP molecule, although it cannot be entirely ruled out that two of the DP genes are pseudogenes only in some haplotypes.

The DQ region also seems to contain two pairs of α and β genes [31]. One pair, which encode the DQ molecule, occur only 12 kb apart [28]. The localization of the two other DQ genes, which have tentatively been called DXα [14] and DXβ, has not been firmly established, but indirect evidence suggest that they are close to each other, and one may speculate that they occur in the vicinity of the expressed DQ α and β genes. Sequence analyses of the CX α [14] and β genes (G. Andersson, unpublished observations) have not revealed any obvious characteristics that make them pseudogenes, but expressed products of these genes have not yet been identified. In contrast to the DQ α and β genes proper, the DX genes exhibit a very low degree of polymorphism.

The structural similarity between the DQ and DX genes is considerably greater than, for example, the similarity between the homologous DP genes. While the latter are approximately 75%–80% identical, the DQ and DX genes are as similar to each other as are alleles of a single segregant series. This great similarity suggests that hybrid molecules of the types DQαDXβ and DXαDQβ may exist, provided all genes are expressed. Accordingly, each haplotype would be able to manufacture four different DQ molecules. Since both DQ α and β genes are extensively polymorphic, heterozygosity at the DQ locus should give rise to a minimum of four but possibly as many as 16 DQ antigens.

As noted above, the number of DR β chain genes varies with the haplotype. While DR8 and DR4 may exhibit one and four genes respectively, most DR haplotypes appear to contain three β genes. Invariably, a single DR α gene has been found. The precise location of the genes is not yet established, but preliminary evidence suggest that at least one β gene is adjacent to the DR α gene. The number of expressed β genes is not yet firmly documented. While polypeptide chain analyses have suggested that two DR β chains may be derived from a single haplotype, it is conceivable that this number will vary with the haplotype. In the DR4 haplotype at least one of the four genes is a pseudogene, as shown by sequence analysis [29]. Thus, a minimum of one and a maximum of three DR antigens may be expressed by a haplotype, and since the DR α chain is largely invariant, these numbers will of course double in the heterozygous state.

The occurrence of a novel β chain gene, homologous to $A\beta_2$ of the mouse [35], was recently discovered. This gene appears to display some genetic polymorphism, but is more conserved than DQ and DR β genes. Its location and expression have not yet been examined but structural analyses suggest that it should not be grouped together with the DP, DQ, or DR β genes and may therefore be derived from a hitherto unidentified locus. It is tempting to suggest that this gene is a member of the same locus as the DZ α gene, which is most likely expressed in the form of the previously mentioned DO α chain [9, 15].

The enumeration and structural analyses of HLA-D α and β chains have revealed an unexpected complexity. It is clear that an individual heterozygous for all loci in the D region will express a minimum of eight different class II molecules. Depending on the degree of polymorphism of the relatively conserved genes and on which genes are expressed, the number of unique class II antigens of a heterozygous individual may in fact be as high as 30. Should hybrid molecules of the DQαDRβ type exist, this number will increase considerably.

Origin of the Class II Antigen Polymorphism

The reasons for the extensive genetic polymorphism exhibited by several genes of the MHC are enigmatic. The simplest way to account for the polymorphism is to assume that it has arisen by natural selection, i.e., that the polymorphism provides a selective advantage. This notion may gain some support from the observation that only a few of the many class I genes of the MHC are extensively polymorphic [36]. The differences in tissue distribution between polymorphic and nonpolymorphic class I genes do indeed suggest separate functions for the two types of proteins, which accordingly may have provided the genes with different evolutionary constraints. The three HLA-D loci which contain genes whose expression has been unambiguously documented, all harbor polymorphic entities. Although it is presently not obvious why the DQ locus contains an extensively polymorphic α gene, in contrast to the DP and DR loci, current information does not allow a functional distinction between the three types of class II antigens. Therefore, it seems reasonable to conclude, at least provisionally, that the class II antigen polymorphism has indeed been acquired by natural selection.

The observations that the genetic polymorphism is largely confined to the exons encoding the N-terminal domains of DQ α and DP, DQ, and DR β chains raise the possibility that selective forces may operate on these exons. The variability among immunoglobulins is similarly distributed, but it is obvious that class II genes do not undergo somatic rearrangements, so other mechanisms must be responsible for the class II antigen polymorphism. Several such mechanisms can be proposed. One possibility is that sequence-specific mutagenic events occur more frequently in the polymorphic exons than in other portions of the genes [16]. Another mechanism which may account for the restricted distribution of the polymorphism is gene-conversion-like events [37, 38], which may operate on the polymorphic exons with high frequency. In gene conversion events longer or shorter DNA segments are copied from one homologous gene to another [39]. Gene conversions of short DNA segments will usually increase the polymorphism. Alternatively, the conservation of other regions of the genes than the polymorphic exon may arise by gene conversions involving long DNA segments, which will homogenize the sequences.

Regardless of mechanism the genetic polymorphism is subject to evolutionary constraints operating on the class II genes and polypeptides. Such selection may be positive and favor polymorphism in one portion of the gene, or negative and conserve existing sequences in other regions. Obviously, both types of selective pressure may be operative simultaneously on discrete sections of a single exon.

Analyses of several class II β gene sequences reveal a consistent pattern in the distribution of the nucleotide substitutions, and it can be concluded that it is unlikely that the mutation rate in the polymorphic exons is significantly greater than in other regions of the genes [19]. Thus, should sequence specific mutational mechanisms exist, their contribution to the overall polymorphism is not major. Nucleotide substitutions that give rise to amino acid replacements are, of course, considerably more frequent in the polymorphic than in the other exons. This is not necessarily due to such substitutions being favored. In fact, it seems more likely to conclude that a conservative selective pressure acts on all exons but the polymorphic ones, thereby eliminating replacement substitutions [40]. Although statistical analyses fail to support the view that the polymorphism is selected for, it should be born in mind that discrete parts of the polymorphic exons may be under positive and negative constraints which have escaped detection.

Further support for the view that it is selection, rather than specific mutational mechanisms, that is the main generator of the polymorphism was obtained by analyses of a DR β pseudogene. Since this gene will not give rise to any translation product, it can be assumed to be relieved of most structural constraints. In keeping with this notion, all exons exhibit similar degrees of "replacement" substitutions. Thus, in the absence of a conservative selective pressure, which eliminates replacement substitutions, all exons seem to attain polymorphism to similar extents [40].

The fact that the class II antigen polymorphism may be accounted for by multiple, independent point mutations does not mean that all point mutations in a given sequence have originated within that sequence. A mutation may arise in one gene but subsequently be copied to another homologous gene by a gene-conversion-like event. Such an event most easily explains the emergence of a mutant murine class II gene [41–43]. This observation strongly suggests that gene conversion, or a mechanism similar to gene conversion, operates on class II genes.

In conclusion, it seems reasonable to assume that different evolutionary constraints have operated on the different portions of the polymorphic class II genes. The exons encoding the N-terminal domains may have acquired amino acid replacements by selective mechanisms that either favor such replacements or at least do not impose constraints against them. Such constraints seem to be operative on the other exons. These types of selective pressures operate independently of whether substitutions occur by point mutations or by gene-conversion-like events.

Biosynthesis of Class II Antigens

Like other membrane proteins, class II antigen α and β chains are manufactured by membrane-bound ribosomes. Concomitant with their transport across the membrane of the endoplasmic reticulum, the signal sequence of the precursor chains is cleaved off. Heterodimer formation occurs rapidly [44]. However, a third chain, denoted γ, associates with the class II antigens in the endoplasmic reticulum [45]. The ternary complex is transported to the Golgi complex, where terminal glycosylation occurs. At this stage in the intracellular transport the γ chain dissociates from the heterodimer, which becomes expressed on the cell surface [46, 47]. The γ chain seems also to be expressed on the surface, if only transiently [47].

Elucidation of the structure of the γ chain revealed that it is composed of 216 amino acid residues and contains two asparagine-linked carbohydrate moieties [48, 49]. There is no obvious sequence similarity between this chain and the class II antigen subunits. In contrast to class II antigen α and β chains, the γ chain is devoid of an N-terminal signal sequence. This finding and other observations make it likely that the transmembrane γ chain has its N-terminus on the cytoplasmic side of the membrane, while the C-terminal region of the chain is exposed on the cell surface.

The fact that the γ chain is always expressed in class II antigen-producing cells suggests that it is coregulated with α and β chains. This is supported by the observation that all three types of chains are induced by γ-interferon [50, 51]. Unfortunately, these and similar observations do not shed light on the function of the γ chain, which remains elusive. Assembly of α and β chains occurs in the absence of the γ chain [52]. However, a role for this chain in promoting the appropriate pairing of α and β chains from the same locus has not been ruled out. Intracellular transport of class II antigen heterodimers, examined in frog oocytes, proceeds even if the γ chain is not present. Under such circumstances the α chain appears to be aberrantly glycosylated (L. Claesson-Welsh, personal communication). Whether the situation is similar in human cells remains to be explored.

Association Between HLA-D Antigens and Disease

The well-established association between certain alleles of the HLA-D region and various autoimmune diseases is intriguing. Improved methods for analyzing the polymorphism of the class II genes have so far failed to establish a direct relationship between, for example, aberrant genes and disease. Thus, despite the fact that studies on the association between HLA-D region restriction fragment polymorphism and diseases are still in their infancy, it is doubtful whether they will reveal any structural correlates. It seems more likely that the tissue distribution of the class II antigens will turn out to be a key feature in understanding the disease associations. Normally, class II molecules occur on B lymphocytes, macrophages, and other antigen-presenting cells such as epidermal Langerhans cells. However, γ-interferon is a potent inducer of class II antigens [53, 54], and the expression of such molecules on activated T cells and various epithelial cells has been documented [55]. Recently, it was suggested that the aberrant class II antigen expression may be causally related to the induction of autoimmune diseases [56]. It is conceivable that viruses or other agents will induce a primary immune reaction involving the activation of T cells, which secrete γ-interferon. Epithelial cells in the vicinity may respond by synthesizing class II molecules, most likely derived from all three loci [51]. Since antigen presentation is a consequence of the local concentrations both of class II molecules and the antigen, aberrant expression of class II molecules may render several endogenous cell surface molecules, present in low concentrations, autoantigenic. This should be particularly true for molecules which are only transitorily expressed on the cell surface, e.g., membrane constituents of secretory vesicles and some hormone receptors. Due to their low concentrations and restricted tissue distribution, it is unlikely that such components are encompassed by T cell tolerance. If properly presented, such molecules may induce a second immune reaction, eventually activating the effector mechanisms of the immune system [56]. The association between diseases and some HLA-D alleles may accordingly reflect the fact that only certain class II molecules may successfully present a given autoantigen. Alternatively, some HLA-D alleles may be inducible with γ-interferon to a greater extent than others.

Concluding Remarks

Great progress has been made in recent years in unraveling the molecular anatomy of the HLA-D region as regards its genes and products. It seems likely that most genes have been identified, but some may still remain undiscovered. The structures of the genes are well worked out, and the rough outline of the origin of the genetic polymorphism is being unraveled. Work in progress in several laboratories will, before too long, establish a detailed molecular map of the HLA-D region, and this information will most likely allow conclusions to be drawn regarding the emergence during evolution of the various D region loci. Future molecular analyses will undoubtedly reveal the nature and location of controlling genetic elements that confer tissue-specific expression and inducibility by γ-interferon to the class II genes.

The availability of isolated class II genes will prompt an avalanche of studies directed at the expression of transfected genes in appropriate cells. Such studies may be of great clinical importance inasmuch as the specificities of serological and cellular reagents may be standardized. Likewise, transfected cells will allow examination of the possible existence of hybrid class II antigens. Whether DP, DQ, and DR antigens are functionally equivalent may also be approached under such simplified experimental conditions.

The precise molecular role of the class II molecules in the presentation of antigens to T cells should be amenable to examination in view of the structural knowledge recently acquired, not only about class II antigens, but also about T cell receptors. These and related problems will keep molecular biologists busy while, hopefully, succinct molecular concepts concerning the role of class II antigens in tolerance induction and thymus selection are being developed.

Acknowledgments. We are grateful to Ms C. Plöen for patiently typing this manuscript.

References

1. Bodmer WF (1978) The HLA system: introduction. Br Med Bull 34:213–216
2. Ryder LP, Svejgaard A, Dausset J (1981) Genetics of HLA disease association. Ann Rev Genet 15:169–187
3. Cresswell P, Geier SS (1975) Antisera to human B-lymphocyte membrane glycoproteins block stimulation in mixed lymphocyte culture. Nature 257:147–149
4. Klareskog L, Sandberg-Trägårdh L, Rask L, Lindblom JB, Curman B, Peterson PA (1977) Chemical properties of human Ia antigens. Nature 265:248–251
5. Hämmerling GJ (1976) Tissue distribution of Ia antigens and their expression on lymphocyte subpopulations. Transplant Rev 30:64–82
6. Wiman K, Curman B, Forsum U, Klareskog L, Malmnäs Tjernlund U, Rask L, Trägårdh L, Peterson PA (1978) Occurrence of Ia antigens on tissues of non-lymphoid origin. Nature 276:711–713
7. Kaufman JF, Auffray C, Korman AJ, Shackelford DA, Strominger J (1984) The Class II molecules of the human and murine Major Histocompatibility Complex. Cell 36:1–13
8. Spielman R, Lee JS, Bodmer WF, Bodmer J, Trowsdale J (1984) Six HLA-D region α-chain genes on human chromosome 6: Polymorphisms and associations of DCα-related sequences with DR types. Proc Natl Acad Sci USA 81:3461–3465
9. Inoko H, Ando A, Kimura M, Ogala S, Tsuji K (1984) Isolation and characterization of the cDNA clones and the genomic clones of the HLA class II antigen heavy chains. In: Albert ED, Baur MP, Mayr W (eds) Histocompatibility testing 1984. Springer, Berlin Heidelberg New York Tokyo, pp 559–564

10. Larhammar D, Gustafsson K, Claesson L, Bill P, Wiman K, Schenning L, Sundelin J, Widmark E, Peterson PA, Rask L (1982) Alpha chain of the HLA-DR transplantation antigen is a member of the same protein superfamily as the immunoglobulins. Cell 30:153–161
11. Lee JS, Trowsdale J, Travers PJ, Carey J, Grosveld F, Jenkins J, Bodmer WF (1982) Sequence of an HLA-DR α-chain cDNA clone and intron-exon organization of the corresponding gene. Nature 299:750–752
12. Auffray C, Korman AJ, Roux-Dosseto M, Bono R, Strominger JL (1982) cDNA clone for the heavy chain of the human B cell alloantigen DC1: strong sequence homology to the HLA-DR heavy chain. Proc Natl Acad Sci USA 79:6337–6341
13. Schenning L, Larhammar D, Bill P, Wiman K, Jonsson A-K, Rask L, Peterson PA (1984) Both α and β chains of HLA-DC class II histocompatibility antigens display extensive polymorphism in their aminoterminal domains. EMBO J 3:447–432
14. Auffray C, Lillie J, Arnot D, Grossberger D, Kappes D, Strominger JL (1984) Isotypic and allotypic variation of human class II antigen α chain genes. Nature 308:327–333
15. Trowsdale J, Young JAT, Kelly AP, Austin PJ, Carson S, Meunier H, So A, Ehrlich HA, Spielman RS, Bodmer J, Bodmer WF (1985) Structure, sequence and polymorphism in the HLA-D region. Immunol Rev 85:5–43
16. Benoist CO, Mathis DJ, Kanter MR, Williams VE, McDevitt HO (1983) Regions of allelic hypervariability in the murine Aα immune response gene. Cell 34:169–177
17. Larhammar D, Schenning L, Gustafsson K, Wiman K, Claesson L, Rask L, Peterson PA (1982) The complete amino acid sequence of an HLA-DR antigen-like β chain as predicted from the nucleotide sequence: similarities with immunoglobulins and HLA-A, B, C antigens. Proc Natl Acad Sci USA 79:3687–3691
18. Long EO, Wake CT, Gorski J, Mach B (1983) Complete sequence of an HLA-DR β chain deduced from a cDNA clone and identification of multiple non-allelic DR β chain genes. EMBO J 2:389–394
19. Gustafsson K, Wiman K, Emmoth E, Larhammar D, Böhme J, Hyldig-Nielsen J-J, Ronne H, Peterson PA, Rask L (1984) Mutations and selection in the generation of class II histocompatibility antigen polymorphism. EMBO J 3:1655–1661
20. Gustafsson K, Emmoth E, Widmark E, Böhme J, Peterson PA, Rask L (1984) Isolation of a cDNA clone coding for an SB β-chain. Nature 309:76–78
21. Roux-Dosseto M, Auffray C, Lillie J, Boss J, Cohen D, DeMars R, Mawas C, Seidman J, Strominger JL (1983) Genetic mapping of a human classs II antigen β-chain cDNA clone to the SB region of the HLA complex. Proc Natl Acad Sci USA 80:6036–6040
22. Kappes DJ, Arnot D, Okada K, Strominger JL (1984) Structure and polymorphism of the HLA class II SB light chain genes. EMBO J 3:2985–2993
23. Böhme J, Owerbach D, Denaro M, Lernmark Å, Peterson PA, Rask L (1983) Human class II major histocompatibility antigen β-chains are derived from at least three loci. Nature 301:82–84
24. Kämpe O, Larhammar D, Wiman K, Schenning L, Claesson L, Gustafsson K, Pääbo S, Hyldig-Nielsen J-J, Rask L, Peterson PA (1983) Molecular analyses of MHC antigens. In: Möller E, Möller G (eds) Genetics of the immune response. Plenum, New York, pp 61–87
25. Korman AJ, Auffray C, Schamboeck A, Strominger J (1982) The amino acid sequence and gene organization of the heavy chain of the HLA-DR antigen: homology to immunoglobulins. Proc Natl Acad Sci USA 79:6013–6017
26. Larhammar D, Hyldig-Nielsen J-J, Servenius B, Andersson G, Rask L, Peterson PA (1983) Exon-intron organization and complete nucleotide sequence of a human major histocompatibility antigen DC β gene. Proc Natl Acad Sci USA 80:7313–7317
27. Servenius B, Gustafsson K, Widmark E, Emmoth E, Andersson G, Larhammar D, Rask L, Peterson PA (1984) Molecular map of the human HLA-SB (HLA-DP) region and sequence of an SBα (DPα) pseudogene. EMBO J 3:3209–3213
28. Jonsson A-K (in preparation) The polymorphic human MHC class II DQ α and β genes are located in close proximity to each other
29. Larhammar D, Servenius B, Rask L, Peterson PA (1985) Characterization of an HLA DRβ pseudogene. Proc Natl Acad Sci USA 82:1475–1479
30. Peterson PA, Andersson G, Bill P, Böhme J, Denaro M, Emmoth E, Gustafsson K, Hammerling U, Hyldig-Nielsen J-J, Jonsson A-K, Kalm B, Larhammar D, Schenning L, Servenius B, Widmark E, Rask L (1983) Features of class I and II antigens of the

major histocompatibility complex at the DNA and protein level. Prog Immunol 5:171–186
31. Böhme J, Andersson M, Andersson G, Möller E, Peterson PA, Rask L (1985) HLA-DR β genes vary in number between different specificities, whereas the number of DQ β genes is constant. J Immunol 135:2149–2155
32. Trowsdale J, Kelly A, Lee J, Carson S, Austin P, Travers P (1984) Linkage map of two HLA-SBβ and two HLA-SBα-related genes: an intron in one of the SB β genes contains a processed pseudogene. Cell 38:241–249
33. Gorski J, Rollini P, Long E, Mach B (1984) Molecular organization of the HLA-SB region of the human major histocompatibility complex and evidence for two SB β-chain genes. Proc Natl Acad Sci USA 81:3934–3938
34. Hurley C, Shaw S, Nadler L, Schlossman S, Capra J (1982) Alpha and beta chains of SB and DR antigens are structurally distinct. J Exp Med 156:1557–1562
35. Larhammar D, Hammerling U, Denaro M, Lund T, Flavell R, Rask L, Peterson PA (1983) Structure of the murine immune response I-A_α locus: sequence of the I-A_β gene and an adjacent β-chain second domain exon. Cell 34:179–188
36. Steinmetz M, Hood L (1983) Genes of the major histocompatibility complex in mouse and man. Science 222:727–733
37. Pease LR, Schulze DH, Pfaffenbach GM, Nathenson SG (1983) Spontaneous H-2 mutants provide evidence that a copy mechanism analogous to gene conversion generates polymorphism in the major histocompatibility complex. Proc Natl Acad Sci USA 80:242–246
38. Weiss EH, Golden L, Zahert R, Mellor A, Fahrner K, Kvist S, Flavell RA (1983) The DNA sequence of the H-2K^b gene: Evidence for gene conversion as a mechanism for the generation of polymorphism in histocompatibility antigens. EMBO J 2:453–462
39. Jackson AJ, Fink GR (1981) Gene conversion between duplicated genetic elements in yeast. Nature 292:306–310
40. Rask L, Gustafsson K, Larhammar D, Ronne H, Peterson PA (1985) Generation of class II antigen polymorphism. Immunol Rev 84:113–133
41. McIntyre KR, Seidman JG (1984) Nucleotide sequence of mutant I-A_β^{bm12} gene is evidence for genetic exchange between mouse immune response genes. Nature 308:551–553
42. Denaro M, Hammerling U, Rask L, Peterson PA (1984) The E^b gene may have acted as the donor gene in a gene conversion-like event generating the A_β^{bm12} mutant. EMBO J 3:2029–2032
43. Widera G, Flavell RA (1984) The nucleotide sequence of the murine I-Eβ^b immune response gene: evidence for gene conversion events in class II genes of the major histocompatibility complex. EMBO J 3:1221–1226
44. Kvist S, Wiman K, Claesson L, Peterson PA, Dobberstein B (1982) Membrane insertion and oligomeric assembly of HLA-DR histocompatibility antigens. Cell 29:61–69
45. Charron DJ, McDevitt HO (1979) Analysis of HLA-D region-associated molecules with monoclonal antibody. Proc Natl Acad Sci USA 76:6567–6571
46. Machamer CE, Cresswell P (1982) Biosynthesis and glycosylation of the invariant chain associated with HLA-DR antigens. J Immunol 129:2564–2569
47. Claesson L, Peterson PA (1983) Association of human γ chain with class II transplantation antigens during intracellular transport. Biochemistry 22:3206–3213
48. Claesson L, Larhammar D, Rask L, Peterson PA (1983) Human invariant (γ) chain of class II MHC antigens has an unusual membrane orientation and is devoid of an amino-terminal signal sequence. Proc Natl Acad Sci USA 80:7395–7399
49. Strubin M, Mach B, Long EO (1984) The complete sequence of the mRNA for the HLA-DR-associated invariant chain reveals a polypeptide with an unusual transmembrane polarity. EMBO J 3:869–872
50. Koch N, Wong GHW, Schrader JW (1984) Ia antigens and associated invariant chain are induced simultaneously in lines of T-dependent mast cells by recombinant interferon-γ. J Immunol 132:1361–1369
51. Collins T, Korman AJ, Wake CT, Boss JM, Kappes DJ, Fiers W, Ault KA, Gimbrone MA, Strominger J, Pober JS (1984) Immune interferon activates multiple class II major histocompatibility complex genes and the associated invariant chain gene in human endothelial cells and dermal fibroblasts. Proc Natl Acad Sci USA 81:4917–4921

52. Long EO, Strubin M, Wake CT, Gross N, Carrel S, Goodfellow P, Accolla RS, Mach B (1983) Isolation of cDNA clones for the p33 invariant chain associated with HLA-DR antigens. Proc Natl Acad Sci USA 80:5714–5718
53. Steeg P, Moore RN, Johnson HM, Oppenheim JJ (1982) Regulation of murine macrophage Ia antigen expression by a lymphokine with immune interferon activity. J Exp Med 156:1780–1793
54. Rhodes JM, Stokes P (1982) Interferon-induced changes in the monocyte membrane: inhibition by retinol and retinoic acid. Immunology 45:531–536
55. Barclay AN, Masen DW (1983) Graft rejection and Ia antigens – paradox resolved? Nature 303:382–383
56. Bottazzo GF, Pujol-Borrell R, Hanafusa T, Feldman M (1983) Role of aberrant HLA-DR expression and antigen presentation in induction of endocrine autoimmunity. Lancet 8359:1115–1119

Physiologic Regulation of Class II Major Histocompatibility Complex Gene Expression *

T. Collins, J. S. Pober, and J. L. Strominger

Table of Contents

Introduction

T inducer (helper) cells can only recognize antigen in association with class II major histocompatibility complex (MHC) antigens on the surface of an antigen-presenting cell [11]. The T cell antigen receptor, in addition to recognizing polymorphic self-class II determinants modified by nominal antigen, can recognize foreign polymorphic (allogeneic) class II determinants, with or without nominal antigen [107]. Recognition of foreign class II determinants generates alloactivated T helper cells which are involved in generating specific effector cells. Inducible expression of class II antigens may confer accessory capacity upon cells not generally thought of as components of the immune system. Such cells could either present nominal antigen or, in the case of transplantation, stimulate an allogeneic response. Therefore, mechanisms regulating the expression of these proteins may play a crucial role in modulating immune responsiveness. To understand possible regulatory mechanisms, a knowledge of the general structural features of these proteins and the coresponding genes is important.

* This work was supported by National Institutes of Health grants HL27642, HL22602, AM13230, AM30241, and 5T32 HL07066. J.S.P. is a Searle Scholar

Structural Aspects of MHC Products

All class II antigens are noncovalently associated heterodimers consisting of an α (33–35 kd) and a β (26–29 kd) chain. Each chain consists of four domains (reviewed in [59]; Fig. 1 a): (a) An N-terminal domain (α1 or β1 domain) of 85–95 amino acids (aa). The β1 domains and some α1 domains (in DQ and I-A) are polymorphic. (b) A membrane proximal domain (α2 or β2 domains) of 95 aa which is homologous to the constant regions of immunoglobulins. (c) A connecting peptide (11–13 aa) and a transmembrane region (23 aa). (d) A small intracytoplasmic domain (8–15 aa) [51, 52]. HLA-DR antigen structure consists of two domains (α1 and β1) which are linked to two immunoglobulin-like domains (α2 and β2). It is thought that the HLA-DR heterodimeric molecule is organized such that the immunoglobulin-like domains interact (Fig. 1). The homology of the various domains of the class II MHC antigens with class I MHC antigens or constant region

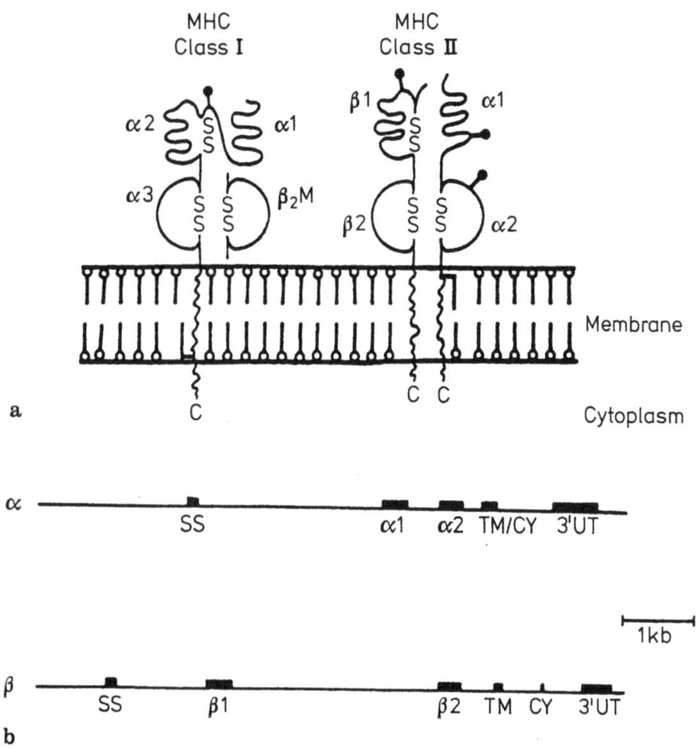

Fig. 1. a Models of the class I and class II MHC antigens illustrating their structural homology. *Circles,* segments of the class II antigens related to immunoglobulin constant region domains; *S-S,* disulfide bonds between cysteine residues folding the chains into domains; *C* C-terminus; ●, N-linked carbohydrate side chains [53]. **b** Genomic architecture of the class II genes. The arrangement of exons and introns comprising typical α and β chain genes is illustrated. The α chain gene consists of five exons: the signal sequence exon (*SS*) contains the leader peptide and the first few amino acids of the mature protein; the α1 and α2 exons encode the corresponding protein domains; the TM/CY exons encode the connecting peptide, the transmembrane region (*TM*), the intracytoplasmic domain (*CY*), and part of the 3′ untranslated region (*3′UT*); the final exon encodes the remainder of the 3′UT sequence. The variations between the α and the similarly arranged β chain genes are discussed in the text (see also [53, 59])

domains of immunoglobulins is reviewed in detail by Kaufman et al. [53] and Korman et al. [59]. Biosynthetic intermediates, but not mature cell surface forms, of the class II antigens are associated with a nonpolymorphic glycoprotein whose gene is encoded outside the MHC (referred to as invariant chain) [21]. The mouse class II MHC antigens have also been called immune response-associated (Ia) antigens; human class II gene products can also be referred to as Ia.

Structural analysis of the class II genes has been extended to the DNA sequence level [53, 59, 66]. Figure 1 b presents representative genomic structures of class II α and β chains. An α chain gene consists of five exons encoding: (a) the 5′ untranslated region and signal sequence, (b) the $\alpha 1$ domain, (c) the $\alpha 2$ domain, (d) the connecting peptide, transmembrane region, cytoplasmic tail, and part of the 3′ untranslated region, and (e) the remainder of the 3′ untranslated region. A β chain gene consists of six exons. Although the β chain gene is similar in organization to an α chain gene, there is an extra intracytoplasmic exon between the transmembrane exon and the exon encoding the last four amino acids of the protein and the entire 3′ untranslated region. The introns between the signal sequence and the $\alpha 1$ or $\beta 1$ exons, and between the $\beta 1$ and $\beta 2$ exons, are very large in class II genes. These large introns may contain sequences important to regulation (see below). Functional protein domains in the class II antigens correlate with the location of intron/exon boundaries. This observation is also correct for those other members of the immunoglobulin family whose genomic structures are known (class I α chain, $\beta 2$-microglobulin, β chain of the T cell receptor, T8, and Thy 1; reviewed in [45, 59, 73]).

Multiple control mechanisms are involved in the expression of these antigens. In general these can be divided into two categories: those probably acting at the level of transcription, e.g., regulatory lymphokines [7] and trans-acting regulatory factors which may act at conserved 5′ structural elements of the class II genes, and those acting post-transcriptionally or at the level of antigen assembly, e.g., the invariant chain and its possible role in α/β pairing. The molecular basis for the regulation of class II gene expression will be examined prior to a discussion of the physiologic mediators regulating Ia antigen expression.

Transcriptional Regulation of Class II MHC Genes

Some of the factors involved in the transcriptional regulation of class II MHC gene expression have become apparent from (a) analysis of somatic cell mutants failing to express HLA-DR, (b) results of class II gene transfection experiments, and (c) direct comparison of the class II gene sequences [53, 59].

Somatic Cell Genetics

Antisera directed against class II determinants and complement have been used to generate cell lines with altered class II expression [2, 38, 94]. Some of these immunoselected somatic cell variants are defective in the regulation of all class II MHC genes [38, 69]. Selection against DR antigens also resulted in mutants which also failed to express DQ(DC) antigens [2]. This lack of surface expression of class II antigens correlates with decreased mRNA content [74, 76]. The regulatory mutants contain essentially no detectable transcripts for DR$\alpha+\beta$, DQ(DC)β, or

DP(SB)$\alpha+\beta$, although the genes for these transcripts are intact. Additionally, the mutants have reduced amounts of class II-associated invariant chain [70, 76]. However, changes in class I surface expression or mRNA content were not observed in the mutants.

Formation of somatic cell hybrids between the regulatory mutants and other B cell lines results in reexpression of the class II specificities of the mutant [3, 38]. This suggests that there is a trans-acting factor required for regulation of the class II genes [3, 49, 69]. Positive trans-acting regulation of class II gene expression is also suggested by the results of somatic cell fusion between class II-negative T cell lines and class II-positive B cell lines; in these hybrids both T and B cell class II specificities are expressed [49]. Since T-B hybrids randomly lose chromosomes at high rates, it should be possible to map these B cell regulatory factors by selecting chromosome loss variants which do not express class II antigens. The concept of a positive regulatory element coordinately regulating a set of class II genes is also consistent with observations on the immune-interferon-mediated induction of class II antigens. DR $\alpha+\beta$, DQ(DC)$\alpha+\beta$ and DP(SB)$\alpha+\beta$, as well as the associated invariant chain, are coordinately induced by immune interferon [23].

Transfection of Class II Antigen Genes

Another potential approach to the analysis of class II regulation has been to examine the expression of transfected class II antigens. Murine class II genes have been transfected into murine B cell and macrophage lines, and the expressed surface proteins are functional in presentation of antigen to T cell hybridomas [12, 32, 35, 79, 80]; additionally, murine class II genes transferred to L cells also express functional Ia antigens on their surface [80, 89]. DNA-mediated gene transformation has also been utilized to express HLA-DR antigens in L cells [98]. Austin et al. [6] and Okada et al [92] have reported the transfection of DP(SB)2 and 3α and β containing cosmids into the same LTK-cells. Although the DP(SB)3 transfectants have not been able to present measles virus to DP(SB)3-restricted measles-virus-specific cytotoxic T cells (CTL) (unpublished data), the DP(SB)2-expressing cells were capable of presenting influenza neuraminidase (either after virus infection or addition of neuraminidase protein) to DP(SB)2-restricted neuraminidase-specific T cell clones [6].

Cotransfection with the invariant chain has not been required for surface expression of the transfected class II antigens. Since the invariant chain has been observed to associate with class II antigens intracellularly, it is believed to be required for surface expression (see below). However, the cell lines used in previous transfections may themselves express the invariant chain. The DR α chain, several DR β chains, and the γ (invariant) chains have also been introduced into cells in retrovirus vectors [58, 59] and are being used to examine the mechanism of class II expression.

The importance of the quantitative aspect of accessory cell Ia expression has been demonstrated by correlating levels of Ia expression with T cell activation. The degree of stimulation of Ia-restricted antigen-specific T cells correlates with the product of the number of Ia molecules and antigen concentration [83]. This proposal has recently been confirmed by obtaining three populations of L cells arising from the same cotransfection of I-A α genes and I-A β genes by successively sorting for different levels of Ia expression [68]. The level of Ia expression by the transfected L cell populations is relatively stable in culture, in contrast to the antigen-presenting cells used in previous work. The three populations of transfected L cells were used in cell or antigen dose-response studies, which confirmed the relationship between the Ia antigen product and the level of T cell activation [68].

The regions of the transfected class II gene responsible for constitutive as well as inducible expression of class II genes have begun to be determined. A 22-kb fragment of the I-E β gene and flanking sequences has been transferred into a macrophage line (P388DI) and shown to be inducible by culture supernatants from concanavalin A-stimulated T cells [32]. The inducible expression of this transfected class II gene indicates that at least some of the sequences responsible for regulated expression of the gene are probably associated with the transfected gene. A "tissue-specific" enhancer active in a lymphoma cell line, but inactive in an L cell line and a myeloma line, was identified in an upstream region of the E β gene [37]. This orientation-independent sequence, which is distinct from the conserved 5′ flanking regions (see below) has been mapped on transfected E β genomic fragments, by enhancer-dependent plasmid transformation, to a 2-kb region upstream of the Eβ promoter. It is possible that this enhancer element itself is an indirect target for the inducing action of immune interferon.

Comparison of the 5′ Flanking Sequences of the Class II Genes

The 5′ ends of the human DRα and murine I-Eα are nearly identical except for a single 15-bp gap [82, 105]. Comparison of E α, DR α, and E β genes revealed two conserved sequences of 10 and 14 bp located between 90 and 120 bp upstream from the startpoint of transcription of Eβ [104]. A comparison of the promotor regions from 11 different class II antigen genes [58, 92] shows extensive sequence conservation of the two elements, as well as the distance between them (19 bp for β and 20 bp for α). Some sequences, i.e., between the two elements and following the 10-bp element, may be specific for α and β chain genes. The conservation of these promoter elements suggests they have a functional role in the coordinate control of expression of the α and β chain genes of class II antigens, possibly in their induction by γ-interferon, and possibly as binding sites for positive trans-acting regulatory elements.

Additional conserved upstream sequences have also been identified by comparing interferon-responsive gene sequences. Because α-interferon regulates transcription of both class I and the metallothionein genes, the upstream sequences were examined for structural homologies [34]. The only significant upstream homology between the HLA-A3 gene and the metallothionein gene is found in a region which is also homologous to the class II DR α chain gene. Alignment of the sequences reveals that the core of the consensus sequences [AGTTTCTC(C/T)TCTC] is nearly invariant. The consensus sequence lies 142 bp upstream of the TATA box in the class I sequence; it is 567 and 600 bp upstream of the HLA-DRα and metallothionein TATA boxes respectively. This consensus sequence may be involved in regulating transcription of interferon-induced genes [34].

Examination of chromatin structure changes following immune interferon induction is consistent with the proposal that sites flanking the first exon of HLA-DR are involved in differential expression. Cloned genomic probes were utilized

		-110*	-98		-78 -69	
Consensus α and β		CCYAGNRACNGATG			CTGATTGGYY	
	DQ2β	--C--AG--A----		AGGTCCTTCAGCTCCAGTG	---------TT	CCTT
	DQ3β	--T--AG--A---T		AGGTCCTTCAGCTCCAGTG	---------TT	CCTT
	DXβ	--C--AGG-A----		AGGTCCTTCAGCTCCAGTG	---------TT	CCTT
	I-Aβ	--C--AG--A----		ACAGACTTCAGGTCCAATG	---------TT	CCTC
	DPβ	--T--TG-GCA---		ACTCATACAAAGCTCAGTG	TCC------TT	CTTT
	SXβ	--C--TG-GCA---		ACTCATACAAAGCTCAGTG	CCC------TT	CTTT
	I-Eβ	A-T--CA--T----		ATGCTGGACTCCTTTGATG	---------CT	CCCA
	▼ DRβ	A-C--CA--T----		ATGCTATTGAACTCAGACG	------CATT	CTCC
Consensus β only				ANRYYNYYCAGCTCCARTG		CYYY
	DQα	G-T--TA--T--GA		TGTCACCATGGGGG ATTTTT	--A------CC	AAAA
	DXα	A-TG-CA-ACA--A		TGTCACCATAGGGG ATTTTT	---------CC	AAAA
	DRα	--T--CA--A----		CGTCA TCTCAAAATATTTTT	---------CC	AAAG
	I-Eα	--T--CA--A----		TGTCAGTCT GAAACATTTTT	---------TT	AAAA
	DPα	--C--CA--A--GA		ATGTCAG CTCTATG ATTTCT	------A--TG	AATC
	DZα	--C--CA--A---A		CATTCA CTCAGAGAATTTCT	G--------CT	GAAG
Consensus α only				TGTCANYCTNRRRRNATTTTT		AAAA

* Bases upstream from the initiation of transcription of DQ2β

Fig. 2. Comparison of the 5′ flanking sequences common to class II genes. Upstream DNA sequences are aligned so that maximum homology is achieved. Consensus sequences which are shared between α and β promoters are shown at the top of the table. Sequences common to either α or β promoters are shown below their respective groups. *N*, any nucleotide; *Y*, pyrimidine; *R*, purine. *DQ2β*, Boss and Strominger [14]; *DQ3β*, Larhammar et al. [64]; *DXβ, DQα, DXα*, Okada et al. [91, 92]; *I-Aβ*, Larhammar et al. [65]; *DPβ* [50 a]; *I-Eβ*, Saito et al. [104]; *DRβ*, Larhammar et al. [63, 67]; *DRα*, Schamboeck et al. [105]; *I-Eα*, Mathis et al. [83]; *DPα, DZα*, Kelley and Trowsdale [54]

to map HLA-DRα-specific, DNAse I-hypersensitive sites in various cell lines which differed in their ability to express HLA-DR [93]. In all cell lines, a DNAse I-hypersensitive site was localized to the conserved sequences in the 5′ flanking promoter region just described. In an inducible cell line (HL-60), however, the administration of immune interferon leads to the appearance of a DNAse I-hypersensitive site in the first intron. Interestingly, viral enhancer core sequences are located in this region of the large first intron of the DRα sequence [93].

Post-Transcriptional Control of Class II Expression

Post-transcriptional regulatory events may also play a role in controlling surface expression of MHC antigens. Surface expression is not entirely a function of mRNA level, because withdrawal of immune interferon leads to rapid disappearance of mRNA, but not to surface expression of class II antigens [23]. In contrast to class II antigens expressed by murine macrophages [10], the apparent stability of the induced class II antigen (in human dermal fibroblasts) may be involved in sustaining an ongoing immune response in the peripheral tissues (see below). Immune interferon increases class I MHC and class II MHC mRNA levels out of proportion to the increase in antigen expression [23, 31, 103]. Possible explanations for this quantitative discrepancy are that interferon promote the appearance of altered MHC molecules at the cell surface which cannot be recognized by anti-MHC monoclonal antibodies, or that post-transcriptional control may modulate surface expression. Recent experiments by Weis and colleagues [116, 117] support the latter proposal. They produced a fusion gene by replacing the normal murine H-2 promoter with the promoter of the metallothionein gene. Since the promoter of the metallothionein gene is much "stronger" than the promoter of the H-2 gene, cells expressing the metallothionein–H-2 fusion gene contain much greater amounts of H-2 mRNA than do cells transformed with normal H-2 genes. Surprisingly, these cells do not have extremely large amounts of H-2 antigens on the cell surface. It is possible that this failure to increase H-2 surface expression by increasing transcription is due to post-translational competition for a limiting amount of β2-microglobulin. Previous studies of mutant cell lines that fail to express any β2-microglobulin also suggest that class I antigens cannot be made in cells lacking β2-microglobulin (reviewed in [53]).

Similar post-transcriptional control mechanisms may exist to regulate surface expression of the class II MHC antigens. The induction of multiple class II MHC antigens by immune interferon occurred together with the invariant chain [23, 56]. The human invariant chain is not linked to the class II gene complex [21]. Both α and β chains of class II antigens interact with invariant chains during biosynthesis prior to formation of the heterodimer [60]. The invariant chain remains associated with the class II dimer prior to appearance at the cell surface. The temporal correlation of the invariant chain and the class II antigen induction by immune interferon is consistent with the proposal that the invariant chain is involved in assembly and intracellular transport of both class II chains to the cell surface. Limiting amounts of invariant chain could, therefore, determine the nature and extent of the class II surface expression induced by interferon. There is no direct evidence, however, that invariant chain levels do in fact regulate either constitutive or inducible class II antigen expression.

Post-translational regulation of Ia expression may also involve α and β chain pairing, possibly mediated by the invariant chain. As yet there is no evidence that one chain of a class II molecule can be expressed without a companion subunit. However, recent data from L cells transfected with murine class II antigens suggest that hybrid class II molecules can be generated and that the level of expression of the haplotype-mismatched pairs varies [36]. Cotransfection of $A\beta^d$ with $E\alpha^k$ leads to surface Ia reactive with monoclonal antibodies recognizing I-A and I-E, indicating production of a mixed isotope ($A\beta E\alpha$) heterodimer. Expression of hybrid I-A molecules is highly dependent upon the alleles involved. Control of expression of hybrid I-A appears to map to the highly polymorphic N-terminal domain of the A β chain [36]. Thus isotype pairing may also regulate class II surface expression by altering the nature, as well as regulating the amount, of expressed class II antigen.

Regulation of Class II Expression by Immune Mediators

To initiate and sustain an immune response, an antigen-processing cell must express class II molecules, process and present antigen, and secrete immunoregulatory molecules which promote effector lymphocyte development. There are important quantitative effects of the Ia density (as well as antigen concentration) on T cell activation, and, as just discussed, the expression of class II molecules involves both transcriptional as well as assembly control mechanisms.

Ia expression in peripheral tissues may be regulated by at least two groups of mediators [114]: First, products of antigen-stimulated T cells can increase class II antigen expression. Immune interferon increases Ia expression on a variety of cells generally not thought of as components of the immune system. Another T cell product, B cell growth factor, can induce a selective increase in the expression of Ia antigens on small resting B cells [88, 102]. Additionally, growth factors such as platelet-derived growth factor (PDGF) and epidermal growth factor (EGF) may regulate immune interferon production by T cells, which, in turn, modulates class II levels on antigen-presenting cells [4, 50]. Second, a number of inhibitory molecules have been reported which diminish Ia expression on some antigen-presenting cells.

Inducible Expression of Class II MHC Antigens by Lymphokine

Class II MHC antigen expression was at first thought to be restricted to bone-marrow-derived cells. The human class II molecules were first identified on peripheral B cells and were found to disappear when these B cells differentiated further to become plasma cells. Class II antigens are expressed on committed stem cells for both granulocyte-monocyte (CFU-GM) and erythroid precursors, but are not present on mature granulocytes, eosinophils, or red blood cells; they are found, however, on macrophages, the mature progeny of CFU-GM [106]. The transient expression of class II molecules on erythroid and granulocyte precursor cells suggests a general role for these molecules in cell interactions during development [22].

Expression of the class II MHC gene products can be modulated by T cell products. The low levels of class II antigen expressed by murine macrophages could be augmented by T cell factors present in crude lymphokine preparations [110]. Subsequently, this inducing factor was identified as immune interferon and the observations were extended to human monocytes. Although virtually all human monocytes and macrophages display framework and polymorphic HLA-DR antigens, only a subset of monocytes express HLA-DQ(DC) antigens [40, 41, 57, 71, 90]. When peripheral blood monocytes were separated into two categories based upon their reactivity with the monoclonal antibody Mac 120, only those which were Mac 120-positive could present antigen. Interestingly only Mac 120-positive cells displayed HLA-DQ [41]. Treatment of monocytes with immune interferon increases expression of HLA-DR [40, 55, 57, 112] and HLA-DQ (DC) [40].

Expression of class II antigens, however, is not confined to traditional cellular components of the immune system. Initially, it was noted that several human tumor cell lines of non-bone-marrow origin also expressed class II antigens (notably melanoma cells), and that this expression could be increased by immune interferon [9]. Normal cultured human large and small vessel endothelial cells, as well as human dermal fibroblasts, could be induced to express HLA-DR, and this effect could be mediated by activated T cell products or by recombinant immune interferon [23, 95, 96]. In fact, recent studies have demonstrated that cultured cells from virtually every organ and embryonic germ layer can be induced to express HLA-DR in response to immune interferon, although a few tumor cell lines, such as teratocarcinomas and neuroblastomas, do not express class II antigens in response to this lymphokine [46].

The dramatic increase in class II antigen surface expression induced by immune interferon is controlled in part through regulation of mRNA levels. When steady-state levels of RNA from immune-interferon-treated human endothelial cells and dermal fibroblasts were analyzed by Northern blot hybridization, mRNAs for the α and β chains of DR, DQ, and DP(SB), were induced, as well as mRNA for the invariant chain; under basal conditions, class II mRNAs were not detected. The level of HLA-DR induction was about ten times greater than for HLA-DQ. Treatment of human lymphoblastoid and myeloma cell lines with immune interferon increases HLA-DR α and β chain mRNA [103]. Furthermore, addition of γ-interferon to cultures of mouse macrophages results in at least a ten fold increase in I-region-encoded mRNA [86]. The dramatic induction is believed to occur at the level of RNA synthesis, although mechanisms relating to RNA processing and stability have not been eliminated.

The expression of class II MHC antigens upon non-bone-marrow-derived cells is now well established. However, the role of these Ia-positive cells in immune responses is a less resolved issue. The HLA-DR induced on human endothelial cells and fibroblasts [95, 96], as well as other cell types, has the typical two-chain structure characteristic of lymphocyte HLA-DR [53, 58]. Although there are no data comparing endothelial HLA-DR structure with the autologous fibroblast or lymphocyte antigen, comparison of HLA-DR antigens of autologous melanoma and B lymphoblastoid cell lines revealed differences in glycosylation, but not in protein structure [5]. Therefore it is possible that, as sugested for allogeneic accessory cells and B cells [26], the expressed class II antigen may be post-translationally altered (i.e., differently glycosylated), and thus exhibit different T cell reactivity. Since studies of the function of murine homologues of the HLA-D region genes suggests that the I-A and I-E loci function independently in the generation of an immune response [87], it is possible that differential expression of induced class II antigens may result in participation of those Ia-positive cells in some but not all immune functions. Thus, although most cells may be induced to express class II MHC antigens, their ability to function as accessory cells in immune responses may be limited by the nature of the induced class II antigens, as well as by their ability to produce the soluble factor interleukin-1 (IL-1) required to support T-cell responses.

Nonetheless, the HLA-DR induced on human umbilical vein endothelium (HUVE) and human dermal fibroblasts (HDF) have been shown to function in immune responses in a variety of ways: First, induced DR antigens on immune-interferon-treated HUVE and HDF are recognized by DR-restricted human CTL clones with subsequent target cell cytolysis [24, 95]. Minor contaminating populations of traditional Ia-positive accessory cells could not account for the effects, since there is no bystander effect in these assays.The array of accessory molecules used by the cloned CTL in the recognition of Ia-positive human fibroblasts and endothelial cells is qualitatively similar to that used in the recognition of a lymphoid target cell [24].

Second, HLA-DR-positive HUVE and HDF can present nominal antigen to resting or activated memory T cells. Traditionally, cells in the mononuclear phagocyte lineage have been considered to be the major antigen-presenting cells, although Langerhans cells of the skin and dendritic cells of lymphoid organs may also function as accessory cells [11, 72]. Although nominal antigen presentation by HUVE was reported [17, 18, 43, 44], contamination by traditional antigen presenting cells was not eliminated in the early work. More convincingly, Burger and coworkers [115] have found that cloned endothelial cells could present nominal antigen to T cell clones. In addition, cultured endothelial cells may secrete a factor that has IL-1-like activity [115]. Isolated human thyroid cells [75], Ia-positive murine vascular smooth muscle cells [85], as well as isolated Ia-positive murine astrocytes [33], also present nominal antigen. Umetsu et al. [113] have reported that in the long term, multiply passaged cultures of HDF, when treated with immune interferon, will also present nominal antigen in an MHC-restricted manner to autologous T cell clones and resting T cells. Murine cells transfected with class II antigens will also present nominal antigen. Thus, a variety of cells can present antigens which require processing;this sugests that perhaps all cells can perform antigen-processing events. The extent to which cells can function as accessory cells may be determined by the efficiency of antigen uptake and processing, as well as the level of Ia expression or the presence of accessory molecules.

Third, HUVE can stimulate naive T cells in a primary allogeneic response [43, 96]. In these responses, it does not matter whether the endothelial cells are pretreated with immune interferon to express DR antigens; presumably, the normal peripheral blood T cells in these cocultures are partly activated and the activated subpopulation rapidly induces endothelial cells to become HLA-DR-positive. HDF are markedly less stimulatory than HUVE, however, whether or not HLA-DR is induced by immune interferon pretreatment and whether or not purified IL-1 is added to supplement the cultures [95]. Why the endothelial cells are immunogenic while HDF fail to generate an allogeneic response is not clear, but it supports the concept that Ia expression is necessary but not sufficient to produce a fully competent accessory cell.

The T cell proliferation generated in an allogeneic response is, at best, only an indirect measure of helper T cell (Th) function. Since not all class II-bearing cells can stimulate a primary allogeneic proliferative response [39] (a measure of Th activation), more relevant questions relate to the ability of these Ia-positive vascular and stromal cells to induce specific effector cell subsets. For example, there is no direct evidence that nonlymphoid cells induced by immune interferon to express Ia will generate both suppressor and helper T cell subsets. Naive resting Th may require different signals from an accessory cell than from previously stimulated Th [20]. In fact, there is a growing body of evidence suggesting that Ia-positive accessory cells are heterogeneous, in that the in vitro function of many accessory cells is restricted to the activation of some, but not all, T cell functions [30, 100]. For instance, Ia-positive murine B cell lymphomas can act as accessory cells to stimulate antigen-specific T cell proliferation. However, these cells did not significantly activate T cell help, but rather efficiently stimulated only suppressor T cells [99]. More surprising, however, is the finding that the activity of dendritic cells may also be restricted to the induction of a limited range of T cell functions which excludes generation of T cell help [30]. Thus, it may be the exception rather than the rule that cells induced to express Ia antigens are capable of activating *all* T cell subsets, as well as participating in T-B cooperation.

T cells, as well as macrophages, secrete factors that alter B cell growth and differentiation [48]. One such B cell growth factor (BCGF I) is derived from supernatants of cultured T cells. This factor has recently been shown to induce a selective increase in the expression of Ia antigens on small resting B cells [88, 102]. B cells may specifically bind antigen via surface immunoglobulin, process it, and present it to T cells. The induced increase in B cell Ia expression by the T cell product may facilitate the process of specific antigen presentation to highly efficient levels [47].

Suppression of Ia Expression

Increased expression of class II MHC gene products may be a mechanism to enhance immunologic responsiveness. Diminishing immune reactivity, however, is at times equally as important. Decreasing Ia expression may play an important role in suppressing immune reactions. The restricted basal expression of class II antigens may represent one mechanism to control lymphocyte responsiveness. The low levels of Ia-positive macrophages in all tissues (except the thymus) may contribute to the ease of inducing tolerance to foreign antigens during neonatal life [77, 78]. However, since most cells can be induced to express class II antigens, it is likely that additional negative control mechanisms exist to suppress development of immune responses. In the murine macrophage, γ-interferon-induced expression of Ia my be opposed by several agents. E class prostaglandins have been shown to diminish expression of Ia antigens on cultured mouse macrophages and on macrophages induced by lymphokines [108]. Bacterial endotoxin [110, 111] and glucocorticosteroids [1] have been shown to diminish expression of Ia on mouse macrophages and epidermal Langerhans cells respectively. It was suggested that LPS inhibits immune interferon regulation of macrophage Ia expression by stimulating macrophage prostaglandin E_2 production [110, 111]. These regulatory agents are probably not part of a general control mechanism, since they do not appear to be active in other cell types.

Physiologic Significance of Inducible Class II MHC Expression

The issue of which cells in vivo actually function as antigen presenting cells with low antigen concentrations remains largely unexplored. The physiological significance of inducible class II MHC antigen expression is unknown, but it is possible that expression of these antigens may confer some of the functions of traditional accessory cells to the vascular or stromal cells in a local immune response. A model (Fig. 3) for such a peripheral immune response illustrates the importance of such an induction [e.g. 97]. Antigen responsiveness may be initiated in the peripheral tissues when a stromal macrophage or antigen-specific B cell processes and presents a foreign antigen in combination with self-class II polymorphic determinants to a T cell. Burger and Vetto [16] have postulated that nominal antigen presentation by vascular endothelium might be the initial mechanism of Th activation. The activated T cell, through release of mediators (e.g., immune interferon) could modulate the endothelium or the nearby microvasculature and neighboring stromal cells to express class II antigens. The endothelium, because of its anatomic position, could recruit blood-borne antigen specific T cells by processing the nominal antigen and presenting it in combination with the newly induced class II molecules. Additionally, the presence of antigen and class II molecules, or other induced antigens [13], on the luminal surface of the vessel wall may promote the adherence of both antigen-specific and naive lymphocytes and

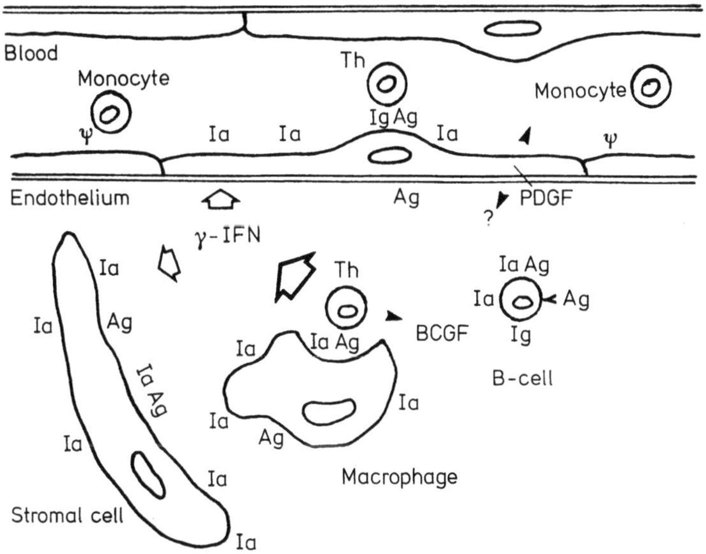

Fig. 3. Induction of class II antigens and the generation of a peripheral immune response. Native antigen (*Ag*) introduced into peripheral tissue is captured by a resident tissue macrophage or bound by B cell Ig receptors. Both these cells can internalize and process antigen and re-present it in the form of peptide fragments (*Ag*) to MHC-restricted T helper cells (*Th*). The T cell receptor recognizes the complex of processed antigen and class II MHC molecules (*Ia*) on either the macrophage or B cell surface and activates the Th cell. Activation results in release of lymphokines, including *BCGF*, which increases Ia antigens on surrounding B cells, as well as immune interferon (γ-*IFN*), which induces Ia expression on surrounding vascular and stromal cells. Increased expression of Ia makes presentation of low concentrations of antigen to responding T cells more efficient. The Ia-positive fibroblasts and endothelial cells can bind native antigen, process it, and re-present the antigen fragment to Th in association with the induced Ia. The relative stability of induced Ia on vascular and stromal cells may serve to sustain the ongoing immune response. Expression of Ia and antigen by the endothelial cell within the vascular lumen may recruit antigen-specific Th cells to the area of the ongoing response. Chemotactic agents produced by the endothelial cells (such as PDGF) may recruit unsensitized PMN or monocytes to the tissues, as well as having additional effects on the cells involved in the immune response. Additionally, monokines (e.g., IL-1) produced by locally activated macrophages may induce antigens on the surface of the endothelial cells (ψ) which facilitate monocyte or naive lymphocyte attachment and transmigration across the vascular wall. In addition to being antigenically different, endothelial cells are morphologically and possibly physiologically altered by their interactions with the traditional cellular components of the immune system and their products. Although these differences may facilitate transmigration of cells to the area of a normal stromal immune response, they may increase recognition and subsequent endothelial destruction by CTL during allograft rejection

mononuclear cells to the endothelium and facilitate their traffic from the blood stream to extravascular sites of inflammation. Stromal cells, similarly induced to express class II antigens, now function as antigen-presenting cells to amplify or sustain the ongoing tissue response. Additionally, stromal B cells, induced to express more surface Ia by the BCGF released from activated T cells, may also process and present antigen to T cells [19, 62, 81, 101]. Since the vascular endothelium can synthesize a PDGF-like mitogen [25, 28], release of this protein may stimulate the ongoing stromal immune response [4, 50], as well as recruit additional monocytes and neutrophils to the area of the response. The interactions between mononuclear cells and endothelium may alter vascular permeability as well as changing regional blood flow patterns [42]. These vascular effects may be responsible for the heterogeneity of the cellular response in many inflammatory infiltrates (as well as in a rejecting allograft).

Evidence is accumulating to support this model of an immune response in the peripheral tissues. The recent observations that microvascular endothelial cell Ia antigens increase prior to inflammatory cell infiltration in guinea pig experimental encephalitis, a model of T cell-mediated autoimmune disease, suggests that in vivo modulation of endothelial cell class II molecules may, in fact, be an important aspect of the local immune response [109]. Additionally, focal microvascular expression of HLA-DR in human skin can be markedly augmented by immunologic reactions. Similarly, Ia antigens have been induced on human epidermal cells (keratinocytes) in pathological conditions where activated T cells are known to be present [8, 15, 61].

Although the normal role of inducible class II antigens may be to recruit T cells and augment developing responses to foreign antigen, in those instances where the endothelium is perceived as foreign (such as in an allograft), the presence of class II antigens may make the endothelium an initiator as well as a target of a pathological immune response. Class II molecules are potent transplantation antigens, as evidenced by their ability to stimulate allogeneic T cell proliferation in vitro and cause rejection of class II incompatible grafts in vivo. The inducible expression of class II antigens on the luminal surface of vessels in allograft organs may activate T cells and make the donor endothelium a prime target for host T cells [27, 84]. In fact, the major site of immunologic attack in an allografted organ is often the vasculature [29]. It is possible, then, that T cell recognition of immune-interferon-induced class II antigens on endothelial as well as a variety of stromal cells may have both physiologic functions in a normal immune response and pathological consequences during immune-mediated injury of an allogeneic transplant.

Acknowledgments. We would like to thank Drs. A. Abbas, J. Boss, D. Dialynas, L. Glimcher, and especially A. Korman for comments on the manuscript, and A. Furumoto-Dawson for manuscript preparation and editing.

References

1. Aberer W, Stingl L, Pogantsch S, Stingl G (1984) Effect of glucocorticosteroids on epidermal cell-induced immune responses. J Immunol 133:792–796
2. Accolla RS (1983) Human B cell variants immunoselected against a single Ia antigen subset have lost expression of several Ia antigen subsets. J Exp Med 157:1053–1058
3. Accolla RS, Carra G, Guardiola J (1985) Reactivation by a trans-acting factor of human MHC-Ia gene expression in interspecies hybrids between an Ia-negative human B cell variant and an Ia-positive mouse B cell lymphoma. Proc Natl Acad Sci USA 82:5145–5149
4. Acres RB, Lamb JR, Feldman M (1985) Effects of PDGF and EGF on antigen-induced proliferation of human T-cell lines. Immunol 54:9–16
5. Alexander S, Hubbard SC, Strominger JL (1984) HLA-DR antigens of autologous melanoma and B lymphoblastoid cell lines: differences in glycosylation but not protein structure. J Immunol 133:315–320
6. Austin P, Trowsdale J, Rudd C, Bodmer W, Feldmann M, Lamb J (1985) Functional expression of HLA-DP genes transfected into mouse fibroblasts. Nature 313:61–64

7. Baglioni C (1985) Mechanism of action of interferons. In: Streilein et al. (eds) Advances in gene technology: molecular biology of the immune system. Cambridge University Press, Cambridge, pp 53–55
8. Barclay AN, Mason DW (1982) Induction of Ia antigen in rat epidermal cells and gut epithelium by immunologic stimuli. J Exp Med 156:1665–1676
9. Basham TY, Merigan TC (1983) Recombinant interferon-γ increases HLA-DR synthesis and expression. J Immunol 130:1492–1494
10. Beller DI, Unanue ER (1981) Regulation of macrophage populations. II. Synthesis and expression of Ia antigens by peritoneal exudate macrophages is a transient event. J Immunol 126:263–269
11. Benacerraf B (1981) Role of MHC gene products in immune regulation. Science 212:1229–1238
12. Ben-Nun A, Glimcher LH, Weis JH, Seidman JG (1984) Functional expression of a cloned I-Aβ^k gene in B-lymphoma cells. Science 223:825–827
13. Bevilacqua MF, Pober JS, Wheeler ME, Mendrick D, Cotran RS, Gimbrone MD (1985) Interleukin-1 acts on vascular endothelial cells to increase their adhesivity for blood leukocytes. J Clin Invest 76:2003–2011
14. Boss JM, Strominger JL (1984) Cloning and sequence analysis of a DC-3β gene. Proc Natl Acad Sci USA 81:5199–5203
15. Breathnach SM, Katz SI (1983) Keratinocytes synthesize Ia antigen in acute cutaneous graft-vs-host disease. J Immunol 131:2741–2745
16. Burger DR, Vetto RM (1982) Vascular endothelium as a major participant in T-lymphocyte immunity. Cell Immunol 70:357–361
17. Burger, DR, Vetto RM, Hamblin A, Dumonde DC (1982) T-lymphocyte activation by antigen presented by HLA-DR compatible endothelial cells. In: Nossel, Vogel (eds) Pathobiology of the endothelial cell. Academic, London, pp 387–407
18. Burger DR, Vetto RM, Hamblin A, Goldstein A, Hubbard M, Dumonde DC (1981) Endothelial cell presentation of antigen to human T cells. Hum Immunol 3:209–230
19. Chesnut RW, Colon SM, Grey HM (1982) Antigen presentation by normal B cells, B cell tumors and macrophages: functional and biochemical comparison. J Immunol 128:1764–1768
20. Chu ET, Lareau M, Rosenwasser LJ, Dinarello CA, Geha RS (1985) Antigen presentation by EBV-B cells to resting and activated T celles: role of interleukin 1. J Immunol 134:1676–1681
21. Claesson-Welsh L, Barker PG, Larhammar D, Rask L, Ruddle FH, Peterson PA (1984) The gene encoding the human class II antigen-associated γ-chain is located on chromosome 6. Immunogenetics 20:89–93
22. Cline J, Golde DW (1979) Cellular interactions in haematopoiesis. Nature 277:177–181
23. Collins T, Korman AJ, Wake CT, Boss JM, Kappes DJ, Fiers W, Ault KA, Gimbrone MA, Strominger JL, Pober JS (1984a) Immune interferon activates multiple class II MHC genes and the associated invariant chain gene in human endothelial cells and dermal fibroblasts. Proc Natl Acad Sci USA 81:4917–4921
24. Collins T, Krensky AM, Clayberger C, Fiers W, Gimbrone MA, Burakoff SJ, Pober JS (1984b) Human cytolytic T lymphocyte interactions with vascular endothelium and fibroblasts: role of effector and target cell molecules. J Immunol 133:1878–1884
25. Collins T, Ginsburg D, Boss JM, Orkin SH, Pober JS (1985) Cultured human endothelial cells express platelet derived growth factor B chain: cDNA cloning and structural analysis. Nature 316:748–750
26. Cowing C, Chapdelaine JM (1983) T cells discriminate between Ia antigens expressed on allogeneic accessory cells and B cells: a potential function for carbohydrate side chains on Ia molecules. Proc Natl Acad Sci USA 80:6000–6004
27. deWaal RMW, Bogman MJJ, Maass CN, Cornelissen LMH, Tax WJM, Koene RAP (1983) Variable expression of Ia antigens on the vascular endothelium of mouse skin allografts. Nature 303:426–429
28. DiCorleto PG, Bowen-Pope DF (1983) Cultured endothelial cells produce a platelet-derived growth factor-like protein. Proc Natl Acad Sci USA 80:1919–2023
29. Dvorak HF, Mihm MC, Dvorak AM, Barnes BA, Manscav EJ, Galli SJ (1979) Rejection of first-set skin allografts in man. The microvasculature is the critical target of the immune response. J Exp Med 150:322

30. Erb P, Ramila G, Studer S, Loeffler H, Cecka JM, Conscience JF, Feldman M (1984) Heterogeneity of accessory cells. Immunobiology 168:141¹53
31. Fellous M, Nir U, Wallach D, Merlin G, Rubinstein M, Revel M (1982) Interferon-dependent induction of mRNA for the major histocompatibility antigens in human fibroblasts and lymphoid cells. Proc Natl Acad Sci USA 79:3082–3086
32. Folsom V, Gold DP, White J, Marrack P, Kappler J, Tonegawa S (1984) Functional and inducible expression of a transfected murine class II MHC gene. Proc Natl Acad Sci USA 81:2045–2049
33. Fontana A, Fierz W, Wekerle H (1984) Astrocytes present myelin basic protein to encephalitogenic T-cell lines. Nature 307:273–276
34. Friedman RL, Stark GR (1985) α Interferon-induced transcription of HLA and metallothionein genes containing homologous upstream sequences. Nature 314:637–639
35. Germain RN, Norcross MA, Margulies DH (1983) Functional expression of a transfected murine class II MHC gene. Nature 306:190–194
36. Germain RN, Lechler RI, Norcross MA, Bentler DM, Margulies DH (1985) Ia expression, structure, and function analyzed by DNA-mediated gene transfer. In: Streilein et al. (eds) Advances in gene technology: molecular biology of the immune system. Cambridge University Press, Cambridge, pp 167–168
37. Gillies SD, Folsom V, Tonegawa S (1984) Cell-type specific enhancer element associated with a mouse MHC gene, Eβ. Nature 310:594–597
38. Gladstone P, Pious D (1980) Identification of a trans-acting function regulating HLA-DR expression in a DR-negative B cell variant. Somatic Cell Genet 6:285–298
39. Glimcher LH, Kim KJ, Green I, Paul WE (1982) Ia antigen-bearing B cell tumor lines can present protein antigen and alloantigen in a MHC-restricted fashion to antigen-reactive T cells. J Exp Med 155:445–459
40. Gonwa TA, Stobo JD (1984) Differential expression of Ia molecules by human monocytes. J Clin Invest 74:859–866
41. Gonwa TA, Picker LJ, Raff HV, Goyert SM, Silver J, Stobo JD (1983) Antigen-presenting capabilities of human monocytes correlates with their expression of HLA-DS, an Ia determinant distinct from HLA-DR. J Immunol 130:706–711
42. Hanto DW, Hopt UT, Hoffman R, Simmons RL (1982) Lymphocyte recruitment, regional blood flow, and vascular permeability at sites of allogeneic cellular interactions. J Immunol 129:2437–2443
43. Hirschberg H, Evensen SA, Henriksen T, Thorsby E (1975) The human mixed lymphocyte-endothelium culture interaction. Transplantation 19:495–507
44. Hirschberg H, Bergh OJ, Thorsby E (1980) Antigen vascular presenting properties of human endothelial cells. J Exp Med 152:249s–255s
45. Hood L, Kronenberg M, Hunkapiller T (1985) T cell antigen receptors and the immunoglobulin supergene family. Cell 40:225–229
46. Houghton AN, Thomson TM, Gross D, Oettgen HF, Old LJ (1984) Surface antigens of melanoma and melanocytes. Specificity of induction of Ia antigens by human γ-interferon. J Exp Med 160:255–269
47. Howard JC (1985) Immunological help at last. Nature 314:494–495
48. Howard M, Paul WE (1983) Regulation of B-cell growth and differentiation by soluble factors. Annu Rev Immunol 1:307–333
49. Howell DN, Berger AE, Cresswell P (1982) Human T-B lymphoblast hybrids express HLA-DR specificities not expressed by either parent. Immunogenetics 15:199–206
50. Johnson HM, Torres BA (1985) Peptide growth factors PDGF, EFG, and FGF regulate immune interferon production. J Immunol 134:2824
50a. Kappes DJ, Arnot D, Okada K, Strominger JL (1984) Structure and polymorphism of the HLA class II SB light chain genes. EMBO J 3:2985–2993
51. Kaufman JF, Strominger JL (1982) HLA-DR light chain has a polymorphic N-terminal region and a conserved Ig-like C-terminal region. Nature 297:694–697
52. Kaufman JF, Strominger JL (1983) The extracellular region of light chains from human and murine MHC class II antigens consists of 2 domains. J Immunol 130:808–817
53. Kaufman JF, Auffray C, Korman AJ, Shackelford DA, Strominger JL (1984) The class II molecules of human and murine major histocompatibility complex. Cell 36:1–13

54. Kelley A, Trowsdale J (1985) Complete nucleotide sequence of a functional HLA-DPβ gene and the region between the DPβ1 and DPα1 genes: Comparison of the 5′ ends of the HLA class II genes. Nucleic Acids Res 13:1607–1621
55. Kelley VE, Fiers W, Strom TB (1984) Cloned human interferon-gamma, but not interferon beta or alpha induces expression of HLA-DR determinants by fetal monocytes and myeloid leukemic cell lines. J Immunol 132:240–245
56. Koch N, Wong GH, Schrader JW (1984) Ia antigens and associated invariant chain are induced simultaneously in lines of T-dependent mast cells by immune interferon. J Immunol 132:1361–1369
57. Koeffler HP, Ranyard J, Yelton L, Billing R, Bohman R (1984) γ-interferon induces expression of the HLA-D antigens on normal and leukemic human myeloid cells. Proc Natl Acad Sci USA 81:4080–4084
58. Korman AJ (1985) Structure and expression of human class II MHC antigens. PhD thesis, Harvard University
59. Korman AJ, Boss JM, Spies T, Sorrentino R, Okada K, Strominger JL (1985) Genetic complexity of human class II histocompatibility antigens. Immunol Rev (in press)
60. Kvist S, Wiman K, Claesson L, Peterson PA, Dobberstein B (1982) Membrane insertion and oligomeric assembly of HLA-DR histocompatibility antigens. Cell 29:61–69
61. Lampert IA, Suitters AJ, Chisholm PM (1981) Expression of Ia antigens on epidermal keratinocytes in graft-versus-host disease. Nature 293:149–151
62. Lanzavecchia A (1985) Antigen-specific interaction between T and B cells. Nature 314:537–539
63. Larhammar D, Schenning L, Gustafsson K, Wiman K, Claesson L, Rask L, Peterson PA (1982) Complete amino acid sequence of an HLA-DR antigen-like β chain as predicated from the nucleotide sequence: similarities with immunoglobulins and HLA-A, -B, and -C antigens. Proc Natl Acad Sci USA 79:3687–3691
64. Larhammar D, Hyldig-Nielsen JJ, Servenius B, Anderson G, Rask L, Peterson PA (1983) Exon-intron organization and complete nucleotide sequence of a human major histocompatibility antigen DCβ gene. Proc Natl Acad Sci USA 80:7313–7317
65. Larhammar D, Hammerling U, Denaro M, L und T, Flavell RA, Rask L, Peterson PA (1983) Structure of the murine immune response I-Aβ locus: sequence of the I-Aβ gene and an adjacent β chain second domain exon. Cell 34:179–188
66. Larhammar D, Anderson G, Bill P, Bohme J, Claesson L, Denaro M, Emmoth E, Gustafsson K, Hammerling U, Heldin E, Hyldig-Nielsen JJ, Und P, Schenning L, Servenius B, Widmark E, Rask L, Peterson P (1983) Molecular analysis of human class II transplantation antigens and their genes. Hum Immunol 8:95–100
67. Larhammar D, Servenius B, Rask L, Peterson PA (1985) Characterization of an HLA-DRβ pseudogene. Proc Natl Acad Sci USA 82:1475–1479
68. Lechler RI, Norcross MA, Germain RN (1985) Qualitative and quantitative studies of antigen presenting cell function using I-A transfected cells. In: Streilein et al. (eds) Advances in Gene Technology: molecular biology of the immune system. Cambridge University Press, Cambridge, pp 223–224
69. Levine F, Pious D (1984) Revertants from the HLA class II regulatory mutant 6.1.6: implications for the regulation of Ia gene expression. J Immunol 132:959–962
70. Levine F, Erlich HA, Mach B, Pious D (1985) Transcriptional regulation of HLA class II and invariant chain genes. J Immunol 134:637–640
71. Linch DC, Nadler LM, Luther EA, Lipton JM (1984) Discordant expression of human Ia-like antigens on hematopoietic progenitor cells. J Immunol 132:2324–2329
72. Lipsky PE, Kettman JR (1982) Accessory cells unrelated to mononuclear phagocytes and not of bone marrow origin. Immunol Today 3:36–42
73. Littman DR, Thomas Y, Maddon PJ, Chess L, Axel R (1985) The isolation and sequence of the gene encoding T8: a molecule defining functional classes of T lymphocytes. Cell 40:237–246
74. Loosmore S, Gladstone P, Pious D, Jerry LM, Tamaoki T (1982) Control of HLA-DR antigen gene expression at the pretranslational level: comparison of an HLA-DR-positive B lymphoblastoid cell line and its HLA-DR-negative variant. Immunogenetics 15:139–150

75. Londei M, Lamb JR, Bottazzo GF, Feldman M (1984) Epithelial cells expressing aberrant MHC class II determinants can present antigen to cloned human T cells. Nature 312:639–641
76. Long EO, Mach B, Accolla RS (1984) Ia-negative B-cell variants reveal a coordinate regulation in the transcription of the HLA class II gene family. Immunogenetics 19:349–353
77. Lu CY, Calamai EG, Unanue ER (1979) A defect in the antigen-presenting function of macrophages from neonatal mice. Nature 282:327–329
78. Lu CY, Beller DI, Unanue ER (1980) During ontogeny, Ia-bearing accessory cells are found early in the thymus but late in the spleen. Proc Natl Acad Sci USA 77:1597–1601
79. Malissen B, Steinmetz M, McMillan M, Pierres M, Hood L (1983) Expression of I-A^k class II genes in mouse L cells after DNA-mediated gene transfer. Nature 305:440–443
80. Malissen B, Price MP, Goverman JM, McMillan M, White J, Kappler J, Marrack P, Pierres M, Pierres A, Hood L (1984) Gene transfer of H-2 class II genes: antigen presentation by mouse fibroblast and hamster B-cell lines. Cell 36:319–327
81. Malynn BA, Wortis HH (1984) Role of antigen-specific B cells in the induction of SRBC-specific T cell proliferation. J Immunol 132:2253–2258
82. Mathis DJ, Benoist CO, Williams V, Kanter MR, McDevitt HO (1983) The murine E immune response gene.Cell 32:745–754
83. Matis LA, Glimcher LH, Paul WF, Schwartz RH (1983) Magnitude of response of histocompatibility-restricted T cell clones is a function of the product of the concentrations of antigen and Ia molecules. Proc Natl Acad Sci USA 80:6019–6023
84. Milton AD, Fabre JW (1985) Massive induction of donor type class I and class II MHC antigens in rejecting cardiac allografts in the rat. J Exp Med 161:98–112
85. Moyer CF, Reinisch CL (1984) Ia expression and antigen presentation by vascular smooth muscle cells. Fed Proc 43:972
86. Nakamura M, Manser T, Pearson G, Daley MJ, Gefter ML (1984) Effect of immune IFN on the immune response in vivo and on gene expression in vitro. Nature 307:381–382
87. Nepom JT, Benacerraf B, Germain RN (1981) Analysis of Ir gene function using monoclonal antibodies: independent regulation of GAT and GLPhe T cell response by I-A and I-E subregion products on a single accessory cell population. J Immunol 127:31
88. Noelle R, Krammer PH, Ohara J, Uhr JW, Vitetta ES (1984) Increased expression of Ia antigens on resting B cells: an additional role for B-cell growth factor. Proc Natl Acad Sci USA 81:6149–6153
89. Norcross MA, Bentley DM, Margulies DH, Germain RN (1984) Membrane Ia expression and antigen-presenting accessory cell function of L cells transfected with class II major histocompatibility complex genes. J Exp Med 160:1316–1337
90. Nunez G, Giles RC, Ball EJ, Hurley CK, Capra JD, Stastny P (1984) Expression of HLA-DR, MB, MT, and SB antigens on human mononuclear cells: identification of two phenotypically distinct monocyte populations. J Immunol 133:1300–1306
91. Okada K, Boss J, Prentice H, Spies T, Mengler R, Auffray C, Lillie J, Grossberger D, Strominger JL (1985) Gene organization of the DC and DX subregions of the human major histocompatibility complex. Proc Natl Acad Sci USA 82:3410–3414
92. Okada K, Prentice H, Boss J, Levy D, Kappes D, Spies T, Raghupathy R, Mengler R, Auffray C, Strominger JL (1985) SB subregion of the human major histocompatibility complex: gene organization, allelic polymorphism and expression in transformed cells. EMBO J 4:739–748
93. Peterlin BM, Hardy KJ (1985) Changes in chromatin structure associated with HLA-DR alpha gene activation. Fed Proc 44:783
94. Pious D, Hawley P, Forrest G (1973) Isolation and characterization of HLA variants in cultured human lymphoid cells. Proc Natl Acad Sci USA 70:1397–1401
95. Pober JS, Collins T, Gimbrone MA, Cotran RS, Gitlin JD, Fiers W, Clayberger C, Krensky AM, Burakoff SJ, Reiss CS (1983) Lymphocytes recognize human vascular endothelial and dermal fibroblast Ia antigens induced by recombinant immune interferon. Nature 305:726–729

96. Pober JS, Gimbrone MA, Cotran RS, Reiss CS, Burakoff SJ, Fiers W, Ault K (1983) Ia expression by vascular endothelium is inducible by activated T cells and by human immune interferon. J Exp Med 157:1339–1353
97. Pober JS, Gimbrone MA, Collins T, Cotran RS, Ault KA, Fiers W, Krensky AM, Clayberger C, Reiss C, Burakoff SJ (1984) Interactions of T lymphocytes with human vascular endothelial cells: role of endothelial cell surface antigens. Immunobiology 168:483–494
98. Rabourdin-Combe C, Mach B (1983) Expression of HLA-DR antigens the surface of mouse L cells co-transfected with cloned human genes. Nature 303:670–674
99. Ramila G, Erb P (1983) Accessory cell-dependent T selection of specific T cell functions. Nature 304:442–445
100. Ramila G, Studer S, Mischler S, Erb P (1983) Evaluation of Ia^+ tumor cell lines and peritoneal exudate macrophages as accessory cells: differential requirements for the activation of certain T cell functions. J Immunol 131:2714–2718
101. Rock K, Benacerraf B, Abbas A (1984) Antigen presentation by hapten specific B lymphocytes. I. Role of surface immunoglobulin receptors. J Exp Med 160:1102–1112
102. Roehm NW, Leibson HJ, Zlotnik A, Kappler J, Marrack P, Cambier JC (1984) Interleukin-induced increase in Ia expression by normal mouse B cells. J Exp Med 160:679–694
103. Rosa F, Hatat D, Abadie A, Wallach D, Revel M, Fellous M (1983) Differential regulation of HLA-DR mRNAs and cell surface antigens by interferon. EMBO J 2:1585–1589
104. Saito H, Maki RA, Clayton LK, Tonegawa S (1983) Complete primary structures of the Eβ chain and its gene of the mouse MHC. Proc Natl Acad Sci USA 80:5520–5524
105. Schamboeck A, Korman AJ, Kamb A, Strominger JL (1983) Organization of the transcriptional unit of a human class II histocompatibility antigen: HLA-DR heavy chain. Nucleic Acids Res 11:8663–8674
106. Schlossman SF, Chess L, Humphreys RE, Strominger JL (1976) Distribution of Ia-like molecules on the surface of normal and leukemic human cells. Proc Natl Acad Sci USA 73:1299–1303
107. Schwartz R (1985) T-lymphocyte recognition of antigen in association with gene products of the MHC. Ann Rev Immunol 3:237–261
108. Snyder DS, Beller DI, Unanue ER (1982) Prostaglandins modulate macrophage Ia expression. Nature 299:163–165
109. Sobel RA, Blanchette BW, Bhan AK, Colvin RB (1984) The immunopathology of experimental allergic encephalomyelitis. II. Endothelial cell Ia increases prior to inflammatory cell infiltration. J Immunol 132:2402–2407
110. Steeg PS, Moore RN, Johnson HM, Oppenheim JJ (1982) Regulation of murine macrophage Ia antigen expression by a lymphokine with immune interferon activity. J Exp Med 156:1780–1793
111. Steeg PS, Johnson HM, Oppenheim JJ (1982) Regulation of murine macrophage Ia antigen expression by an immune interferon-like lymphokine: inhibitory effect of endotoxin. J Immunol 129:2402–2406
112. Sztein MB, Steeg PS, Johnson MM, Oppenheim JJ (1984) Regulation of human peripheral blood monocyte or antigen expression in vitro by lymphokines and recombinant interferons. J Clin Invest 73:556–565
113. Umetsu DT, Pober JS, Jabara HJ, Fiers W, Yunis E, Burakoff SJ, Reiss CS, Geha RS (1985) Human dermal fibroblasts present tetanus toxoid antigen to antigen specific T cell clones. J Clin Invest 76:254–260
114. Unanue E, Beller E, Lu E, Allen PM (1984) Antigen presentation: comments on its regulation and mechanism. J Immunol 132:1–5
115. Wagner CR, Vetto RM, Burger DR (1984) The mechanism of antigen presentation by endothelial cells.Immunobiology 168:453–469
116. Weis JH, Seidman JG (1985) The expression of major histocompatibility antigens under metallothionein gene promotor control. J Immunol 134:1999–2003
117. Weis JH, Murre C (1985) Differential expression of H-2D^d and H-2L^d MHC antigens. J Exp Med 161:356–365

Epitopes Are the Functional Units of HLA Class II Molecules and Form the Molecular Basis for Disease Susceptibility *

J. Silver and S. M. Goyert

Table of Contents

Introduction

The incidence of many autoimmune diseases has for many years been known to be associated with certain HLA class II types. For example, 70% of rheumatoid arthritis (RA) patients type as DR4, compared with only 28% of the normal population. Similarly, 59% of multiple sclerosis (MS) patients express DR2, against only 26% of the normal population. Other autoimmune diseases, such as myasthenia gravis and juvenile diabetes, have also been shown to be associated with certain HLA class II types (Table 1). These associations are presumed to reflect the effect of particular class II gene products on an individual's ability to respond immunologically to an exogenous pathogen, or alternatively on his ability to regulate his response to endogenous autoantigens. This ability to respond would in turn play an important role in the etiology or pathogenesis of the disease. However, the most puzzling feature of these analyses is the lack of absolute association of the disease with a particular class II type, i.e., why many individuals with other class II types and therefore different class II gene products also develop the disease. For example, 30% of individuals with RA do not express DR4, and 41% of individuals with MS do not express DR2. Two proposals have been put for-

* This work was supported by grants from the National Institutes of Health

Table 1. The association between disease susceptibility and HLA class II type

Disease	HLA class II type	Antigen frequency (%)		Relative risk[a]	Reference
		Patients	Controls		
Rheumatoid arthritis	DR4	70	28	6.0	[41]
Multiple sclerosis	DR2	59	26	4.1	[42]
Myasthenia gravis	DR3	50	28	2.5	[42]
Insulin – dependent	DR3	56	28	3.3	[42]
diabetes	DR4	32	6	6.4	
Goodpasture's syndrome	DR2	88	32	15.9	[41]

[a] Incidence of disease among individuals with a particular class II Ia type/incidence of disease among individuals without it

ward to explain the presence of the disease in individuals with the inappropriate class II type. One is that the lack of absolute association of disease susceptibility with HLA class II type is due to the fact that the serologically detectable class II gene product does not in fact represent the real disease susceptibility gene, but is merely closely linked to it, and that if there were a means of detecting this other gene, a stronger association with the particular disease would be obtained. This logic has provided the impetus for restriction fragment length polymorphism (RFLP) studies in which the aim is to define just such a gene [1]. Although these studies have very often shown that certain class II gene fragments correlate strongly with the incidence of a particular disease, they have failed to demonstrate a substantially higher association than is normally found using serologic methods. Indeed, the result of these studies has often been to demonstrate a "splitting" of the classically defined class II types into subtypes. The second proposal that has been put forward to explain the lack of absolute association between disease susceptibility and class II type is that the disease being analyzed is in reality a heterogeneous mixture of diseases with multiple etiologies, only one or a few of which are associated with a particular class II type. This theory predicts that if one divides these complex autoimmune diseases into more homogeneous entities one should be able to demonstrate a stronger association. RA is a good example where such an approach has been used. For example, Nepom et al. [2] analyzed the expression of Ia types among juvenile RA patients who were seropositive for rheumatoid factor and found a strong association with certain subtypes of DR4. However, despite the fact that the patient population was carefully selected, there was still a lack of absolute association.

Hypothesis

We would like to propose an alternative hypothesis to explain this lack of absolute association of disease susceptibility with HLA class II type. This hypothesis contains five important components:

1. There are no disease susceptibility genes, only disease susceptibility epitopes. Thus, the association of RA with DR4 is actually an association with a class II epitope which is commonly found in DR4 individuals.

2. The conventional serologically defined DR allotype represents a conglomeration of epitopes, only one or a few of which predispose an individual to a particular disease.
3. The disease susceptibility epitope normally found in association with one DR allotype can occasionally be found associated with other DR allotypes. For example, the RA susceptibility epitope normally associated with DR4 can occasionally be found in non-DR4 individuals. This would explain the apparent lack of absolute association of RA with DR4.
4. The presence of the disease susceptibility epitope in the inappropriate DR allotype may be the result of unusual genetic mechanisms such as gene conversion or nonhomologous recombination operating between different class II loci and/or haplotypes.
5. These epitopes determine disease susceptibility by virtue of the fact that they influence immune function or, more specifically, immune responsiveness of the individual to antigens.

We will attempt to describe below the observations made by us and by several other groups which have led us to formulate this hypothesis.

The Conventional Serologically Defined DR Allotype Represents a Conglomeration of Epitopes

Three important elements combine to lead to the conclusion that the conventional, serologically defined DR allotype in fact represents a conglomeration of epitopes: (1) The MHC encodes multiple HLA class II gene loci. (2) Many of these gene loci are polymorphic. Furthermore, the products of these polymorphic loci are complex rather than simple alleles, i.e., they differ by multiple amino acid substitutions. Thus, a single class II gene product has the potential to encode multiple allodeterminants or epitopes. (3) Several class II gene loci are in strong linkage disequilibrium with each other and are consequently inherited as if they were a single genetic unit. The evidence supporting each of these tenets is summarized below.

The MHC Encodes Multiple HLA Class II Gene Loci

One of the earliest studies to demonstrate the existence of multiple HLA class II gene products involved the use of several different monoclonal antibodies (MoAbs) in immunoprecipitation and two-dimensional (2D) gel analysis. Three separate MoAbs could be shown to immunoprecipitate three different class II products from a consanguineous HLA-homozygous cell line, thus demonstrating the existence of at least three class II gene loci (Fig. 1). More recently, recombinant DNA studies have shown that there are at least seven β chain gene loci and five α chain gene loci (Fig. 2) [3–7]. These class II gene loci can be divided into three groups, DP (formerly designated SB), DQ (formerly designated DS and DC), and DR, on the basis of structural similarities and differences. Thus, the three β chain genes that comprise the DR group are approximately 95% identical, while those belonging to different groups are only 60% identical (Figs. 3 and 4). The DR and DQ molecules are the human homologues of murine I-E and I-A molecules respectively [8, 9].

The isolation of cDNA clones encoding class II molecules [4, 7, 10–14] and 2D gel analysis of class II molecules isolated from HLA-homozygous cell lines [15,

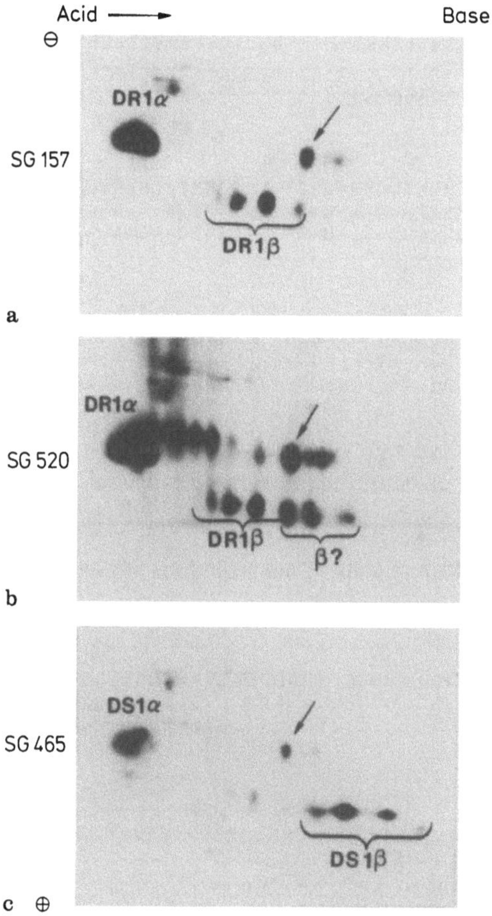

Fig. 1. Two-dimensional gel profiles of HLA class II molecules isolated from a consanguineous HLA-homozygous DR1 cell line, LG2, with three MoAbs, SG157, SG520, and SG465. The *arrow* designates the major spot of the invariant chain that was used to align the three profiles. The MoAb SG520 (panel *b*) precipitates two β chains, one identical to that in panel *a* and a second unidentifiable one different from the DQ β chain present in panel *c*

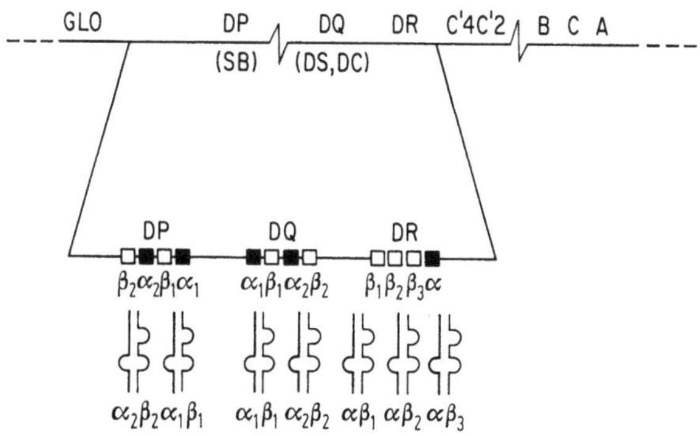

Fig. 2. Genetic organization of the human HLA class II region. The genes for three major families of class II molecules, DP, DQ, and DR are located between the genetic loci for several complement components and glyoxylase (*GLO*). They encode five α subunits (two DP, two DQ, one DR) and seven β subunits (two DP, two DQ, three DR) which associate to form $\alpha\beta$ heterodimers. The α and β subunits are both glycoproteins and contain protein moieties of approximately 235 amino acids which can be subdivided into two domains of 95 amino acids each and transmembrane and intracytoplasmic segments. The *jagged lines* between the class I loci (*A, B, C*) and the complement components (*C'4, D'2*), and between the DP and DQ loci indicate sites of frequent recombination. In contrast, no recombinational event between DQ and DR has ever been confirmed

```
        1       10        20        30        40        50       59
DP           NYLFQGRQECYAFNGTQR  FLERYIYNREEFARFDSDVGEFRAVTELGRPAAE
DQ      RDSPEDFVY-FKGM--FT---E-VRLVT--------Y--------VY----P--P----
DR      GDTRPRF-ELLKS--HF----E-VR----HFH-Q--Y---------Y---R-----D--

        60        70        80        90       100       110      118
DP      YWNSQKDILEEKRAVPORMCRHNYELGGPMTLQRRVQPKVNVSPSKKEPLNHHNLLVCH
DQ      -N----EV--RT--ELDTV-----Q-ELRT------E-T-TI---RT-A---------S
DR      -------L--Q--GQVDNY-----GVVESF-V----H-Q-T-Y-A-TQ--Q-------S

        119        130       140       150       160       170     177
DP      VTDFYPGSIEVRWFLNGQEETAGVVSTNLIRNGDWTFEILVMLEMTPQEGDVYICQVEH
DQ      ------AQ-K--M-R-D----T-----P---------Q----------R----T-H---
DR      -SG-----------R-----K------G--Q------QT-----TF-RS-E--T-----

        178         190       200       210       220       230      237
DP      TSLDSP  VEWKAQSDSARSKTLTGAGGFVLGLIICGVGIFMHRRSKKVQRGSA
DQ      P--QNPII---G---E--Q--M-S-I--------FL-L-LII-H--Q-GLLH
DR      P-VT--LT--MS-R-E--Q--M-S-V-------LFL-A-L-IYF-NQ-GHS-LQPTGFLS
```

Fig. 3. Protein sequences of DP, DQ, and DR β subunits. (Data taken from [4, 10])

```
          1       10        20        30        40        50     56
DP         IKADHVSTYAA FVQTHRPTGEFMFEFDEDEMFYVDLDKKETVWHLEEFGQAFSFE
DQ       ED-V-----ASCGVNLY-FYG-S-QYTH---G--Q-----ER---A-RWP--SKFGG-D
DR         --EE--IIQ-E -YLNPDQS-----D--G--I-H--MA------R-----RFA---

         57 60        70        80        90       100       110 114
DP       AQGGLANIAILNNNLNTLIQRSNHTQATNDPPEVTVFPKEPVELGQPNTLICHIDKFF
DQ       P--A-R-M-VAKH---IM-K-Y-S-A---EV------S-S--T---------LV-NI-
DR       ---A-----VDKA--EIMTK---Y-PI--V------LTNS----RE--V---F----T

         115 120       130       140       150       160       170
DP       PPVLNVTWLCNGELVTEGVAESLFLPRTDYSFHKFGYLTFVPSAEDFYDCRVEHWGLD
DQ       ---V-I---S--QS---D-S-TS--SKS-H--F-IS----L---DEI---K-------
DR       ---V-----R--KP--T--S-TV----E-HL-R--H--P-L--T--V-----------

         173     180       190       200       210       220       230
DP       QPLLKHWEAQEPIQMPETTETVLCALGLVLGLVGFIVGTVLIIKSLRSGHDPRAQGTL
DQ       --------PEI-AP-S-L----V-----SV--M-IV----F--QG---VGAS-H--P-
DR       E-------FDA-SPL-----N-V-----TV----I-I--IF---G--KSNAAERR-P-
```

Fig. 4. Protein sequences of DP, DQ, and DR α subunits. (Data taken from [12, 45])

16] has enabled estimation of the number of genes actually expressed. Thus, it appears that at least two of the DR β genes, two DQ β genes, and one DP β gene are expressed. A homozygous individual, therefore, can express at least five different β chain genes, and a heterozygous individual may express as many as ten.

Many HLA Class II Gene Loci Are Polymorphic

DNA sequence analysis of DR β chain genes has shown that this is an extremely polymorphic system; each individual with a different DR type encodes a different

```
        1        10        20        30        40        50        59
DR3,6   GDTRPRFLEYSTSECHFFNGTERVRYLDRYFHNQEENVRFDSDVGEFRAVTELGRPDAE
DR3,6   ----------EVKF-----------L-E-RV-----YA-Y------Y------------
DR4,6   ----------LLK------------F-E-H------YA--------Y---R--------
DR2/2   ---------WQPKR-----------F-----Y----S----------------------

        60        70        80        90        100       110      118
DR3,6   YWNSQKDLLEQKRGRVDNYCRHNYGVVESFTVQRRVHPKVTVYPSKTQPLQHHNLLVCS
DR3,6   ----------RR-AA--T--------G---------Q----------------------
DR4,6   --------------Q-----------------------Q-----A--------------
DR2/2   -------I---A-AA--T------------I-----Q----------------------

        120       130       140       150       160       170      177
DR3,6   VSGFYPGSIEVRWFRNGQEEKTGVVSTGLIHNGDWTFQTLVMLETVPRSGEVYTCQVEH
DR3,6   -N----------------------------Q----------------Q-----------
DR4,6   ---------------------A--------Q--------------F-------------
DR2/2   --------------L------A-G------QD---------------------------

        178        190       200       210       220       230      237
DR3,6   PSVTSPLTVEWRARSESAQSKMLSGVGGFVLGLLFLGAGLFIYFRNQKGHSGLQPRGFLS
DR3,6   ---M-------------------------------------------------P-T----
DR4,6   -----------S-------------------------------------------T----
DR2/2   ---------------------
```

Fig. 5. Structural polymorphism of DR β subunits. (Data taken from [10])

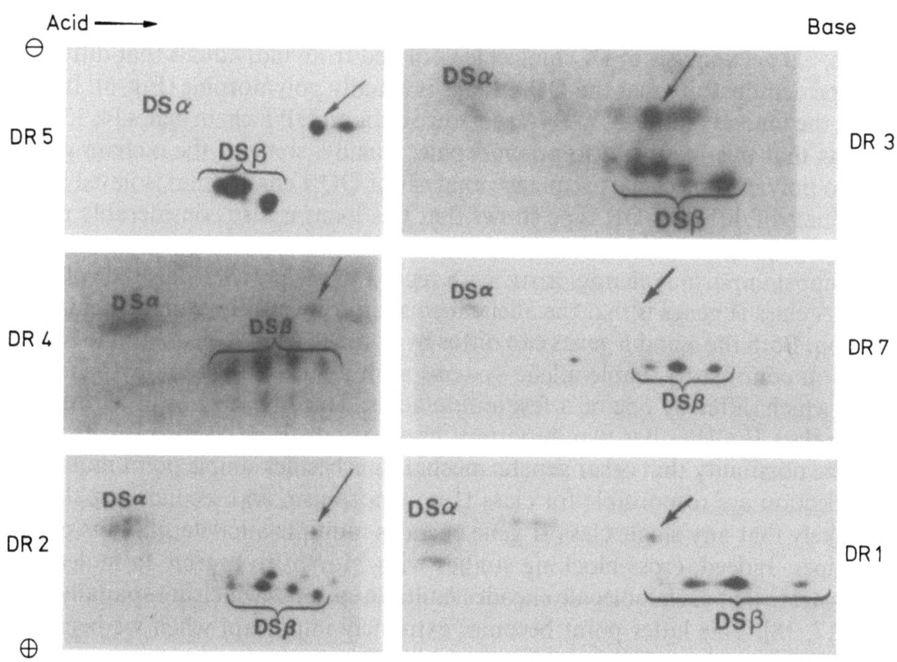

Fig. 6. Polymorphism of DQ subunits. DQ molecules were isolated from cell lines of differing DR type and analyzed by 2D gel electrophoresis. Panels are arranged according to the charge of the β chain (from more acidic to more basic) using the invariant chain (*arrow*) as a reference point. As can be seen, the DQ β subunit from a DR5 cell line is the most acidic, while that from a DR1 cell line is the most basic

```
     1        10        20        30        40        50      58
DQ4  EDIVADHVASYGVNLYQSYGPSGQYSHEFDGDEEFYVDLERKETVWQLPLFRRFRRFD
DQ7  -----------------------FT---------------------K----H-LR --
DQ9      ------------------------------------------------------
DQ6  ----------C------F-------T-------Q----------A-RW-E-SK-GG--

     59        70        80        90       100       110     116
DQ4  PQFALTNIAVLKHNLNIVIKRSNSTAATNEVPEVTVFSKSPVTLGQPNTLICLVDNIF
DQ7  ----------------------------------------------------------
DQ9  ----------------------------------------------------------
DQ6  --G--R-M--A------M---Y------------------------------------

     117 120       130       140       150       160       170 174
DQ4  PPVVNITWLSNGHSVTEGVSETSFLSKSDHSFFKISYLTFLPSADEIYDCKVEHWGLD
DQ7  ----------------------------------------------------------
DQ9  -------------------------------------------D--------------
DQ6  ------------Q----D----------------------------------------

     175  180       190       200       210       220         232
DQ4  EPLLKHWEPEIPTPMSELTETVVCALGLSVGLVGIVVGTVLIIRGLRSVGASRHQGPL
DQ7  ------------A---------------------------------------------
DQ9  ----------------------------------------------------------
DQ6  Q-------------------------------M-------F--Q--------------
```

Fig. 7. Structural polymorphism of DQ α subunits. (Data taken from [26])

DR β chain gene (Fig. 5). However, this polymorphism is not restricted to the DR β locus; 2D gel analysis of DQ molecules isolated from individuals that differ by DR type demonstrate that the DQ β locus is equally polymorphic (Fig. 6). In addition, the limited amount of DNA sequence data on DP β chain genes [4, 13, 14] suggests that this locus is also polymorphic. Finally, some of the α chain genes are also polymorphic; DNA sequence analysis of DQ α chain genes isolated from individuals of differing DR type shows that this locus is also considerably polymorphic (Fig. 7).

The most important characteristic with regard to the polymorphism displayed by HLA class II genes is that the allelic forms differ by multiple amino acid substitution. Both the α and β genes can differ by as much as 10% or 25 amino acids. This is in contrast to simple allelic systems such as the globin and cytochrome genes, which differ by one or a few amino acids. This high degree of variability among class II alleles has two important implications. First, it forces us to consider the possibility that other genetic mechanisms besides simple point mutation and selection are responsible for class II polymorphism and second, it makes it very likely that any single class II gene encodes multiple allodeterminants or alloepitopes. Indeed, cross-blocking studies with MoAbs to murine Ia molecules demonstrate that each molecule encodes multiple epitopes which are spatially distinct [17, 18]. This latter point becomes extremely important when we begin to consider the number of alloepitopes that a single individual can express.

Several HLA Class II Genes Are in Strong Linkage Disequilibrium

Several studies employing various techniques have suggested that at least three genetic loci, DQα, DQβ, and DRβ are in strong linkage disequilibrium and con-

```
        <-- L|1D -->
           -1|1                                        20
DQ4  S P C G G|E D I V A D H V A S Y G V N L Y Q S Y G P S G Q Y S H E F D G D E E F
DQ7  - - - - - - - - - - - - - - - - - - - - - - - - - - - - - F T - - - - - - - - -
DQ9  - - - - (         ) - - - - - - - - - - - - - - - - - - - - - - - - - - - - - -
DQ6  - - - - - - - - - - - - - - - C - - - - - - F - - - - - - - T - - - - - - - Q -

           40                                      60
DQ4  Y V D L E R K E T V W Q L P L F R R F R R F D P Q F A L T N I A V L K H N L N I
DQ7  - - - - - - - - - - - K - - - - H - L ( ) - - - - - - - - - - - - - - - - - - -
DQ9  - - - - - - - - - - - - - - - - - - - - - - - - - - - - - - - - - - - - - - - -
DQ6  - - - - - - - - - A - R W - E - S K - G G - - - - G - - R - M - - A - - - - - -

                  <-- 1D|2D -->
           80                                          100
DQ4  V I K R S N S T A A T N|E V P E V T V F S K S P V T L G Q P N T L I C L V D N I
DQ7  L - - - - - - - - - - - - - - - - - - - - - - - - - - - - - - - - - - - - - - -
DQ9  - - - - - - - - - - - - - - - - - - - - - - - - - - - - - - - - - - - - - - - -
DQ6  M - - - Y - - - - - - - - - - - - - - - - - - - - - - - - - - - - - - - - - - -

           120                                     140
DQ4  F P P V V N I T W L S N G H S V T E G V S E T S F L S K S D H S F F K I S Y L T
DQ7  - - - - - - - - - - - - - - - - - - - - - - - - - - - - - - - - - - - - - - - -
DQ9  - - - - - - - - - - - - - - - - - - - - - - - - - - - - - - - - - - - - - - - -
DQ6  - - - - - - - - - - - - - Q - - - - D - - - - - - - - - - - - - - - - - - - - -

                                              <-- 2D|CP -->           <-- CP|
           160                                     180
DQ4  F L P S A D E I Y D C K V E H W G L D E P L L K H W|E P E I P T P M S E L T E|T
DQ7  - - - - - - - - - - - - - - - - - - - - - - - - - - - - - - - A - - - - - - - -
DQ9  - - - - D - - - - - - - - - - - - - - - - - - - - - - - - - - - - - - - - - - -
DQ6  - - - - - - - - - - - - - - - - - - - Q - - - - - - - - - - - - - - - - - - - -

                                     <-- TM|CY -->
           200                                 220
DQ4  V V C A L G L S V G L V G I V V G T V L I I|R G L R S V G A S R H Q G P L
DQ7  - - - - - - - - - - - - - - - - - - - - - - - - - - - - - - - - - - - - -
DQ9  - - - - - - - - - - - - - - - - - - - - - - - - - - - - - - - - - - - - -
DQ6  - - - - - - - - - - - M - - - - - - - F - - Q - - - - - - - - - - - - - -
```

Fig. 8. Protein sequences of DQ α subunits belonging to the MT3 (DR4, 7, and 9) and MT1 (DR6) serologic groups. Sequences are identical unless otherwise indicated. *Parentheses* indicate deletions required to align the sequence. The DQ α subunit and the other class II subunits are organized into a leader (*L*) region (signal peptide), two extracellular domains (*1D, 2D*), a connecting peptide (*CP*), a transmembrane region (*TM*), and an intracytoplasmic region (CY)

sequently are virtually always inherited together. The first evidence that DQβ and DRβ rarely segregate came from early studies in which the 2D gel profiles of DQ β chains isolated from two different DR7 individuals were compared. It was found that the two DR7 cell lines, which expressed the same DR β chain, also expressed identical DQ β chains [19]. More recently, it has been shown by RFLP analysis that DNA fragments corresponding to the DQ β gene segregate together with the DR β genes [20].

RFLP and DNA sequence analysis have also been used to demonstrate strong linkage disequilibrium between DQ α genes and DR β genes. Several studies have demonstrated that DNA fragments corresponding to the DQ α gene segregate in a pattern that is reminiscent of the serologic specificities known as MT1, MT2, and MT3 [21] which are associated with HLA class II molecules [5, 6]. Two of these specificities, MT2 and MT3, have been shown to be carried by DR β chains [22, 25]. More recently, it has been shown that cell lines which express the MT3 determinant, i.e., DR4, DR7, and DR9, have DQ α genes that are virtually identical in sequence but which differ substantially from the sequence of DQ α genes isolated from cells which express the MT1 serologic specificity, i.e., DR1, DR2,

Table 2. Quantitative differences between DQ α subunits belonging to the MT3 (DR4, 7, 9) and MT1 (DR6) serologic groups[a]

	Protein					
	4×7	4×9	7×9	4×6	7×6	9×6
α1 domain	7	1	8	18	19	19
α2 domain	0	1	1	3	3	4
Total	8	2	10	24	26	26
	DNA					
	4×7	4×9	7×9	4×6	7×6	9×6
α1 domain	10	2	10	13	12	31
α2 domain	0	2	2	9	9	9
Total	12	4	14	51	48	49

[a] The number of amino acid and nucleotide differences between each pair of DQ α subunits was determined for each of the two domains. The total number of differences includes those observed in the remainder of the molecule, including the connecting peptide, the transmembrane portion, and the cytoplasmic portion

and DR 6 (Fig. 8, Table 2) [25]. Since the MT3 specificities are carried on DR β chains, it is difficult to reconcile the sequence and serologic data unless one proposes that the DQ α gene is in strong linkage disequilibrium with the DR β gene and that the two genes have evolved together. Indeed, this appears to be the case in mice, where it has been shown that the A α, A β, and E β loci, which are analogous to the human DQ α, DQ β, and DR β loci, are inherited together as a single genetic unit with a very low frequency of recombination.

The strong linkage disequilibrium among DQ α, DQ β, and DR β genes has important implications in terms of the numbers of alloepitopes which may be detected when individuals with different DR types are cross-immunized. Clearly, since all three loci are polymorphic and each locus very probably encodes multiple alloepitopes, alloantisera produced by cross-immunizing DR-disparate individuals will contain antibodies against multiple alloepitopes. Indeed, because of the strong linkage disequilibrium among DQ α, DQ β, and DR β genes it will be virtually impossible to distinguish alloepitopes encoded by each of these genes using conventional typing alloantisera. Thus, DR allotypes as conventionally defined using alloantisera very probably represent a conglomeration of alloepitopes encoded by at least three genetic loci.

Distribution of Epitopes Among Different HLA Class II Haplotypes

Initial attempts at HLA class II typing clearly demonstrated that alloantisera could distinguish different class II haplotypes, which were then given different DR designations. Subsequent studies, however, showed that some alloantisera detected particular antigenic determinants or epitopes that were shared by several different haplotypes [21, 27]. For example, it was found that individuals who were typed as DR1, DR2, or DR6 shared a determinant known as MB1 (Table 3).

Table 3. Association of MB and MT serologic specificities with DR type

MT		MB	
MT1	DR1 DR2 DR6	MB1	DR1 DR2 DR6
MT2	DR3 DR5	MB2	DR3 DR7
MT3	DR4 DR7 DR9	MB3	DR4 DR5

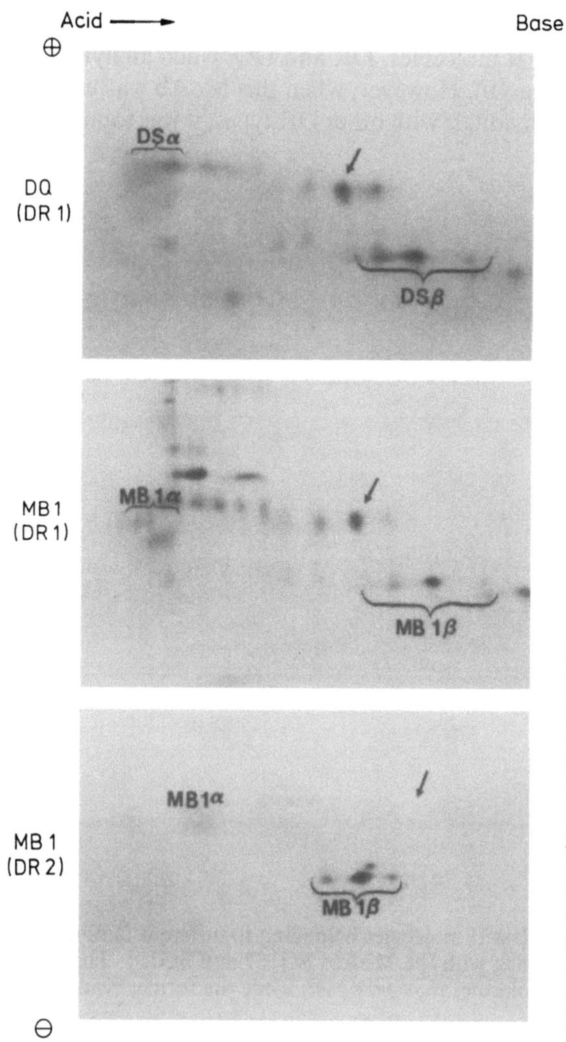

Fig. 9. Identification of MB1 molecules. DQ molecules immunoprecipitated from a DR1 cell line (*top panel*) with the DQ-specific heterologous rabbit antiserum RB03 and MB1 molecules immunoprecipitated from DR1 (*middle panel*) and DR2 (*bottom panel*) cell lines with the MB1-specific MoAb SDR1.2 were analyzed by 2D gel electrophoresis. The MB1 molecule from a DR1 cell line is much more basic than that from a DR2 cell line. The *arrows* designate the invariant spot

Similarly, individuals who are DR4 or DR5 share a determinant known as MB3 and individuals who type as DR3 or DR7 share one known as MB2. The issue of whether these common epitopes, also referred to as "supertypic specificities", were present on a common class II molecule which was structurally identical in individuals of different class II type or represented common epitopes on structurally distruct class II molecules was first resolved by 2D gel analysis using MoAbs which displayed activity for "supertypic specificities" [28]. Thus, analysis of the MB1 specificity on DR1 and DR2 cells (Fig. 9) and the MB3 specificity on DR4 and DR5 cells [28, 29] revealed that the MB1 specificity was present on structurally distinct DQ molecules isolated from DR1 and DR2 cells and that the MB3 specificity is present on structurally distinct DQ molecules isolated from DR4 and DR5 cells. The MB series of "supertypic" specificities therefore represent common epitopes expressed by structurally distinct class II molecules.

Additional insight into the way in which epitopes can be distributed among different class II haplotypes came from a series of studies employing MoAbs which did not display the patterns of reactivity characteristic of DR type or supertypic specificity, but which nevertheless could distinguish various class II molecules. For example, it could be shown that one epitope detected with the MoAb SG171 was present on two different class II molecules, DR and DQ, when analyzed on individuals who typed as DR7 (Fig. 10). However, when this MoAb was used to analyze class II molecules from individuals with other DR types, it was found that

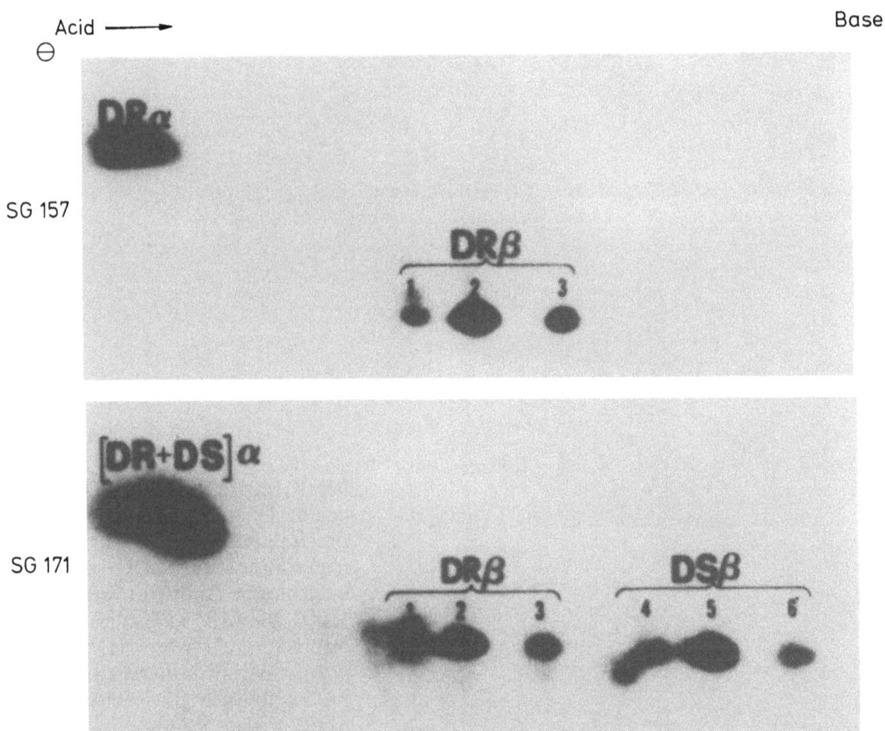

Fig. 10. Sharing of epitopes by HLA class II molecules belonging to different families. 2D gel analysis of class II molecules reacting with the MoAbs SG157 and SG171. The latter reacts with both DR and DQ (*DS*) molecules (*bottom panel*) while the former reacts only with DR molecules (*top panel*)

Table 4. Reactivity of MoAbs products of different class II loci

DR type of cell line	SG171	SG465	SG520
DR1	DR	DQ	DR + third locus product
DR2	DR	DR + DQ	DR + third locus product
DR3	DR	DR + DQ	DR + DQ
DR4	DR	DQ	DR + third locus product
DR5	DR	DQ	DR
DR7	DR + DQ	DQ	DQ

it only reacted with DR molecules (Table 4). Thus, sometime during the evolution of the HLA class II system, an epitope which was present solely on DR molecules was transferred to a DQ molecule, but only in DR7 individuals. Similar evidence for the "mobility" of epitopes came from studies using other MoAbs (Table 4) [28].

"Mobile" Epitopes and Their Effect on the Immune Response

The distribution of HLA class II epitopes on different gene products as a function of class II haplotype suggests that the class II region is in a state of dynamic flux and that certain genetic mechanisms may be operational in translocating epitopes between different class II gene loci and haplotypes. Indeed, recent studies involving bm12 mice, a spontaneous mutant of C57Bl/6 mice, suggest that gene conversion or homologous but unequal crossing-over play an important role in translocating epitopes between different class II gene loci. The bm12 mutant was initially detected because it rejected skin grafts from C57Bl/6 mice. Fine structure genetic analysis localized the mutation to the I region (encoding class II molecules) of the MHC [30] and peptide map analysis of class II molecules from both strains of mice showed that the bm12 mutant had an A β subunit (analogous to the human DQ β subunit) that was structurally distinct from the A β subunit isolated from C57Bl/6 mice [31]. When the entire protein structure of the two A β subunits was determined by recombinant DNA analysis, it was found that they differed by three amino acids at positions 68, 71, and 72 [32–34] (Fig. 11). These three amino acid substitutions are due to three nucleotide substitutions. The fact that the bm12 mutant is the result not of a single point mutation, but in fact of multiple nucleotide substitutions clustered within a very small region, suggests that other genetic mechanisms besides simple mutation are responsible for the generation of this mutant. Indeed, when the nucleotide and protein sequences of the E β subunit (analogous to the DR β subunit in man) are compared to the mutant and normal A β sequences, it is observed that the three nucleotide substitutions in the bm12 A β subunit correspond precisely to the nucleotide sequence of the E β subunit (Fig. 11). This observation suggests that a small stretch of genetic information (a maximum of 44 nucleotides in this case) has been transferred from the E β gene to the A β gene in the generation of the bm12 mutant. Similar transfers of genetic information, presumably due to gene-conversion-like events, have been observed among other multigenic systems including the globin genes [35], immunoglobulin genes [36], and, more importantly, the class I genes of the MHC [37].

		50									60							
	CGC	GCG	GTG	ACC	GAG	CTG	GGG	CGG	CCA	GAC	GCC	GAG	TAC	TGG	AAC	AGC	CAG	CCG	GAG
Aβ[b]	Arg	Ala	Val	Thr	Glu	Leu	Gly	Arg	Pro	Asp	Ala	Glu	Tyr	Trp	Asn	Ser	Gln	Pro	Glu
Aβbm12																			
Eβ[b]													A Asn						

			70										80					
	ATC	CTG	GAG	CGA	ACG	CGG	GCC	GAG	CTG	GAC	ACG	GTG	TGC	AGA	CAC	AAC	TAC	GAG
Aβ[b]	Ile	Leu	Glu	Arg	Thr	Arg	Ala	Glu	Leu	Asp	Thr	Val	Cys	Arg	His	Asn	Tyr	Glu
Aβ[bm12]	[T Phe]			[A Gln	A Lys]													
Eβ[b]	[T Phe]			[A Gln	A Lys]				C Val								T	

Fig. 11. Nucleotide and predicted protein sequences of A β (murine homologue of DQ β) subunits from C57Bl/6 mice (*top line*) and bm12 mice (*middle line*) and E β (murine homologue of DR β) subunit from C57Bl/6 mice (*bottom line*). The sequences of the three subunits are identical unless indicated otherwise. The boxed residues at amino acid positions 68, 71, and 72 represent part of the C57Bl/6 E β subunit which presumably was transferred to the C57Bl/6 A β subunit in the generation of the bm12 mutant. (Adapted from [33])

The changes conferred on the A β subunit by these three amino acid substitutions has a profound effect on the immune responsiveness of bm12 mice to several antigens. These mice are not able to develop T cell responses to the HY antigen or antibody responses to beef insulin, in contrast to normal C57Bl/6 mice, which are able to respond to both [38–40]. Thus, the presence of a particular epitope whose structure is determined by three amino acids is sufficient to drastically alter the immune responsiveness of bm12 mice. It should also be pointed out that although the genetic information for this epitope is also present in the E β subunit of C57Bl/6 mice, they are unable to express this particular epitope on the cell surface due to a structural defect of the E α subunit. Thus, this particular gene conversion event has had the effect of transferring a "silent" epitope to a now expressed gene product.

The occurrence of such gene conversion events in the HLA class II system has profound implications for disease susceptibility analyses. Clearly, if genetic information encoding single epitopes is capable of "migrating" from one class II haplotype and/or locus to another, it is easy to see how individuals who might appear to be class II-identical by conventional serologic typing (which looks at the entire conglomeration of epitopes) might in fact differ by a single epitope. If such an epitope were indeed to make an individual susceptible to a particular disease, individuals would develop the disease who appear to have the inappropriate disease-susceptible class II haplotype.

Epitope Typing as a Predictor of Disease Susceptibility

If the functionally important components of HLA class II molecules are indeed epitopes, and if some of these epitopes determine disease susceptibility, then we should be able to identify epitopes that are better predictors of disease susceptibility than those identified by conventional class II typing. That is, these epitopes should be present not only in patients with the appropriate class II haplotype, but

Table 5. Frequency of HLA class II allotypes and epitopes in rheumatoid arthritis patients and normal Causcasoid controls (adapted from [43])

Class II type	Normal Caucasoids	Adult RA patients	Relative risk
DR4	0.290	0.741	7.0
Class II epitope			
MB3	0.503	0.838	5.1
MT3	0.468	0.838	5.9
MC1	0.47	0.935	16.1

Table 6. Association of an epitope detected with the MoAb 109d6 and rheumatoid arthritis (from [44])

	Rheumatoid arthritis ($n=58$)	Controls[a] ($n=60$)	Relative risk
109d6	81%	43%	5.4
DR4	55%	23%	3.9

[a] Ethnically matched with the patient population

also in patients with the inappropriate haplotype. Indeed, several recent studies performed with carefully selected alloantisera or MoAbs have demonstrated that epitopes detected with such reagents can show a stronger association with RA than can conventional DR typing. For example, individuals expressing an epitope(s) detectable with an alloantiserum designated MC1 have a stronger likelihood of developing RA than those displaying the conventional DR4 type (Table 5). This is because this alloantiserum is capable of detecting those rare DR1 individuals who will develop the disease. Similarly, the MoAb 109d6 shows a stronger association and a higher relative risk with RA than does the DR4 type (Table 6). Although neither of these reagents show a 100% association with RA, it is likely that as additional antibodies, as well as allospecific T cell clones, are generated and analyzed such reagents will be found.

Conclusion

The studies described above provide strong support for the hypothesis that epitopes represent the functionally important components of HLA class II molecules. Class II epitopes strongly influence immune responsiveness and very likely represent the "susceptibility genes" associated with some autoimmune diseases. Furthermore, biochemical and recombinant DNA studies suggest that the class II system is much more dynamic than previously envisioned, with genetic information "migrating" between different class II gene loci and haplotypes. Therefore, if we are to understand the molecular basis of "disease-susceptibility genes" associated with the class II system, it will be necessary to define "disease-susceptibility epitopes," to determine how many different protein and nucleotide sequences can encode such epitopes, and to examine the mechanisms and determine the frequency with which nucleotide sequences encoding such epitopes can be transmitted from one class II haplotype and/or gene locus to another.

This work was supported by grants from the National Institutes of Health.

References

1. Owerbach D, Lernmark A, Platz P, Ryder LP, Rask L, Peterson PA, Ludvigssdon J (1983) HLA-D region β-chain DNA endonuclease fragments differ between HLA-DR identical healthy and insulin-dependent diabetic individuals. Nature 303:815–817
2. Nepom BS, Nepom GT, Mickelson E, Schaller JG, Antonelli P, Hansen JA (1984) Specific HLA-DR4-associated histocompatibility molecules characterize patients with seropositive juvenile rheumatoid arthritis. J Clin Invest 74:287–291
3. Servenius B, Gustafsson K, Widmark E, Emmoth E, Andersson G, Larhammar D, Rask L, Peterson PA (1984) Molecular map of the human HLA-SB (HLA-DP) region and sequence of an SBα (DPα) pseudogene. EMBO J 3:3209–3214
4. Gorski J, Rollini P, Long E, Mach B (1984) Molecular organization of the HLA-SB region of the human major histocompatibility complex and evidence for two SB β chain genes. Proc Natl Acad Sci USA 81:3934–3938
5. Spielman RS, Lee J, Bodmer WF, Bodmer JG, Trowsdale J (1984) Six HLA-D region α-chain genes on human chromosome 6: polymorphisms and associations of DCα-related sequences with DR types. Proc Natl Acad Sci USA 81:3461–3465
6. Auffray C, Kuo J, DeMars R, Strominger JL (1983) A minimum of four human class II α chain genes are endoded in the HLA region of chromosome 6. Nature 304:174–177
7. Long EO, Wake CT, Gorski J, Mach B (1983) Complete sequence of an HLA-DRβ chain gene. EMBO J 2:389–394
8. Allison JP, Walker LE, Russell WA, Pellegrino MA, Ferrone S, Reisfeld RA, Frelinger JA, Silver J (1978) Murine Ia and human DR antigens: homology of amino terminal sequences. Proc Natl Acad Sci USA 74:5135–5139
9. Goyert SM, Shively JE, Silver J (1982) Biochemical characterization of a second family of human Ia molecules, HLA-DS, equivalent to murine I-A subregion molecules. J Exp Med 156:550–556
10. Schenning L, Larhammar D, Bill P, Wiman K, Jonsson AK, Peterson PA (1984) Both α and β chains of HLA-DC class II histocompatibility antigens display extensive polymorphism in their amino terminal domains. EMBO J 3:447–452
11. Larhammar D, Schenning L, Gustafsson K, Wiman K, Claesson L, Rask L, Peterson P (1982) Complete amino acid sequence of an HLA DR antigen like β chain as predicted from the nucleotide sequence similarities with immunoglobulins and HLA-A, B, and C antigens. Proc Natl Acad Sci USA 79:3687–3691
12. Auffray C, Korman AJ, Roux-Dosseto M, Bono R, Strominger JL (1982) cDNA clone for the heavy chain of the human B cell alloantigen DC1: strong sequence homology to the HLA DR heavy chain. Proc Natl Acad Sci USA 79:6337–6341
13. Roux-Dosetto M, Auffray C, Lillie JW, Boss JM, Cohen D, DeMars R, Mawas C, Seidman JG, Strominger JL (1983) Genetic mapping of a human class II antigen β chain cDNA clone to the SB region of the HLA complex. Proc Natl Acad Sci USA 80:6036–6040
14. Gustafsson K, Emmoth E, Widmark E, Bohine J, Peterson PA, Rask L (1984) Isolation of a cDNA clone coding for an SB β-chain. Nature 309:76–78
15. Karr RW, Kannpell CC, Zangara RJ, Goyert SM, Silver J, Schwartz BD (1983) An HLA-DR5 homozygous cell line expresses two DS (I-A-like) molecules. J Exp Med 158:1374–1379
16. Karr RW, Alber C, Goyert SM, Silver J, Duquesnoy RJ (1984) The complexity of HLA-DS molecules: a homozygous cell line expresses multiple HLA-DS alpha chains. J Exp Med 159:1512–1531

17. Koch N, Hammerling KN, Tada GJ, Kimura S, Hammerling U (1982) Cross blocking studies with monoclonal antibodies against I-A molecules of haplotypes b, d, and k. Eur J Immunol 12:909–914
18. Pierres M, Devaux C, Dosseto M, Marchetto S (1981) Clonal analysis of B and T-cell responses to Ia antigens I Topology of epitope regions on IA^k and IE^k molecules analyzed with 35 monoclonal alloantibodies. Immunogenetics 14:481–495
19. Goyert SM, Shively JE, Silver J (1982) Biochemical characterization of a second family of human Ia molecules HLA-DS equivalent to murine IA subregion molecules. J Exp Med 156:550–566
20. Cohen D, LeGall I, Marcadet A, Font MP, Lalquel JM, Daussett J (1984) Clusters of HLA class IIβ restriction fragments describe allelic series. Proc Natl Acad Sci USA 81:7870–7874
21. Park MS, Terasaki PI, Nakata S, Aoki D (1980) MT1, MT2, and MT3 – alternate allelic candidates for DRw supratypic antigens. In: Terasaki PI (ed) Histocompatibility testing 1980. UCLA Tissue Typing Laboratory, Los Angeles, pp 858–859
22. Markert ML, Cresswell P (1982) Human B cell alloantigens: expressions of MB and MT determinants. J Immunol 128:2004–2008
23. Karr RW, Kannapell CC, Stein JA, Gebel HM, Mann DL, Dusquesnoy RJ, Fuller TC, Rodey GE, Schwartz BD (1982) Molecular relationships of the human B cell alloantigens, MT2, MT3, MT4, and DR5. J Immunol 128:1809–1818
24. Tanigaki N, Tosi R, Sagana K, Minowada J, Ferrara GB (1983) The distribution of DR5, MT2, and MB3 specificities on human Ia subsets. Immunogenetics 17:371–386
25. Hurley CK, Giles RC, Nunez G, DeMars R, Nadler L, Winchester R, Stastny P, Capra JD (1984) Molecular localization of human class II MT2 and MT3 determinants. J Exp Med 160:472–493
26. Moriuchi J, Moriuchi T, Silver J (1985) Nucleotide sequence of an HLA-DQ α chain derived from a DRw9 cell line: genetic and evolutionary implications. Proc Natl Acad Sci USA 82:3420–3424
27. Duquesnoy RJ, Marrari M, Annen K (1979) Identification of an HLA-DR-associated system of B-cell alloantigens. Transplant Proc 11:1757–1761
28. Goyert SM, Silver J (1983) Further characterization of HLA-DS molecules: implication for studies assessing the role of human Ia molecules in cell interactions and disease susceptibility. Proc Natl Acad Sci USA 80:5719–5723
29. Giles RC, Nunez G, Hurley CK, Nunez-Roldan A, Winchester R, Stastny R, Capra JD (1983) Structural analysis of a human I-A homologue using a monoclonal antibody that recognizes an MB3-like specificity. J Exp Med 157:1461–1470
30. McKenzie IFC, Morgan GM, Sandrin MS, Michaelides MM, Melvold RW, Kohn HI (1979) B6C-H-2(bm12), a new H-2 mutation in the I region in the mouse. J Exp Med 150:1323–1338
31. McKean DJ, Melvold RW, David CS (1981) Tryptic peptide comparison of Ia antigen α β polypeptide from the I-A mutant B6-C-H-2(bm12) and its congenic parental strain B6. Immunogenetics 14:41–51
32. McIntyre K, Seidman J (1984) Nucleotide sequence of mutant I-Aβ (bm12) gene is evidence for genetic exchange between mouse immune response genes. Nature 308:551–554
33. Denaro M, Hammerling U, Rask L, Peterson PA (1984) The Eβ gene may have acted as the donor gene in a gene conversion-like even generating the Aβ (bm12) mutant. EMBO J 3(9):2029–2032
34. Mengle-Gaw L, Conner S, McDevitt HO, Fathman CG (1984) Gene conversion between murine class II major histocompatibility complex loci. J Exp Med 160:1184–1194
35. Slightom J, Blechl AE, Smithies O (1980) Human fetal Gγ and Aγ-globin genes: complete nucleotide sequences suggest that DNA can be exchanged between the duplicated genes. Cell 21:627–638
36. Bothwell A, Paskind M, Reth M, Imanishi-Kari T, Rajewsky K, Baltimore D (1981) Multiple differences between the nucleic acid sequences of the IgG2a and IgG2ab alleles of the mouse. Cell 24:625–637
37. Mellor AL, Weiss EH, Ramachandran K, Flavell RA (1984) A potential donor gene for the bm1 conversion event in the C57BL mouse. Nature 306:792–795

38. Michaelides M, Sandrin M, Morgan G, McKenzie IFC, Ashman R, Melvold RW (1981) Ir gene function in an I-A subregion mutant B6C-H-2(bm12). J Exp Med 153:464–469
39. Lin CC, Rosenthal AS, Passmore HC, Hansen TH (1981) Selective loss of an antigen-specific Ir gene function in the I-1 mutant B6.C-H-2(bm12) is an antigen-presenting cell defect. Proc Natl Acad Sci USA 78:6406–6410
40. Hochman PS, Huber BT (1984) A class II gene conversion event defines an antigen-specific Ir gene epitope. J Exp Med 160:1925–1930
41. Stastny P (1978) Association of the B cell alloantigen DRw4 with rheumatoid arthritis. N Engl J Med 298:869–871
42. Svejgaard A, Platz P, Ryder LP (1983) HLA and disease 1982. A survey. Immunol Rev 70:0105–2896
43. Duquesnoy RJ, Marrari M, Hackbarth S, Zeevi A (1984) Serological and cellular definition of a new HLA-DR associated determinant, MC1, and its association with rheumatoid arthritis. Hum Immunol 10:165–176
44. Lee SH, Gregersen PK, Shen HH, Silver J, Winchester RJ (1985) Strong association of rheumatoid arthritis with a polymorphic Ia epitope defined by monoclonal antibody. Comparison with the allodeterminant DR4. Rheumatol Int (in press)
45. Kajimura Y, Toyoda H, Shively JE, Goyert S, Silver and Itakura K (1983) Characterization of a cDNA clone coding for the heavy chain of HLA-DR antigens. DNA 2:175–178

Biochemistry

Structure of Human Class II Antigens Expressed by a Homozygous Lymphoblastoid B Cell Line

H. Kratzin, H. Götz, F. P. Thinnes, T. Kruse, H. U. Barnikol, P. Wernet, and N. Hilschmann

Table of Contents

Introduction

Human class II antigens are, like class I and class III antigens, encoded by the MHC on the short arm of chromosome 6. While class III antigens represent serum complement factors, class I (HLA-A, -B, and -C) antigens and class II (HLA-D) antigens are the classical histocompatibility or transplantation antigens [43, 44, 73, 83, 87].

Besides their more passive role in transplant rejection or survival, these two latter classes of antigens also play an active role in the immune response as restricting elements in the cooperation with different T cell subsets. Class I antigens are responsible for allogeneic restriction, in which cytotoxic or T killer (Tc) cells recognize the foreign antigen together with the HLA antigen and destroy it [4, 32, 61]. Class II antigens have a more regulatory function, determining whether an immune response is of a high or a low order (high or low responder), depending on the cooperation of the B cell with a T helper (Th) or a T suppressor (Ts) cell [5, 60, 77].

Class II antigens, which can be divided into the HLA-DR, -DQ and -DP subclasses, represent heterodimeric molecules. The subunits are designated α and β chains, or heavy and light chains, respectively. Both are intrinsic and highly polymorphic membrane glycoproteins which occur in close association with the cell surface [7, 33, 41, 79, 88].

Class I antigens are also composed of two subunits. The heavy chain is also membrane-bound and polymorphic. The light chain, or β_2-microglobulin, however, is not anchored in the membrane, is presumably not polymorphic, and is also not encoded in the MHC [1, 6, 24, 67]. While class I antigens are found on nearly every nucleated cell, the distribution of class II products is restricted to mainly lymphoid cells, indicating a specialized function. Within lymphoid cells they are predominantly expressed by B cells, monocytes, and activated T cells, but not by resting T cells.

In the following we describe the isolation, characterization, and amino acid sequence analysis of class II antigens and compare our results with data from other laboratories.

Isolation

The class II antigens were isolated [19, 85] from the cell line H2LCL, a lymphoblastoid B-cell line, transformed by Epstein-Barr virus, and kept in long-term culture. The serological and cellular characterization demonstrated homozygosity at all class I and class II HLA loci (A3, B7, DR2, Dw2, DQw1, DPw4). The cells were maintained at 37 °C in RPMI 1640 supplemented with 10% fetal calf serum, penicillin, and streptomycin. Usually they were harvested at 10^6 cells/ml and a crude membrane fraction was prepared by differential centrifugation. After solubilization in 0.02 *M* sodium acetate at pH 5.0 made 2% in Nonidet P-40 and 5% in 2-mercaptoethanol, the isolation was an exclusively chemical, three-step procedure.

First, a considerable enrichment was achieved by chromatography on CM cellulose employing the solubilization buffer. At pH 5.0 the 34/29-kd complex of class II molecules was not bound by the ion exchanger, and was therefore separated from the majority of other membrane proteins, including class I molecules. Second, in gel filtration on Sephacryl S-300, low- and high-molecular-weight contaminants were separated from the class II α/β complex. In the third and final step, this complex was separated into heavy and light chains by chromatography on hydroxyapatite. The last two steps had to be carried out in the presence of sodium dodecyl sulfate.

The α and β chain fractions were characterized by one- and two-dimensional polyacrylamide gel electrophoresis, isoelectric focusing, and manual Edman degradation. The first two procedures demonstrated heterogeneity in both chains, more pronounced in the β chain than in the α chain. By Edman degradation, however, one main sequence was deduced for the light as well as for the heavy chain fraction. Since at that time specific antisera and monoclonal antibodies were not available and chemical or physical methods were not promising for further separation of these glycoproteins, the α and β chain fractions were subjected to sequence analysis without further purification.

Amino Acid Sequence Determination

Prior to digestion with trypsin, α-chymotrypsin, or SV-8 protease, the α and β polypeptides were reduced with dithiothreitol (DTT) and alkylated with iodoacetic acid. The enzymatic digests were separated by reverse-phase high-performance liquid chromatography (RP-HPLC) on Hypersil ODS employing a previously described chromatography/rechromatography system [46, 89]. All peptides were isolated, checked for purity by amino acid analysis, and afterwards subjected to manual sequence analysis [11].

The Primary Structure of the α Chain Fraction

These classical procedures combined with the high resolving power of RP-HPLC not only resulted in the complete primary structure of the DR α chain [49, 90], but additionally allowed the alignment of 180 amino acids of the DQw1 α chain [23, 48] (Fig. 1). From peptides isolated by HPLC we have to conclude that the DR α and the DQw1 α chains represent 80% and 20% of the total α fraction, respectively.

The overall structure of both α chain types is similar. They are almost the same length, having 229 (DR) and 232 (DQ) amino acids. They can be subdivided into three parts: a long extracellular part [positions 1-191 (DR), 1-194 (DQw1)], a short membraneous segment of exclusively hydrophobic amino acids, and a short

```
            1                 10                  20                  30
DR2α        I K E E H V I I - Q A E F Y L N P D Q S G E F M F D F D G D E I F H V D M A
DQw1α   E D I V A D H V A S C G V N L Y Q F Y G P S G Q Y T H E F D G D E Q F Y V D L E

            40                50                  60                  70
DR2α    K K E T V W R L E E F G R F A S F E A Q G A L A N I A V D K A N L E I M T K R S
DQw1α   R K E T A W R W P E F S K F G G F D P Q G A L R N M A V A K H               R Y

            80                90                 100                   110
DR2α    N Y T P I T N V P P E V T V L T N S P V E L R E P N V L I C F I D K F T P P V V
DQw1α   N S T A A T N E V P E V T V F S K S P V T L G Q P N T L I C L V D N I F P P V V

          120                130                 140                 150
DR2α    N V T W L R N G K P V T T G V S E T V F L P R E D H L F R K F H Y L P F L P S T
DQw1α                             G V S E T S F L S K S D H S F F K I S Y L T F L P S A

          160                170                 180                 190
DR2α    E D V Y D C R V E H W G L D E P L L K H W E F D A P S P L P E T T E N V V C A L
DQw1α   D E I Y D C K V E H W G L D Q P L L K H W E P E I P A P M

          200                210                 220               229
DR2α    G L T V G L V G I I I G T I F I I K G   R K S N A A E R R G P L
DQw1α                                             S V G A S R H Q G P L
```

Fig. 1. Comparison of DR2 α and DQw1 α chains isolated from H2LCL. The amino acid sequences are depicted according to the one-letter notation [36]. For maximal homology the DR2 α chain N-terminal lisoleucine residue had to be placed over position 3 of the DQw1 α chain and a single gap had to be introduced between positions 8 and 9 of the DR2 α chain. The N-linked carbohydrate moieties are depicted as ♀, the cysteines forming the disulfide bridges are marked by *arrows*, and the 23 hydrophobic amino acids responsible for imbedding into the lipid bilayer are *underlined*. In position 124 of the DR2 α chain the previously determined D is replaced by N hydrophilic tail of 15 residues protruding into the cytoplasm. Posttranslational modifications such as disulfide formation and the comparison between both α chain types reveal a two-domain structure for the extracellular parts.

The extracellular portion of the DR α chain consists of two domains comprising residues 1-85 and 86-191. While both are glycosylated, only the membrane proximal domain is stabilized by a disulfide loop, including 55 amino acids between the cysteins. The carbohydrates are both *N*-glycosidically linked to positions 78 and 118. They represent, however, a high mannose type in the N-terminal and a complex type in the membrane-proximal domain. All these characteristics seem to be identical in the DQw1 α chain and in other class II α chains.

The Primary Structure of the β Chain Fraction

As expected from isoelectric focusing, our β fraction was more heterogeneous than the α fraction [23]. This was also observed by others investigating immunoprecipitated class II antigens [17, 18, 38]. From the completely determined amino acid sequence of the DR2 β_1 chain [47] (Kratzin et al., in prep.), major parts of a second DR2 β chain designated DR2β_2, and of a DQw1 β chain, at least three class II β chain isotypes [23] were identified (Fig. 2). Among additionally isolated peptides, a characteristic tryptic glycopeptide indicated a second β chain of the DQw type. The classification of other fragments isolated in addition to those which were assigned to DR2β_1, DR2β_2, and DQw1β is still an open question.

The primary structure of the DR2β_1 chain also shows the division into three parts that is characteristic for intrinsic membrane proteins in general and has already been described for heavy chains.

There is a hydrophilic extracellular part with two domains. In contrast to α chains, each has a disulfide loop but only the N-terminal domain (1-95) has a carbohydrate side chain attached to asparagine in position 19. While the N-terminal disulfide loop includes 63 amino acids, the loop of the second domain comprises 55 amino acids between the two cysteines (positions 117 and 173). This is exactly the same length as that detected in the α chain. The extracellular two domains are followed by 23 exclusively hydrophobic amino acid residues representing the membrane anchor. Imbedding into the lipid bilayer is achieved by these hydrophobic amino acids alone. In vivo labeling with radioactive palmitic acid [40], in contrast to α chains, indicated that fatty acid is not attached to the hydrophobic sequence. The membrane segment is followed by the third part. This consists of 16 amino acids which are hydrophilic. They represent the C-terminus of the β chain and protrude into the cytoplasm. In contrast to α chains, both regions flanking the hydrophobic membraneous part are predominantly basic (*R*A*R*SESAQS*K*M ..... 23 ..... *R*NQ*K*GHSGLQPTGFLS).

The lipid bilayer – at least of red blood cells and probably also of other cells (e.g., H2LCL) – has an asymmetrical distribution of phospholipids, with the negatively charged phosphatidylserins mainly at the cytoplasmic half [10]. Therefore, the basic residues of the cytoplasmic portion of integral membrane proteins, like the α and β chains of class II antigens, probably interact with the negatively charged headgroups of the phospholipids. In the so-called connecting peptide – the amino acid sequence preceding the hydrophobic membrane segment at the extracellular part – α and β chains are differently charged. These opposite charges

```
        1                 10                  20                  30                  40
DR2β1   G D T R P R F L W Q P K R E C H F F N G T E R V R F L D R Y F Y N Q E E S V R F
DR2β2   G D T R P R F L Q Q D K Y E C H F F N G T E R V R F L H R D I Y N Q E E D L R F
DQw1β   R D S P E D F V F Q F K G M C Y F T N G T E R V R L V T R Y I Y N R E E Y A R F

                          50                  60                  70                  80
DR2β1   D S D V G E F R A V T E L G R P D A E Y W N S Q K D I L E Q A R A A V D T Y C R
DR2β2   D S D V G E Y R A V T E L G R P D A E Y W N S Q K D F L E D R R A A V D T Y C R
DQw1β   D S D V G V Y R A V T P Q G R P D A E Y W N S Q K E V L E G T R A E L D T V C R
                                               Y W N S Q K D E
                                               Y W N S Q M D F L E
                                               Y W N S Q M D I L E
                                               Y W N S Q K D F V E

                          90                  100                 110                 120
DR2β1   H N Y G V V E S F T V Q R R V Q P K V T V Y P S K T Q P L Q H H N L L V C S V S
DR2β2   H N Y G V G E S F T V Q R R V E P K V T V Y P A R T Q T L E H H N L L V C S V
DQw1β   H N Y E V A F R G I L Q R R V E P T V T I S P S R T E A L N H H N L L V C S V T

                          130                 140                 150                 160
DR2β1   G F Y P G S I E V R W F L N G Q E E K A G M V S T G L I Q D G D W T F Q T L V M
DR2β2                     V R W F R N S Q E E K A G V V S T G L I Q
DQw1β   D F Y P G Q I K V R W F R N D Q E E T A G V V S T P L I R

                          170                 180                 190                 200
DR2β1   L E T V P R S G E V Y T C Q V E H P S V T S P L T V E W R A R S E S A Q S K M L
DQw1β                   G D V Y T C H V E H P S L Q S P I T V E W R A Q S E S A Q S K

                          210                 220                 230           237
DR2β1   S G V G G F V L G L L F L G A G L F I Y F R N Q K G H S G L Q P T G F L S
DQw1β                                                                     G L L H
```

Fig. 2. Comparison of class II light chains isolated from H2LCL. Symbols as in Fig. 1

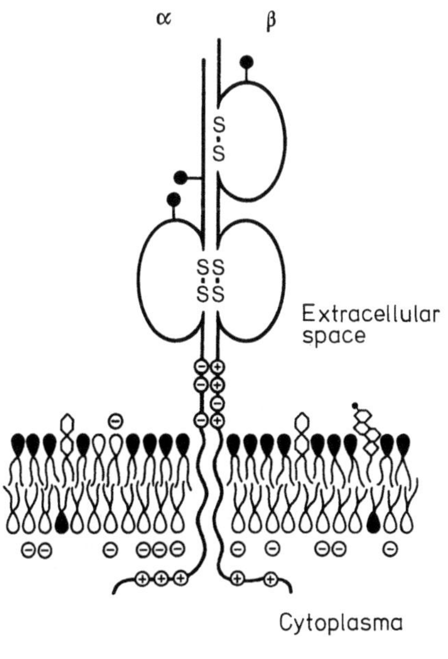

Fig. 3. Schematic representation of the HLA-DR2 antigen. The peptide backbone is shown as a *solid line*, disulfide-containing domains are depicted as *loops*, and the charges of either basic or acidic amino acids flanking the hydrophobic transmembrane segment are included in *circles*. The plasma membrane region with the different phospholipids is not true to scale

may lead to an electrostatic α/β interaction facilitating an α/β association (Fig. 3).

Comparison of α and β Chains

In order to reveal the homology between the heavy and light chains, the N-terminus of the α chain has to be shifted ten residues to the right of the β chain (Fig. 4). Without insertion of gaps this alignment shows identical amino acids in 45 positions, representing 19.8% homology. Furthermore, this homology divides the extracellular section into two parts: a scarcely homologous N-terminal half (11 of 95 identical) and a significantly homologous second half (29 of 92 identical) [90]. The break between the first and the second domain is according to the now known exon boundaries [45, 55], in positions 85 and 95 of the DR α and DR β chain, respectively. Consequently, the ends of the second domains are in positions 179 (α) and 189 (β). Based on this alignment, the remaining C-terminal parts, including connecting peptide, membrane segment, and cytoplasmic tail, share only five amino acids, indicating 9.8% homology, which is also found among unrelated proteins.

Here we briefly refer to the division into three parts – extracellular, transmembrane, and cytoplasmic – of the mature class II proteins. This division (depicted

```
                                1                 10                  20                  30
DR2α                            I K E E H V I I Q A E F Y L N P D Q S G E F M F D F D G D E
DR2β1       G D T R P R F L W Q P K R E C H F F N G T E R V R F L D R Y F Y N Q E E S V R F
            1                 10        └─►     • 20                  30                  40

                              40                  50                  60                  70
DR2α        I F H V D M A K K E T V W R L E E F G R F A S F E A Q G A L A N I A V D K A N L
DR2β1       D S D V G E F R A V T E L G R P D A E Y W N S Q K D I L E Q A R A A V D T Y C R
                              50                  60                  70            ◄─┘ 80

                          ↑   80                  90                  100         ┌─► 110
DR2α        E I M T K R S N Y T P I T N V P P E V T V L T N S P V E L R E P N V L I C F I D
DR2β1       H N Y G V V E S F T V Q R R V Q P K V T V Y P S K T Q P L Q H H N L L V C S V S
Ig                                                                                C
                              90                  100                 110         └─► 120

                          ↑   120                 130                 140                 150
DR2α        K F T P P V V N V T W L R N G K P V T T G V S E T V F L P R E D H L F R K F H Y
DR2β1       G F Y P G S I E V R W F L N G Q E E K A G M V S T G L I Q D G D W T F Q T L V M
Ig                              W
                              130                 140                 150                 160

                          160◄─┐                  170                 180                 190
DR2α        L P F L P S T E D V Y D C R V E H W G L D E P L L K H W E F D A P S P L P E T T
DR2β1       L E T V P R S G E V Y T C Q V E H P S V T S P L T V E W R A R S E S A Q S K M L
Ig                                  C
                          170◄─┘                  180                 190                 200

                              200                 210                 220               239
DR2α        E N V V C A L G L T V G L V G I I I G T I F I I K G   R K S N A A E R R G P L
DR2β1       S G V G G F V L G L L F L G A G L F I Y F R N Q K G H S G L Q P T G F L S
                              210                 220                 230           237
```

Fig. 4. Comparison of the DR2 antigen heavy (α) and light (β) chains. The N-terminus of the α chain starts at position 11 of the β chain, resulting in 19.8% homology. Amino acid residues which are identified in all V- and C-terminal domains of immunoglobulin heavy and light chains [29] are shown below the amino acid sequences. Symbols as in Fig. 1

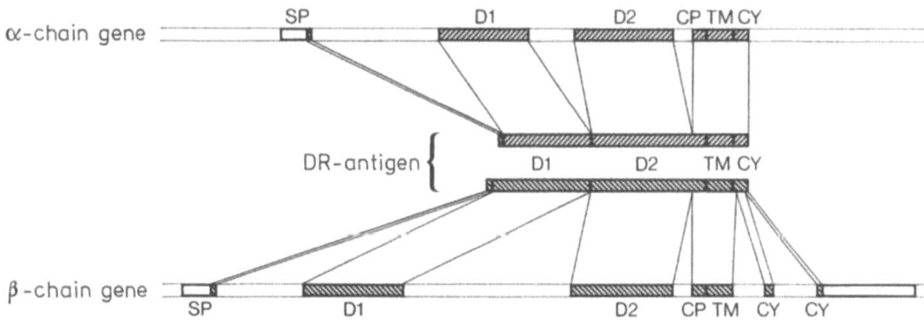

Fig. 5. Comparison of HLA-DR antigen heavy and light chains with their corresponding genes. *SP*, signal peptide; *D1*, first domain; *D2*, second domain; *CP*, connecting peptide; *TM* transmembrane region; *CY* cytoplasmic tail

for DR α and DR β chains in Fig. 5) is not observed in α and β genes discussed in detail elsewhere in this volume. The amino acid sequence is encoded in four and six exons for α and β chains, respectively [45, 55]. While the first two amino acids of the N-terminal α domain are encoded together with the signal sequence in exon 1, the remainder of the first domain is included in exon 2. The sequence of the second α domain is found entirely in exon 3, while the rest of the extracellular part – the already mentioned "connecting peptide" – is at the beginning of exon 4. Exon 4 also contains the transmembrane and cytoplasmic regions of the α chains, thereby including at least segments of all three protein parts [16, 45].

Deduced from a recently characterized pseudogene [55], the DR β chain extracellular part is found in exons 1, 2, and 3, and, with the connecting peptide, also at the beginning of exon 4. Exon 4 contains the complete transmembrane region, but only the outset of the cytoplasmic tail. Two more exons are necessary for the remaining 11 amino acids of the DR β chain. Because of an aberrant splicing site in all DQ β chains, the fifth exons, encoding eight amino acids, are spliced out together with the flanking introns [9, 53, 54]. Nevertheless, two points should be emphasized. First, the fourth exon in all class II genes includes, at least partially, codons of all three protein parts. The connecting peptide represents the end of the extracellular part and deserves a special designation only because it is separately encoded; structurally, it is indistinguishable from other hydrophilic peptides except for its high proline content. This, however, is not characteristic for all intrinsic membrane proteins.

The significance of the homology in the second domains is underlined by the fact that there is an extensive homology to immunoglobulin-constant regions [50, 51, 90]. This was also calculated for the DR2 β_1 chain [73]. Furthermore, homology is evident to the third domain of human and mouse class I antigens, to β_2-microglobulin, to the Thy antigen [31], the secretory piece [20, 62], and various chains of the T cell receptor [28]. The sequence homology between these proteins supports the hypothesis that all of their domains are derived from a single common ancestral gene. The diversity arose by gene duplications and subsequent point mutations during evolution.

Secondary Structure

Concerning the folding of the class II polypeptide chains, only faint ideas exist for the N-terminal part and for the cytoplasmic part. Only for the second domain have computer programs based exclusively on the amino acid sequence resulted in concepts which can be interpreted, especially by analogy to immunoglobulins. In Fig. 6a a schematic view of the DR2 α and DR2 β_1 chain second domains is presented. This type of illustration has already been used for immunoglobulin domains [29]. As for immunoglobulin constant domains (C_H), seven strands (A-G) of β-pleated sheet structure are connected by more or less characteristic β turns. The stretches A, C, E, and G are in one layer, while B, D, and F form a three-stranded layer. The carbohydrate of the heavy chain in position 118 is in the upper three-strand layer, leaving as contact area to the corresponding β domain only the four-stranded layer. By analogy to immunoglobulins, it may be assumed that

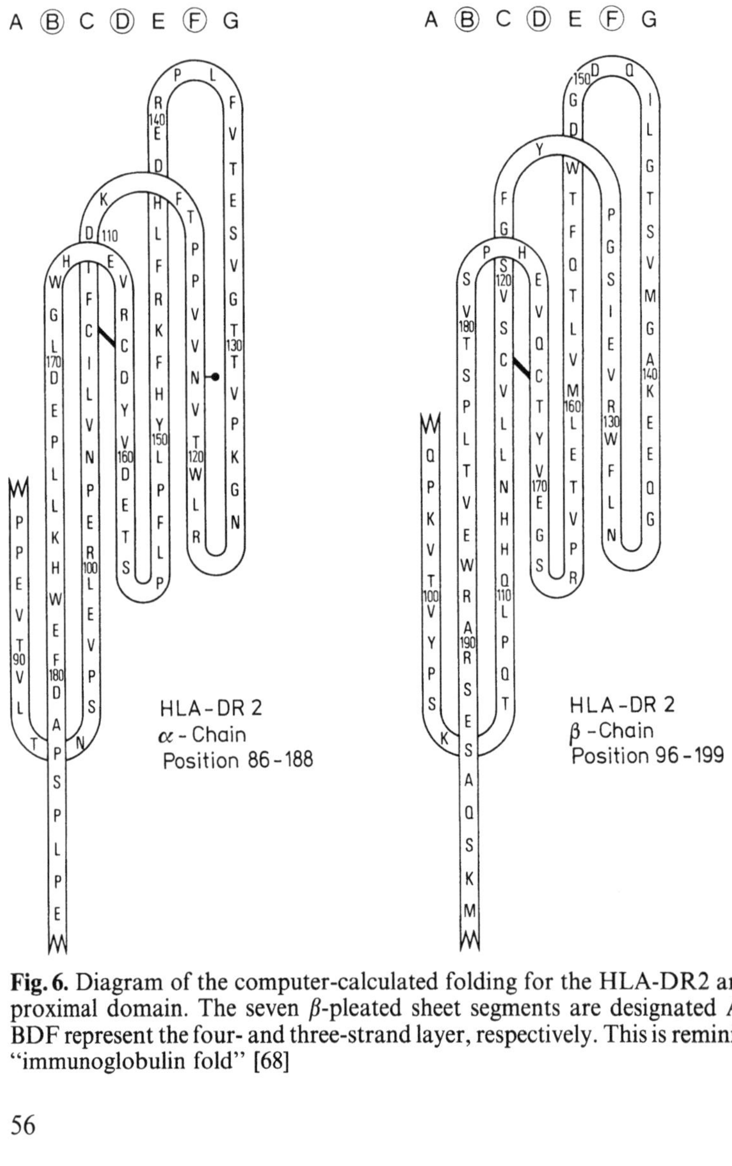

Fig. 6. Diagram of the computer-calculated folding for the HLA-DR2 antigen membrane proximal domain. The seven β-pleated sheet segments are designated A-G. ACEG and BDF represent the four- and three-strand layer, respectively. This is reminiscent of the basic "immunoglobulin fold" [68]

the β chain also uses the four-stranded layer. Our model is based on data calculated according to computer programs [13, 14, 69] kindly provided by Prof. Dr. G. Schulz and Dr. U. Heinemann and adapted by J. Friedrich.

With minor variations, this prediction is identical to those of Novotny and Auffray [64] and Travers et al. [86]. They extended their model to the transmembrane region and combined α and β chains to computer-based stereo presentations. According to existing proposals [84], they assumed α-helical structures for the α/β transmembrane segment. Because of characteristic glycine residues in the hydrophobic core, they proposed a more parallel packing of the α and β helices than usual.

Isotypic Heterogeneity

The isotypic heterogeneity of H2LCL class II molecules, as identified from our chemically prepared material, comprises two α types, DR2α and DQw1α, and at least three β types, which are discussed below.

To maximize the homology between the DR2 α chain and the DQw1 α chain (Fig. 1), the N-terminal amino acid of DR2α had to be placed beyond position 3 of DQw1α and a gap had to be introduced between positions 8 and 9 of DR2α. In this way the DQw1 α chain is three residues longer than the DR2 α chain. The carbohydrates of both α chain types occupy homologous positions (78 and 118 in DR2α, 81 and 121 in DQw1α) as do the cysteines of the low loops (107 and 163 in DR2α, 110 and 166 in DQw1α). Furthermore, from this comparison the two-domain structure is evident. The two chains are not only identical according to posttranslational modifications, they also share 40 of 88 amino acids in the disulfide loop free N-terminal domain and 60 of 93 in the second disulfide bridged domain, representing 45.5% and 64.5% homology, respectively. Since the exon/intron organization of class II α genes [16, 45, 56] roughly reflects this domain structure, the boundaries for calculating the homology were chosen according to this genetic information.

The amino acid sequence comparison between the three β chain isotypes of H2LCL unambiguously elucidates characteristics observed and already described for α chains. All three chain types – DR2β_1, DR2β_2, and DQw1β – have a more variable N-terminal domain and a more conserved second domain [23, 48].

Table 1 demonstrates that the homology between DR2β_1 and DR2β_2 is higher than between either DR2β_1 or DR2β_2 and DQw1β. This is valid for both extracellular domains. Hence DR2β_1 and DR2β_2 represent two light chains of the same subclass, while DQw1β belongs to another subclass, as anticipated using the DR/DQ nomenclature. Furthermore, these data divide the three β isotypes into only two subclasses, as with α chains. The difference, however, is that there are two DRβ isotypes as opposed to only one DRα type. From the yields of the α and β chains of H2LCL, we have to assume that the DRα combines with DRβ, and the DQw1α with the DQw1β. Since intermingling has never been observed and heterotrimeric molecules can be excluded, since in cross-linking experiments only heterodimers could be identified [42, 81], we have to assume that the DR α chain associates with either the DR2 β_1 chain or the DR2β_2 chain [23, 48]. It was estimated from peptide yields that DR2β_2 represents only 25% of the amount of DR2β_1. If these values really reflect the concentrations of the two DRβ isotypes

Table 1. Homology of H2LCL light chains

	Homology (%)	
	Domain 1	Domain 2
$DR2\beta_1/DR2\beta_2$	86.3	82.2
$DR2\beta_1/DQw1\beta$	61.1	75.3
$DR2\beta_2/DQw1\beta$	62.1	75.6

Exon structures used as domain boundaries

on the cell surface of H2LCL, the expression of the corresponding genes must occur in a coordinated fashion.

Another interesting question is the elucidation of the function of these molecules. As discussed, the more constant second domains are involved in mediating the contact between the α and β chains, probably via their four-stranded layer of the β-pleated sheet. They are not primarily responsible for recognizing foreign structures; this function is presumably performed by the more variable N-terminal domains. During evolution, numerous point mutations, and probably other genetic mechanisms such as gene conversion, generated class II diversity dedicated to specialized and restricted functions.

Comparable to the aforementioned more constant domains is the Fc part of immunoglobulins. While the immunoglobulin-constant region is believed to represent the complement-fixing region, no adequate function for class II antigen second domains is yet known. Before functions can be assigned to single domains, the role of class II antigens in general, and the different subclasses in particular, remains to be elucidated.

The $DR2\alpha/DR2\beta_1$, $DR2\alpha/DR2\beta_2$, and $DQw1\alpha/DQw1\beta$ and, probably, the $DQw1\alpha/DQw1\beta_2$ antigens so far isolated from H2LCL cells are certainly not representative of the whole class II phenotype. No DP-type antigens could be detected. This might be due to our isolation procedure or to low amounts of DP antigens on the cell surface. The DP antigen must, however, be present, since H2LCL types DPw4. In the literature only rough estimates exist of the amount of DP in the total class II pool [80].

Since our H2LCL cell line has been typed homozygous, the findings described above added a new dimension to the heterogeneity of class II antigens. In DR antigens from different cell lines, variation had been attributed to the heavy as well as the light subunit. Our findings from a homozygous cell line not only allowed a subclassification of class II antigens in DR and DQ, they also demonstrated a constant DR heavy chain, but two different DR light chains. At least between class II isoantigens, the light chain carries the alloantigenic specificity irrespective of whether it is a primary structural determinant of the $DR\beta$ chain alone or a tertiary structural epitope formed with both α and β chains in common. That a homozygous cell line can indeed express at least two $DR\beta$ chains has in the meantime been confirmed with monoclonal antibodies [74]. As discussed later, even three DR β genes have to be assumed per haplotype [57]. How many are expressed in which cells remains to be ascertained.

Comparison with Amino Acid Sequences of Other Authors

A comparison of H2LCL-derived amino acid sequences with data determined directly from proteins is only possible for the N-terminal regions. These data, however, obtained by N-terminal sequencing subsequent to immunoprecipitations, revealed the distinction between subclasses and showed which light chain type is associated with which heavy chain type.

Fragmentary N-termini represent the only protein-derived basis for the classification of DP DNA sequences [34]. The comparison with N-terminal amino acid sequences of metabolically labeled murine class II (Ia) antigens suggested homology between DR and I-E/C as well as DQ and I-A antigens [48, 83, 90]. This homology is valid for both light and heavy chains, demonstrating that each human subclass identified by primary structural analysis from H2LCL has its murine homologue. No murine counterpart has so far been observed for the cellularly defined DP specificity. The best hybridization of DPβ DNA was with the I-Eβ_2 sequence [58]. The elucidation of the sequence, however, revealed that it is not more homologous to DPβ than are I-Eβ and I-Aβ (Braunstein and Germain, cited in [58]).

Class II α Chain Heterogeneity and Polymorphism

Except for the H2LCL data, the complete amino acid sequences shown in Fig. 7 are deduced from human genomic and cDNA clones. These data confirm and extend the results gained from H2LCL. In class II antigen α chains more isotypes than detected with H2LCL have to be distinguished, and at present, the existence of at least five α isotypes is accepted. The amino acid sequences of four are known and are depicted in Fig. 7, ordered according to homology and subclass affiliation.

Irrespective of the DR specificity shown in the left margin, the DRα amino acid sequences are identical. Hence, the DRα has neither isotypic nor allotypic variation: it is invariant. This result is supported by investigations with restriction endonucleases. No restriction fragment length polymorphism (RFLP) could be detected. The significance of the single amino acid substitution observed in the cytoplasmic portion of the DRw6-derived chain [45] remains to be resolved.

In contrast to DRα, all DQ α chains show amino acid substitutions. Since they are derived from different cell lines, they vary from allotype to allotype. With the exception of the upper two, all amino acid sequences in the DQ block are different. The identity of the DRw6- and DR2-derived DQ α chains is presumably due to the fact that both represent the same allele. Population studies have revealed a strong linkage disequilibrium of the DQw1 allele with both the DR2 allele and the DRw6 allele.

Added to the DQ block is the amino acid sequence of the DX α chain. The spatial separation illustrates that this is an independent isotype present in addition to a DQ α chain on the same haplotype. Figure 7 shows, however, the strong homology to the other DQα sequences. This is especially evident in the second domain, which is subclass-conserved.

Thin boxes in Fig. 7 represent subtype specific residues. DXα [3] has 63 thin boxes in common with the DQα subclass, and consequently has to be considered

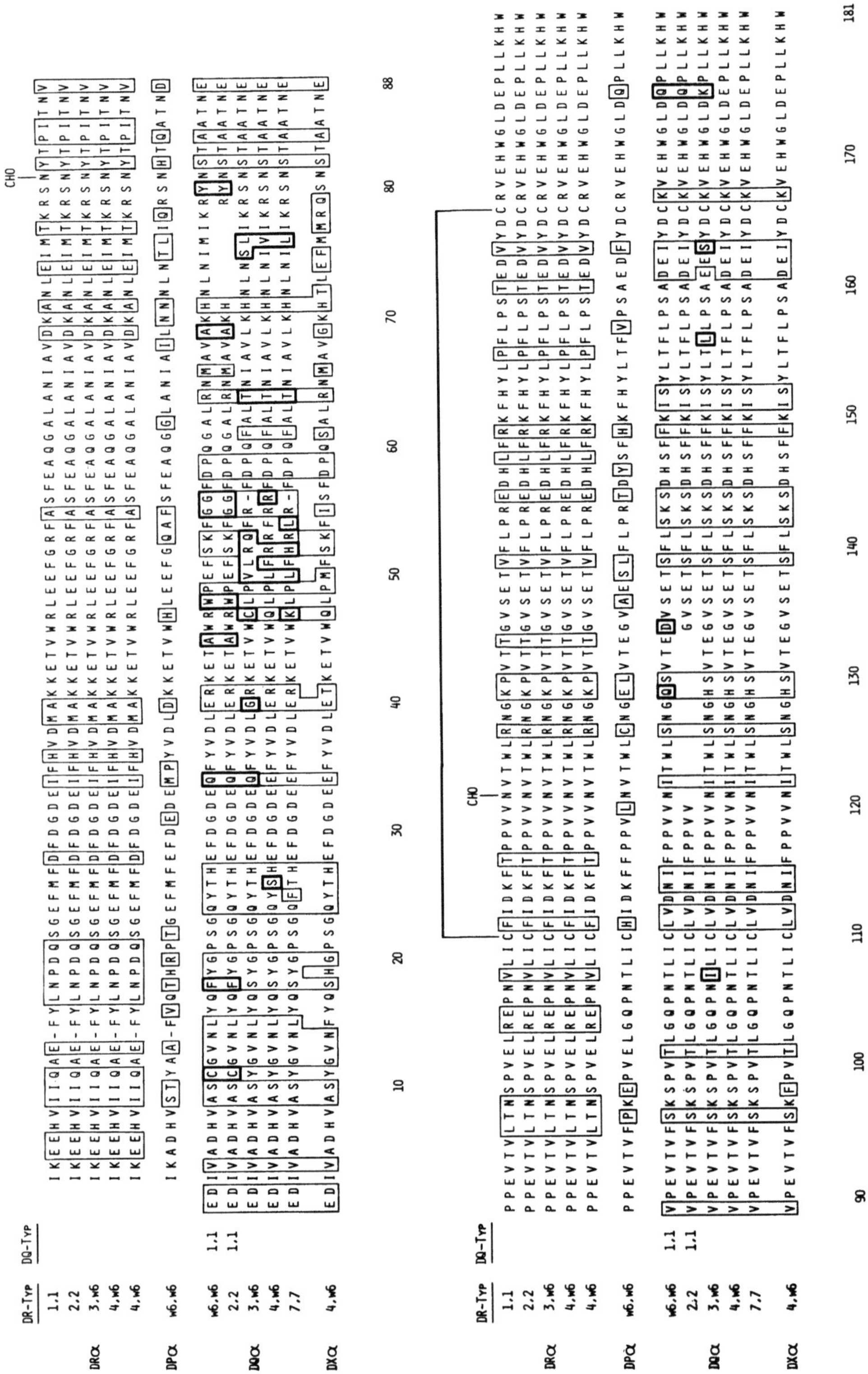
DRα
DPα
DQα
DXα
DR-Typ
DQ-Typ
CHO
10
20
30
40
50
60
70
80
88
90
100
110
120
130
140
150
160
170
181

as a second DQα isogenotype [8, 49]. Meanwhile the existence of two DQ α genes per haplotype is generally accepted [59]. Therefore, heavily boxed amino acids simply mark differences and cannot be attributed to either allotypic or isotypic substitutions. In other words, classification into isotypes and/or allotypes by simply comparing DQα amino acid sequences is difficult unless more data of the same haplotype uncover a DQ subdivision.

From five to six cellularly defined DP allotypes [75, 76], only one complete DP heavy chain sequence has been established so far [3]. Recently, 73 amino acids of another DP α chain N-terminal domain and 22 amino acids from the end of the second and the beginning of the third domain have been published [35]. Amino acid substitutions occur in the N-terminal domain which, in contrast to DRα, demonstrates DPα variation. This variation, however, is less pronounced than that between DQ α chains. In summary, class II heavy chain amino acid sequences of the DR, DP, and DQ types are invariant, slightly variant, and clearly variant, respectively. The heterogeneity found for DQα is reminiscent of the murine system, where the DQ homologue, I-A, also represents the highest variability [39,

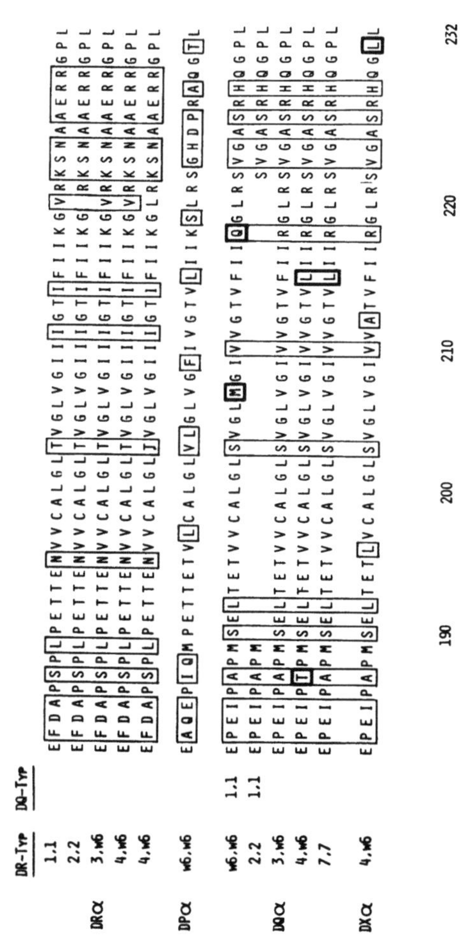

Fig. 7. Comparison of published human class II HLA antigen α chain amino acid sequences. The sequences are depicted in three blocks essentially according to the known exon structures. The *upper block* comprises the N-terminal domain, the *middle block* encompasses the second domain with the single disulfide bridge, and the *lower block* includes the connecting peptide, transmembrane region, and cytoplasmic tail. The carbohydrates attached to asparagine are shown as *CHO* above the corresponding residues. *Thin-boxed* amino acids indicate subclass specific residues, *heavily boxed* residues mark amino acid substitutions. DRα: 1,1 [56]; 2,2 [90]; 3,w6 [27a, 51]; 4,w6 [16, 45]; 4,w6 [45, 70a]. DPα: [3]. DQα: w6,w6 [3]; 2,2 [23]; 3,w6 [71]; 4,w6 [2, 3]; 7,7 [12]. DXα: [3]

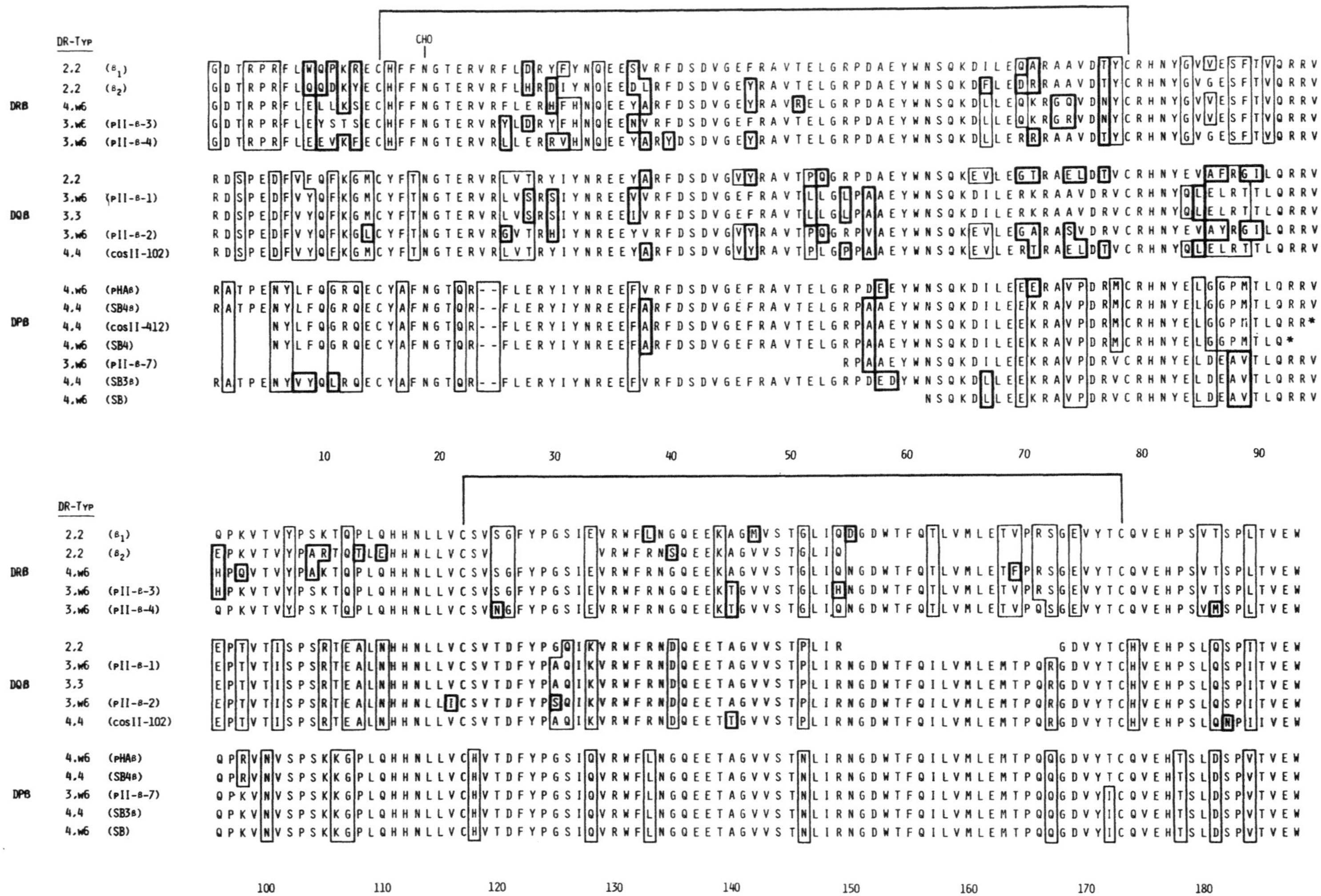

82]. As discussed for DQ, we have to assume two DPα isogenotypes [8, 59]. Up to now, however, nucleotide sequencing indicates one functional and one pseudo DP gene [65, 72]. Whether or not the second DPα chain is expressed in at least some cell lines cannot be decided.

Quantitative comparisons have shown that the DP α chain is as closely related to DRα as it is to DQα [3]. From Fig. 7 we would deduce a slightly closer relationship between DRα and DPα, based on the number of amino acids which DPα shares with DRα and DQα in positions to which either DQ or DR subclass-specific residues were assigned. Counted were residues opposed to thin-boxed, subclass-specific residues, e.g., the first lysine in position 2 of DRα represents a DR/DP identity. Residues identical between all α chains were not considered. While 15, 13, and 5 of the above-described DR/DP identities are found in the first, second, and third domain respectively, only 10, 10, and 7 DQ/DP identities appear

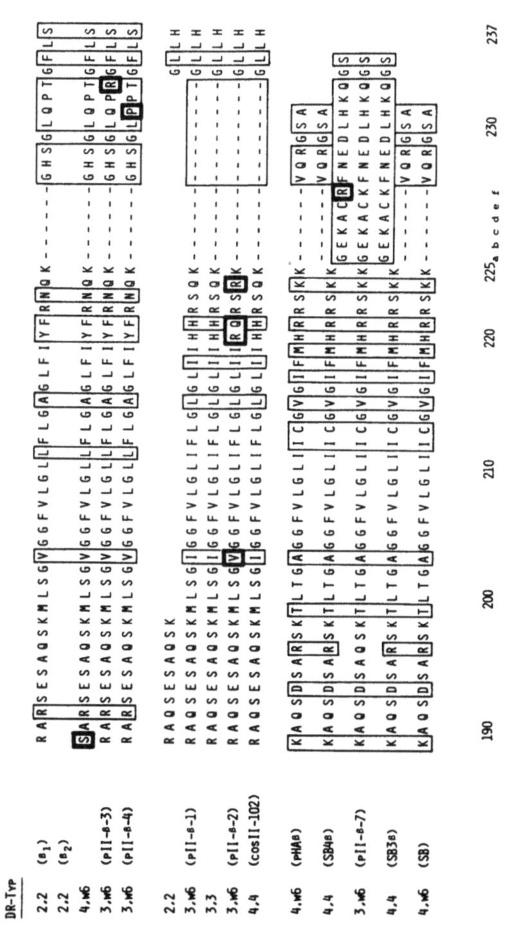

Fig. 8. Comparison of published human class II HLA antigen β chain amino acid sequences. The sequences are depicted in three blocks, essentially according to the known exon structures. The *upper and middle blocks* comprise the N-terminal and membrane proximal extracellular domains respectively. In each domain the disulfide bridge is indicated and the single carbohydrate side chain at asparagine in position 19 is shown as *CHO*. *Thin-boxed* and *heavily boxed* residues represent subclass-specific amino acid residues and amino acid substitutions respectively. Additionally to the subclass affiliation, the DR type and author-specific designations are shown on the left. DRβ: 2,2 (β_1) [47, 49]; 2,2 (β_2) [23]; 4,w6 [57]; 3,w6(pII-β-3) and 3,w6(pII-β-4) [27]. DQβ: 2,2 [23]; 3,w6(pII-β-1) [52]; 3,3 [9]; 3,w6(pII-β-2 [53]; 4,4 [54]. DPβ: 4,w6(pHAβ) [37, 39, 70], 4,(w53) (SB4β [37]; 4,4 [26]; 4,w6(SB4) [25]; 3,w6 [26]; 4, (w53) (SB3β) [37]; 4,w6 [25, 58]. * characterizes partial sequences. For SB4β and SB3β genes the two possible translation products are shown.

in the corresponding domains. The evolutionary and functional relevance of this relationship remains to be elucidated.

Considering the amino acid substitutions in Fig. 7, the most striking features are the accumulations of heavily boxed amino acids: first in DQ, second in the N-terminal domain, and third in the region between positions 45 and 56. This unambiguously assigns specialized functions to the different subclasses, and within the subclasses to the N-terminal domain of DQ. The concentration of amino acid substitutions between positions 45 and 56 could identify this region as one part of the "DQ combining site."

Class II β Chain Heterogeneity and Polymorphism

As deduced from H2LCL, homozygous cell lines express β chains of different subclasses [23, 48]. Two members of the DR type and reliably one, but presumably two, of the DQ type were identified. If all known class II light chain amino acid sequences are ordered according to homology, at the present time a subdivision into three subclasses is reasonable. This division into three subclasses reflects the situation observed for heavy chains. DNA typing reveals at least three or even multiple DR β genes, two DQ β genes, and two DP β genes [57]. Therefore, at least two β isotypes may be included in the amino acid sequences of each subclass depicted in Fig. 8.

Generally, the amino acid substitutions are unequally distributed in all β chains. An accumulation is observed in the first domains of all three subclasses. Within the subclasses, however, the substitutions are located at different sites. While thin-boxed, subtype-specific residues cluster between positions 1 and 18 in all three subclasses, heavily boxed amino acid substitutions occur only in the corresponding DRβ positions concentrated between position 9 and 13. Other more variable regions exist in DR β and DQ β chains (i.e., 26–38, 47, 52–58, and 66–77). These "hypervariable" regions are probably important for the class II "combining site."

Another interesting observation which can be made from Fig. 8 is the subdivision of all subclasses into two subtypes. In positions 84–89, DR β chains have either GVVESF or GVGESF, DQ β chains either EVAFRGI or QLELRTT, and DP β chains either ELDEAV or ELGGPM. Since DR2β_1 and DR2β_2 have been shown to represent isotypes, one can assume that the subdivision of the other chains is also based on isotypic variation. This might also be valid for DP β chains, since primed lymphocyte stimulation studies suggest that at least in some cell lines, a second DP-like antigen may be expressed [66].

In contrast to DR β chains, two of the DQ β chains are identical [9, 52]. The only difference betwen the DR3,w6-derived pII-β-1 chain and the DR 3,3-derived DQ β chain is in position 37, where valine is substituted for isoleucine and simply represents a point mutation. Whether or not this identity indicates a lower degree of isotypic variation for DQ light chains than for DR light chains remains to be determined. Considering the complexity of class II β chains, the difficulty in declaring one amino acid to represent an allelic substitution is obvious. At this time, we recognize the subclass affiliation, but no rules for differentiating between isotypes and allotypes have emerged. To approach this problem more data are necessary, especially from homozygous cell lines.

Heterogeneity of Complete Class II Molecules

In addition to the observed α and β chain isotypy and allotypy, random association of heavy and light chains may contribute to class II heterogeneity. Intermingling of heavy chains with light chains from different loci, e.g., DRα + DQβ, may be possible, but so far it has not been observed. Since two heavy and two light chain genes have been detected in the DQ and DP subclasses, we have to consider the possibility that – as for DR – each α chain may associate with either β_1 or β_2. This expands the class II repertoire of each cell, irrespective of whether they are homozygous or heterozygous.

Transcomplementation, however, is confined to heterozygotes. Since DR antigens consist of the very same α chain, transcomplementation is not detectable in the DR subclass, in contrast to DQ and DP. In both of these latter subclasses, allotypic α chain variation exists in addition to β chain variability, and consequently, transcomplementation should become obvious. First results indicate DQ transcomplementation [21, 22] which, interestingly, is proven for murine I-A antigens representing the DQ homologue [15, 78]. Based on transcomplementation, the heterogeneity of class II molecules varies between homo- and heterozygotes, heterozygotes having potentially twice the number of complete antigens in subclasses with both α and β variation.

Considering this immense heterogeneity, one can easily imagine the problems encountered with investigations concerning disease associations of class II antigens or their functional role in general.

The described isotypic and allotypic variation implies different functions for these antigens [30, 63]. In cell-cell interactions, each subclass may be responsible for generating the contact to a certain type of cell. After this primary contact via unknown receptors for class II antigens has been prepared, subsequent reactions may be initiated. The cooperation of HLA class II-positive B cells and class II-negative Th cells commencing the T cell-dependent humoral immune response might be only one class II-restricted reaction.

Acknowledgments. We would like to thank Mrs M. Praetor and Mr W. Sinn for performing the amino acid analyses, and gratefully acknowledge the expert technical assistance of Mrs I. Anders, Mrs C. Buchhagen, Mrs B. Wehle, Mrs H. Wicher-Ptak, Mrs I. Zywietz, and Mr. R. Merker. We also acknowledge the skillful secretarial services of Mrs E. Kontokollias and Mrs H. Schmidt and the experienced preparation of the illustrations by Mrs U. Pruchniewicz and Mr L. Kolb.

References

1. Appella E, Sawicki JA (1984) β_2-microglobulin. Methods Enzymol 108:494–504
2. Auffray C, Korman AJ, Roux-Dosseto M, Bono R, Strominger JL (1982) cDNA clone for the heavy chain of the human B cell alloantigen DC1: strong sequence homology to the HLA-DR heavy chain. Proc Natl Acad Sci USA 79:6337–6341
3. Auffray C, Lillie JW, Arnot D, Grossberger D, Kappes D, Strominger JL (1984) Isotypic and allotypic variation of human class II histocompatibility antigen α-chain genes. Nature 308:327–333
4. Bach FH, Bach ML, Sondel PM (1976) Differential function of major histocompatibility complex antigens in T lymphocyte activation. Nature 259:273–281

5. Benacerraf B (1981) Role of MHC gene products in immune regulation. Science 212:1229–1238
6. Berggård J, Bearn AG (1968) Isolation and properties of a low molecular weight β_2-globulin occurring in human biological fluids. J Biol Chem 243:4095–4103
7. Billing R, Safani M, Lesch J (1977) Two chain subunit structure of HLA-D antigens. Tissue Antigens 10:267–272
8. Bodmer WF (1984) The HLA system. In: Albert ED, Baur MP, Mayr WR (eds) Histocompatibility testing 1984. Springer, Berlin Heidelberg New York Tokyo, pp 11–22
9. Boss JM, Strominger JL (1984) Cloning and sequence analysis of the human major histocompatibility complex gene DC-3β. Proc Natl Acad Sci USA 81:5199–5203
10. Bretscher M (1973) Membrane structure: some general principles. Science 181:622–629
11. Chang JY, Creaser EH, Bently KW (1976) 4-*N,N*-dimethylaminoazobenzene-4′-isothiocyanate. A new chromophoric reagent for protein sequence analysis. Biochem J 153:607–611
12. Chang HC, Moriuchi T, Silver J (1983) The heavy chain of human B-cell alloantigen HLA-DS has a variable N-terminal region and a constant immunoglobulin-like region. Nature 305:813–815
13. Chou PY, Fasman GD (1974) Conformational parameters for amino acids in helical, β-sheet, and random coil regions calculated from proteins. Biochemistry 13:211–221
14. Chou PY, Fasman GD (1974) Prediction of protein conformation. Biochemistry 13:222–245
15. Cook R, Vitetta E, Uhr J, Capra JD (1980) Structural studies on the murine Ia alloantigens VII. Further evidence for two-gene control of the E/C alloantigens. J Immunol 124:1594–1598
16. Das HK, Lawrance SK, Weissman SM (1983) Structure and nucleotide sequence of the heavy chain gene of HLA-DR. Proc Natl Acad Sci USA 80:3543–3547
17. de Kretser TA, Crumpton MJ, Bodmer WF (1982) Two-dimensional gel analysis of the polypeptides precipitated by a polymorphic HLA-DR1, 2, and w6 monoclonal antibody. Eur J Immunol 12:600–606
18. de Kretser TA, Crumpton MJ, Bodmer JG, Bodmer WF (1983) Biochemical analysis of the polymorphism of three HLA-D region antigens. Mol Biol Med 1:59–76
19. Egert G, Thinnes FP, Götz H, Pauly E, Kratzin H, Yang CY, Kölbel S, Altevogt P, Wernet P, Hilschmann N (1984) Primärstruktur der menschlichen Histokompatibilitätsantigene der Klasse II (HLA-D). II. Trennung der α- von den β-Ketten des HLA-D einer homozygoten, lymphoblastoiden B-Zell-Linie, H2LCL (HLA-A3,3; B7,7; Dw2,2; DR2,2; MT1,1; DC1,1; MB1,1) und Charakterisierung der isolierten Ketten. Hoppe Seyler's Z Physiol Chem 365:1291–1308
20. Eiffert H, Quentin E, Decker J, Hillemeir S, Hufschmidt M, Klingmüller D, Weber MH, Hilschmann N (1984) Die Primärstruktur der menschlichen freien Sekretkomponente und die Anordnung der Disulfidbrücken. Hoppe Seyler's Z Physiol Chem 365:1489–1495
21. Giles RC, Capra JD (1985) Biochemistry of MHC class II molecules. Tissue Antigens 25:57–68
22. Giles RC, de Mars R, Chang CC, Capra JD (1985) Allelic polymorphism and trans-association of molecules encoded by the HLA-DQ subregion. Proc Natl Acad Sci USA 82:1776–1780
23. Götz H, Kratzin H, Thinnes FP, Yang CY, Kruse T, Pauly E, Kölbel S, Egert G, Wernet P, Hilschmann N (1983) Primary structure of human class II histocompatibility antigens. 3rd communication. Hoppe Seyler's Z Physiol Chem 364:749–755
24. Goodfellow PN, Jones EA, van Heyningen V, Solomon E, Bobrow M, Miggiano V, Bodmer WF (1975) The β_2-microglobulin gene is on chromosome 15 and not in the HL-A region. Nature 254:267–269
25. Gorski J, Rollini P, Long E, Mach B (1984) Molecular organization of the HLA-SB region of the human major histocompatibility complex and evidence for two SB β-chain genes. Proc Natl Acad Sci USA 81:3934–3938
26. Gustafsson E, Emmoth E, Widmark E, Böhme J, Peterson PA, Rask L (1984) Isolation of a cDNA clone coding for an SB β-chain. Nature 309:76–78

27. Gustafsson K, Wiman K, Emmoth E, Larhammar D, Böhme J, Hyldig-Nielsen JJ, Ronne H, Peterson PA, Rask L (1984) Mutations and selection in the generation of class II histocompatibility antigen polymorphism. EMBO J 3:1655–1661
27a. Gustafsson K, Wiman K, Larhammar D, Rask L, Peterson PA (1984) Signal sequences distinguish class II histocompatibility antigen β chains of different loci. Scand J Immunol 19:91–97
28. Hedrick SM, Nielsen EA, Kavalier J, Cohen DJ, Davis MM (1984) Sequence relationships between putative T-cell receptor polypeptides and immunoglobulins. Nature 308:153–158
29. Hilschmann N, Barnikol HU, Kratzin H, Altevogt P, Engelhard M, Barnikol-Watanabe S (1978) Genetic determination of antibody specificity. Gene translocation and fusion, the molecular basis of the differentiation of the antibody producing cell. Naturwissenschaften 65:616–639
30. Hilschmann N, Kratzin H, Götz H, Kruse T, Thinnes FP, Wernet P (1985) Genetic und Struktur von Transplantationsantigenen. Nova Acta Leopoldina (in press)
31. Hood L, Steinmetz M, Malissen B (1983) Genes of the major histocompatibility complex of the mouse. Ann Rev Immunol 1:529–568
32. Hood L, Kronenberg M, Hunkapillar T (1985) T cell antigen receptors and the immunoglobulin superfamily. Cell 40:225–229
33. Humphreys RE, McCune JM, Chess L, Herrman HC, Malenka DJ, Mann DL, Parham P, Schlossman SF, Strominger JL (1976) Isolation and immunologic characterization of a human B-lymphocyte specific cell surface antigen. J Exp Med 144:98–112
34. Hurley CK, Shaw S, Nadler L, Schlossman S, Capra JD (1982) The α and β chains of SB and DR antigens are structurally distinct. J Exp Med 156:1557–1562
35. Inoko H, Ando A, Kimura M, Ogata S, Tsuji K (1984) Isolation and characterization of the cDNA clones and the genomic clones of the HLA class II antigen heavy chains. In: Albert ED, Baur MP, Mayr WR (eds) Histocompatibility testing 1984. Springer, Berlin Heidelberg New York Tokyo, pp 559–564
36. IUPAC-IUB Commission on Biochemical Nomenclature (1969) A one-letter notation for amino acid sequences. Biochem J 113:1–4
37. Kappes DJ, Arnot D, Okada K, Strominger JL (1984) Structure and polymorphism of the HLA Class II SB light chain genes. EMBO J 3:2985–2993
38. Kaufman JF, Andersen RL, Strominger JL (1980) HLA-DR antigens have polymorphic light chains and invariant heavy chains as assessed by lysin-containing tryptic peptide analysis. J Exp Med 152:37s–53s
39. Kaufman JF, Auffray C, Korman AJ, Shackelford DA, Strominger JL (1984) The class II molecules of the human and murine major histocompatibility complex. Cell 36:1–13
40. Kaufman JF, Krangel MS, Strominger JL (1984) Cysteines in the transmembrane region of major histocompatibility complex antigens are fatty acylated via thioester bonds. J Biol Chem 259:7230–7238
41. Klareskog L, Sandberg-Trägårdh L, Rask L, Lindblom JB, Curman B, Peterson PA (1977) Chemical properties of human Ia antigens. Nature 265:248–251
42. Klareskog L, Trägårdh L, Rask L, Peterson PA (1979) Isolation and characterization of detergent solubilized human HLA-DR transplantation antigens. Biochemistry 18:1481–1489
43. Klein J (1977) Evolution and function of the major histocompatibility system: facts and speculations. In: Götze D (ed) The major histocompatibility system in man and animals. Springer, Berlin Heidelberg New York, pp 339–378
44. Klein J (1979) The major histocompatibility complex of the mouse. Science 203:516–521
45. Korman AJ, Auffray C, Schamboeck A, Strominger JL (1982) The amino acid sequence and gene organization of the heavy chain of the HLA-DR antigen: homology to immunoglobulins. Proc Natl Acad Sci USA 79:6013–6017
46. Kratzin H, Yang CY (1981) Separation of enzymatic hydrolysates by reverse-phase HPLC. The primary structure of a monoclonal L-chain of κ-type, subgroup I (Bence Jones protein Wes). In: Lottspeich F, Henschen A, Hupe KP (eds) High performance liquid chromatography in protein and peptide chemistry. De Gruyter, Berlin, pp 269–282

47. Kratzin H, Yang CY, Götz H, Pauly E, Kölbel S, Egert G, Thinnes FP, Wernet P, Altevogt P, Hilschmann N (1981) Primärstruktur menschlicher Histokompatibilitätsantigene der Klasse II, 1. Mitt.: Aminosäuresequenz der N-terminalen 198 Reste der β-Kette des HLA-Dw2,2; DR2,2 Alloantigens. Hoppe Seyler's Z Physiol Chem 362:1665–1669
48. Kratzin H, Yang CY, Götz H, Thinnes FP, Kruse T, Egert G, Pauly E, Kölbel S, Wernet P, Hilschmann N (1983) Heterogeneity of class II histocompatibility antigens isolated from a human lymphoblastoid B cell line homozygous at the HLA loci. Hum Immunol 8:65–73
49. Kratzin H, Götz H, Thinnes FP, Kruse T, Egert G, Wernet P, Hilschmann N (1985) Struktur und Funktion von Klasse II Transplantationsantigenen. Allergologie 8:145–152
50. Larhammar D, Wiman K, Schenning L, Claesson L, Gustafsson K, Peterson PA, Rask L (1981) Evolutionary relationship between HLA-DR antigen β-chains, HLA-A, B, C antigen subunits and immunoglobulin chains. Scand J Immunol 14:617–622
51. Larhammar D, Gustafsson K, Claesson L, Bill P, Wiman K, Schenning L, Sundelin J, Widmark E, Peterson PA, Rask L (1982) Alpha chain of HLA-DR transplantation antigens is a member of the same protein superfamily as the immunoglobulins. Cell 30:153–161
52. Larhammar D, Schenning L, Gustafsson K, Wiman K, Claesson L, Rask L, Peterson PA (1982) Complete amino acid sequence of an HLA-DR antigen-like β chain as predicted from the nucleotide sequence: similarities with immunoglobulins and HLA-A, -B, and -C antigens. Proc Natl Acad Sci USA 79:3687–3691
53. Larhammar D, Andersson G, Andersson M, Bill P, Böhme J, Claesson L, Denaro M, Emmoth E, Gustafsson K, Hämmerling U, Heldin E, Hyldig-Nielsen JJ, Lind P, Schenning L, Servenius B, Widmark E, Rask L, Peterson PA (1983) Molecular analysis of human class II transplantation antigens and their genes. Hum Immunol 8:95–103
54. Larhammar D, Hyldig-Nielsen JJ, Servenius B, Andersson G, Rask L, Peterson PA (1983) Exon-intron organization and complete nucleotide sequence of a human major histocompatibility antigen DCβ gene. Proc Natl Acad Sci USA 80:7313–7317
55. Larhammar D, Servenius B, Rask L, Peterson PA (1985) Characterization of an HLA DRβ pseudogene. Proc Natl Acad Sci USA 82:1475–1479
56. Lee JS, Trowsdale J, Travers PJ, Carey J, Grosveld F, Jenkins J, Bodmer WF (1982) Sequence of an HLA-DR α chain cDNA clone and intron-exon organization of the corresponding gene. Nature 299:750–752
57. Long E, Wake CT, Gorski J, Mach B (1983) Complete sequence of an HLA-DRβ chain deduced from a cDNA clone and identification of multiple non-allelic DRβ chain genes. EMBO J 2:389–394
58. Long E, Gorski J, Mach B (1984) Structural relationship of the SB β-chain gene to HLA-D-region genes and murine I-region genes. Nature 310:233–235
59. Mach B (1984) The human D region as a multigene family. Scand J Immunol 20:473–477
60. McDevitt HO, Benacerraf B (1969) Genetic control of specific immune responses. Adv Immunol 11:31–74
61. Möller G (1978) Acquisition of the T cell repertoire. Immunol Rev 42:1–270
62. Mostov KE, Friedlander M, Blobel G (1984) The receptor for transepithelial transport of IgA and IgM contains multiple immunoglobulin-like domains. Nature 308:37–43
63. Navarrete C, Jaraquemada D, Hui K, Awad J, Okoye R, Festenstein H (1985) Different functions and associations of HLA-DR and HLA-DQ (DC) antigens shown by serological, cellular, and DNA assays. Tissue Antigens 25:130–141
64. Novotny J, Auffray C (1984) A programm for prediction of protein secondary structure from nucleotide sequence data: application to histocompatibility antigens. Nucleic Acids Res 12:243–255
65. Okada K, Prentice HL, Boss JM, Levy DJ, Kappes D, Spies T, Raghupathy R, Mengler RA, Auffray C, Strominger JL (1985) SB subregion of the human major histocompatibility complex: gene organization, allelic polymorphism and expression in transformed cells. EMBO J 4:739–748
66. Pawelec G, Shaw S, Wernet P (1982) Analysis of the HLA-linked SB gene system with cloned and uncloned alloreactive T-cell lines. Immunogenetics 15:187–198

67. Peterson PA, Cunningham BA, Berggård I, Edelman GM (1972) β_2 microglobulin – a free immunoglobulin domain. Proc Natl Acad Sci USA 69:1697–1701
68. Poljak RJ, Amzel LM, Avey HP, Chen BL, Phizackerley RP, Saul F (1973) Three-dimensional structure of the Fab' fragment of a human immunoglobulin at 2.8-Å resolution. Proc Natl Acad Sci USA 70:3305–3310
69. Rose GD (1978) Prediction of chain turns in globular proteins on a hydrophobic basis. Nature 272:586–590
70. Roux-Dosseto M, Auffray C, Lillie JW, Boss JM, Cohen D, De Mars R, Mawas C, Seidman JG, Strominger JL (1983) Genetic mapping of a human class II antigen β-chain cDNA clone to the SB region of the HLA complex. Proc Natl Acad Sci USA 80:6036–6040
70a. Schamboeck A, Korman AJ, Kamb A, Strominger JL (1983) Organization of the transcriptional unit of a human class II histocompatibility antigen: HLA-DR heavy chain. Nucl Acids Res 11:8663–8675
71. Schenning L, Larhammar D, Bill P, Wiman K, Jonsson AK, Rask L, Peterson PA (1984) Both α and β chains of HLA-DC class II histocompatibility antigens display extensive polymorphism in their aminoterminal domains. EMBO J 3:447–452
72. Servenius B, Gustafsson K, Widmark E, Emmoth E, Andersson G, Larhammar D, Rask L, Peterson PA (1984) Molecular map of the human HLA-SB (HLA-DP) region and sequence of an SBα (DPα) pseudogene. EMBO J 3:3209–3214
73. Shackelford DA, Kaufman JF, Korman AJ, Strominger JL (1982) HLA-DR antigens: structure, separation of subpopulations, gene cloning and function. Immunol Rev 66:133–187
74. Shackelford DA, Lampson LA, Strominger JL (1983) Separation of three class II antigens from a homozygous human B cell line. J Immunol 130:289–296
75. Shaw S, Johnson AH, Shearer GM (1980) Evidence for a new segregant series of B cell antigens that are encoded in the HLA-D region and that stimulate secondary allogeneic proliferative and cytotoxic responses. J Exp Med 152:565–580
76. Shaw S, Duquesnoy RJ, Smith PL (1981) Population studies of the HLA-linked SB antigens. Immunogenetics 14:153–162
77. Shreffler DC, David CS (1974) The H-2 histocompatibility complex and the I immune response region: genetic variation, function, and organization. Adv Immunol 20:125–195
78. Silver J, Swain SL, Hubert JJ (1980) Small subunit of I-A subregion antigens determines the allospecificity recognized by a monoclonal antibody. Nature 286:272–274
79. Snary D, Barnstable C, Bodmer WF, Goodfellow P, Crumpton MJ (1976) Human Ia antigens – purification and molecular structure. Cold Spring Harbor Symp Quant Biol 41:379–386
80. Sogn JA, Robinson MA, Kulaga H (1984) Functional distinctions among the products of different class II subregions. Scand J Immunol 20:478–483
81. Springer TA, Kaufman JF, Siddoway LA, Mann DL, Strominger JL (1977) Purification of HLA-linked B lymphocyte alloantigens in immunologically active form by preparative sodium dodecyl sulfate-gel electrophoresis and studies on their subunit association. J Biol Chem 252:6201–6207
82. Steinmetz M, Malissen M, Hood L, Örn A, Maki RA, Dastoornikoo GR, Stephan D, Gibb E, Romaniuk R (1984) Tracts of high or low sequence divergence in the mouse major histocompatibility complex. EMBO J 3:2995–3003
83. Strominger JL, Engelhard VH, Fuks A, Guild BC, Hyafil F, Kaufman JF, Korman AJ, Kostyk TG, Krangel MS, Lancet D, Lopez de Castro JA, Mann DL, Orr HT, Parham PR, Parker KC, Ploegh HL, Pober JS, Robb RJ, Shackelford DA (1980) Biochemical analysis of products of the MHC. In: Dorf ME (ed) The role of the major histocompatibility complex in immunbiology. Garland, New York, pp 115–281
84. Tanford C (1978) The hydrophobic effect and the organization of living matter. Science 200:1012–1018
85. Thinnes FP, Egert G, Götz H, Pauly E, Altevogt P, Kölbel S, Wernet P, Kratzin H, Yang CY, Hilschmann N (1984) Primärstruktur der menschlichen Histokompatibilitätsantigene der Klasse II (HLA-D). I. Isolierung, Reinigung und Charakterisierung des α/β-Ketten-Komplexes des HLA-D einer homozygoten, lymphoblastoiden B-Zell-Linie, H2LCL (HLA-A3,3; B7,7; Dw2,2; DR2,2; MT1,1; DC1,1; MB1,1). Hoppe Seyler's Z Physiol Chem 365:1277–1289

86. Travers P, Blundell TL, Sternberg MJE, Bodmer WF (1984) Structural and evolutionary analysis of HLA-D-region products. Nature 310:235–238
87. Van Someren H, Westerveld A, Hagemaijer A, Mees JR, Meerakhan P, Zaalberg OB (1974) Human antigen and enzyme markers in man–Chinese hamster somatic cell hybrids: evidence for synteny between the HL-A, PGM, ME, and IPO-B loci. Proc Natl Acad Sci USA 71:962–965
88. Wernet P (1976) Human Ia-type alloantigens: Methods of detection, aspects of chemistry and biology markers for disease states. Transplant Rev 30:271–298
89. Yang CY, Kratzin H (1981) Chromatography and rechromatography of peptide mixtures by reverse-phase HPLC. In: Lottspeich F, Henschen A, Hupe KP (eds) High performance liquid chromatography in protein and peptide chemistry. De Gruyter, Berlin, pp 283–292
90. Yang CY, Kratzin H, Götz H, Thinnes FP, Kruse T, Egert G, Pauly E, Kölbel S, Wernet P, Hilschmann N (1982) Primärstruktur menschlicher Histokompatibilitätsantigene der Klasse II. 2. Mitteilung: Aminosäuresequenz der N-terminalen 179 Reste der α-Kette des HLA-Dw2/DR2 Alloantigens. Hoppe Seyler's Z Physiol Chem 363:671–676

The Complexity of HLA-DQ Molecules

R. Sorrentino and G. Corte

Table of Contents

Introduction

The existence of an allelic system coded in the MHC but different from HLA A, B, and C was first recognized by studying the reactivity in a mixed lymphocyte culture (MLC) of cells obtained from individuals identical at the A, B, and C loci. The locus responsible for this stimulation mapped on the short arm of chromosome 6 at a position centromeric to the HLA A, B, C loci. It was therefore named HLA D. Later, in the serum of pregnant women antibodies were found directed against polymorphic determinants present on the surface of B cells. These alloantisera were able to block a mixed lymphocyte reaction (MLR) and defined an allelic system that correlated with the MLC-defined D antigens.

As the correlation was not complete, the locus coding for these molecules was named DR (D related) [4, 18, 61]. Similar antigens were known to be coded in the I region of the murine H-2, the so called Ia antigens. Recombination between congenic strains led to the recognition of five loci in the I region of the mouse: I-A, I-B, I-J, I-E, I-C [34, 35, 52]. Molecular genetics studies later showed that only two subregions are present in the mouse I region, I-E and I-A, both containing one alpha and two beta genes. A third I-A beta gene has been identified but shown to be a pseudogene (for more details see chapter by M. Steinmetz in this volume and [42]). In man, the analysis of the region could rely only on the pattern of reactivity of the available alloantisera. In the seventh International Histocompatibility Workshop most alloantisera could be grouped in clusters defining alloantigenic specificities which gave a rather good fit with the population distribution expected by Hardy-Weinberg equilibrium and that could all be accomodated in a single segregant series.

These results led most investigators to conclude that in contrast with the mouse Ia region, a single locus existed in the D region of the human MHC. However, a small percentage of alloentisera reacted with two or more of the defined alleles. At first they were classified as recognizing so-called supertypic specificities. In 1978, a careful study of the reactivity of some of these antisera with purified human Ia molecules led to the discovery of a second locus of the D region coding for antigens different from DR, which carried one of the supertypic specificities, namely DC1 [58]. In that study it was clearly demonstrated that the DC1 determinant was carried by molecules different from those carrying DR determinants. DC1, like MB1, MT1, LB12 supertypic specificities, shows a strong association with DR1, 2, and w6 alleles. Eventually all these determinants were shown to be carried by the same subset of molecules.

Recently, at the Ninth International Histocompatibility Workshop, the nomenclature of the HLA D region was changed, and the HLA DC subregion was provisionally named DQ. Table 1 reports the alternative nomenclature, indicating the DQ specificities together with the associated DR specificities. This new nomenclature will be adopted throughout this review except when, for clarity, the nomenclature used in the original papers will be maintained. When monoclonal antibodies directed against DQw1 (DC1) became available, the differences between DQ and DR molecules could be fully appreciated. Using one of these monoclonal antibodies, BT3/4, DQw1 molecules were isolated and compared to DR molecules by microfingerprinting analysis [16]. Both DQw1 alpha and beta chains had a higher mobility in $NaDodSO_4$ gel electrophoresis than did DR molecules and a distinct peptide pattern from that of DR subunits. The two-dimensional peptide map of DQw1 alpha chains is indeed strikingly different from that of DR alpha chain, completely lacking a cluster of peptides with low electrophoretic mobility which are the major spots present in the DR alpha chain pattern. Two-dimensional gel electrophoresis of two beta chains obtained from either DR2- or DRw6-homozygous cell lines revealed a difference in their isoelectric points [50]. These results definitively established that DQw1 is a supertypic determinant carried by DQ alleles in linkage disequilibrium with DR1, 2, w6. Different DQ beta chains were even found associated with the same DR allele (DRw6) [51]. More recently, it has been shown that at least three distinct DQw3 molecules [29, 44] and at least five distinct DR4 molecules are detectable in several

Table 1. New provisional designation for HLA-DQ specificities

New	Previous equivalents			Associated DR specificities
DQw1	DC1	MB1	MT1	1, 2, w13(w6), w10
DQw2	DC3	MB2	–	3[a], 7[a]
DQw3	DC4	MB3	MT4	4, 5, 7[a], w9, w12(5)
DC5				4[a], 5, w12(5)
DCα3				3[a], 5, w12(5)
DC HON				4, w9

Drw13 and Drw14 are splits of DRw6: see Nomenclature for factors of the HLA system 1984. *Tissue Antigens* 24:73 for further details. DC5, DCα3, and DC HON are new specificities recently described by Tanigaki et al. [56, 57] and Tosi et al. [60]. See text for comments

[a] Partial association only

DR4-homozygous cell lines [5, 43]. The latter correspond to the "D" typing, indicating that a number of biochemically distinct molecules fall under one single serological specificity that can be more finely dissected on the basis of recognition by T cells. Examples of this more sophisticated discriminating power of T cells versus alloantisera have also been reported for class I antigens, where in some cases the site of the molecule involved in the cell-cell interaction has been identified [6, 36].

The General Organisation of the Two Subunits Composing DQ Molecules is Apparently Very Similar to That of DR Molecules

In a study of the structure of DR and DQ molecules, it was shown that the light chains of DR and DQ molecules both consist of two external domains, analogous to the murine I-E and I-A light chains [33]. Both DR and DQ beta chains have a chymotryptic cleavage site that generates an N-terminal fragment of 12 kd. A major tryptic fragment of 20 kd is immunoprecipitated by the DQw1-specific monoclonal antibody Genox 3.53, but only poorly by an anti-DR monoclonal antibody.

One major difference between DR and DQ beta chains is that the DQ beta chain intracytoplasmic region lacks eight C-terminal amino acids [27] which are encoded in a single exon in I-E and I-A and DR. This could be due to the presence of an aberrant splice site eliminating an exon in the DC beta genes [9, 38].

No difference could be detected in the glycosilation pattern of DR and DQ molecules. DQ alpha chain, like DR alpha chain, has one complex type and one high mannose type oligosaccharide, and the beta chain has one complex-type oligosaccharide, as determined by the sensitivity of the molecule to endoglycosidases H and D [49]. DNA sequence analysis of several genes coding for either alpha or beta chain has confirmed the existence of two glycosilation sites for the alpha chain and one glycosilation site for the beta chain. It is not known, however, whether the composition of the carbohydrate moieties is the same in DR and DQ molecules.

The N-terminal amino acid sequence analysis of DQw1 alpha chain, as well as that of DQw1 beta chain [8], revealed a striking homology to the murine I-A molecule, while DR molecules are more homologous to the I-E molecules. This finding indicates that DQ molecules are the human counterpart of the murine I-A while DR antigens correspond to the murine I-E molecules, suggesting that the two subregions originated before the separation of the two species.

Serological studies have identified three DQ specificities: DQw1 in linkage disequilibrium with DR1, 2, w6; DQw2 in linkage disequilibrium with DR3 and 7; and DQw3 linked to DR4 and 5 [55]. Recently, three additional DQ specificities have been described. DC5, in linkage disequilibrium with DR5, DRw12, and some DR4 [56], is likely to be the same specificity recognized by the monoclonal antibody TA10 [40]. DC HON is in linkage disequilibrium with DR4 and DRw9 [57]. The third specificity, named DCα3, resides on the alpha chain and is associated with DR5, DR12, and some DR3 [60].

It has been previously discussed that DQ molecules from DR1-, DR2-, and DRw6-homozygous cell lines share an identical alpha chain but have structurally distinct beta chains. A recent report [5a] showing that the primary structure of

```
                                 10        20        30        40        50
                        ↓        .         .         .         .         .
DC3 (DR3)               RDSPEDFVYQFKGMCYFTNGTERVRLVSRSIYNREEIVRFDSDVGEFRAV
pII-β-1 (DR3,w6)        ------------------------------------V-------------
pII-β-2 (DR3,w6)        -------------L-----------G-T-H------Y--------VY---
DC4 (DR4)               ---------------------------T-Y------YA-------VY---
DC1 (DR2)               --------F------------------T-Y------YA-------VY---
DX   (DR4)              .....--LV----------------G-A-Y------YG---------Q--

                                 60        70        80        90    ↓   100
                                 .         .         .         .         .
DC3                     TLLGLPAAEYWNSQKDILERKRAAVDAVCRHNYQLELRTTLQRRVEPTVT
pII-β-1                 --------------------------------------------------
pII-β-2                 -PQ-R-V--------EV--GA--S---------EVAY-GI----------
DC4                     -P--P----------EV---T--EL-T-----------------------
DC1                     -PQ-R-D--------EV--GT--EL-T------EVAF-GI----------
DX                      -E--R SI-D--NY--F--QE-----K------EA--------Q

                                110       120       130       140       150
                                 .         .         .         .         .
DC3                     ISPSATEALNHHHNLLVCSVTDFYPAQIKVRWFANDQEETAGVVSTPLIRN
pII-β-1                 ---------------------------------------------------
pII-β-2                 ---------------I--------S--------------------------
DC4                     ----------------------------------------T----------
DC1                     -------------------------G-------------------------

                                160       170       180       190       200
                                 .         .         .        ↓.         .
DC3                     GDWTFQILVMLEMTPQRGDVVYTCHVEHPSLQSPITVEWRAQSESAQSKML
pII-β-1                 ---------------------------------------------------
pII-β-2                 ---------------------------------------------------
DC4                     --------------------------------N--I---------------
DC1                     .................--------------------------------..

                                210       220
                                 .         .
DC3                     SGIGGFVLGLIFLGLGLIIHHRSQK
pII-β-1                 -------------------------
pII-β 2                 --V----------------RQ--R-
DC4                     -------------------------
DC1                     .........................
```

Fig. 1. Comparison of published complete amino acid sequences of DQ beta chains. DC3: DR3,3 cells [9]; pII-β-1 and pII-β-2: Raji cells (DR3,w6) [27]; DC4: cosII-102 [39]; DC1: DR2,2 cells [24]; DX beta: DR4,4 cells [47]. *Arrows,* intron-exon boundaries

```
                           10        20        30        40        50
                            .         .         .         .         .
DC1 (DRw6)         EDIVADHVASCGVNLYQFYGPSGQYTHEFDGDEQFYVDLERKETAWRWPE
DC4 (DR4,w6)       ----------Y------S-------S-------E----------V-QL-L
DX  (DR4,w6)       ----------Y---F--SH------T-------E------T---V-QL-M
pII-α-5            ----------Y------S---------------------G----V-CL-V
DS7(DR7)           ----------Y------S------F--------E----------V-KL-L

                           60        70        80        90       100
                            .         .         .       ↓ .         .
DC1                FSKFGGFDPQGALRNMAVAKHNLNIMIKRYNSTAATNEVPEVTVFSKSPV
DC4                -RR-RR----F--T-I--L------V---S--------------------
DX                 -SK-IS----S--R-N--G--T-EFHMRQS-----------------F--
p-II-α-5           LRQ-R.----F--T-I--L-----SL---E--------------------
DS7                -HRLR.----F--T-I--LL-----L---S--------------------

                          110       120       130       140       150
                            .         .         .         .         .
DC1                TLGQPNTLICLVDNIFPPVVNITWLSNGQSVTEDVSETSFLSKSDHSFFK
DC4                ----------------------------H----G----------------
DX                 ----------------------------H----G----------------
pII-α-5            ------I---------------------H----G----------------
DS7                ----------------------------H----G----------------

                          160       170       180       190       200
                            .         .         . ↓       .         .
DC1                ISYLTFLPSADEIYDCKVEHWGLDQPLLKHWEPEIPAPMSELTETVVCAL
DC4                ------------------------E-----------T--------L----
DX                 ------------------------E--------------------L----
pII-α-5            -----L----E-S-----------K-------------------------
DS7                ------------------------E-------------------------

                          210       220       230
                            .         .         .
DC1                GLSVGLMGIVVGTVFIIQGLRSVGASRHQGPL
DC4                ------V-------L--R--------------
DX                 -------A--F--A------------------
pII-α-5            ------V----------R--------------
DS7                ------V-------L--R--------------
```

Fig. 2 Comparison of complete sequences of DQ alpha chains. DC1: HB20 cDNA clone from DRw6,w6 cells [3]; DC4 and DX are from JY cells (DR4,w6 [47]; DS7: DR7 cell line [11]. *Arrows,* intron-exon boundaries

DQw1 beta chain from a DR1-homozygous cell line (LG2) is identical to that of DQw6$^+$ cell line (Raji) would seemingly contradict the above statement. However, these data would be explained if the correct typing of Raji is DR1, 3 rather than DR3, w6, as has indeed been reported [56]. A study of DQ beta chains from DR4- and DR5-homozygous cell lines made with a monoclonal antibody preferentially recognizing DQw3 molecules demonstrated the existence of two different beta chains. The DQw3 beta chain associated with DR4 lacks the tyrosine residue at position 26 present in the DR5-associated DQw3 molecules [20] (see Fig. 4).

Moreover, six different DQ beta chains could be identified in cell lines homozygous for DR1, 2, 3, 4, 5, and 7, and were called DS (D secondary) [25, 26]. The existence of at least six different beta chains could suggest that the determinants defining the observed supertypic specificities were carried by the alpha subunits. However, the polymorphism of DQ alpha chains follows a different pattern. For instance, DQ alpha alleles associated with DR3 and DR5 have an identical genomic restriction map [1], and the corresponding proteins were shown to be identical in their peptide map [60]. Furthermore, a similar analysis showed that DR4- and DR7-associated DQ alpha chain genes have the same restriction pattern [53]. Although the number of beta chain alleles is higher than that of alpha chain, the polymorphism of DQ beta genes does not seem to be more extensive than that of the DQ alpha genes. In both cases the substitutions are concentrated in the first domain [48]. It might be worth noting that DQw1 beta chain has a conserved stretch of amino acids (84 to 90) that may be part of DQw1-specific allodeterminant (Figs. 1 and 2).

There is no obvious genetic explanation for the fact that DQ alpha and beta alleles are independently linked to DR alleles. However, one should bear in mind that class II molecules must act as a functional set on the surface of antigen-presenting cells. Thus, DQ alpha and beta may have sorted independently in response to a selective pressure to generate the best possible combination of antigen-presenting molecules. Looking at the published amino acid sequences deduced from DQ alpha genes (Fig. 2), it is evident that DC4 and DS7 alpha gene products share a higher homology (only eight substitutions) to each other than to DC1 alpha gene (26 and 25 substitutions, respectively) and also that the DC3 alpha gene sequence (pII-α-5) is more similar to DC4 and DS7 (13 and 18 substitutions respectively) than to DC1 (27 substitutions). Furthermore, DQw1 alpha gene from a DR2 cell line [24] shows no detectable differences with DQw1 from a DRw6 cell line. In this view, this pattern of homology suggests a higher probability of transassociation between products of DQw2 and DQw3 haplotypes, even though transassociation between DQw1 alpha chain and some products of the other subregions has already been demonstrated in some cases (see below).

The Multigenic Nature of the DQ Subregion

Southern blot analysis with a cDNA probe specific for DC1 alpha chain gene has uncovered the existence of a second DC-like hybridizing sequence that was identified as an intact gene named DX [2]. The derived amino acid sequence of the DX gene from the JY cell line (DR4, w6) differs in only 25 residues from both DC1 and DC4 alpha chains (Fig. 2). However, although no abnormal feature was found in the sequence that would prevent the DX alpha gene from being translated, its expression has never been formally proven.

However, the expression of two DC-like subsets in homozygous cell lines was demonstrated by several independent biochemical studies. Karr et al. [31] described in a DR5-homozygous cell line a second DQ subset which could be isolated using a specific rabbit antiserum. This subset has a beta chain clearly distinguishable by two-dimensional gel electrophoresis from the known DQ beta chain. More recently the same group described two subsets of DQ molecules, each one with its own distinct alpha and beta chains. The authors also postulated the ex-

```
                                 10                  20
DC1 (DRw6)     E D I V A D - V A Q L G V N L Y Q F Y G P - G Q Y/F--E
DC1 (DR4,w6)   E D I V A D H V A - - G V N L Y Q F Y G P
DS7 (DR7)      E D I V A D H V A A Y G V N L Y Q S Y G
DS2 (DR2)          I V       V               Y     Y
MB3 (DR4)          I V       V     Y   V   L Y     Y           Y

33.1(DR1)                                    Y   F Y           Y   F
33.1(DR2)                                    Y   F Y           Y   F
33.1(DR4)                          Y         Y     -           Y   F
33.1(DR5)                          Y         Y     Y           Y   F
33.1(DRw6)                                   Y   F Y           F   F
33.1(DR7)                          Y         Y     Y           F   F
```

Fig. 3. Comparison of N-terminal sequences of DQ alpha chains determined by radioactive or conventional techniques. DC1 is from either DRw6 [7] or JY (DR4,w6) [8]; DS7 and DS2 are from cell lines homozygous for DR7 and DR2 respectively [26]; MB3 is from Priess cell line (DR4,4) [21]; 33.1 are from cell lines homozygous for DR1, 2, 4, 5, 6, and 7 [37]

istence of a third alpha chain, but the evidence provided is far from being definitive [32]. Studying a large number of typed individuals and a panel of homozygous cell lines with several anti-DQw1 monoclonal antibodies, Johnson and Wank [30] have obtained strong evidence for the expression of two distinct DQ beta molecules and showed that each of these carries distinct alloantigenic specificities that can be defined by monoclonal antibodies. Finally, the monoclonal antibody 33.1 has been shown to react with a subset of molecules having a high degree of homology to murine I-A molecules but different from previously described DQ molecules [41]. This second DQ subset is likely to be the same as the one described by Karr et al. [31], even though a direct comparison of the two molecules has never been made. The partial N-terminal sequence of this DQ-like subset shows the existence of a structurally distinct beta chain, although the sequence available is too limited to exclude the possibility that the two molecules are allelic products of the same DQ subset. No differences were found between the limited available sequence of the alpha chain and the published DQ alpha chain sequences (Figs. 3 and 4) [37]. Comparison of the published sequences of 33.1 antigen with the sequence of DX alpha and beta genes does not indicate a gene-product relationship between them since the 33.1 sequence from a DR4-homozygous cell line shows a tyrosine in position 9 where the DX sequence indicates the presence of a valine. Moreover, the phenylalanine in position 15 that differentiates DX alpha gene from both DC1 and DC4 alpha genes in a DR4,w6 cell line would have been detected, if present, in the radiochemical sequence based on phenylalanine and tyrosine of 33.1 alpha chains.

Recently, by using a DC alpha probe, a new alpha chain gene has been discovered and named DO [53]. Assuming that there is a beta counterpart expressed, this new antigen can be a candidate for bearing the 33.1 determinant.

There is then sufficient evidence in favor of the existence of at least two DQ subsets, although there are not enough data to establish a gene-product relationship between the known genes and proteins. However, it remains to be seen to which extent the two subsets are polymorphic and whether the two DQ alpha and beta chains associate only in a given combination, i.e., $alpha_1$ with $beta_1$ and $alpha_2$ with $beta_2$. A partial answer to the first question comes from a Southern blot analysis of 88 haplotypes with a DQ beta probe that shows the existence of two

										10										20										30	
DC1(DR4,w6)	R	D	S	P	E	D	F	V	Y	Q	F	K	G	M	-	Y	F	T	N	G	T	E	R	V	R	L	V	-	R		
MB3 (DR4)							F	V	Y		F					Y	F							V			V			Y	Y
MB3 (DR5)									Y							Y										Y				Y	Y
33.1 (DR1)							F		Y		F					Y	F														Y
33.1 (DR2)							F		F		F					Y	F													Y	Y
33.1 (DR2)							F		F		F					Y	F													Y	Y
33.1 (DR2)							F	V	Y		F					Y	F							V			V				F
33.1 (DR4)							F		Y		F					Y	F													Y	Y
33.1 (DR5)							F		Y		F					Y	F													Y	Y
33.1 (DRw6)							F		Y		F					Y	F													-	Y
33.1 (DR7)							F		Y		F					Y	F													Y	Y

Fig. 4. Comparison of N-terminal sequences of DQ beta chains determined by radioactive or conventional techniques. DC1: DR4,w6 cells [8]; MB3: DR4- and DR5-homozygous cell lines [21]; 33,1 from cell lines homozygous for DR1, 2, 4, 5, 6, and 7 [37]; DS2 and DS7: DR2- and DR7-homozygous cell lines [26]. *Blanks,* no assignment

allelic series of DQ genes: one that follows the DQw1, 2, and 3 distribution, and a second that follows more closely the DR allelic series [14a]. Some evidence of transassociation of different alpha and beta DQ alleles has been obtained very recently in heterozygous cell lines. Using two monoclonal antibodies specific for either DC1 (G25a) or DS7 (SG171) beta chains, it could be demonstrated that the DS7 beta chain associated to both DS7 and DC1 alpha chains. DC1 beta chains was always found associated only with DC1 alpha chain [13]. Giles et al. [22] have obtained similar results supported by N-terminal sequence analysis. These two reports indicate that the number of antigenically different DQ molecules that can be expressed by a single cell is likely to be higher than expected. However, as these experiments also imply, it is likely that only certain combinations are allowed. For instance, DC1 beta chain was not found associated to DS7 alpha chain.

The polymorphism of DQ alpha chain is a unique feature that characterizes these molecules among human class II antigens. The functional and the evolutionary implications of this phenomenon are unknown. An obvious consequence is the potentially greater number of combinatorial determinants that may enable these molecules to interact with a wider "pool" of different T cells.

Do Biochemical Differences Between DQ and DR Molecules Reflect Different Functions?

The few available data do not point so far to a striking different role or even to a different tissue distribution of DQ and DR molecules. Few reports seem to indicate that the expression of DQ molecules on human monocytes differs from that of DR molecules. Indeed, two populations in human peripheral blood monocytes have been described, one DQ-positive and one DQ-negative [45] and only the DQ-positive population is able to induce T cell proliferation in response to the antigen *C. albicans* [23]. However these data need to be confirmed using more sensitive techniques, since it is known that DQ molecules are always expressed in much lower amounts than DR molecules. A drop in the level of expression of both antigens linked to a transient, physiological state of the monocyte could bring the amount of DQ molecules below the limit of a relatively insensitive method such as immunofluorescence. It is in fact known that products of cell of the immune system, like γ-interferon, can increase the level of expression of DR and DQ antigens [15] suggesting that the concentration of Ia molecules on the cell membrane can be rapidly changed in response to physiological stimuli. However, the monoclonal antibody 33.1 does not stain monocytes, while it reacts readily with B cells [41]. This differential distribution of this putative DQ subset correlates with the distribution of a second I-A beta chain which has been recently described in the mouse [38]. This molecule is not inducible by γ-interferon in mouse macrophages [60 a].

A differential expression of DR and DQ molecules has also been reported in a patient with hairy cell leukemia [19]. The leukemic cells did not express any DQ molecule on their surface. Treatment with either 5-azacytidine or sodium butyrate restored the expression of DQ molecules.

In a study of the inhibitory effect of anti-Ia antibodies on human T cells, it was shown that the monoclonal antibody BT3/4, directed against DC1, can effectively block the generation of cytotoxic T cells. However, neither proliferation of T cells in response to allo- or soluble antigens nor the production of Ig after pokeweed mitogen stimulation were affected. In contrast, anti-DR monoclonal antibodies blocked all T cell functions tested [17]. This is an indication of a possible differential function of DQ and DR molecules. However, only one monoclonal antibody directed to DQ molecules was used. It would be desirable, now that more monoclonal antibodies are available, to confirm this study by the use of several monoclonals and haplotypes.

A number of diseases have been reported to have a preferential association with some HLA haplotypes. A preferential association of DQ molecules with some diseases, such as celiac disease [59], chronic lymphocytic leukemia [46], and multiple sclerosis [14] has also been reported. In some cases, as for celiac disease, the association with a DQ allele, DQw2, is so strong as to suggest a direct involvement of this antigen in the pathogenesis of the disease.

Many laboratories are currently involved in biochemical and serological studies aimed at pinpointing differences in MHC genes or their products between patients and normal individuals carrying the same haplotype or at discovering new determinants that fit better to the associations described. For instance, celiac disease was first thought to be linked to DR3 and DR7, while it is now clear that the closest association is with the more recently described DQw2 specificity [60]. Other diseases, such as juvenile diabetes, are known to be linked to one or more D haplotypes. However, the actual allele to which they are associated has not yet been found.

It is likely that the identification of the factors, either HLA-related or T cell-related, to which these diseases are linked will provide insight not only into the pathogenesis of the diseases, but also into the mechanisms underlying antigen recognition.

Acknowledgments. We thank Oreste Acuto, Alan Korman, and Roberto Tosi for critical reading of the manuscript, and Jack Strominger and the members of his laboratory for making data available before publication.

References

1. Auffray C, Kuo J, DeMars R, Strominger JC (1983) A minimum of four human Class II alpha genes are encoded in the HLA region of chromosome 6. Nature 304:174
2. Auffray C, Ben-Nun A, Roux-Dosseto M, Germain RN, Seidman JG, Strominger JL (1983) Polymorphism and complexity of the human DC and murine I-A alpha chain genes. EMBO J 2:121
3. Auffray C, Lillie JW, Arnot D, Grossberger D, Kappes D, Strominger JC (1984) Isotypic and allotypic variation of human class II histocompatibility antigens alpha chain genes. Nature 308:327
5. Bach FH, van Rood JH (1976) The major histocompatibility complex: genetics and biology. N Engl J Med 295:806
5. Bach FH, Watson AJ (1983) Dw/LD associated molecular polymorphism of DR4 beta chains: intramolecular localization of polymorphic sites. J Immunol 131:1622

5a. Bell JI, Estess P, John TS, Saiki R, Watling DL, Erlich HA, McDevitt HO (1985) DNA sequence and characterization of human class II major histocompatibility complex beta chains from the DR1 haplotype. Proc Natl Acad Sci USA 82:3405

6. Biddison WE, Ward FE, Shearer GM, Shaw S (1980) The self determinants recognised by human virus-immune T cell can be distinguished from the serologically defined HLA antigens. J Immunol 124:548
7. Bono MR, Strominger JC (1981) Direct evidence of homology between human DC1 antigen and murine I-A molecules. Nature 291:455
8. Bono MR, Strominger JC (1983) Amino-terminal sequence of the alpha and beta chains of human DC1 antigen isolated from the JY cell line. Homology with murine I-A molecules. Immunogenetics 18:455
9. Boss JM, Strominger JC (1984) Cloning and sequence analysis of the human major histocompatibility complex gene DC3 beta. Proc Natl Acad Sci USA 81:5199
10. Deleted in production
11. Chang HC, Moriuchi T, Silver J (1983) The heavy chain of human B cell alloantigen HLA-DS has a variable N-terminal region and a constant immunoglobulin-like region. Nature 305:813
12. Deleted in production
13. Charron D, Lotteau V, Turmel P (1984) Hybrid HLA-DC antigens provide molecular evidence for gene trans-complementation. Nature 312:157
14. Cohen D, Cohen O, Marcadet A, Massart C, Lathcop M, Descchamps I, Hors I, Schuller E, Dausset J (1984) Class II HLA-DC beta chain DNA restriction fragments differentiate among HLA-DR2 individuals in insulin dependent diabetes and multiple sclerosis. Proc Natl Acad Sci USA 81:1774

14a. Cohen D, LeGall I, Marcadet A, Font MP, Lalouel JM, Dausset J (1984) Clusters of HLA class II β restriction fragments describe allelic series. Proc Natl Acad Sci USA 81:7870

15. Collins T, Korman AJ, Wake CT, Boss JM, Kappes DS, Firs W, Ault KA, Gimbrone MA, Strominger JL, Pober JS (1984) Immune interferon activates multiple Class II MHC genes and the associated invariant chain gene in human endothelial cells and dermal fibroblasts. Proc Natl Acad Sci USA 81:4917
16. Corte G, Calabi F, Damiani G, Bargellesi A, Tosi R, Sorrentino R (1981) Human Ia molecules carrying DC1 determinants differ in both alpha and beta subunits from Ia molecules carrying DR determinants. Nature 292:357
17. Corte G, Moretta A, Cosulich ME, Ramarli D, Bargellesi A (1982) A monoclonal anti DC1 antibody selectively inhibits the generation of effector T cells mediating specific cytolytic activity. J Exp Med 156:1539
18. Dausset J (1981) The major histocompatibility complex in man. Science 213:1469

19. Faille A, Turmel P, Charron DJ (1984) Differential expression of HLA-DR and HLADC/DS molecules in a patient with hairy cell leukemia: restoration of HLADC/DS expression by (12-0-tetradecanoyl phorbol-13-acetate), 5-azacytidine, and sodium butyrate. Blood 64:33
20. Giles RC, Nunez G, Hurley Katovich C, Nunez Roldan A, Winchester R, Stastny P, Capra DJ (1983) Structural analysis of human I-A homologue using a monoclonal antibody that recognizes a MB3-like specificity. J Exp Med 157:1461
21. Giles RC, Hurley Katovich C, Capra JD (1984) Primary structural variation among serologically indistinguishable DS antigens; the MB3-bearing molecule in DR4 cells differs from the MB3-bearing molecule in DR5 cells. J Immunol 133:1
22. Giles RC, DeMars R, Chang CC, Capra JD (1985) Allelic polymorphism and trans-complementation of molecules encoded by the HLA-DQ subregion. Proc Natl Acad Sci USA 82:1776
23. Gonwa TA, Picker LJ, Raff HV, Goyert S, Silver J, Stobo JD (1983) Antigen presenting capabilities of human monocytes correlates with their expression of HLA-DS, an Ia determinant distinct from HLA-DR. J Immunol 130:706
24. Gotz H, Kratzin H, Thinnes FP, Yang CY, Kruse T, Pauley E, Kolbel S, Egert G, Wernet P, Hilschmann N (1983) Primary structure of human class II histocompatibility antigens. Hoppe-Zeylers Z Physiol Chem 364:749
25. Goyert S, Silver J (1983) Further characterization of HLA-DS molecules, implications for studies assessing the role of human Ia molecules in cell interactions and disease susceptibility. Proc Natl Acad Sci USA 80:5719
26. Goyert S, Shively JE, Silver J (1982) Biochemical characterization of a second family of human Ia molecules, HLA-DS, equivalent to murine I-A subregion molecules. J Exp Med 155:550
27. Gustafsson K, Wiman K, Emmoth E, Larhammar D, Bohne J, Hyldig-Nielson JJ, Ronne H, Peterson PA, Rask L (1984) Mutation and selection in the generation of class II histocompatibility antigen polymorphism. EMBO J 3:1655
28. Deleted in production
29. Ikeda H, Kasahara M, Ogasawara K, Takemouchi T, Okuyama T, Ishikawa N, Wakisaka A, Kikuchi Y, Aizawa M (1984) Evidence for polymorphism of MB3 antigens among three HLA-D clusters associated with HLA-DR4. Immunogenetics 19:381
30. Johnson JP, Wank R (1984) Identification of two cis-encoded HLA-DR molecules that carry distinct alloantigenic specificities. J Exp Med 160:1350
31. Karr RW, Kannagel CC, Langare RJ, Goyert S, Silver J, Schwartz BD (1983) An HLA-DR5 homozygous cell line expresses two DS (Ia-like) molecules. J Exp Med 158:1374
32. Karr RW, Alber C, Goyert S, Silver J, Duquesnoy RJ (1984) The complexity of HLA-DS molecules: a homozygous cell line expresses three HLA-DS alpha chains. J Exp Med 159:1512
33. Kaufman JF, Strominger JL (1983) The extracellular region of light chains from human and murine MHC Class II antigens consists of two domains. J Immunol 130:808
34. Klein J (1975) Biology of the mouse. Histocompatibility complex. Springer, Berlin Heidelberg New York
35. Klein J (1979) The major histocompatibility complex of the mouse. Science 203:516
36. Krangel MS, Taketani S, Biddison WE, Strominger JL (1982) Comparative structural analysis of HLA-A2 antigens indistinguishable by cytotoxic T lymphocytes: variants MT and DR1. Biochemistry 21:6313
37. Kuo MC, Li XM, Marti GE, Sachs JA, Sogu JA, Coligan JE, Kindt YJ (1984) Primary structural sequence polymorphism in the human Class II MHC antigen 33.1. Immunogenetics 19:27
38. Larhammar D, Hammerling U, Denaro M, Lund T, Flavell RA, Rask L, Peterson PA (1983 a) Structure of the murine immune response I-A beta locus: sequence of the I-A beta gene and an adjacent beta chain second domain exon. Cell 34:179
39. Larhammar D, Hyldig-Nielsen JJ, Servenius B, Anderson G, Rask L, Peterson PA (1983 b) Exon-intron organization and complete nucleotide sequence of a human major histocompatibility antigen DC beta gene. Proc Natl Acad Sci USA 80:7313
40. Maeda H (1984) Mouse monoclonal antibody detects a new polymorphic Ia determinant other than HLA-DR antigen: a possible allele of DC1. Tissue Antigens 23:163

41. Marti GE, Kuo MC, Shaw S, Chang CC, DeMars R, Sogn JA, Coligan JE, Kindt TJ (1983) A novel HLA-D/DR-like antigen specific for human B lymphoid cells. J Exp Med 158:1924
42. Mengle-Glaw, McDevitt HO (1985) Genetics and expression of mouse Ia antigens. Ann Rev Immunol 3:367
43. Nepom BS, Nepom GT, Mickelson E, Antonelli P, Hansen JA (1983) Electrophoretic analysis of human HLA-DR antigens from HLA-DR4 homozygous cell lines: correlation between beta chain diversity and HLA-D. Proc Natl Acad Sci USA 80:6962
44. Nepom GT, Nepom BS, Antonelli P, Mickelson E, Silver J, Goyert SM, Hansen JA (1984) The HLA-DR4 family of haplotypes consists of a series of distinct DR and DS molecules. J Exp Med 156:394
45. Nunez G, Giles RC, Ball EJ, Hurley CK, Capra JD, Stastny P (1984) Expression of HLA-DR, MB, MT, and SB antigens on human mononuclear cells: identification of two phenotypically distinct monocyte populations. J Immunol 133:1300
46. Nunez-Roldan A, Szero I, Toguchi T, Cuttner J, Winchester R (1982) Association of certain Ia allotypes with the occurrence of chronic lymphocytic leukemia. J Exp Med 156:1872
47. Okada K, Boss J, Prentice H, Spiest T, Mengler R, Auffray C, Lillie J, Grossberger D, Strominger JL (1985) Gene organization of the DC and DR subregions of the human major histocompatibility complex. Proc Natl Acad Sci USA 82:3410
48. Schenning N, Larhammar D, Bill P, Wiman K, Jonsson AK, Rask L, Peterson PA (1984) Both alpha and beta chains of HLA-DC class II antigens display extensive polymorphism in their amino-terminal domains. EMBO J 3:447
49. Shackelford DA, Strominger JL (1983) Analysis of two oligosaccharides on the HLA-DR and DC1 B cell antigens. J Immunol 130:274
50. Shackelford DA, Mann DL, van Rood JJ, Ferrara GB, Strominger JL (1981) Human B cell alloantigens DC1, MT1, and LB 12 are identical to each other but distinct from the HLA DR antigen. Proc Natl Acad Sci USA 78:4566
51. Shackelford DA, Eibl B, Strominger JL (1983) Structural polymorphism of the DC1 light chains from DR1, DR2, and DRw6 possible cell lines. Immunogenetics 18:625
52. Snell GD (1981) Studies in histocompatibility. Science 213:172
53. Spielman RS, Lee J, Bodmer WF, Bodmer JG, Trowsdale J (1984) Six HLA-D region alpha chain genes on human chromosome 6: polymorphism and association of DC alpha related sequences with DR types. Proc Natl Acad Sci USA 81:3461
54. Deleted in production
55. Tanigaki N, Tosi R (1982) The genetic control of human Ia alloantigens: a three loci model derived from the immunochemical analysis of supertypic specificities. Immunol Rev 66:537
56. Tanigaki N, Tosi R, Centis D, Ferrara GB (1985) DR5-associated DC molecules carry three different allospecifities. Hum Immunol 12:47–57
57. Tanigaki N, Tosi R, Katagiri M, Ferrara GB (1985) A new allodeterminant on HLA-DQ molecules carrying the DQw3 specificity. Hum Immunol (in press)
58. Tosi R, Tanigaki N, Centis D, Ferrara GB, Pressman D (1978) Immunological dissection of human Ia molecules. J Exp Med 148:1592
59. Tosi R, Vismara D, Tanigaki N, Ferrara GB, Ciccimarra F, Buffolano W, Follo D, Auricchio S (1983) Evidence that coeliac disease is primarily associated with a DC locus allelic specificity. Clin Immunol Immunopathol 28:395
60. Tosi R, Tanigaki N, Sorrentino R, Centis D, Ferrara GB (1984) Serologically detectable polymorphism of the HLA-DC alpha subunit. J Immunol 132:277
60a. Wake CT, Flavell RA (1985) Transcription of a novel murine immune response gene, Aβ2. Cell (in press)
61. Winchester RJ, Kunkel HG (1979) The human Ia system. Adv Immunol 28:221

HLA-DP: Current Status

M. Sanchez-Perez and S. Shaw

Table of Contents

Overview

HLA class II molecules (Ia) are highly polymorphic cell surface glycoproteins encoded on the short arm of chromosome 6. They have a characteristic dimeric structure formed by two transmembrane glycoproteins of molecular weight about 29 kd(β) and 35 kd(α). Like HLA class I molecules, class II molecules play a critical role in recognition by T cells, but their tissue distribution is restricted primarily to B cells, antigen-presenting cells, and certain activated cells. Three different families of class II molecules have been defined, have strong structural homologies, and are presumed to have had a common evolutionary origin: DR, DQ, and DP. DP behaves as genetic "outsider" in the D region: (a) recombination occurs relatively frequently between DP and DR/DQ (which have not been clearly distinguished by recombination); (b) linkage disequilibrium between DP and DR (or DQ) is much weaker than between DR and DQ. Less DP is found on the cell surface than DR. Like DR, DP induces proliferative and cytotoxic T cell (CTL) responses, but DP-specific responses are often weaker. Finally, an important historical feature which distinguishes DP from DR and DQ is that even now, 5–7 years after its definition, its alleles are defined by cellular techniques rather than by antisera. This review summarizes the current status of studies regarding the function, genetics, structure, and expression of DP; some of the data show differences between DP and other class II molecules but many of them emphasize the similarities. We have tried to be as complete as possible in our reference citations on DP, but have been sparing in other citations.

Nomenclature

The designation HLA-DP was formally adopted by the HLA Nomenclature Committee (operating under the auspices of the World Health Organization) following the Ninth International Histocompatibility Workshop in 1984 [1]. This group serves the essential function of deciding a uniform international nomenclature for histocompatibility determinants. The new designation replaces principally the designation "SB", which had been coined in 1980 to indicate alleles of a proposed *S*econdary *B* cell locus [2]. "SB" had become a de facto standard nomenclature by 1982 [3], largely because of extensive sharing of reagents between laboratories. There is a substantial body of literature which antedates the "SB" terminology and uses a variety of terminologies for lymphocyte-activating determinants which relate, in whole or in part, to products of the DP region [e.g., 4–11]. The best-developed independent nomenclature ("PL3") [12, 13] was graciously replaced with "SB" after direct comparison between laboratories [3, 14].

Cellular Recognition

Products of the DP locus were first defined by allogeneic T cell recognition. Phenotyping of donors for alleles of this locus continues to be done by "cellular typing" rather than serotyping. Furthermore, it is widely believed that T cell recognition of class II molecules in general (and of DP in particular) is central to their physiologic function [15]. Therefore, cellular recognition of DP products will be discussed in detail.

Cellular Typing for DP

Primed Lymphocyte Typing

Phenotyping of a donor for DP is generally done by using his peripheral blood mononuclear leukocytes (PBML) to stimulate proliferation of primed T cells, in an assay known as primed lymphocyte typing (PLT) [16]. Since T cell proliferation is antigen-specific, T cells primed to a particular cellular antigen will specifically proliferate again only when they are restimulated with the same antigen. For example, if a donor's PBML induce proliferation from "DPw1-specific" primed T cell populations, the PBML must express the DPw1 antigen.

Polyclonal Reagents. As in any assay, the reliability of the test is largely determined by the quality of the reagents used. The typing reagents generally used to define DP alleles are "bulk" populations of primed T cells which are functionally monospecific. Rapid progress in the study of the DP antigens was made possible by creation and distribution of a standard set of DP typing reagents [16] generated by priming T cells between allogeneic donors who were exhaustively matched for all the other known HLA markers [2, 16, 17]. Five DP antigens were described using two independent reagents to define each. These reagents, together with DPw6-specific reagents identified subsequently [18], have become the benchmark for the definition of DP for various practical reasons: (a) they are remarkably monospecific (i.e., there is minimal proliferation induced by other antigens); (b) there is excellent concordance in the proliferative responses of the two reagents used to identify each DP antigen [16, 19]; (c) the proliferative responses of these T cells to the relevant DP antigen are strong and relatively independent of experimental protocol; (d) the reagents are cryopreserved in aliquots and are unaffected by shipping to other laboratories and by several years of storage in liquid nitrogen; (e) the reagents can be amplified at least several hundred fold without apparent alteration in specificity by restimulation in the presence of exogenous interleukin-2 (IL-2) [20]; (f) many laboratories have had difficulties in generating reagents which are as sensitive and specific (however, other laboratories have succeeded in generating some discriminatory "bulk" reagents [14, 21–23] whose reactivity has generally correlated well with that of the standard reagents); (g) serologic detection has proven difficult (see Antibodies which Relate to DP, p. 89). These reagents have been used in more than 40 different laboratories, either by direct collaboration or via the Ninth International Histocompatibility Workshop [19].

Technical Considerations with Polyclonal Reagents. Although *generation* of the DP-specific reagents is relatively difficult, *use* of the reagents in PLT assays is relatively simple. Standard techniques used in many different laboratories are satisfactory; however, more stimulator cells may be required than for DR-specific PLT (unpublished observations), presumably because of the relatively low-level expression of the DP antigens (see Detection with MoAb, p. 100). To obtain data suitable for statistical analysis it is essential that at least 20 stimulator cells be assayed simultaneously. Assays must include control stimulator cells for each of the DP antigens being tested (to validate reactivity of the typing reagent). Assays must also include a control condition to document the stimulatory capacity of each stimulator cell population tested; in our lab we use the response of a pool of T cells from different donors, each of which has been primed against a pool of allogeneic stimulator cells. The most common cause of failure to type a donor for DP alleles is poor stimulator cell function.

It is also possible to type lymphoblastoid B cell lines (LCL) for DP antigens in a similar assay [24] using a lower number of stimulator cells and inactivating the stimulator with mitomycin C or a high dose of gamma irradiation. However, some additional reactivities may be seen, particularly with DPw4 reagents.

Cloned T Cell Reagents. T cell clones are highly discriminatory reagents which are the cellular typing equivalent of monoclonal antibodies (MoAb). A number of laboratories have succeeded in generating discriminatory DP-specific T-cell clones [11, 25–29]. Moen and coworkers have demonstrated the feasibility of doing extensive population studies with T cell clones [25]; Nose and coworkers report the definition of a putative new DP allele with T cell clones [29]. A number of laboratories are analyzing genetic complexity of the defined alleles with DP-specific T cel clones [11, 26, 27, 30]. The advantages of cloned reagents are self-evident. However, there are some real and potential disadvantages: (a) longevity of clones has been a problem in some laboratories [26]; (b) idiosyncratic cross-reactions of individual clones can be misleading [31]; (c) some laboratories report a low frequency of discriminatory clones [< 12%) even in carefully chosen priming combinations [11].

Assignment of DP Phenotype. Although the results of PLT assays are usually unambiguous enough to allow assignment of DP antigens by visual inspection, we believe that objective statistical algorithms should be used. We prefer a modified cluster analysis approach [16], although other approaches also work [32]. However, approaches which assume that antigens will be present in less than half of the stimulator cell donors (including most normalization schemes) are inappropriate for DPw4 or any allele present in high frequency in a particular experiment. Assignment of phenotype should always be based on more than one discriminatory reagent specific for each antigen.

Cell-Mediated Cytotoxicity

Early studies of DP [2] demonstrated that cell-mediated cytotoxicity was generated against determinants indistinguishable from the DP antigens detected by T cell proliferation. Cytotoxicity can be used instead of PLT to assay for the presence of the relevant DP allele [31]. This is generally not satisfactory for bulk T cell populations, which may be functionally monospecific for DP by proliferation but include CTL specific for other antigens [20] (including minor histocompatibility antigens [33]). However, we have found that when T cell clones are used for the assignment of DP antigens, the results are more consistent when LCL from the donor are used as targets in a cell-mediated lympholysis (CML) assay than when PBML or LCL from the donor are assayed as the stimulator cells in a proliferative assay (unpublished observations).

Allogeneic T Cell Recognition

Primary Proliferative Response

Available evidence suggests that the DP antigens can stimulate primary proliferative responses, although the strength of the response is weak relative to primary allogeneic proliferation to other class II alloantigens. The lack of a strong primary response caused DP to be overlooked in early studies of allogeneic proliferation and prompted our designation "*S*econdary *B* cell" antigens. However, the ability of antigens in the DP region to induce some primary allogeneic proliferation suggested the existence of a new (DP) subregion of the HLA complex in studies of a family with a recombinant HLA haplotype [5]. Similarly, a very weak (but consistent) primary allogeneic proliferation between "HLA-identical" siblings was the impetus for our own investigations of DP [34]. In our analyses of donors matched for HLA-A1, 2, B7, 8, the mean relative response among donors mismatched for DP was only 8%, compared to 3% for autologous responses and 48% for D/DR-mismatched combinations [2]. Termijtelen's studies of responses among A1, B8, DR3 cells also indicate little stimulation among DP-matched combinations, but a mean of 26% stabilized relative response (SRR) was observed among DP-mismatched cells [13]; these figures are somewhat higher than ours, but the difference is more apparent than real because of the SRR normalization of their data. Matsui et al. [35] observed a higher response between "DP-only" mismatched stimulating cells – about 40% of a random allogeneic response. In our experience, comparisons between the strength of primary proliferative responses to DP alone and the response to a full haplotype depend strongly on time and conditions of the assay, since the former peaks on about day 7 while the latter peaks on about day 5 (unpublished results). DP-specific proliferative responses may be weaker than those to DR (and perhaps DQ), because: (a) there are differences in the level of expression of the antigens on stimulator cells (DP is expressed at a much lower level than DR; (see Detection with MoAB, p. 100), and (b) there is a lower frequency of DP-specific precursor cells. This has been suggested by the results of studies by Bach and coworkers of T cell clones isolated following bulk sensitization against a full HLA haplotype: 11% are DP-specific, while 45% are DR-specific [36].

DP and HLA-D Typing

Do differences in DP type affect the results of HLA-D typing? Yes, but Termijtelen et al. find that the influence of matching for DP has only a marginal effect on the results of HLA-D typing [37]. However, it is interesting that when Hartzman DP-typed cells which had been selected as "good" homozygous typing cells (HTC), he found more DPw4-positive cells than would be predicted from gene frequencies in control populations (R. Hartzman, unpublished observations). This suggests that DP disparity contributes to "noise" in HTC typing and that the presence of DPw4 on a typing cell would decrease such "noise" for the majority of the population (which is DPw4-positive). DP typing of HTC reported by Wernet et al. [38] is consistent with that interpretation, although the distribution of DP antigen frequency is not radically different from that found in population studies of Caucasians. However, it is clear that DP differences do not explain most of the dramatic proliferative responses between DR-matched cells [39].

Secondary Proliferative Responses to DP

Although primary allogeneic proliferative responses to DP are weak, secondary proliferative responses are very robust. Indeed, in our experience priming and restimulation against a DP-only disparty is usually stronger (i.e., greater yield of viable cells and greater ^{3}H-thymidine incorporation) than: (a) priming and restimulation against a whole HLA haplotype disparity; (b) priming and restimulation against a DR/DQ-only disparity (supported by the findings of the Ninth International Histocompatibility Workshop [19] that DP-specific PLT responses were much stronger than those of other class II specificities); and (c) priming against a whole haplotype and restimulation with DP only! We have postulated that this may reflect the generation of relatively little suppression in DP-specific responses, but have not tested this hypothesis experimentally. IL-2 is generated by DP-specific clones [28], but it has not been determined whether more IL-2 is produced than in responses to other class II molecules.

Allogeneic Cell-Mediated Cytotoxicity

Early studies described the generation of DP-specific CML [2]. Like the proliferative responses, cytotoxic responses are marginal in primary stimulation but are markedly amplified in secondary responses. T cell responses to other class II antigens also generate CTL; however, results from cloning of DP-specific T cells [40, 41] (unpublished observations) have surprised us in two respects: a high frequency of CTL, and a predominance of helper-independent CTL. The findings are as follows: (a) Among T cells we have cloned by limiting dilution from DPw1- and DPw2-specific tertiary bulk cultures, there was a high frequency of clones (approximately 30% of those which grew) which had DP-specific cytotoxic activity. Some, though not all, of Ohta et al.'s findings [28, 41] support the hypothesis that a high proportion of the DP response is by cytotoxic cells. In a response against LCL, most DP-specific clones had cytotoxic activity [41], but in a sensitization against PBML, only one of 15 DP-specific proliferative T cell clones was cytotoxic [28]. It should be noted that Ohta et al.'s sensitizations differ from ours, since they include priming against DP and determinants other than DP. (b) All 20 DP-specific cytotoxic T cell clones which we have generated proliferate in a helper-independent fashion [40]. The DP-specific CTL clones described by Ohta et al. [28, 41] are also all helper-independent. He demonstrated that the two DP-specific CTL clones studied can both produce IL-2 [28].

Allogeneic Recognition of DP as a Model System

DP-specific T cell recognition has been used as a model system in which to analyze mechanisms of T-cell recognition. The phenotype of DP-reactive cells is largely OKT4+. Bulk populations of cell primed to DP are generally comprised of >85% OKT4+ cells [42]. Furthermore, studies of antibody and complement elimination demonstrate that the vast majority of the DP-specific CTL activity in bulk DP-primed populations is mediated by T4+ cells [42]. Indeed, when analyzed at the clonal level, all of Ohta's 15 DP-specific T cell clones [28] and all but one of our 20 DP-specific CTL clones are OKT4+ [40] (unpublished observations). However, one of our DPw2-specific CTL clones is OKT8+ OKT4-. Both the preponderance of T4+ cells and the rare occurrence of T8+ cells are consistent with the pattern seen with other class II-specific T cell responses.

Biddison and coworkers have used DP-specific CTL to analyze the role of the T4 molecule in T cell recognition [40, 42–46]. The data demonstrate that the T4 molecule can facilitate class II-specific T cell interactions at the stage of conjugate formation with the target, but also suggest that the requirement for the T4-interaction may be greater for "low-affinity" clones than for "high-affinity" clones.

HLA Restriction

Two cardinal feature of class II (as well as class I) antigens of the major histocompatibility complex (MHC) are that: (a) T cells recognize foreign antigens in association with them (i.e., they "restrict" foreign antigen recognition), and (b) their recognition by allogeneic T cells is independent of (i.e., not "restricted" by) other MHC molecules. The lack of restriction by other MHC loci of DP-specific allogeneic recognition was established by early studies with DP-specific proliferative and CTL responses [2]. Subsequent studies indicate that DP region products can act as restricting elements for T cell recognition of foreign antigens. Eckels and coworkers [47] identified two virus-specific proliferative T cell clones whose pattern of reactivity on panels of virus-infected stimulator cells was associated with the donor's DP alleles, and not with their other class II specificities. One clone, specific for a neuraminidase antigen of influenza virus, was restricted by an antigen indistinguishable from DPw2 (corrected $p < 0.005$). This clone was stimulated by a mouse L cell only after transfection with DP genes [48]. The other clone, specific for herpes simplex virus, had a pattern of recognition consistent with restriction by DPw4 ($p \simeq 0.05$ if one corrects for testing the relationship to six autologous class II antigens). Qvigstad et al.'s analysis of T cell clones reactive with *Chlamydia trachomatis* [49] showed that one of 17 tested was restricted by an antigen associated with DPw4 in all but one stimulator cell (corrected $P \simeq 0.05$). Studies of trinitrophenyl (TNP)-specific T cells also suggested restriction by a DPw4-associated determinant [50]. Studies on these clones demonstrate restriction by a determinant in linkage disequilibrium with DP, but only the transfection studies demonstrate that it is the DP region products themselves that mediate restriction.

Antibodies Which Relate to DP

Many questions regarding DP could be more easily approached if there were good serological tools to identify DP; in particular, one would like antibodies which detect (a) determinants shared by all DP alleles (i.e., monomorphic determinant), but not by other molecules ("DP-specific alloindifferent" antibodies), and (b) determinants unique to each allele of DP ("DP-specific allospecific" antibodies). The first section below outlines approaches to define the specificity of an antibody for DP products, and the second comments in more detail on the findings for some of the more interesting antibodies.

Approaches to Analysis of Specificity of Antibodies for DP

Inhibition of DP-Specific T Cell Function

Since the standard for definition of DP antigens is cellular recognition, the most direct demonstration that an antibody binds DP is that it inhibits DP-specific T cell responses. Many preparations of anti-class II MoAb inhibit DP-specific proliferation by bulk populations [51–54] or cloned T cells [51]. However, MoAB inhibition of proliferation does not always indicate that the MoAB binds to the DP antigen on the stimulator cell [53]; the inhibition may be nonspecific (due to contaminating substances in the antibody preparation tested), or due to action of the antibody on the responder cell [55]. Consequently, inhibition of proliferation must be done under carefully controlled circumstances, preferably with antibody preparations that have been dialyzed against culture media. In our experience, the ability of a MoAb to inhibit DP-specific cytotoxicity is the most specific indicator that the MoAb binds to the product recognized by T cells [53]. Although this assay is very specific, it is not very sensitive, and DP-binding antibodies may fail to inhibit because they are present below saturating levels or because they bind to the DP molecule in a way which does not interfere with T-cell recognition. A number of studies have been performed of MoAb inhibition of DP-specific cytotoxicity mediated by bulk populations [53] or by cloned T cells [28, 30, 41, 56]. One complicating feature is that some MoAb which bind to all HLA haplotypes tested only inhibit CML specific for particular DP alleles [51, 53].

Classical Genetics

Classical genetic approaches can help identify and characterize antibodies which bind to a polymorphic determinant on DP. The two reports of alloantisera with putative specificity for DP [57, 58] were based on population analyses showing very strong association between the pattern of binding of the antibodies to panels of donors' cells and the presence of a particular DP allele on those donors. Similar analysis has been possible only for one allospecific DP-binding MoAb [52]. For an alloindifferent MoAb the approach can be extended by using it to immunoprecipitate a class II molecule and then showing [e.g., by isoelectrofocusing (IEF)] that polymorphism of the product correlates with DP alleles [59, 60]. Obviously, such approaches cannot distinguish between binding to DP and binding to products of genes in strong linkage disequilibrium with DP.

Somatic Cell Genetics

The recent development of panels of HLA deletion mutant cell lines [61], particularly those which have completely lost expression of some but not other class II subregions, has provided a powerful tool for the analysis of the subregion specificity of anti-class II MoAb [52, 62–64]. The availability of mutant lines expressing DPw2 but not DR or DQ (e.g., 721.82) has made this technology particularly helpful in analyzing MoAb binding to DPw2. The ability of a MoAB to bind to line 721.82 (and other similar mutants) is necessary, but not sufficient, to establish that it binds DPw2; even after loss of DQ and DR expression, DP may not be the only remaining class II molecule (see subsection below on MHM4, p. 92). Studies of MoAb binding to panels of HLA deletion mutants demonstrate [63]: (a) many anti-class II MoAb bind to DP region determinants, but (b) there is extraordinary complexity of cross-reactions of such MoAb on DR and DQ, and (c) MoAb raised against mouse class II molecules have complex patterns of cross-reaction on human class II molecules, which does not correlate well with the intraspecies class II homology determined by sequence analysis (e.g., anti-I-A does not react exclusively on its structural homologue, DC) [63]. Transfection is another tool of somatic cell genetics which promises to provide definitive evidence regarding binding of particular MoAb to products of defined genes. There are already two studies of MoAb binding to cells transfected with DP genes [48, 65]. The binding of a MoAb like B7/21 to the transfected lines confirms expectations in both directions: that the MoAb is DP-specific, and that the transfected genes are DP.

Other Approaches

Three other approaches deserve mention:

1. Immunochemical approaches cannot, by themselves, assign specificity of a MoAb to DP. However, recent collaborative studies of B7/21 have, by exclusion of its reactivity with DR and DQ, strengthened the inference of its reactivity with DP [66].

2. Differences in tissue distribution have been useful for distinguishing DR- and DQ-reactive antibodies, but lack of known differences between the tissue distribution of DR and DP has precluded similar approaches for DP [67].

3. Once the DP specificity of a MoAb has been established (e.g., B7/21 or ILR1), that MoAb can be used for cross-blocking or lyso-stripping to help establish the DP specificity of other antibodies (G. Nunez and P. Stastny, personal communication).

Individual Anibodies of Interest

Alloantisera

Many laboratories involved in serotyping have been attempting to identify alloantisera which detect DP. However, only two studies [57, 58] have documented alloantisera with specificity for determinants highly associated with DP (see Detection with Antisera, p. 100), for unexpected findings on tissue distribution). Although DP is expressed at lower levels than DR, it is not clear whether this alone is enough to explain the great difficulty in identifying DP-specific sera.

B7/21 (FA)

The MoAb which promises to be most useful in future studies of DP is one generated (and generously distributed) by I. Trowbridge called B7/21. It has also been referred to as "FA" by Bach and coworkers in their extensive studies of this antibody. B7/21 is so useful not because it binds DP, but because it binds so *exclusively* to DP. Watson [60, 62] demonstrated that this antibody selectively immunoprecipitates a class II molecule distinct from DR and DQ (see Biochemical Characterization, p. 96); that selectivity has been confirmed in an extensive collaborative study [66]. That this new molecule is the DP product recognized by T cells had been strongly suggested by findings that (a) B7/21 is a potent inhibitor of DP-specific CTL responses [28, 30], (b) structural polymorphism of the molecule immunoprecipitated by B7/21 correlates well (although not exactly) with DP alleles [59], and 3) B7/21 continues to bind to mutant cell lines which have lost DR and DQ but retain expression of DP [62]. We are now using this antibody extensively in our laboratory and expect it to be central to studies of DP in many laboratories in the near future.

ILR1

ILR1, like B7/21 was shown to bind to a new subset of class II molecules: first by sequential immunoprecipitation [68], and subsequently by amino acid sequencing [69]. Its specificity for DP was indicated by (a) its ability to inhibit DP-specific T cell responses, (b) population studies correlating its binding with DP alleles present on the target cells, and (c) its binding to HLA deletion mutants which have lost DR and DQ but not DP [52]. However, analyses of its pattern of binding in population studies [52] and amino acid sequencing of the precipitate (C. Hurley, personal communication) show that in addition to some alleles of DP (at least DPw2 and DPw3), it also binds to DR5. The reacticity with only some DP alleles and the cross-reactivity with DR5, together with poor performance in complement fixation and as an immunoprecipitating antibody, make it not ideal. However, when used carefully, as for example in studies of tissue distribution [70, 71], it is a useful reagent.

Other MoAb Which Bind DP

We know of no other DP-specific MoAb. However, many include DP binding in their reactivities [63]. Tu39 is one in which DP binding is prominent [59, 63] and which is particularly potent as an inhibitor of DP-specific T cell function [51]. Of the broad anti class II MoAb which we have tested, three – DA6.121, DA6.231, and IVA 12 – are potent inhibitors of DP-specific CTL directed at *all* of the five DP alleles we have tested [53].

MHM4

Some findings suggest that MHM4 might bind DP: this MoAb immunoprecipitates a class II-like molecule distinct from DR and DQ [72] and it binds to HLA deletion mutant cell lines which have lost DR and DQ [63]. However, it is also retained by an HLA deletion mutant cell line [73] which has lost the DP $\alpha1$ and $\beta1$ genes (R. DeMars, unpublished observations) and the expression of DP (by cellular analysis and studies of B7/21 and ILRI binding). It also does not inhibit DP-specific responses, and indeed, appears to enhance them [53]. This has convinced us that MHM4 binds to a molecule distinct from the "classic" DP molecule bound by B7/21. There are conflicting results as to whether it binds to the products of cell lines transfected with DP$\alpha1$, $\beta1$, and $\alpha2$ [48, 65]. If DP$\alpha2$ and $\beta2$ are pseudogenes (see Expression, p. 98), it is hard to explain the MHM4-binding protein as a DP region product.

Classical Genetics

Defined Alleles

The HLA-DP designation [1] was accepted for six antigens thought to be alleles of a single locus (where locus is used in the broad sense of at least two genes, α and β). Five of these antigens were identified in the original description of "SB" [2, 16] and a sixth was described subsequently [18]. One additional allele (Cp63) has been clearly identified by three T cell clones with similar reactivity [29], and another one has been suggested by studies with bulk T cell populations [74]. Most of the available data support the conclusion that all these antigens are allotypic markers on a single molecule: (a) the distribution of DP phenotypes fits Hardy-Weinberg equilibrium [e.g., 16]; (b) no cell has been convincingly demonstrated to express three DP "alleles" [19]; (c) no haplotypes have been convincingly demonstrated to encode more than one DP product [17, 75]. However, such studies always have difficulty distinguishing between alleles and pseudoalleles; therefore, it cannot be completely excluded that some of these antigens are encoded by another gene (i.e., not DPα or β) whose alleles are in strong linkage disequilibrium with alleles of DP.

Complexities

Two types of complexity have been observed in population studies. First, there is heterogeneity within some of the DP antigens, particularly when analysis is performed with T cell clones. Little heterogeneity has been observed for DPw1, w2, w3, w5 [11, 27, 31], (although one laboratory has observed possible heterogeneity within DPw1 [76]. DPw4 is notorious for its complexity both as detected by T cells [16, 26] and by MoAb [77]. On the basis of such data it has been postulated that the complexity within the DP region (presumably the number of expressed genes) may be as great as that within DR [76]. We find the alternate hypothesis equally plausible: it postulates that only DPα1/β1 are expressed, and that complexities in the phenotyping of the DP antigens reflect (a) the existence of more than one polymorphic epitope on individual DP molecules (at least one of which may vary between donors assigned a particular DP specificity), (b) complementation of DP genes on opposite haplotypes [78], and (c) perhaps even complementation of DP α and β chains with DR or DQ α and β chains.

Second, new antigenic determinants have been described which have been proposed to be related to DP [30, 79]. Although it is possible that they are on a product encoded by the DPα2/β2 (postulated by others to be pseudogenes; see Expression, p. 98), we favor the possibility that they relate to yet another class II gene product distinct from DP. The inference that they were related to DP was based on two lines of reasoning: (a) lack of relation to DR and DQ, and (b) inhibition of the response by MbAb Tu39, which is known to bind to DP and inhibit DP-specific responses. However, we find this insufficient to implicate DP molecules, since Tu39 binds to a wide spectrum of class II molecules. Furthermore, these new determinants were found not to be highly associated with DP in population studies [30, 79].

Ethnic Variation

Population studies of DP have been reported in a variety of Caucasian populations [16, 19, 21, 22, 25, 29, 39] and in Japanese [29, 80]. The results demonstrate that there is good general agreement among the seven studies of different Caucasian subgroups. The estimated gene frequency (gf) for DPw1 varies from 5% to 12% (except 2% in Israelis); for DPw2 from 11% to 18% (except 7% in the Workshop study); for DPw3 from 8% to 13%; for DPw4 from 35% to 50% (except 23% in southern France); and for DPw5 from 0% to 2% (except 6% in the midwestern USA). Limited studies with DPw6 and Cp63 [29] suggest that they are present on only 2% and 4% respectively of Caucasian haplotypes. The method for estimating gene frequency of blanks is the least direct, and the results vary widely between studies, from 15% to 43%.

There are marked variations between the frequency distributions of DP antigens among Caucasians and Japanese [29, 80]. The most frequent allele in Japanese, DPw5, (gf about 30%) is the least frequent among Caucasians (gf about 1%)!. The DPw4 antigen is much more frequent among Caucasians (gf about

40%) than among Japanese (gf about 10%). Unpublished studies by R. Hartzman and by H. Festenstein and their respective coworkers suggest that DPw 4 is also much less frequent among Negroes. Thus, DP polymorphism resembles that of other HLA loci in the extensive differences in allele frequency between different racial subgroups.

Linkage Disequilibrium

The lack of strong linkage disequilibrium between DP and DR/DQ contrasts with the extraordinarily strong linkage disequilibrium found between DR and DQ. The only DP and DR alleles which have been observed to be in linkage disequilibrium (in more than one study) are DR3 and DPw1[16, 21, 22, 35]. The strength of the association between these two alleles is of the same order of magnitude as that between B8 and DR3. It is noteworthy that this association is part of an extended HLA haplotype A1-B8-DR3-DPw1-SC01 (note: SC01 is a shorthand for the alleles of the complement genes found on this haplotype) and that there is reported to be an association of DPw4 with the extended haplotype A26-Bw38-Dw10-DR4-SC21 [35]. The lack of strong linkage disequilibrium between DR/DQ and DP is consistent with the following possibilities: (a) the DP region is located quite some distance centromeric to the DR/DQ region; (b) there is a "hot spot" of recombination between DR/DQ and DP which disrupts linkage disequilibrium; or (c) genetic regulatory mechanisms which contribute to linkage disequilibrium within the rest of HLA may not include the DP region.

Mapping

DP has been mapped between GLO and DR/DQ by analysis of (a) HLA deletion mutant cell lines [24], and (b) HLA recombinant haplotypes in families. Data have been published on four DR/DP recombinant haplotypes clearly identified in family studies [77, 23, 82]. But we have also been informed of the probable identification of three additional recombinant haplotypes by R. Hartzman, M. Pollack, J. Hansen, and their respective coworkers, and another four potential recombinants have been identified by studies in the Ninth International Histocompatibility Workshop [75]. Unfortunately, since the data were not collected for this purpose, accurate estimates cannot be made about the frequency of recombination between DP and DR/DQ from the recombinant haplotypes described above, since (a) the selection of families was biased to include ones expected to have recombination within the class II region, and (b) for the families studied, the number of recombinants is a minimal estimate because some recombinations would not be observed due to shared alleles or blanks at the marker loci (the distribution of markers for DP suggest about half would be missed). As a working hypothesis, we continue to estimate that the recombination frequency between DR and DP is 1%–2%. One complementary approach for estimation of recombination frequency has been the study of cells presumed to be genetically homozygous for HLA because of (a) descent from a marriage of first cousins, and (b) homozygosity for HLA-A, B, C, D, DR. The finding that three of 19 such cells were heterozygous for DP favors the interpretation of a significant recombination frequency between DR and DP, perhaps as high as 3.3% (see detailed discussion in [83]).

Disease Association

From a theoretical viewpoint, DP is an attractive candidate for studies of HLA and disease association: (a) it is a highly polymorphic marker and therefore potentially informative; (b) because there is weak linkage disequilibrium between DR and DP, typing for DP provides information on a new subregion of HLA. However, DP typing is technically more demanding than serotyping, and reagents are less available. Largely as a result of such technical limitations, there are only a few published studies on DP and disease association. The most intriguing results come from Hoffman and coworkers, who observed an increase in DPw2 (67% vs 32% in controls) in pauciarticular juvenile rheumatoid arthritis (JRA) with iridocyclitis [84]. This finding is particularly interesting because the increase in DPw2 does not appear to be explained by its linkage disequilibrium with DRw5, which is known to be associated with the disease. The only other statistically significant alteration of DP antigen frequency was found in a study of patients with dermatitis herpetiformis [85]. There was a significant elevation in the frequency of DPw1 (42% vs 11% in controls), along with a trend of increased DPw3 and decreased DPw2. The increase in DPw1 is largely (but perhaps not completely) explained by the known linkage disequilibrium between DPw1 and DR3 (which is known to be markedly increased in patients with dermatitis herpetiformis).

Essentially negative findings have emerged from published and unpublished studies in four other diseases. De Jongh and coworkers found no marked difference between patients with insulin dependent diabetes and healthy controls in their distribution of DP antigens [86]. These data indicate that DP is a useful marker of different DR3 haplotypes: DPw1 is apparently present on many of the DR3 haplotypes which confer risk for dermatitis herpitiformis, but on few of the DR3 haplotypes involved in diabetes.

Moen and coworkers' study of multiple sclerosis (MS) failed to find statistically significant alterations in DP antigen frequency but showed a trend of decreased DPw1 and increased DPw4 [87]. This increase in DPw4 was explained by linkage disequilibrium between DPw4 and DR2 (which was associated with MS in this and other studies). Our studies of MS patients also showed no striking shift in DP antigen distribution (H. McFarland and S. Shaw, unpublished observations). Limited studies of patients with systemic lupus erythematosis (J. Balow and S. Shaw, unpublished observations), rheumatoid arthritis, and myasthenia gravis (G. Pawelec and P. Wernet, unpublished observations) have also failed to detect any strong associations with DP antigens.

The diseases studied have all been ones with known strong association with DR alleles. With the probable exception of the study of pauciarticular JRA, associations with DP appear to be largely secondary to linkage disequilibrium between DP and the DR allele of interest. This suggests either that DP does not have strong association with many diseases, or that the DP-associated diseases will generally be ones not already known to be DR-associated.

Protein Structure

There is relatively little information on the biochemical characterization of the DP α and β polypeptides, largely because (a) the amount of DP expressed on the cell surface is much lower than the amount of DR, (b) until recently there were no DP-specific MoAb generally available, and (c) the DP polypeptides are difficult to identify on two-dimensional gels because the α chain often labels poorly with ^{125}I and the β chain focuses poorly on IEF. In general, however, their characteristics are similar to those of other class II molecules [88].

Amino Acid Sequencing

Hurley and coworkers [69] are the only group to have reported amino acid sequence data on DP molecules. They found that both the α and β chains from the molecule immunoprecipitated by the "DP-specific" MoAb ILR1 (see p. 91) differed in partial N-terminal amino acid sequences of the DR α (mismatch at 2/6 residues) and β (mismatch at 8/10 residues) chains immunoprecipitated from the same cell line.

Biochemical Characterization

Watson, Bach, and coworkers [59, 60, 62, 89] identified class II-like molecule distinct from DR and DQ which was specifically immunoprecipitated by MoAb B7/21, and dubbed both the antigen and MoAb "FA". It is now evident that B7/21 is the only widely available MoAb which is specific for DP (see p. 91) and that FA is probably DP [66]. Studies with FA demonstrated three peculiar characteristics: (a) The α chain is not labeled with ^{125}I, but is demonstrable with ^{35}S-methionine metabolic labeling. Crumpton's description of collaborative studies conducted in the Ninth International Histocompatibility Workshop [66] confirms the difficulties in surface-labeling the DPα chain with ^{125}I, but this has not been found in all laboratories (R. Knowles, personal communication). (b) There are differences in the molecular weight of DPβ (25 kd vs 27 kd) between different alleles [62]. This difference might result from variability in the number of N-linked carbohydrate moieties, particularly since the DP β gene has a second potential site for glycosylation. Alternatively, this could be due to a difference in mRNA splicing which might result from an alternate splice site found in DPβ (see Features which Distinguish DP from DR/DQ, p. 97). (c) It is difficult to focus the DP β chain by IEF. However, when the β chain is cleaved by chymotrypsin into 16-kd (N-terminal) and 13-kd (C-terminal) fragments, the N-terminal fragment can be focused readily and polymorphism in isoelectric point is observed which generally (but not always) correlates with cellular typing for DP [59].

An additional complexity has been observed in the DP molecule. In a two-dimensional gel electrophoretic analysis of molecules immunoprecipitated by B7/21 from a DPw2-homozygous cell line (derived from consanguinous mating), Crumpton et al. [66] report two β spots with the same molecular weight but a small difference in charge. Since these spots persists following neuraminadase treatment, Crumpton et al. inferred that they might be products of two separate genes. However, molecular genetic studies indicate that one of the two DP β genes is a pseudogene (see Expression, p. 98). Heterogeneity of iodination is one technical problem which could explain charge variation in a single gene product labeled with ^{125}I.

Molecular Genetics

Molecular genetic approaches have rapidly provided insights into the diversity and complexity of the human class II molecules in general, and of DP in particular. Since the molecular genetics of class II is covered in detail elsewhere in this volume (P. A. Peterson and L. Rask, T. Collins et al., H. Kratzin et al., R. Sorrentino and G. Corte) the following is a simplified summary for DP. We start with the assumption that the genes designated "DP" encode the product which stimulates DP-specific T cells, but return to address that question later (correlation of DP Gene Products with DP Function, pp. 98).

Genomic Organization of the DP Region

Two α and two β genes have been identified in the DP region, occurring in the order DPα1, DPβ1, DPα2, DPβ2 [65, 90, 91] (Terminology is potentially confusing, since these genes are still referred to as SB instead of DP, and because some investigators use "SXα" to refer to DPα2 and "SXβ" for DPβ2.) Gene order has been fully established for DP but not DR or DQ, apparently because the DP genes are spaced close to each other: the four DP genes are contained within a 70-kb region (which has been isolated in overlapping clones from three different haplotypes [65, 91]). The orientation of this region has been established to be DPα1/β1 closest to DR, and DPα2/β2 closest to GLO, on the basis of hybridization studies mapping deletions in mutant LCL [73]. The DP region has not yet been linked by overlapping cosmids to the DR or DQ regions; it remains to be seen whether there is an extended region of DNA which separates them or whether the relatively high recombination frequency between DP and DR/DQ reflects a hot spot of recombination similar to that observed in the murine Ia region [88]. The DP α and β genes are oriented in opposite polarities in a "head-to-head" manner which could allow coordinate regulation of α and β from a central promoter [92]. This orientation has not been found in any of the other class II α/β genes studied: I-A, I-E, DQ (both DC and DX) [65].

Features Which Distinguish DP from DR/DQ

The exon/intron organization of the DP α and β genes is similar to the other class II genes [93]. However, there are at least three features which, at present, distinguish DP products. First, there is an alternate splice site near 3′ end of the DP β1 gene which, in theory, would allow the production of two alternate forms of the β chain which differ by ten amino acids in their cytoplasmic tail [94, 95]. Second, the DPβ1 gene has apparently undergone a six-nucleotide deletion at the beginning of the first domain [95]. Third, the DPβ1 sequence has a second potential glycosylation site (not present in DRβ or DQβ) at the beginning of the second domain [95].

Polymorphism

DP α and β genes are both polymorphic. Comparison of the two available DPα1 cDNA sequences show variations in three of 120 amino acids compared, most of which map in the first protein domain [96]. This degree of DP α gene polymorphism is greater than that for DRα but less than that for DQα1 [66]. The DP β1 gene has more extensive polymorphism than the DP α1 gene, but less than that for DRβ and DQβ [95]. Comparisons of six different DPβ1 DNA sequences from four different DP alleles show that the amino acid polymorphism is predominantly in the first domain [65, 95]. There are nucleotide variations elsewhere, but most of these are silent changes (i.e., which have not changed the amino acid at that position). This difference between the first domain and the rest of the molecule suggests that there has been an evolutionary selective pressure *for* allelic variation in the first domain (possibly for interaction with variable regions on the T cell receptor and a diversity of environmental antigens) and *against* variation in the rest of the molecule (possibly for conserving sites of interaction with other T cell structures, such as perhaps T4 [42]).

Restriction fragment length polymorphisms (RFLP) have been found in the DP region, in some cases associated with DP alleles [65, 96, 97]. More RFLP have been identified in the DP "pseudogenes" (α2 and β2) than in the expressed genes (α1 and β1) [65]. However, such differences are not necessarily useful in making functional interpretations, because (a) many RFLP do not affect the expressed protein, and (b) RFLP are sometimes hard to find in areas of substantial amino acid polymorphism, like exon 1 of DPβ1 [65].

Expression

Are the DP genes expressed? The DPα1 and DPβ1 genes are expressed; the DPα2 and DPβ2 genes probably are not. The evidence is as follows:

1. cDNA clone isolation: clones have been repeatedly isolated for α1 and β1, but not for α2 and β2 [95–99].
2. Genomic sequence: the nucleotide sequences for α1 and β1 are consistent with normal expression, while the nucleotide sequences for both α2 [65, 91] and β2 [65, 95] are apparently inconsistent with expression in the lines studied.
3. Northern analysis: there are no published studies which analyze expression of DP mRNA with probes which would discriminate α1 from α2 and β1 from β2. However, E. Long and coworkers failed to find expression of β2 using a probe specific for β2 (personal communication).
4. Transfection: the DPβ2 gene is not necessary for DP expression, since human class II molecules were detected by DP-reactive MoAb at the cell surface of mouse L cells [48] or a macrophage cell line [65] which had been transfected with two different cosmids containing DPα1, β1, and α2.

Are there functional DP genes on all haplotypes? DP products have been defined by cellular typing on about 70% of Caucasian haplotypes (see Ethnic Variations, p. 93). In two donor combinations where allosensitization was attempted against a DP "blank" haplotype, two new DP alleles have been detected (see Defined Alleles, p. 92). It remains to be determined whether any of the remaining blanks could represent haplotypes with no expressed DP product.

Correlation of DP Gene Products with DP Function

Are the products of the DP genes identical to those that are recognized by DP-specific T cells? Almost undoubtedly yes. There are some studies relating molecular genetic studies and cellular recognition directly, and some in which they are related by intermediate reagents: MoAb. Among the former are the following:

1. A DP-restricted influenza virus-specific T cell clone was stimulated by the DP transfectant mentioned above [48]; controls indicated that the stimulation was dependent on DP-transfection and antigen-specific. This would appear to be the most direct possible proof of the relationship between DP genes and DP-specific T cell responses. However, studies with DP-specific CTL clones have failed to demonstrate recognition of the same lines (M. Sanchez-Perez and P. Austin, unpublished observations). This failure may relate to a postulated requirement for other human molecules on the target cell for such CTL recognition [100]. But it is possible that the DP-allospecific T cells and the influenza-specific DP-restricted T cells recognize distinct but related gene products.

2. RFLP of genomic DNA probed with DPα [96] and DPβ [97] probes correlates in populations with DP alleles and not with other class II specificities.

3. RFLP of genomic DNA probed with DPβ segregates with DP alleles in two DP/DR recombinant families [77, 97].

4. There is a correlation between loss of DP genes in mutant LCL and their loss of expression of DP products recognized by T cells [73].

Evidence via intermediate reagents, MoAbs, includes (a) identity between amino acid residues predicted from DNA sequences and those found in the limited N-terminal sequence of α and β chains from a "DP" molecule precipitated by the MoAb ILR1 [69], and (b) expression of molecules on DP-transfected cells which are bound by MoAb which bind DP, but not by four class II-specific MoAb which fail to bind DP [48, 65] (except for MHM4; see p. 92).

Surface Expression and Tissue Distribution

Although there are many studies of class II antigen expression on cells from different tissues, there is little reliable information on expression of DP. There have been technical limitations in the three approaches used to assess expression: (a) cellular typing is not well suited to studies in situ or to studies of many different types of cells; (b) DP locus-specific antibodies have not been widely available (see Antibodies which Relate to DP, p. 89). (c) Northern blotting for mRNA expression required the development of probes which are exquisitely specific for individual genes.

Cellular Recognition

The initial inference that DP was a "B cell" antigen was based on the observation that DP-specific CTL were able to kill LCL well, but killed phytohemagglutinin-induced lymphoblasts (largely T cells) rather poorly [2]. Limited studies of lysis of target cell populations enriched for subpopulations of PBML demonstrated better lysis of B cells and macrophages than T cells, but the experiments were technically imperfect (unpublished observations). Analysis of hybridization between resting T cells and B cell lines demonstrate that the DP genes of the T cells can be expressed in such hybrids [101]. Studies by Pawelec et al. [102] indicated that activated T cells expressed DP, since DP-specific CTL were able to lyse T cells which had been activated and propagated in IL-2. However these studies suggested that the expression of DP an activated T cells might not be sufficient to trigger DP-specific proliferation (when they are used as stimulator cells). Pollack and coworkers [103] demonstrated that melanoma cells generally expressed DP (as well as DR) antigens, since they were able to stimulate DP-specific responses.

Serologic Detection

Detection with Antisera

Van Leeuwen and coworkers [57] described several alloantisera which identified DPw4-associated determinants. These antisera were cytotoxic to macrophages from DPw4-positive donors, but failed to consistently lyse their peripheral blood B cells [57]. Results of typing on LCL were inconsistent (personal communication). This apparent difference in tissue distribution could be artifactual (reflecting, for example, greater resistance of the B cells to the action of the antibody and complement), or could indicate that this serologically defined product is distinct from DP (although in linkage disequilibrium with it). Johnson and colleagues identified a DPw1-associated specificity on peripheral blood B cells with an alloantisera [58]. One unique finding was the loss of serologically detectable expression of this antigen (but not DR) from B cells stored for 2 days at room temperature.

Detection with MoAb

Studies with ILR1 (which is largely DP-specific but has occasional cross-reactions or DR; see p. 91) confirmed that DP was expressed on peripheral blood B cells and monocytes, but not resting T cells [70, 104]. DP is also not expressed on unstimulated endothelial cells [70]. Linch et al. [71] detected ILR1 binding on both granulocyte/monocyte and erythroid progenitor cells. Steele and coworkers [105–107] have extensively studied the patterns of reactivity of a MoAb with broad anti-class II binding (DA6.231, which binds DP as well as DR) and a DR-specific MoAb (DA6.164). They have made inferences regarding DP expression from differences in binding of these two antibodies; we believe that such inferences must be interpreted very cautiously. B7/21 promises to be a much more useful DP-specific reagent (see p. 91), but studies of tissue distribution have not yet been published with this antibody.

How much DP is expressed on cell surfaces? Our studies indicate that the expression of DP on LCL is about 10%–30% of that of DR. There are data from two approaches in which an antibody serves as its own control. First, binding of ILR1 to DPw2- or DPw3-positive lines is only 20% on average of its binding to cells via its cross-reaction on DR5 (S. Shaw and C. Hurley, unpublished observations). Second, binding of broad anti-class II antibodies to mutant LCL expressing only DPw2 is about 10%–25% of that to the parental line expressing DR (and DQ). Studies of antibody binding to T cell clones have not been done with the same rigorous internal controls, but comparisons between binding of SG171 (broad anti-class II) and B7/21 (DP only) suggest that DP is well expressed but that it represents perhaps 15% of total class II (unpublished observations).

Detection of mRNA

Quantitation of mRNA expression by Northern blot analysis using class II locus-specific probes can help solve the technical problems of DP detection. Collins et al. [108) have exploited this technology to demonstrate that endothelial cells and dermal fibroblasts do not have detectable levels of mRNA for DP (DR, DQ, or invariant chain) in the resting state. However, they can be induced to transcribe each of these mRNAs by treatment with gamma-interferon.

Summary

Thus, the expression of DP is qualitatively indistinguishable from that of DR, although expression of both may not always correlate with expression of DQ. Quantitatively, DP is expressed at lower levels than DR, and may be lost more easily by B cells during in vitro culture.

Evolutionary Considerations

It was postulated on the basis of very limited N-terminal amino acid sequencing that DP is more similar to DR [69]. And class II-specific MoAb cross-reactions more frequently include DP and DR than DP and DQ [63]. However, comparisons between the available sequences of DP, DR, and DQ indicate that they are "equidistant" from each other [95, 109, 110]. Thus, structural comparisons suggest that DP is not derived from either DR or DC by recent gene duplication.

Comparisons between murine and human class II molecules, first by DNA hybridization and later by nucleotide sequencing, demonstrated unequivocal preferential homology of DR to I-E and DC to I-A, but failed to find a homologue of DP [88, 95]. In addition, I-A and DC α chains are both polymorphic, but DR and I-E α chains are essentially nonpolymorphic [93]. Is there a DP equivalent in the mouse? A murine pseudogene I-Eβ2 became a candidate for the DPβ homologue on the basis of its preferential cross-hybridization with DPβ probes [110]; however, this conclusion has not been supported by subsequent comparisons of nucleotide sequence [111]. The isolation and partial sequencing of a new murine β gene "IAβ3" appears to resolve the issue [112]. The homology between the nucleotide sequences in the second exons of this gene and DPβ is as high (83%) as the homology found between the same exons of I-A vs DQ and I-E vs DR. Southern blot hybridization studies suggest that this gene is present in all of the six haplotypes tested, but the structure of the gene suggests that it cannot be expressed as a functional product in either of the two haplotypes analyzed in detail. This gene, like DP in man, is the most centromeric class II gene in the murine MHC. It remains to be determined whether there is an α chain gene in the mouse which is homologous to DPα. If so, one might expect it to be oriented head-to-head with IAβ3.

Conclusions

We find no basis in the foregoing data for far-reaching conclusions regarding functional differences between DP and other human class II molecules. On the contrary, we are impressed that in most respects DP behaves in a qualitatively similar way to DR. Perhaps the only strong evidence for qualitative differences among class II molecules relates to distinct patterns of tissue distribution for DQ compared with DP/DQ. Quantitatively, however, it appears that T cell and antibody responses to DP are lower in magnitude than responses to DR and perhaps DQ. The overall amount of DP expressed per cell is clearly lower than that of DR and probably DQ. Polymorphism of DP is somewhat less than for DR and DQ. So far, disease association with DP alleles is less striking than with DQ/DR.

If DP molecules play the same functional role as DR and DQ molecules, and do so apparently in a less striking manner, why has DP expression been preserved in most (or perhaps all) HLA haplotypes? We suspect that retention of DP relates to the selective advantage of having a diverse ensemble of class II molecules present on cell surfaces to facilitate T cell interactions for the recognition of foreign antigen. Diversity is created by the combined effects of: (a) expression of multiple families of class II molecules; (b) polymorphism of α and β genes in the population (which results in heterozygosity of most individuals); (c) codominant expression; and (d) α/β complementation for each locus (and potentially among loci). On the other hand, we are inclined to believe that each subregion product will have some unique functional properties; however, if this is true, it remains to be shown what these are for DP.

Acknowledgments. We thank Drs. F. Bach, R. DeMars, H. Festenstein, R. Hartzman, A. Johnson, E. Long, J. Lee, Y. Matsui, G. Pawelec, P. Peterson, M. Pollack, J. Strominger, K. Tsuji, and G. Widera for providing data before its publication. We thank Drs. W. Biddison, E. Long, J. Lunney, and R. Hoffman for careful review of this manuscript.

References

1. Bodmer WF, Albert E, Bodmer JG, Dausset J, Kissmeyer-Nielsen F, Payne R, Van Rood JJ, Trnka Z, Walford RL (1984) Nomenclature for factors of the HLA system 1984. Hum Immunol 11:117–125
2. Shaw S, Johnson AH, Shearer GM (1980) Evidence for a new segregant series of B cell antigens that are encoded in the HLA-D region and that stimulate secondary allogeneic proliferative and cytotoxic responses. J Exp Med 152:565–580
3. Termijtelen A, Van Leeuwen A, Van Rood JJ (1982) HLA-linked lymphocyte activating determinants. Immunol Rev 66:79–101
4. Mawas C, Charmot D, Mercier P (1980) Split of HLA-D into two regions alpha and beta by a recombination between HLA-D and GLO. I. Study in a family and primed lymphocyte typing for determinants coded by the beta region. Tissue Antigens 15:458–466
5. Mawas C, Charmot D, Sivy M, Mercier P, North ML, Hauptmann G (1978) A weak human MLR locus mapping at the right of a crossing over between HLA-D, Bf, and GLO. J Immunogenet 5:583–595
6. Charmot D, Mawas C, Kristensen T, Mercier P (1981) The HLA-D system: at least two loci and four distinct phenotypic traits per haplotype. Introduction to component typing in families and population by primed lymphocyte typing. Immunogenetics 13:57–84

7. Wank R, Schendel DL, Blanco ME, Dupont B (1979) Secondary MLC responses of primed lymphocytes after selective sensitization to non-HLA-D determinants. Scand J Immunol 9:499–505
8. Zier KS, Gross-Wilde H, Huber C, Braunsteiner H, Albert ED (1978) Restimulation in secondary MLC by a non-D-locus determinant within the MHC. Immunogenetics 6:459–369
9. Sasportes M, Nunez-Roldan A, Fradelizi D (1978) Analysis of products involved in primary and secondary allogeneic proliferation in man. III. Further evidence for products different from Ia-like, DRw antigens, activating secondary allogeneic proliferation in man. Immunogenetics 6:55–68
10. Wank R, Schendel DJ, Hansen JA, Dupont B (1978) The lymphocyte restimulation system: evaluation by intra-HLA-D group priming. Immunogenetics 6:107–115
11. Bach FH, Reinsmoen N (1982) Cloned cellular reagents to define antigens encoded between HLA-DR and glyoxylase. Hum Immunol 5:133–138
12. Termijtelen A, Bradley BA, Van Rood JJ (1980) A new determinant, defined by PLT, coded for in the HLA region and apparently independent of the HLA-D and DR loci. Tissue Antigens 15:267–274
13. Termijtelen A, Van Rood JJ (1981) The role in primary MLC of the non HLA-D/DR determinant PL3A. Tissue Antigens 17:57–63
14. Termijtelen A, Shaw S, Van Rood JJ (1983) Identity of PL3A and SB1. Tissue Antigens 21:400–401
15. Benacerraf B (1981) Role of MHC gene products in immune regulation. Science 212:1229–1238
16. Shaw S, Duquesnoy RJ, Smith PL (1981) Population studies of the HLA-linked SB antigens. Immunogenetics 14:153–162
17. Shaw S, Pollack MS, Payne SM, Johnson AH (1980) HLA-linked B cell alloantigens of a new segregant series: population and family studies of the SB antigens. Hum Immunol 1:177–185
18. Robbins FM, Hartzman RJ, Phillips E (1985) A new allele of DP: DPw6. Hum Immunol (submitted)
19. Wank R, Schendel DJ (1984) Genetic analysis of HLA-D region products defined by PLT. In: Albert ED, Baur MP, Mayr WR (eds) Histocompatibility testing 1984. Springer, Berlin Heidelberg New York Tokyo, pp 289–299
20. Hartzman RJ, Shaw S, Robbins FM (1984) Origin and expansion of SB-specific reagents characterized in the Ninth International Workshop. In: Albert ED, Baur MP, Mayr WR (eds) Histocompatibility testing 1984. Springer, Berlin Heidelberg New York Tokyo, pp 303–305
21. Bourgue F, Charmot D, Mercier P, Tongio MM, Shaw S, Mawas C (1982) HLA-SB in the south of France. Correlation between locally derived and reference typing reagents. Tissue Antigens 20:254–259
22. Cohen N, Shaw S, Amar A, Oksenberg J, Brautbar C (1984) HLA-linked SB antigens in Israel: Population study, analysis of homozygous typing cells and generation of local SB reagents. Tissue Antigens 24:1113–120
23. Morling N, Hartzman RJ, Jakobsen BK, Oedum N, Platz P, Ryder LP, Shaw S, Svegaard A (1984) Typing for DP-like determinants. In: Albert ED, Baur MP, Mayr WR (eds) Histocompatibility testing 1984. Springer, Berlin Heidelberg New York Tokyo, p 469
24. Kavathas P, DeMars R, Bach FH, Shaw S (1981) SB: A new HLA-linked human histocompatibility gene defined using HLA-mutant cell lines. Nature 293:747–749
25. Moen T, Bratlie A, Kiss E, Bruserud O, Thorsby E (1983) Identification of four SB antigens by cloned cells. Population studies of Norwegians. Tissue Antigens 22:298–309
26. Pawelec G, Shaw S, Wernet P (1982) Analysis of the HLA-linked SB gene system with cloned and uncloned alloreactive T-cell lines. Immunogenetics 15:187–198
27. Pawelec G, Shaw S, Schneider M, Rehbein A, Wernet P (1983) Homogeneity of the HLA-linked SB2 and SB3 specificities demonstrated by cloned alloreactive T-cells. Immunogenetics 17:179–188
28. Ohta N, Reinsmoen NL, Bach FH (1984) Cellular basis of the anti-SB response. Hum Immunol 11:127–141

29. Nose Y, Nakatsuji T, Tsuji K, Reinsmoen NL (1985) A new HLA-DP(SB) specificity (Cp63) defined in Japanese and Caucasian cell populations by cloned PLT cells. 13:145–149
30. Ohta N, Bach FH (1985) An HLA-DP region encoded determinant not associated with the DPw segregant series. (in preparation)
31. Biddison WE, Shaw S (1984) SB-specific CTL clones exhibit functional heterogeneity in their susceptibility to blocking by anti-T3 and anti-T4 antibodies. In: Feldman M (ed) Human T cell clones: a new approach to immune regulation. Humana, London
32. Bickert K, Morling N, Schendel DJ, Jennert W, Wank R (1984) Median stabilization of PLT data for the central workshop analysis. In: Albert ED, Baur MP, Mayr WR (eds) Histocompatibility testing 1984: Springer, Berlin Heidelberg New York Tokyo, pp 301–302
33. Tekolf WA, Shaw S (1983) In vitro generation of cytotoxic cells specific for human minor histocompatibility antigens by lymphocytes from a normal donor potentially primed during pregnancy. J Exp Med 157:2172–2177
34. Shaw S, O'Neill GJ, Shearer GM (1979) Immunogenetic analysis of an unusual HLA region recombination by intrafamilial MLR, PLT, and CMC. Transplant Proc 11:1804–1808
35. Matsui Y, Alosco SM, Awdeh Z, Duquesnoy RJ, Page PL, Hartzman RJ, Alper CA, Yunis EJ (1985) Linkage disequilibrium of HLA-SB1 with the HLA-A1; B8, DR3, SCO1, and of HLA-SB4 with the HLA-A26, Bw38, Dw10, DR4, SC21 extended haplotypes. Immunogenetics 20:623
36. Bach FH, Anichini A, Reinsmoen N, Groner J, Watson A, Segall M (1983) Genetic and molecular analyses of lymphocyte-defined HLA-D region specificities. Hum Immunol 8:25–32
37. Termijtelen A, Den Berge SN, Suwandii-Thung L, Van Rood JJ (1984) The influence of matching for SB on MLC typing is significant but marginal. Scand J Immunol 19:265–268
38. Wernet P, Shaw S, Brautbar C, Westphal E, Pawelec G (1983) SB types of HLA-D homozygous typing cells. Immunogenetics 18:547–551
39. Pawelec G, Shaw S, Schneider M, Blaurock M, Frauer M, Brackertz D, Wernet P (1982) Population studies of the HLA-linked SB antigens and their relative importance in primary MLC-typing: analysis of HLA-D homozygous typing cells and normal heterozygous populations. Hum Immunol 5:215–223
40. Biddison WE, Rao PE, Talle MA, Goldstein G, Shaw S (1984) Possible involvement of the T4 molecule in T cell recognition of class II HLA antigens: evidence from studies of CTL-target cell binding. J Exp Med 159:783–797
41. Ohta N, Anichini A, Reinsmoen NL, Strassmann G, Wernet P, Bach FH (1985) Analysis of human class II antigens by cloned cytolytic T cell reagents: a study using HLA loss mutant lymphoblastoid cell lines and monoclonal antibodies detecting the HLA-DP product(s). Hum Immunol 13:21–32
42. Biddison WE, Rao PE, Talle MA, Goldstein G, Shaw S (1982) Possible involvement of the OKT4 molecule in T cell recognition of class II HLA antigens: evidence from studies of cytotoxic lymphocytes specific for SB antigens. J Exp Med 156:1065–1076
43. Biddison WE, Rao PE, Talle MA, Goldstein G, Shaw S (1983) Possible involvement of the T4 molecule in T cell recognition of class II HLA antigens: evidence from studies of proliferative responses to SB antigens. J Immunol 131:152–157
44. Biddison WE, Shaw S (1983) Possible involvement of the OKT4 molecule in T-cell recognition of class II HLA antigens. J Diagn Immunol 1:112–115
45. Biddison WE, Shaw S (1984) Antibodies to the T4 (Leu 3) molecule block CTL-target cell binding but do not inhibit the lytic phase of cytotoxicity. In: Sercarz E, Cantor H (eds) Regulation of the immune system. Liss, New York, p 221
46. Shaw S, Goldstein G, Springer TA, Biddison WE (1985) Susceptibility of cytotoxic T lymphocyte (CTL) clones to inhibition by anti-T3 and anti-T4 (but not anti-LFA-1)monoclonal antibodies varies with the avidity of CTL-target interaction. J Immunol 134:3019–3026
47. Eckels DD, Lake P, Lamb Jr, Johnson AH, Shaw S, Woody JN, Hartzman RJ (1983) SB-restricted presentation of influenza and herpes virus antigens to human T-lymphocyte clones. Nature 301:716–718

48. Austin P, Trowsdale J, Rudd C, Bodmer W, Feldmann M, Lamb J (1985) Functional expression of HLA-DP genes transfected into mouse fibroblasts. Nature 313:61
49. Qvigstad E, Moen T, Thorsby E (1984) T-cell clones with similar antigen specificity may be restricted by DR, MT(DC), or SB class II HLA molecules. Immunogenetics 19:455–460
50. Hanke JH, Brown MF, Pollack MS, Rich RR (1985) Class II determinants recognized by TNP-specific cloned human T cell lines. Hum Immunol 14:59–76
51. Pawelec G, Shaw S, Ziegler A, Muller C, Wernet P (1982) Differential inhibition of HLA-D or SB-directed secondary lymphoproliferative responses with monoclonal antibodies detecting human Ia-like determinants. J Immunol 129:1070–1075
52. Shaw S, DeMars R, Schlossman SF, Smith PL, Lampson LA, Nadler LM (1982) Serologic identification of the human secondary B cell (SB) antigens: correlations between function, genetics, and structure. J Exp Med 156:731–741
53. Shaw S, Sanchez-Perez M, DeMars R (1984) Analysis of DP region products by T cells and monoclonal antibodies: blocking of DP-specific proliferation and cell-mediated cytotoxicity. In: Baur MP, Albert ED, Mayr WR (eds) Histocompatibility testing 1984. Springer, Berlin Heidelberg New York Tokyo, pp 465–468
54. Wernet P, Ziegler A, Shaw S, Blaurock M, Pawelec G (1983) Monoclonal antibodies against Ia-like antigens inhibit HLA-D and/or SB-directed secondary proliferative responses. Transplant Proc 15:94–98
55. Accolla RS, Moretta A, Cerottini JC (1981) Allogeneic mixed lymphocyte reactions in humans: Pretreatment of either the stimulator or the responder cell with monoclonal anti-Ia antibodies leads to an inhibition of proliferation. J Immunol 127:2438–2442
56. Ohta N, Reinsmoen NL, Anichini A, Bach FH (1985) Analysis of cytolytic clones directed at class I and class II antigens using HLA loss mutants of a lymphoblastoid cell line. (submitted)
57. Van Leeuwen A, Termijtelen A, Shaw S, Van Rood JJ (1982) The recognition of a polymorphic monocyte antigen in HLA. Nature 298:565–567
58. Johnson AH, Thorsby E, Nakatsuji T, Fang T, Moen T, Hartzman RJ (1985) Recognition of polymorphic HLA-DPw1 alloantiserium raised by planned immunization. Immunogenetics (in press)
59. Linner KM, Bach FH (1984) HLA-FA: a non-DR, non-DQ HLA class II product. In: Baur MP, Albert ED, Mayr WD (eds) Histocompatibility Testing 1984. Springer, Berlin Heidelberg New York Tokyo, pp 538–539
60. Watson AJ, Bach FH (1985) Structural polymorphism of FA: An HLA class II antigen with unusual molecular properties. (submitted)
61. DeMars R, Chang CC, Rudersdorf RA (1983) Dissection of the D-region of the human major histocompatibility complex by means of induced mutations in a lymphoblastoid cell line. Hum Immunol 8:123–139
62. Watson AJ, DeMars R, Trowdrige IS, Bach FH (1983) Detection of a novel human class II HLA antigen. Nature 304:358–361
63. Shaw S, Ziegler A, DeMars R (1985) Specificity of monoclonal antibodies directed against human and murine class II histocompatibility antigens as analyzed by binding to HLA-deletion mutant cell lines. Hum Immunol 12:191–212
64. Shaw S, DeMars R (1984) Binding specificity of anti-human Ia monoclonal antibodies analyzed with HLA-deletion mutant cell lines: patterns of binding to products of two different HLA haplotypes and of three subregions of a single haplotype. Dis Markers 2:183–195
65. Okada K, Prentice HL, Boss JM, Levy DJ, Kappes D, Spies T, Raghupathy R, Mengler RA, Auffray C, Strominger JL (1985) SB subregion of the human major histocompatibility complex: gene organization, allelic polymorphism and expression in transformed cells. EMBO J 3:2985
66. Crumpton MJ, Bodmer JG, Bodmer WF, Heyes JM, Lindsay J, Rudd CE (1984) Biochemistry of class II antigens: workshop report. In: Baur MP, Albert ED, Mayr WR (eds) Histocompatibility testing 1984. Springer, Berlin Heidelberg New York Tokyo, pp 29–37

67. Bodmer J, Kennedy L, Aizawa M, Dawkins R, Lepage V, Mazzilli MC, Richiardi P (1984) HLA-D region monoclonal antibodies. In: Albert ED, Baur MP, Mayr WR (eds) Histocompatibility testing 1984. Springer, Berlin Heidelberg New York Tokyo, pp 217–236
68. Nadler LM, Stashenko P, Hardy R, Tomaselli KJ, Yunis EJ, Schlossman SF, Pesando JM (1981) Monoclonal antibody identifies a new Ia-like (p 29, 34) polymorphic system linked to the HLA-D/DR region. Nature 290:591–593
69. Hurley CK, Shaw S, Nadler L, Schlossman S, Capra JD (1982) The alpha and beta chains of SB and DR antigens are structurally distinct. J Exp Med 156:1557–1562
70. Neppert J, Nunez G, Stastny P (1984) HLA-A, B, C; -DR; -MT, -MB, and SB antigens on unstimulated human endothelial cells. Tissue Antigens 24:40–47
71. Linch DC, Nadler LM, Luther EA, Lipton JM (1984) Discordant expression of human Ia-like antigens on hematopoeitic progenitor cells. J Immunol 132:2324–2329
72. Makgoba MW, Hildreth JEK, McMichael AJ (1983) Identification of a human Ia antigen that is different from HLA-DR and DC antigens. Immunogenetics 17:623–635
73. DeMars R, Chang CC, Shaw S, Reitnauer PJ, Sondel PM (1984) Homozygous deletions that simultaneously eliminate expressions of class I and class II antigens of EBV-transformed B-lymphoblastoid cells. I. Reduced proliferative responses of autologous and allogeneic T cells to mutant cells that have decreased expression of class II antigens. Hum Immunol 11:77–97
74. Pollack MS, Moshief RD, Maurer DH (1985) Evidence for detection of a new allele in the DP(SB) system. Hum Immunol 12:103–103
75. Schendel DJ, Hartzman R, Jaraquamada D, Kristensen T, Morling N, Ollier W, Termijtelen A, Wank R (1984) Segregation analysis of PLT reagents in families. In: Baur MP, Albert ED, Mayr WR (eds) Histocompatibility testing 1984. Springer, Berlin Heidelberg New York Tokyò, pp 300–301
76. Eckels DD, Johnson AH, Hartzman RJ, Dacek D (1985) Quantitative variation in the expression of HLA-DPw1-associated alloantigens: analysis with human T cell clones (abstract). Hum Immunol 12:110–110
77. Robinson MA, Long EO, Johnson AH, Hartzman RJ, Mach B, Kindt TJ (1984) Recombination with the HLA-D region: correlation of molecular genotyping with functional data. J Exp Med 160:222–238
78. Eckels DD, Johnson AH, Hartzman RJ, Dacek D (1985) Clonal analysis of HLA-DPw1-(SB1)-associated allodeterminants: a novel example of transcomplementation? Hum Immunol 12:103–104
79. Pawelec G, Wernet P, Rosenlund R, Blaurock M, Schneider EM (1984) Strong lymphoproliferative suppressive function of PLT clones specific for SB-like antigens. Hum Immunol 9:145–157
80. Nishimura Y, Yasuda N, Sasazuki T, Shaw S (1984) The gene frequency of SB alleles in the Japanese population. Tissue Antigens 23:314–315
81. Shaw S, Kavathas P, Pollack MS, Charmot D, Mawas C (1981) Family studies define a new histocompatibility locus, SB, between HLA-DR and GLO. Nature 293:745–747
82. Termijtelen A, MeraKhan P, Shaw S, Van Rood JJ (1983) Mapping SB in relation to HLA and GLO1 using cells from first cousing marriage offspring. Immunogenetics 18:503–512
83. Hoffman RW, Shaw S, Francis L, Petersen RA, Chylack LT, Glass DN (1985) HLA-DP (SB) antigens in pauciarticular JRA with iridocyclitis (abstract). Arthritis Rheum 28:535
84. Shaw S, Hall RP, Duquesnoy RJ, Katz SI (1981) Interaction between HLA-SB and HLA-DR phenotype in determining the risk of dermatitis herpitiformis. (abstract) Hum Immunol 3:387
85. de Jongh BM, Termijtelen A, Bruining GJ, DeVries RRP, Van Rood JJ (1984) Relation of insulin-dependent diabetes mellitus (IDD) and the HLA-linked SB system. Tissue Antigens 23:87–93
86. Moen T, Stien R, Bratlie A, Bondevik E (1984) Distribution of HLA-SB antigens in multiple sclerosis. Tissue Antigens 24:126–127

87. Kaufman JF, Auffray C, Korman AJ, Shackelford DA, Strominger J (1984) The class II molecules of the human and murine major histocompatibility complex. Cell 36:1–13
88. Bach FH, Groner J, Watson AJ, Reinsmoen N, Segall M (1985) HLA class II molecules: T cell responses and molecular characterization. (submitted)
89. Trowsdale J, Kelly A, Lee J, Carson S, Austin P, Travers P (1984) Linkage map of two HLA-SB beta and two HLA-SB alpha-related genes: an intron in one of the SB beta genes contains a processed pseudogene. Cell 38:241–249
90. Servenius B, Gustafsson K, Widmar E, Emmoth E, Andersson G, Larhammer D, Rask L, Peterson PA (1985) Molecular map of the human HLA-SB region. EMBO J 3:3209
91. Gorski J, Rollini P, Long E, Mach B (1984) Molecular organization of the HLA-SB region of the human major histocompatibility complex and evidence for two SB beta chain genes. Proc Natl Acad Sci USA 81:3934–3938
92. Steinmetz M, Hood L (1983) Genes of the major histocompatibility complex in mouse and man. Science 222:727–733
93. Gustafsson K, Emmoth E, Widmark E, Bohme J, Peterson PA, Rask L (1984) Isolation of a cDNA clone coding for an SB beta chain. Nature 309:76–78
94. Kappes DJ, Arnot D, Okada K, Strominger JL (1984) Structure and polymorphism of the HLA class II SB light chain genes. EMBO J 3:2985–2993
95. Inoko H, Ando A, Kimura M, Ogata S, Tsuji K (1985) Isolation and characterization of the cDNA clones and genomic clones of the HLA-SB antigen heavy chain. (submitted)
96. Roux-Dosseto M, Auffray C, Lillie JW, Boss JM, Cohen D, DeMars R, Mawas C, Seidman JG, Strominger JL (1983) Genetic mapping of a class II antigen beta-chain cDNA clone to the SB region of the HLA complex. Proc Natl Acad Sci USA 80:6063–6040
97. Long EO, Wake CT, Strubin M, Gross N, Accolla RS, Carrel S, Mach B (1982) Isolation of distinct cDNA clones encoding HLA-DR β chains by use of an expression assay. Proc Natl Acad Sci USA 79:7465–7469
98. Inoko H, Ando A, Kimura M, Ogata S, Tsuji K (1984) Isolation and characterization of the cDNA clones and the genomic clones of the HLA class II antigen heavy chains. In: Baur MP, Albert ED, Mayr WR (eds) Histocompatibility testing 1984. Springer, Berlin Heidelberg New York Tokyo, pp 559–564
99. VanDeRijn M, Bernabeu C, Royer-Pokora B, Weiss J, Seidman JG, DeVries J, Spits H, Terhorst C (1984) Recognition of HLA-A2 by cytotoxic T lymphocytes after DNA transfer into human and murine cells. Science 226:1083–1085
100. Howell DN, Hartzman RJ, Cresswell P (1983) Expression of T-lymphoblast-encoded HLA-DR, MT, and SB antigens on human T-B lymphoblast hybrids. Hum Immunol 8:167–175
101. Pawelec G, Blaurock M, Schneider EM, Shaw S, Wernet P (1982) Alloactivated long-term cultured human T lymphocytes express both HLA-DR and SB antigens but lack lymphocyte stimulatory capacity. Eur J Immunol 12:967–972
102. Pollack MS, Chin-Louie J, Moshief RD (1984) Functional characteristics and differential expression of class II DR, DS, and SB antigens on human melanoma cell lines. Hum Immunol 9:75–87
103. Nunez G, Giles RC, Ball EJ, Hurley CK, Capra JD, Stastny P (1984) Expression of HLA-DR, MB, MT, and SB antigens on human mononuclear cells: Identification of two phenotypically distinct monocyte populations. J Immunol 133:1300–1306
104. Van Heyningen V, Guy K, Newman R, Steel CM (1982) Human MHC class II molecules as differentiation markers. Immunogenetics 16:459–469
105. Guy K, Van Heyningen V, Cohen BB, Deane DL, Steel CM (1982) Differential expression and serologically distinct subpopulations of human Ia antigens detected with monoclonal antibodies to Ia alpha and beta chains. Eur J Immunol 12:942–948
106. Brown G, Walker L, Ling NR, Richardson P, Johnson GD, Guy K, Steel CM (1984) T-cell proliferation and expression of MHC class II antigens. Scand J Immunol 19:373–377

107. Collins T, Korman AJ, Wahr CT, Boss JM, Kappes DJ, Fiers W, Ault KA, Ginbrone Jr MA, Strominger JL, Pober JS (1984) Immune interferon activates multiple class II MHC genes and the associated inv chain gene in human endothelial cells and dermal fibroblasts. Proc Natl Acad Sci USA 81:4917–4921
108. Auffray C, Lillie JW, Arnot D, Grossberger D, Kappes D, Strominger JL (1984) Isotypic and allotypic variation of the class II human histocompatibility antigen alpha chain genes. Nature 308:327–333
109. Long EO, Gorski J, Mach B (1984) Structural relationship of the SB beta chain gene to HLA-D region genes and to murine I region genes. Nature 310:233–235
110. Braunstein N, Germain R (1985) The murine E-beta2 gene: structure, sequence, and expression. In: Streilein JW, Ahmad F, Black S, Blomberg B (eds) Advances in gene technology: molecular biology of the immune system. Cambridge University Press, Cambridge, p 119
111. Widera G, Flavell RA (1985) The I-region of the C57BL/10 mouse: characterization and physical linkage to H-2K of an SBbeta-like class II pseudogene, Abeta3. Proc Natl Acad Sci 82:5500–5504

Genes Encoding Mouse Ia

Structural and Functional Studies of Mouse Class II Genes

M. Steinmetz

Table of Contents

Introduction

This review summarizes our current knowledge about the organization, structure, expression, and evolution of the class II genes in the major histocompatibility complex (MHC) of the mouse. Class II genes code for highly polymorphic cell surface molecules, called class II antigens or Ia antigens. The mouse class II antigens are the counterparts to the human HLA-DP, DQ, and DR antigens (previously called SB, DC/DS/MB, and DR, respectively) which are encoded in the D region of the HLA complex. Class II molecules play an important role in the generation of immune responses because they are involved in the recognition of foreign antigens by regulatory T cells (for recent reviews see [28, 65]).

Two different class II antigens called I-A and I-E have been identified in the mouse and are usually found on the cell surface of B cells and macrophages. They are composed of two polypeptide chains, α and β, which are glycoproteins with molecular weights of approximately 34000 and 28000 daltons respectively. The α and β polypeptides are believed to be composed of two extracellular protein domains and a part that spans the cell membrane and extends slightly into the cy-

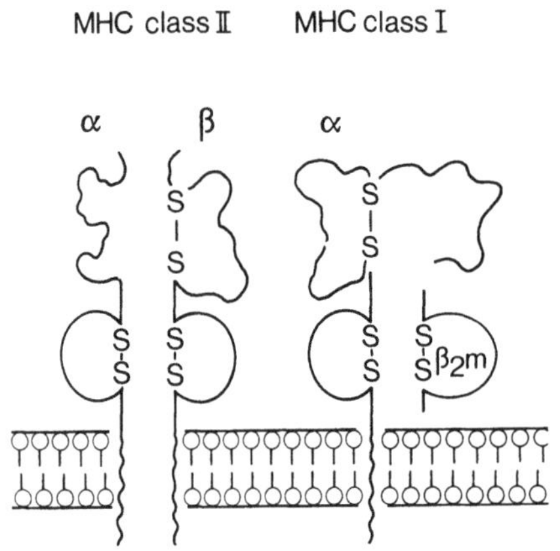

Fig. 1. Domain organization of class I and class II molecules. Extracellular protein domains are indicated by *circles* or *irregular-shaped areas*. Domains shown as circles are virtually conserved between different alleles and display homology to immunoglobulin domains [25]. *S-S*, disulfide bridges; $\beta_2 m$, β_2-microglobulin

toplasm (Fig. 1). Class II molecules therefore appear to have a similar structure to class I molecules, to which they are evolutionarily and functionally related (for a review see [25]).

Class II Gene Organization

Genes encoding class II molecules are located in the I region of the MHC, between the K region, encoding the H-2K class I molecule, and the S region, coding for proteins which are structurally and functionally unrelated to class I and class II molecules (Fig. 2). A major portion of the I region was cloned by chromosome walking experiments from a cosmid library constructed with BALB/c DNA [66, 67]. Figure 3 shows the organization of the class II genes in the cloned portion. Six class II genes were identified, two α genes and four β genes. The A_α, A_β, E_α, and E_β genes code for the polypeptides of the I-A and I-E molecules. Protein products encoded by the $A_{\beta 2}$ and $E_{\beta 2}$ genes have so far not been identified. Both the $A_{\beta 2}$ and $E_{\beta 2}$ genes appear to be transcribed at low levels in spleen cells [10, 71].

Recently two more β genes were found. One, called $A_{\beta 3}$, is located between the K and $A_{\beta 2}$ genes, separated by 80 kb from H-$2K^d$ and by 160 kb from $A_{\beta 2}{}^d$ [76]

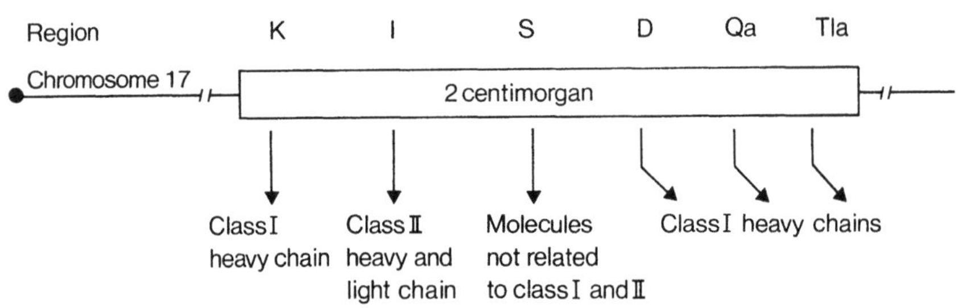

Fig. 2. The MHC of the mouse, divided into six regions called K, I, S, D, Qa, and T1a. The boundaries of these regions are defined by crossing-over events which occurred in certain recombinant mouse strains. The K, D, Qa, and T1a regions code for class I molecules, the I region for class II molecules, and the S region for certain enzymes and some complement components

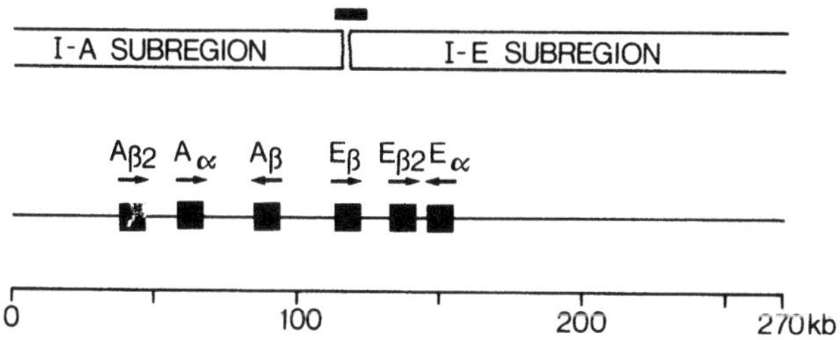

Fig. 3. Organization of six closely linked class II genes in the mouse. The cloning of 270 kb of DNA from the I region of the BALB/c mouse and the identification of the $A_{\beta 2}$, A_β, A_α, E_β, $E_{\beta 2}$, and E_α genes has been reported [66, 67]. The K gene is located to the left about 240 kb upstream from the $A_{\beta 2}$ gene in the BALB/c mouse (Steinmetz et al., submitted). The complement genes are located to the right at an unknown distance away from the E_α gene. Recombination events, which by definition separate the I-A from the I-E subregion, have occurred in nine independently derived intra-I region recombinant mouse strains [B10.A(3R), B10.A(4R), B10.A(5R), B10.GD, B10.HTT, B10.RSB-1, B10.S(8R), B10.S(9R), and B10.TBR-2] in a stretch of DNA 9.8 kb in length [66], as indicated by the *bar*

(Steinmetz et al., submitted). The other, called $E_{\beta 3}$, has been mapped into the S region [71].

More class II genes have been found in man, namely at least six α and seven β genes, although some haplotype-specific variation in the number of β genes appears to occur [9, 38]. The possibility cannot be excluded that more class II genes exist in the mouse which might have escaped detection so far because of insufficient homology to the hybridization probes used.

Class II Gene Structure

The DNA sequences of the class II genes whose protein products have been identified serologically have all been determined, with the exception of the A_α gene, which has only been sequenced at the cDNA level. The exon-intron organization of these class II genes is shown in Fig. 4. As for class I genes, there is a correlation

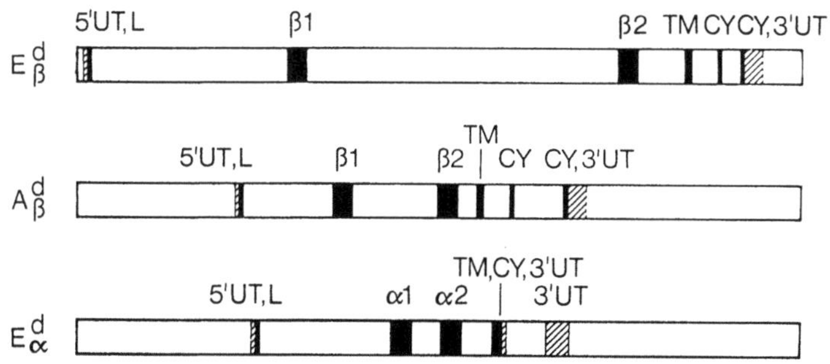

Fig. 4. Exon-intron organization of mouse class II genes. Exons are labeled according to the portion of the protein they encode: *L*, signal or leader peptide; *α1*, *β1*, first external domain of the α or β chain; *α2*, *β2* second external domain; *TM*, transmembrane region; *CY*, cytoplasmic portion; *5′ UT*, *3′ UT*, 5′ and 3′ untranslated regions of the mRNA. Class II gene organizations have been published: E^d_β, Saito et al. [63]; A^d_β, Malissen et al. [40]; E^d_α, Hyldig-Nielsen et al. [26]

between exon-intron organization and protein domain organization. Separate exons encode the leader or signal peptide, the first and second internal domains, the transmembrane region, and the cytoplasmic tail.

An interesting variation is observed at the 3′ end of the genes, where the two β chain genes contain an intron in the coding sequence for the cytoplasmic portion of the protein, whereas the E_α gene has an intron in the 3′ untranslated region (Fig. 4). All human class II α and β chain genes so far sequenced have the same distinctive organization at the 3′ end. Since the β_2-microglobulin gene also shows an intron in the 3′ untranslated region, it has been speculated that the β_2-microglobulin gene is evolutionary more closely related to the class II α genes than to the class II β genes [25]. It is also possible, however, that the occurrence of an intron in the 3′ untranslated region in class II α and β_2-microglobulin genes is the result of independent mutations which placed termination codons in the penultimate coding exons. Such mutations have probably generated similar structures in certain human and rabbit class I genes which show an intron in the 3′ untranslated region [42].

The $E_{\beta2}$ gene, which has been sequenced almost completely, has an exon-intron organization similar if not identical to the other β genes [10]. It shows a leader, $\beta1$, $\beta2$, and transmembrane exon; however, the precise exon-intron organization of the 3′ end of the gene is still unclear. The $A_{\beta2}$ gene has been sequenced partially and is known to possess a $\beta2$ exon [37]; it remains to be seen whether it is a complete β gene and encodes a functional protein. The $A_{\beta3}$ gene appears to be nonfunctional, at least in C57BL/10 mice and in mice of the H-2^k haplotype [71, 76]. It shows a deletion of 8 bp in the $\beta2$ exon, leading to premature termination of translation if the gene is transcribed and translated.

Sequence comparisons of mouse and human class II genes indicate that the $A_{\beta3}$, A_β, and E_β genes are the counterparts to the human DP_β, DQ_β, and DR_β genes respectively (Table 1). This is in complete agreement with sequence com-

Table 1. Nucleotide and amino acid sequence homologies (%) between mouse and human class II β chain exons encoding the second external domain [71]

	Nucleotides			Amino acids		
	DPβ	DQβ	DRβ	DPβ	DQβ	DRβ
$A^b_{\beta3}$	*83*	73	70	*75*	68	60
A^b_β	75	*83*	71	70	*81*	67
E^b_β	78	75	*83*	69	70	*83*
$A^b_{\beta2}$	69	71	73	62	63	65

Table 2. Amino acid sequence homologies (%) between mouse and human class II α chain exons encoding the second external domain [5]

	DPα	DQα	DRα
A_α	60	*68*	55
E_α	63	60	*76*

parison of α chain genes, which shows that the A_α and E_α genes are the mouse equivalents to the human DQ_α and DR_α genes (Table 2).

It appears therefore that the three gene loci, DP, DQ, and DR, were present before speciation separating the mouse and human evolutionary lines occurred. Presumably the counterpart to the DP_α gene has subsequently been lost in mice, although it is possible that a distantly related α gene or the remnants of it are still linked to $A_{\beta 3}$ but have escaped detection so far. It is interesting to note that the gene order DP-DQ-DR with respect to the genes encoding the components is the same in mice and men [9, 76].

Hot Spots for Recombination

Molecular typing of nine different intra-I region recombinant mouse strains by Southern blot analysis led to the unexpected finding that all recombination events had occurred in a small stretch of DNA [66]. This stretch of DNA is at most 9.8 kb in length and covers the E_β gene (Figs. 3 and 5). For two more intra-I region recombinants analyzed recently the recomination site also maps within this region [62]. Thus it appears that this region contains a genetic element, termed a hot spot for recombination, which confines recombination events to a small stretch of DNA. A more detailed analysis of some of these recombinant mouse strains by molecular cloning and restriction mapping has shown that for one of them (B10.GD), the recombination point can be confined to a region of about 2 kb of DNA encompassing the β2 exon and part of the large intron between the β1 and β2 exon of the E_β gene [33] (Fig. 5). DNA sequence determination has narrowed this region down further to a stretch of 1 kb in length located entirely in the large intron (J. Kobori, personal communication).

The presence of a hot spot for recombination in the E_β gene may indicate that other recombinational hot spots will exist elsewhere in the MHC and perhaps also outside in other regions of the genome. One might assume that such hot spots will be found between the I and S regions and between the S and D regions, where respectively over 20 and 80 independent recombination events have been scored [32]. Recent experiments have indicated that certain subspecies of mice *(Mus*

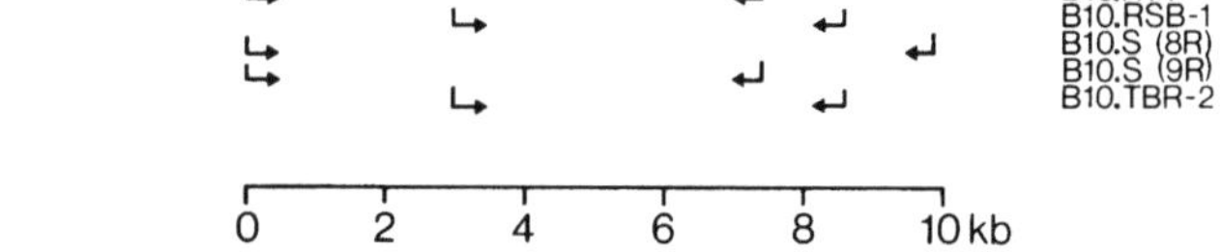

Fig. 5. A hot spot for recombination in the E_β gene. Regions, as indicated by *arrows,* to which the recombination point in nine different intra-I region recombinant mouse strains could be confined are shown with respect to their location in the E_β gene [33, 66]. From these analyses, the maximum distance between the I-A and I-E subregions is 2.0 kb of DNA

musculus molossinus, Mus musculus castaneus) also contain a recombinational hot spot between the K and I regions [64] (Steinmetz et al., submitted). When these mice were crossed to different *Mus musculus domesticus* strains, a 30 to 100-fold increase in recombination frequency was observed between the K and I marker loci, as compared to intraspecies crosses between *Mus musculus domesticus* strains. Thus recombinational hot spots might be present in some strains but missing in others.

The occurrence of hot spots for recombination inside and perhaps even outside the MHC has several important implications. First, there will be no linear correlations between genetic maps measured in recombination frequencies and molecular maps measured in base pairs. In fact, the presence of a hot spot for recombination in the middle of the I region leads to a threefold higher recombination frequency as expected from the molecular distance of the marker loci [66]. Thus frequencies of recombination are determined by molecular distance and presence or absence of recombinational hot spots. Second, linkage disequilibrium observed for certain alleles might in part be explained by result from the presence or absence of hot spots for recombination. Selective forces favoring the linkage or the rapid exchange of certain alleles will either prevent or promote the occurrence of recombinational hot spots between genes that are kept in close physical association for various other reasons. Third, susceptibility to certain human diseases appears to be associated with the presence of certain HLA alleles [61]. In some cases this might be due to a very low recombination frequency between linked genes, the first being responsible for the disease and the second encoding the HLA molecule. For instance, congenital adrenal hyperplasia results from a mutation in the gene coding for 21-hydroxylase, which is found in the HLA complex in two copies closely linked to the C4A and C4B genes [74]. Deficiency in 21-hydroxylase is strongly associated with the Bw47 allele, perhaps because recombinational hot spots are absent between the two genes. Fourth, recombinational hot spots might show different patterns of distribution in different individuals. For instance, high or low recombination frequencies, observed for the same two MHC loci when different combinations of mouse strains are crossed [30, 64], could be due to presence or absence of hot spot for recombination in the different strains.

The I-J Enigma

Specific antisera and monoclonal antibodies have been used to identify a molecule composed of two polypeptide chains in the supernatant of suppressor T cells which exhibits antigen-specific, MHC-restricted suppressive activity [72]. The gene coding for one chain of this molecule was mapped into the I region, more precisely into a subregion called I-J between the I-A and I-E subregions, using recombinant mouse strains, especially B10.A (3R), B10.A (5R), B10.HTT, and B10.S (9R) [49]. The molecular characterization of these and other recombinants, however, showed that the presumptive I-J subregion – if there at all – could be confined to less than 3.4 kb of DNA, part of which is covered by coding sequences for the E_β molecule (see Fig. 5) [66]. This stretch of DNA appeared to be too small to code for the different I-J molecules which had been described, creating a paradox between the serological and molecular genetic findings. In fact, recent DNA sequence data obtained for B10.A (3R) and B10.A (5R) has shown that these two recombinants are identical across the boundary between the I-A and I-E subregions (J. Kobori, personal communication).

The inability to find the I-J genes at their proposed position stimulated a renewed search for their possible chromosomal location. In a series of elegant experiments [22, 23] it has been shown that the I-J^k molecule is controlled by at least two genes, one mapping into the I-E subregion or S region [defined by the recombination events in B10.A (4R) and B10.A (2R)], the other located on chromosome 4. The dual control of the I-J^k molecule by an H-2 gene and a non-H-2 gene appears also to be true for the I-J^b molecule and might be true for I-J^q and I-J^s molecules, although in these cases the controlling genes have not yet been mapped [22]. A number of questions remain concerning the identity of the postulated genes, the observation that although located on different chromosomes, they behave like linked genes in genetic crosses, and their mode of expression. The model currently favored assumes that the H-2 component is expressed on epithelial cells in the thymus where it serves as a recognition element for I-J molecules, expressed on precursor cells for suppressor T cells. I-J molecules might be encoded by a gene located on chromosome 4 or encoded elsewhere, but are modified by a gene(s) on chromosome 4. Proper recognition would be the selective force whereby only suppressor cells, expressing I-J molecules compatible with the polymorphic H-2 component, would be able to differentiate.

Clearly, what is missing at present is more information on the biochemistry of I-J polypeptides. Molecular weights of 25000–30000 daltons for the cellular and soluble forms of I-J have been reported [35, 68]. I-J molecules appear to be part of the antigen receptor on suppressor T cells which has recently been analyzed with molecular probes. Initial studies have failed to show that the T cell receptor β genes (which are expressed in helper and killer T cells) are used to code for one chain of the antigen receptor on suppressor T cell hybridomas [24, 34]. In fact, it appears that a major proportion of these cells have, for unknown reasons, lost both copies of chromosome 6, carrying the β genes from the T cell parent. Recently, an apparently functional β gene rearrangement has been found in a cloned suppressor cell line and antibodies directed against the β chain have been shown to precipitate soluble products with suppressor activity [1]. This indicates that at least some mouse suppressor T cells use the same β genes as helper and killer T cells to code for one chain of the antigen receptor. These latter findings are in agreement with the presence of apparently functional β chain genes in human suppressor T cell clones [60, 69].

Evolution of Diversity

Class I and class II molecules, to which T cells bind in the detection of foreign antigens, are highly polymorphic [31]. This means that many alleles occur at comparable frequencies in the mouse population. It is currently assumed that the different alleles have been established during evolution through selective forces. Since a large number of different pathogens must be recognized by the T cell receptors, a large number of different receptor molecules are needed. On the other hand, certain receptor structures which would be capable of recognizing self-determinants in conjunction with MHC molecules are not allowed. Thus pathogens could evolve which would interact with certain MHC molecules in the same way as self-determinants do, and would therefore escape immune surveillance. The presence in the population of different MHC alleles, however, would assure that at least some members of the species show an immune response against the pathogen. Presumably, a large number of different MHC restriction elements has not been established in individual members of the species because the large number of self-determinants which would then have to be tolerated would result in a small T cell repertoire. Of course, this does not explain why MHC restriction occurs at all.

Not all mouse class II genes show a great degree of polymorphism. Whereas the A_α, A_β, and E_β genes are highly polymorphic, the E_α gene is only slightly polymorphic [8, 31, 65]. The degree of polymorphism correlates with the number of amino acid substitutions found between different alleles. Whereas the A_α, A_β, and E_β molecules encoded by different alleles show 5%–10% amino acid substitutions, only few amino acid differences (less than 1%) have been found for different E_α allomorphs.

At least three different molecular mechanisms create the diversity found between alleles. First, gene duplication will establish multiple loci which can then drift and become different from one another through the accumulation of mutations. Second, recombination events, occurring with high frequencies at recombinational hot spots, will shuffle various alleles and create new linkage groups or haplotypes. Third, gene conversion events occurring between the different genes in a linkage group will transfer small blocks of sequences and create extensive mutations. The selective forces discussed above will then operate on the pool of mutated sequences to establish useful alleles in the species. In the following, some structural evidence that supports the occurrence of these mechanisms is discussed.

Gene Duplication

The order and orientation of the closely linked class II genes in the I region (Fig. 3) appears to reflect the action of at least two duplication events (not to mention the original duplication which yielded α and β genes): one which generated the two β genes in the β-β-α unit, and a second one which duplicated the unit. We do not know which event occurred first. Genetic drift allowed the duplicated genes to diverge from one another. As discussed above, at least some of the duplication events which generated multiple class II genes are probably very old, since evidence for the occurrence of class II genes related to the three different human class II β gene loci, DP, DQ, and DR, has been found in mice.

Comparison of different *Mus musculus domesticus* strains for their gene organization in a portion of the I region has shown that they are all identical, except for some small deletions or insertions outside of class II genes [67]. Even among different subspecies and species of mice the number of class II genes appears to be constant [58]. This is in marked contrast to the numbers of class I genes in different mice, which can change over short periods of evolutionary time [73, 77] (Steinmetz et al., unpublished results). Thus, gene expansion and contraction, presumably by unequal crossing over, occurs frequently among the closely related members of the class I gene family, but only rarely for class II genes. Whether the structural basis for this observation is mainly the more distant relationship between different class II genes, or whether the I region forms a particularly rigid chromosome structure, is not known.

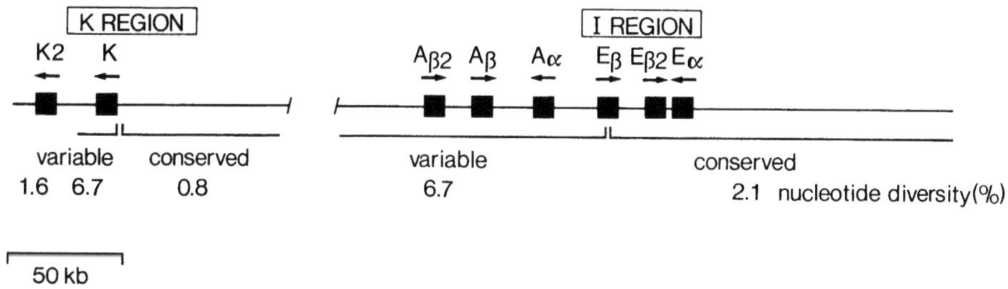

Fig. 6. Variable tracts alternate with conserved tracts of DNA in the MHC. The organization of the two class I genes in the K region and of the six class II genes in the I region is shown together with their location in either variable or conserved tracts of DNA. Restriction map comparisons between two (K region) or three (I region) different mouse inbred strains have shown that the mutation frequency in the variable tracts is three times higher than in the conserved tracts. The same result was obtained when mouse strains were compared by Southern blot analysis with a large number of probes from the different regions and when DNA sequences were compared directly. (Data from Steinmetz et al. [67])

Variable and Homogeneous Tracts of DNA

Comparison of cloned DNA from the K region, the I region, and the S region between different mouse strains has indicated that the MHC is composed of variable tracts alternating with more homogeneous tracts of DNA [67]. Coding *and* noncoding sequences in the variable tracts are mutated to a higher degree than coding and noncoding sequences in homogeneous tracts. On average, these regions differ by a factor of three in mutation frequencies. The variable tract identified in the K region appears to be small, whereas the variable tract in the I region covers at least 120 kb of DNA (Fig. 6). It is interesting to note that the highly polymorphic genes K, A_α, A_β, and E_β, which show extensive allelic variability, are all located in variable tracts, whereas the less variable genes E_α, C4, and Slp are all located in homogeneous tracts. It has been suggested that the variable tracts of DNA were generated through increased mutation rates or gene conversion events occurring simultaneously in coding and noncoding sequences [67]. Alternatively, however, the variable tracts might originate from a pool of sequences which are, evolutionarily speaking, older than the homogeneous tracts and were taken up into the mouse MHC by recombination events. This trans-specific model of evolution, originally proposed by Arden and Klein [3], has gained some support, since recombinational hot spots have indeed been found at two boundaries of the variable tracts, namely between the K and I regions and between the I-A and I-E subregions [67] (Steinmetz et al., submitted).

Gene Conversion

A third mechanism contributes to the diversification of class II genes which leads to the simultaneous mutation of several nucleotides in a small stretch (perhaps up to 50 bp) of DNA. The genetic change is believed to occur through a process termed gene conversion, initially observed in fungi [56], in which a short stretch of sequence from a donor gene is transferred to an acceptor gene, where it replaces the homologous sequence previously present. The precise molecular mechanism by which gene conversion events occur is not known.

In the case of mouse class II genes, the A_β^{bm12} mutant gene appears to be the result of a gene conversion-like event [4, 45, 47, 75]. The A_β^{bm12} mutant gene, which arose spontaneously in a (BALB/c × B6)F_1 mouse, differs from the parent A_β^b gene in 3 individual bp within a stretch of 14 bp. The three mutations in the gene result in three amino acid changes in the first domain of the A_β chain (residues 67, 70, 71), which are obviously responsible for the altered immune response that is observed in the mutant strain compared to its parent. Interestingly, the E_β^b gene is identical in sequence to the A_β^{bm12} gene over a stretch of 44 bp which includes the mutated residues. This finding is consistent with the assumption that the E_β^b gene, as the donor gene, converted the A_β^b gene into the A_β^{bm12} gene. Thus, gene conversion events, leading to the transfer of short DNA sequences between nonallelic genes, appear to contribute to the diversity of class II genes. Gene conversion events apparently generate diversity in class I genes as well [46, 51].

Class II Gene Expression

Class II molecules are normally found on the cell surface of B cells, macrophages, and dendritic cells, indicating that class II gene expression is controlled in a cell-type-specific manner. A priori, this could be achieved by transcriptional, translational, and translocational (transport from cytoplasm to cell surface) control mechanisms. Expression of class II molecules on macrophages is controlled by both positive and negative regulation [70]. Negative regulation has been observed through the action of prostaglandins. Positive regulation is exerted by γ-interferon in human and murine systems through the enhancement of transcription [59]. In fact, γ-interferon has been shown to activate class II gene expression even in cells which normally do not express class II genes, such as human vascular endothelial cells and dermal fibroblasts [11, 54].

Sequences that might be involved in the regulation of class II gene expression have been studied by comparison of 5′ flanking sequences of class II genes to identify conserved sequences possibly involved in regulation of transcription and by transfer into various cell types of class II genes that had or had not been modified in vitro.

Sequence comparisons have indicated the presence of two conserved blocks of sequences (A and B) in the 5′ flanking regions of human and mouse class II α and β chain genes [29, 38, 44, 63]. The A and B sequences are 21 bp and 15 bp in length and are found about 100 bp and 70 bp upstream of the start site of transcription respectively. The function of these elements is not known. Similar blocks of conserved sequences have been found upstream of several other genes, including immunoglobulin and histone genes [15]. In the case of immunoglobulin κ light chain genes, the conserved elements are important for correct transcription. It is interesting to note that two generally conserved sequences, the so-called CCAAT and TATA boxes (located usually about 70 bp and 25 bp upstream of the transcriptional start site), which have been shown to control transcription of many genes, are not particularly conserved in different mouse and human class II genes [29]. This suggests that transcription of class II genes is regulated by different sequences than those important for most other genes, possibly involving the A and B sequences.

Gene transfer experiments have shown that class II genes transfected into mouse fibroblasts with or without viral enhancer sequences can be transcribed and translated even though the endogenous class II genes are transcriptionally inactive [39, 52, 55]. Other studies, however, have indicated that at least the E_β^b gene contains a tissue-specific enhancer element [19]. This enhancer element was mapped to a 2-kb region of DNA about 700 bp upstream from the E_β gene and was shown to enhance transformation frequencies in B cells compared to fibroblasts and myeloma cells (which are inactive with regard to class II gene expression). Transcription of sequences linked to the E_β gene enhancer was also shown to be tissue-specific: no transcription was found in fibroblasts, but high levels of transcription were observed in B cells. This finding seems to contradict the successful transfection of fibroblasts with class II genes mentioned above, and the apparent conflict has not yet been explained.

The transcriptional enhancer sequences of the E_β^d gene map further upstream than the A and B sequences conserved between mouse and human class II genes. It is possible that the enhancer elements are the target sequences for γ-interferon-induced expression of class II genes in macrophage cells. These target sequences can be studied, since it has been shown that the induction by γ-interferon can be reproduced in a gene transfection system: macrophage cells transfected with the E_β^b gene showed expression of exogenous and endogenous class II genes only after induction with supernatants from concanavalin-A-stimulated T cells [16]. Perturbation of the upstream sequences of the E_β gene by in vitro mutagenesis should allow further characterization of the regulatory elements.

Class II Sequences Recognized by T Cells

Hypervariable Regions

Amino acid sequences have now been obtained for a number of allomorphs encoded by A_α, A_β, E_α, and E_β genes. All of these amino acid sequences were derived from the nucleotide sequences of cDNA or genomic clones. Three important points have emerged from sequence comparison in each allelic series. First, as pointed out above, in contrast to the A_α, A_β, and E_β genes, which show extensive variability between alleles, the E_α gene is more homogeneous. If we assume that the polymorphism of the A_α, A_β, and E_β genes has been established through selective forces, then it follows that similar selective forces have not been operating on the E_α gene. Presumably, the mouse can deal with the large number of foreign antigens without the need of polymorphism in the E_α polypeptide. In fact, some haplotypes have lost a functional E_α gene and others have lost both a functional E_α gene and a functional E_β gene [12, 13, 27, 43]. We do not know why similar mutations have never been found for the I-A molecule.

Second, amino acid sequence variability is primarily confined to the first domain of the A_α, A_β, and E_β molecules (Table 3). This finding is currently assumed to mean that the first domain is primarily involved in the associative recognition of foreign antigen by the T cell receptor, whereas other portions of the molecules possess effector functions and/or are important for the proper association of α and β chains. Exon-shuffling experiments support this contention (see below).

Table 3. Amino acid sequence variability (%) in class II α and β chain alleles

No. of alleles compared	Molecule	First domain	Second domain	Transmembrane and cytoplasmic portion
8	A_α	11.8	1.9	0.5
3	A_β	14.7	2.8	1.4
2	E_α	0	1.1	1.9
3	E_β	15.2	0.7	0

The sequence comparisons have all been published: A_α: Landais et al. [36]; A_β, E_α: Steinmetz and Hood [65]; E_β: Widera and Flavell [75]

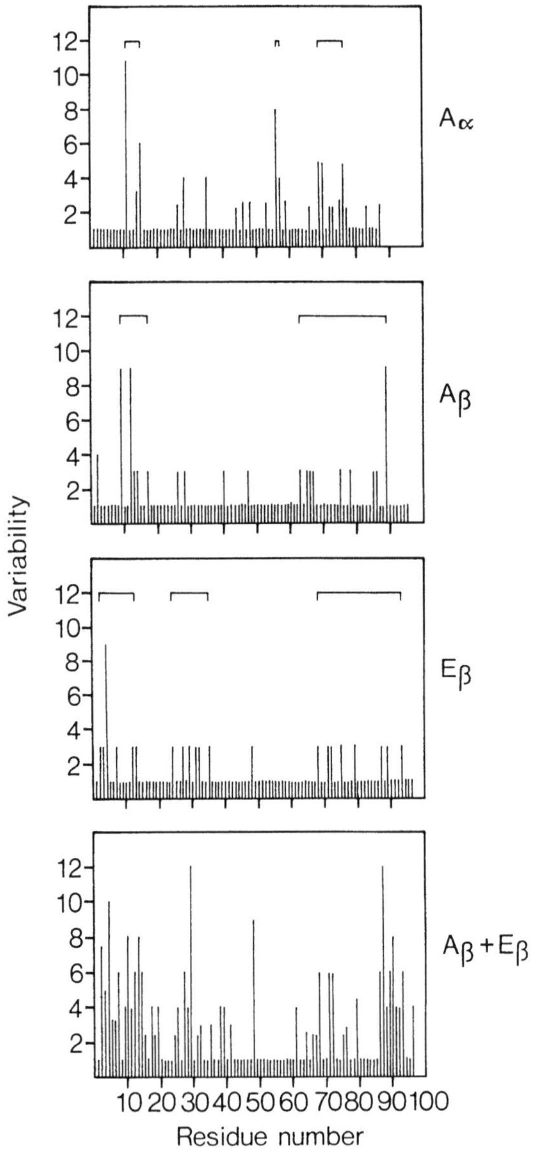

Fig. 7. Variability of amino acid residues in the first domain of A_α, A_β, and E_β chains. The variability was calculated according to Wu and Kabat [78]. Hypervariable regions, tentatively identified, are indicated by *brackets*. The individual plots were obtained by comparing eight A_α alleles [36], three A_β alleles (compiled in [65]), three E_β alleles (compiled in [75]), and all six class II β chain alleles

Third, hypervariable regions alternating with more conserved segments have been identified in the variable domains (Fig. 7). The best evidence stems from a comparison of eight A_α alleles leading to the identification of three hypervariable regions in the first domain: amino acid residues 11–15, 56–57, and 69–76 [8, 36]. Comparison of three A_β alleles [65] and three E_β alleles [14, 75] also indicates clustering of variable residues, although sequences of more alleles are needed to identify hypervariable regions clearly. Interestingly, as shown by a comparison of all six mouse class II β chain sequences available, certain segments in the first domain are conserved even between A_β and E_β molecules (Fig. 7). This indicates that these residues are important either for proper folding of the β chain first domain or for interactions with other protein molecules. Potential glycosylation sites and cysteine residues involved in internal disulfide bridge formation are located in the conserved segments [75]. Conserved sequences in the first domain are also found for A_α and E_α polypeptides [7].

It is reasonable to assume that the hypervariable regions of A_α, A_β, and E_β chains in the first domains are involved in the interaction between T cell receptor, foreign antigen, and class II molecule either by binding directly to receptor or antigen or by changing the conformation of an alternative binding site. In agreement with this assumption is the specificity involved in MHC restriction, the fact that the mutation in the A_β^{bm12} molecule appears to occur in a hypervariable region, and the ability of monoclonal antibodies, which apparently recognize residues in the second and third hypervariable region of the A_α chain [36], to block T cell recognition.

Shuffling of Variable Domains

In order to identify functionally important regions on class II molecules it is desirable to have a series of mutants available with alterations in various parts of the molecule. The in vitro mutagenesis technique allows construction of such mutants in the test tube. To use the technique one needs class II genes, cloned and sequenced, which can be introduced and expressed in cells which do not normally express these genes. Such cells, after they have acquired class II molecules on their surface, should be able to present antigens to T cells.

Intitially, A_α^k and A_β^k genes were introduced into mouse L cells which are fibroblasts derived from C3H (H-2^k) mice [39]. Since fibroblasts do not normally express class II genes (see above), the transfected genes could be analyzed for transcription and expression. It was shown that the introduced genes, which were stably integrated into the genome of the host cell, were transcribed and translated and led to the display of I-A^k molecules on the cell surface which appeared normal by serological analysis and two-dimensional gel electrophoresis. Surprisingly, the transfected L cells were also capable of presenting polypeptide and complex protein antigens to T cell clones and hybridomas together with the I-A^k molecules as a restricting element [41, 52]. These findings indicate that fibroblasts have the capacity to assemble functional class II molecules and to take up, process, and present complex antigens so that they can be recognized by T cells.

Similar class II gene transfer experiments have been carried out with cells normally expressing class II molecules. The E_β^b gene has been transfected into a B lymphoma and a macrophage cell line both of BALB/c (H-2^d) origin [16]. In contrast to the B lymphoma cell, which expresses the transfected gene constitutively, the macrophage cell line needs stimulation by soluble T cell factors to express the introduced class II gene (see above). The transfected cells display an $E_\beta^b\,E_\alpha^d$ complex on the cell surface which is effectively used by $E_\beta^b\,E_\alpha^d$-restricted T helper hybridomas in the recognition of antigen. Furthermore, hamster B-cell lines transfected with A_α^k and A_β^k genes acquire the ability to present certain antigens to I-A^k-restricted T helper hybridomas [41].

These experiments, which showed that class II molecules expressed by genes transfected into B cells, macrophages, or fibroblasts can function as proper restriction elements, offered a way to dissect the structural elements important for T cell recognition by exchanging different portions of the class II molecules. First, experiments were set up in which the proper α chain was exchanged with an α chain encoded by a different allele, in order to determine whether determinants formed exclusively by the polymorphic residues on the β chain were sufficient for T cell recognition. Indeed, I-A^d-bearing B cells transfected with the A_β^k gene can present the antigen L-glutamic acid^{60}-L-alanine^{30}-L-tyrosine^{10} (GAT) to an I-A^k-restricted helper T cell clone [17]. This result indicates that at least some epitopes acting as I-A^k-specific restriction elements are formed by the A_β^k polypeptide alone, independent of allele-specific residues on the A_α^k chain. However, several other I-A^k-restricted helper hybridomas and clones did not respond to the presumptive complex $A_\alpha^d\,A_\beta^k$ and are therefore apparently restricted by epitopes which are formed by allele-specific residues on the A_α^k chain or on the $A_\alpha^k\,A_\beta^k$ complex [6]. In a similar way, some monoclonal antibodies directed against the I-A^k molecule can recognize determinants on the A_β^k chain independent of its association with A_α^k, whereas others cannot [6, 17].

As discussed above, sequence comparisons have shown that the N-terminal domain of the A_β molecule contains most of the polymorphic residues. One might therefore expect that the epitopes recognized by T helper cells on the A_β^k polypeptide map to the first domain. Indeed, exon-shuffling experiments in which the second domain, the transmembrane segment, and the cytoplasmic portion of the A_β^k molecule were replaced with the corresponding sequences from the A_β^d molecule have confirmed this expectation [18]. Mouse fibroblasts transfected with such a hybrid gene together with the A_α^k gene express hybrid class II molecules on the cell surface that are indistinguishable from I-A^k molecules, as tested by a series of monoclonal antibodies and I-A^k-restricted antigen-specific T lymphocytes. Thus the four amino acids that distinguish the second domain of the A_β^k molecule from that of the A_β^d molecule do not contribute to these immunologically relevant determinants displayed by the I-A^k molecule.

Conclusions

During the past 3 years the genes from the I region of the MHC of the mouse which control the recognition of antigen by T cells have been cloned and characterized. Four genes have been identified, coding for the A_α, A_β, E_α, and E_β molecules. In addition, four more β genes have been found ($A_{\beta2}$, $A_{\beta3}$, $E_{\beta2}$, and one gene mapping into the S region). It is currently not known whether the $A_{\beta2}$ and $E_{\beta2}$ genes code for proteins that serve some function, but it has been shown that they are transcribed at low levels in spleen cells. The $A_{\beta3}$ gene is nonfunctional. A complete linkage map has been established for the $A_{\beta3}$, $A_{\alpha3}$, A_β, A_α, E_β, $E_{\beta2}$, and E_α class II genes in the BALB/c mouse at the molecular level [66] (Steinmetz et al., submitted) and has greatly simplified some earlier versions of I region genetic maps. For instance, no evidence has been found for the postulated I-B and I-J subregions, stimulating a renewed search for the chromosomal location of the genes coding for the enigmatic I-J suppressor polypeptides. Since the gap between the K region and the I region of the MHC has been closed by chromosomal walking experiments, all the DNA is at hand to search for the various genes that have been postulated [21, 48] to be located between the K and the I region.

Sequence comparisons of class II genes have revealed the clustering of polymorphic residues in the N-terminal domains of the α and β chains (with the exception of the E_α chain, which appears to be almost invariant). Two findings strongly suggest that these hypervariable regions play an important role in MHC-restricted antigen recognition. First, a spontaneous mutation, which apparently occurs in a hypervariable region of the A_β^b chain, severely affects immune responses restricted by the I-A^b molecule. Second, exon-shuffling experiments show that the polymorphic residues in the first domain of the A_β^k chain form at least some of the elements used for T cell restriction.

Several arguments support the idea that positive selection forces have established the variability of class II alleles during evolution – as opposed to the view that the diversity occurs at positions which are under no selective constraint at all. First, exons encoding variable domains show higher mutation frequencies than introns or noncoding flanking sequences [75]. Second, hypervariable regions show more productive nucleotide changes (those leading to alterations of amino acid residues) than expected from chance alone [20]. Third, allomorphs usually differ from one another in several amino acid residues, as opposed to just one or two residues. Fourth, evolution has placed MHC genes under at least two special mechanisms which generate and maintain variability: gene conversion and enhanced recombination at hot spots.

MHC class I and class II molecules are structurally and functionally related. Both molecules apparently use the N-terminal domains ($\alpha 1$ and $\alpha 2$ of class I, $\alpha 1$ and $\beta 1$ of class II) to restrict the specificity of T cells. Exon-shuffling experiments indicate that at least some of the conserved extracellular domains ($\alpha 3$ of class I, $\beta 2$ of class II) can be exchanged without affecting the specificity of T cell recognition [18, 53, 57], whereas the variable domains can be separated in some cases [17, 50] but not in others [2, 4, 6]. By placing variable domains onto the two separate chains of the I-A class II molecule, nature has apparently invented an efficient way of generating new restriction determinants in heterozygous animals.

In vitro mutagenesis experiments involving changing of the polymorphic residues in the N-terminal domains will have to be done to confirm and extend our current idea that these domains exert T cell restriction. However, it will be difficult to distinguish residues directly involved in binding to the T cell receptor from those important for the proper configuration of the binding site(s). Another problem concerns the antigen which is recognized by the T cell in conjunction with the MHC molecule. We do not know at present whether the foreign antigen interacts with the class II molecule, the T cell receptor, or both. One hopes that the current characterization of the T cell receptor at the molecular level will allow us to devise models that can be tested by in vitro mutagenesis of T cell receptor and MHC genes. In the end, however, X-ray analyses of crystals containing all three components might be required to obtain the final answer.

Acknowledgments. I thank C. Benoist, R. Germain, C. Hayes, J. Kobori, D. Larhammar, D. Singer, and G. Widera for the communication of unpublished results or preprints of their work, Z. Dembić and J. Kaufman for critical comments on the manuscript, L. Gisler for preparation of the manuscript, and H.P. Stahlberger for artwork.

References

1. Adorini L, Palmieri G, Sette A, Appella E, Doria G (1985) Expression of T cell receptor β chain gene products by a mouse monoclonal antigen-specific suppressor T cell line. Curr Top Microbiol Immunol (in press)
2. Allen H, Wraith D, Pala P, Askonas B, Flavell RA (1984) Domain interactions of H-2 class I antigens alter cytotoxic T cell recognition sites. Nature 309:279–281
3. Arden B, Klein J (1982) Biochemical comparison of major histocompatibility complex molecules from different subspecies of Mus musculus: evidence for trans-specific evolution of alleles. Proc Natl Acad Sci USA 79:2342–2346
4. Arnold B, Burgert HG, Hamann U, Hämmerling G, Kees U, Kvist S (1984) Cytolytic T cells recognize the two amino-terminal domains of H-2 K antigens in tandem in influenza A infected cells. Cell 38:79–87
5. Auffray C, Lillie JW, Arnot D, Grossberger D, Kappes D, Strominger JL (1984) Isotypic and allotypic variation of human class II histocompatibility antigen α-chain genes. Nature 308:327–333
6. Ben-Nun A, Glimcher LH, Weis J, Seidman JG (1984) Functional expression of a cloned I-Aβ^k gene in B-lymphoma cells. Science 223:825–828
7. Benoist CO, Mathis DJ, Kanter MR, Williams II VE, McDevitt HO (1983) The murine Ia α chains, E_α and A_α, show a surprising degree of sequence homology. Proc Natl Acad Sci USA 80:534–538
8. Benoist CO, Mathis DJ, Kanter MR, Williams II VE, McDevitt HO (1983) Regions of allelic hypervariability in the murine A_α immune response gene. Cell 34:169–177
9. Bodmer J, Bodmer W (1984) Histocompatibility 1984. Immunol Today 5:251–254
10. Braunstein N, Germain R (1985) The murine $E_{\beta 2}$ gene: structure, sequence and expression. In: Streilein et al. (eds) Advances in gene technology: molecular biology of the immune system. Cambridge University Press, Cambridge, p 119–120
11. Collins T, Korman AJ, Wake CT, Boss JM, Kappes DJ, Fiers W, Ault KA, Gimbrone MA, Strominger JL, Pober JS (1984) Immune interferon activates multiple class II major histocompatibility complex genes and the associated invariant chain gene in human endothelial cells and dermal fibroblasts. Proc Natl Acad Sci USA 81:4917–4921
12. Dembić Z, Singer PA, Klein J (1984) E^o: a history of a mutation. EMBO J 3:1647–1654
13. Dembić Z, Ayane M, Klein J, Steinmetz M, Benoist CO, Mathis DJ (1985) Inbred and wild mice carry identical deletions in their E_α MHC genes. EMBO J 4:127–131
14. Denaro M, Hammerling U, Rask L, Peterson PA (1984) The E_β^b gene may have acted as the donor gene in a gene conversion like event generating the A_β^{bm12} mutant. EMBO J 9:2029–2032
15. Falkner FG, Zachau HG (1984) Correct transcription of an immunoglobulin K gene requires an upstream fragment containing conserved sequence elements. Nature 310:71–74
16. Folsom V, Gold DP, White J, Marrack P, Kappler J, Tonegawa S (1984) Functional and inducible expression of a transfected murine class II major histocompatibility complex gene. Proc Natl Acad Sci USA 81:2045–2049
17. Germain RN, Norcross MA, Margulies DH (1983) Functional expression of a transfected murine class II MHC gene. Nature 306:190–194
18. Germain RN, Ashwell JD, Lechler RI, Margulies DH, Nickerson KM, Suzuki G, Tou JYL (1985) Exon-shuffling maps control of antibody and T cell recognition sites to the NH_2-terminal domain of A_β. Proc Natl Acad Sci USA 82:2940–2944
19. Gillies SD, Folsom V, Tonegawa S (1984) Cell type-specific enhancer element associated with a mouse MHC gene, E_β. Nature 310:594–597

20. Gustafsson K, Wiman K, Emmoth E, Larhammar D, Böhme J, Hyldig-Nielsen JJ, Ronne H, Peterson PA, Rask L (1984) Mutations and selection in the generation of class II histocompatibility antigen polymorphism. EMBO J 3:1656–1661
21. Hayes CE, Bach FH (1980) I-N, a newly described H-2 I subregion between K and I-A. J Exp Med 151:481–485
22. Hayes CE, Klyczek KK (1985) The I-J glycoprotein: Genetic control, biochemistry, and function. Immunol Rev 83:41–59
23. Hayes CE, Klyczek KK, Krum DP, Whitcomb RM, Hullett DA, Cantor H (1984) Chromosome 4 Jt gene controls murine T cell surface I-J expression. Science 223:559–563
24. Hedrick SM, Germain RN, Bevan MJ, Dorf M, Engel I, Fink P, Gascoigne N, Heber-Katz E, Kapp J, Kaufmann Y, Kaye J, Melchers F, Pierce C, Schwartz RH, Sorensen C, Taniguchi M, Davis MM (1985) Rearrangement and transcription of a T-cell receptor β-chain gene in different T-cell subsets. Proc Natl Acad Sci USA 82:531–535
25. Hood L, Steinmetz M, Malissen B (1983) Genes of the major histocompatibility complex of the mouse. Ann Rev Immunol 1:529–568
26. Hyldig-Nielsen JJ, Schenning L, Hammerling U, Widmark E, Heldin E, Lind P, Servenius B, Lund T, Flavell R, Lee JS, Trowsdale J, Schreier PH, Zablitzky F, Larhammar D, Peterson PA, Rask L (1983) The complete nucleotide sequence of the I-E_{α}^{d} immune response gene. Nucleic Acids Res 11:5055–5071
27. Jones PP, Murphy DB, McDevitt HO (1981) Variable synthesis and expression of Eα and Ae (Eβ) Ia polypeptide chains in mice of different H-2 haplotypes. Immunogenetics 12:321–337
28. Kaufman JF, Auffray C, Korman AJ, Shackelford DA, Strominger J (1984) The class II molecules of the human and murine major histocompatibility complex. Cell 36:1–13
29. Kelly A, Trowsdale J (1985) Complete nucleotide sequence of a functional HLA-DPβ gene and the region between the DPβ1 and DPα1 genes: comparison of the 5′ ends of HLA Class II genes. Nucleic Acids Res 13:1607–1621
30. Klein J (1975) Biology of the mouse histocompatibility complex. Springer, Berlin Heidelberg New York
31. Klein J, Figueroa F (1981) Polymorphism of the mouse H-2 loci. Immunol Rev 60:23–57
32. Klein J, Figueroa F, David CS (1983) H-2 haplotypes, genes and antigens: second listing. Immunogenetics 17:553–596
33. Kobori JA, Winoto A, McNicholas J, Hood L (1984) Molecular characterization of the recombination region of six murine major histocompatibility complex (MHC) I-region recombinants. J Mol Cell Immunol 1:125–131
34. Kronenberg M, Goverman J, Haars R, Malissen M, Kraig E, Phillips L, Delovitch T, Suciu-Foca N, Hood L (1985) Rearrangement and transcription of the β-chain genes of the cell antigen receptor in different types of murine lymphocytes. Nature 313:647–653
35. Kumagai Y, Okumura K, Tada T (1984) Photoaffinity labeled hapten-binding T cell receptor on a suppressor T cell hybridoma. Mol Immunol 21:545–559
36. Landais D, Matthes H, Benoist C, Mathis D (1985) A molecular basis for the Ia-2 and Ia-19 antigenic determinants. Proc Natl Acad Sci USA 82:2930–2934
37. Larhammar D, Hammerling U, Denaro M, Lund T, Flavell RA, Rask L, Peterson PA (1983) Structure of the murine immune response I-A_{β} locus: sequence of the I-A_{β} gene and an adjacent β-chain second domain exon. Cell 34:179–188
38. Larhammar D, Servenius B, Rask L, Peterson PA (1985) Characterization of an HLA-DR β pseudogene. Proc Natl Acad Sci USA 82:1475–1479
39. Malissen B, Steinmetz M, McMillan M, Pierres M, Hood L (1983) Expression of I-A^{k} class II genes in mouse L cells after DNA-mediated gene transfer. Nature 305:440–443
40. Malissen M, Hunkapiller T, Hood L (1983) Nucleotide sequence of a light chain gene of the mouse I-A subregion: Aβ^{d}. Science 221:750–754
41. Malissen B, Price MP, Goverman JM, McMillan M, White J, Kappler J, Marrack P, Pierres A, Pierres M, Hood L (1984) Gene transfer of H-2 class II genes: antigen presentation by mouse fibroblast and hamster B-cell lines. Cell 36:319–327

42. Marche PN, Tykocinski ML, Max EE, Kindt TJ (1985) Structure of a functional rabbit class I MHC gene: similarity to human class I genes. Immunogenetics 21:71–82
43. Mathis DJ, Benoist C, Williams II VE, Kanter M, McDevitt HO (1983) Several mechanisms can account for defective Eα gene expression in different mouse haplotypes. Proc Natl Acad Sci USA 80:273–277
44. Mathis DJ, Benoist CO, Williams II VE, Kanter MR, McDevitt HO (1983) The murine Eα immune response gene. Cell 32:745–754
45. McIntyre KR, Seidman JG (1984) Nucleotide sequence of mutant I-A_{β}^{bm12} gene is evidence for genetic exchange between mouse immune response genes. Nature 308:551–553
46. Mellor AL, Weiss EH, Ramachandran K, Flavell RA (1983) A potential donor gene for the bml gene conversion event in the C57BL mouse. Nature 306:792–795
47. Mengle-Gaw L, Conner S, McDevitt HO, Fathman CG (1984) Gene conversion between murine class II major histocompatibility complex loci. J Exp Med 160:1184–1194
48. Monaco JJ, McDevitt HO (1982) Identification of a fourth class of proteins linked to the murine major histocompatibility complex. Proc Natl Sci USA 79:3001–3005
49. Murphy DB (1981) Genetic fine structure of the H-2 gene complex. In: Dorf ME (ed) The role of the major histocompatibility complex in immunobiology. Garland STPM, New York, p 1–32
50. Murre C, Choi E, Weiss J, Seidman JG, Ozato K, Liu L, Burakoff SJ, Reiss CS (1984) Dissection of serologic and cytolytic T lymphocyte epitopes on murine major histocompatibility antigens by a recombinant H-2 gene separating the first two external domains. J Exp Med 160:167–178
51. Nathenson SG, Geliebter J, Geier SS, Mashimo H, Hemmi S, Kumar A, McGovern D, Nakagawa M, Pfaffenbach G, Pontarotti P, Zeff R (1985) The study of H-2 major histocompatibility complex mutants reveals structure-function relationships and mechanisms of generation of diversity and polymorphism. In: Streilein et al. (eds) Advances in gene technology: molecular biology of the immune system. Cambridge University Press, Cambridge, p 37–40
52. Norcross MA, Bentley DM, Margulies DH, Germain RN (1984) Membrane Ia expression and antigen-presenting accessory cell function of L cells transfected with Class II major histocompatibility complex genes. J Exp Med 160:1316–1337
53. Ozato K, Evans GA, Shykind B, Margulies DH, Seidman JG (1983) Hybrid H-2 histocompatibility gene products assign domains recognized by alloreactive T cells. Proc Natl Acad Sci USA 80:2040–2043
54. Pober JS, Collins T, Gimbrone Jr MA, Cotran RS, Gitlin JD, Fiers W, Clayberger C, Krensky AM, Burakoff SJ, Reiss CS (1983) Lymphocytes recognize human vascular endothelial and dermal fibroblast Ia antigens induced by recombinant immune interferon. Nature 305:726–729
55. Rabourdin-Combe C, Mach B (1983) Expression of HLA-DR antigens at the surface of mouse L cells co-transfected with cloned human genes. Nature 303:670–674
56. Radding CM (1978) Genetic recombination: strand transfer and mismatch repair. Ann Rev Biochem 47:847–880
57. Reiss CS, Evans GA, Margulies DH, Seidman JG, Burakoff SJ (1983) Allospecific and virus-specific cytolytic T lymphocytes are restricted to the N or Cl domain of H-2 antigens expressed on L cells after DNA-mediated gene transfer. Proc Natl Acad Sci USA 80:2709–2712
58. Rogers MJ, Germain RN, Hare J, Long E, Singer DS (1985) Comparison of MHC genes among distantly related members of the genus *Mus*. J Immunol 134:630–636
59. Rosa F, Fellous M (1984) The effect of gamma-interferon on MHC antigens. Immunol Today 5:261–262
60. Royer HD, Bensussan A, Acuto O, Reinherz EL (1984) Functional isotypes are not encoded by the constant region genes of the β subunit of the T cell receptor for antigen/major histocompatibility complex. J Exp Med 160:947–952
61. Ryder LP, Svejgaard A, Dausset J (1981) Genetics of HLA disease association. Ann Rev Genet 15:169–187
62. Saha BK, Cullen SE (1985) Molecular analysis of two mouse I-region recombinants. In: Streilein et al. (eds) Advances in gene technology: molecular biology of the immune system. Cambridge University Press, Cambridge, p 281–282

63. Saito H, Maki RA, Clayton LK, Tonegawa S (1983) Complete primary structures of the Eβ chain and gene of the mouse major histocompatibility complex. Proc Natl Acad Sci USA 80:5520–5524
64. Shiroishi T, Sagai T, Moriwaki K (1982) A new wild-derived H-2 haplotype enhancing K-IA recombination. Nature 300:370–372
65. Steinmetz M, Hood L (1983) Genes of the major histocompatibility complex in mouse and man. Science 222:727–733
66. Steinmetz M, Minard K, Horvath S, McNicholas J, Frelinger J, Wake C, Long E, Mach B, Hood L (1982) A molecular map of the immune response region from the major histocompatibility complex of the mouse. Nature 300:35–42
67. Steinmetz M, Malissen M, Hood L, Örn A, Maki RA, Dastornikoo GR, Stephan D, Gibb E, Romaniuk R (1984) Tracts of high or low sequence divergence in the mouse major histocompatibility complex. EMBO J 3:2995–3003
68. Taniguchi M, Tokukisa T, Hoh T, Kanno M (1984) Functional roles of two polypeptide chains that compose an antigen-specific suppressor T cell factor. J Exp Med 159:1096–1104
69. Toyonaga B, Yanagi Y, Suciu-Foca N, Minden M, Mak TW (1984) Rearrangements of T-cell receptor gene YT35 in human DNA from thymic leukemia T-cell lines and functional T-cell clones. Nature 311:385–387
70. Unanue ER, Beller DI, Lu CY, Allen PM (1984) Antigen presentation: comments on its regulation and mechanism. J Immunol 132:1–5
71. Wake CT, Widera G, Flavell RA (1985) Organization and expression of the murine MHC. In: Streilein et al. (eds) Advances in gene technology: molecular biology of the immune system. Cambridge University Press, Cambridge, p 33–36
72. Webb DR, Kapp JA, Pierce CW (1983) The biochemistry of antigen-specific T-cell factors. Ann Rev Immunol 1:423–438
73. Weiss EH, Golden L, Fahrner K, Mellor AL, Devlin JJ, Bullman H, Tiddens H, Bud H, Flavell RA (1984) Organization and evolution of the class I gene family in the major histocompatibility complex of the C57BL/10 mouse. Nature 310:650–655
74. White PC, New MI, Dupont B (1984) HLA-linked congenital adrenal hyperplasia results from a defective gene encoding a cytochrome P-450 specific for steroid 21-hydroxylation. Proc Natl Acad Sci USA 81:7505–7509
75. Widera G, Flavell RA (1984) The nucleotide sequence of the murine I-Eβ^b immune response gene: evidence for gene conversion events in class II genes of the major histocompatibility complex. EMBO J 3:1221–1225
76. Widera G, Flavell RA (1985) The I-region of the C57BL/10 mouse: characterization and physical linkage to H-2 K of a novel, SBβ-like class II pseudogene ψAβ3. Proc Natl Acad Sci USA 82:5500–5504
77. Winoto A, Steinmetz M, Hood L (1983) Genetic mapping in the major histocompatibility complex by restriction enzyme site polymorphisms: most mouse class I genes map to the T1a complex. Proc Natl Acad Sci USA 80:3425–3429
78. Wu TT, Kabat EA (1970) An analysis of sequences of variable regions of Bence-Jones proteins and myeloma light chains and their implications for antibody complementarity. J Exp Med 132:211–250

Cross-reaction Between Various Species

Cross-reactions of Class II Histocompatibility Antigens of Various Species

M. Pla and P. Ivanyi

Table of Contents

Introduction

A major histocompatibility complex (MHC) has been demonstrated in all mammalian and avian species studied and in several fish and amphibian species. Interestingly, the MHC loci occur in a homologous linkage group in various species. Whether such conservation of a linkage group during the evolution of species is due to chance or is of functional (selective) significance is unknown. Recent analyses of cDNA and genomic clones show the similar overall structure and domain organization of the genes coding for class I and class II antigens of the MHC in various species. Biochemical characterization of the histocompatibility antigens has shown their basic molecular structure to be the same in every species so far examined.

Another important characteristic of the MHC class I and class II antigens is their high polymorphism within a species, which has allowed an extensive analysis of their properties to be made by alloantisera. When H-2-specific alloantisera were first tested against evolutionarily distant species (human cells) a considerable amount of cross-reactivity was observed [40, 41]. Many investigators have subsequently studied the serological cross-reactions between the MHC antigens of various species and obtained similar results. This work has been reviewed by Ivanyi [36]. The mechanism of diversification and origin of MHC antigen polymorphism is still disputed. Data on MHC cross-reaction can contribute to the understanding of and/or show the consequences of inter- and intraspecies MHC antigen diversification. The finding that alloantisera (and monoclonal antibodies) cross-react with distantly related species suggests that the histocompatibility polymorphism was in fact conserved during evolution [43], or that allodeterminants of similar nature (as recognized by cross-reactions) developed in various species and were maintained by selection [14, 36]. The latter possibility points to the view that most of the polymorphism developed after speciation from the (limited) pool of genetic material available at the "beginning" of the species. (This possibility is close to, but not identical with, the proposal of one homozygous MHC breeding pair for each species; possibly *Homo sapiens* obtained about 10–20 alleles for the HLA-B locus, as opposed to the about 100 that have already been detected and to the more than 100 B locus alleles that probably exist).

There are numerous other facets of the MHC interspecies cross-reactions. Not only alloimmune but also xenoimmune anti-MHC antibodies cross-react with the histocompatibility antigens of various species. Moreover, some xenoimmune MHC-specific antibodies detect polymorphism among individuals of the species to which the immunized individual belongs (e.g., mouse anti-human or mouse anti-frog antibodies detect polymorphism of H-2 antigens) [36, 76]. The same aspects as mentioned for antibodies were also studied by the cellular technique [mixed lymphocyte reaction (MLR), cell-mediated lympholysis] and provide information about the T cell receptor repertoire which is able to detect allodeterminants across species barriers.

In this review we summarize data about interspecies cross-reactions for class II MHC antigens.

Comparative Interspecies Aspects

Class II Genes in Various-Species

The majority of the data presented in this book were obtained from man and mouse. There is an overall analogous genetic organization of the MHC chromosomal region in these two species (Figs. 1 and 2, Table 1) and there is also structural analogy for class II antigens (see later). As a consequence of the latter analogy, serological and cellular reagents can detect cross-reactivity between class II products of various species. There is also an overally analogy for the functions of class II molecules in different species. Therefore there is frequent reference to the human/mouse MHC model. We tacitly presume that the situation is, in principle, identical in all other species, and in fact, although the data from several other species are much less elaborated, at least the beginnings do not indicate major differences among species (Fig. 3). In rats, the RT1.B and RT1.D antigens are homologous to the A/DQ and E/DR antigens respectively [29].

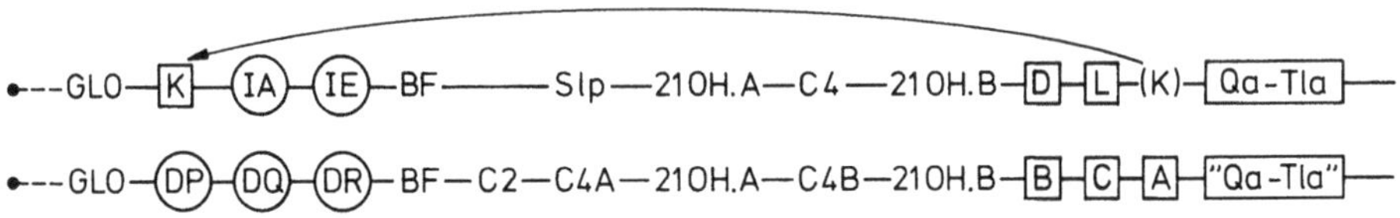

Fig. 1. Schematic map of HLA and H-2 gene orders for MHC products. Presumably a translocational event produced the *Mus musculus* exception for the MHC by placing class I genes on both sides of class II genes (for details see Ivanyi [36]). *GLO*, erythrocyte enzyme glyoxalase I; *21OH*, genes for P-450$_{C21}$; *BF, C2, C4* (and *Slp*), genes for the complement pathway. The relative gene order for class III and class IV (enzyme) genes of the MHC chromosomal region is hypothetical [94, 95]. The human "Qa-T1a" genes are murine Qa-T1a-like genes not yet included in the official HLA nomenclature

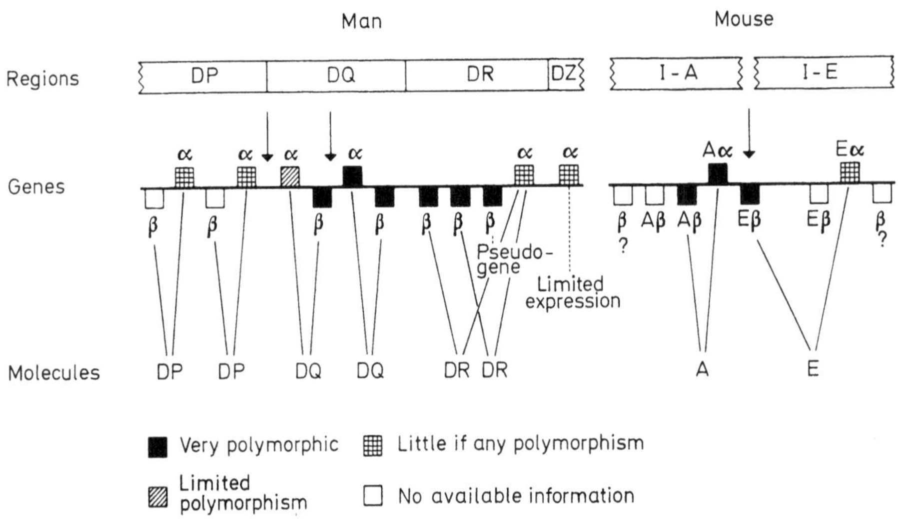

Fig. 2. Schematic map of the class II human and murine regions based on the dates of various authors, reviewed by Hood et al. [34], Lafuse and David [46], and Bodmer and Bodmer [10]

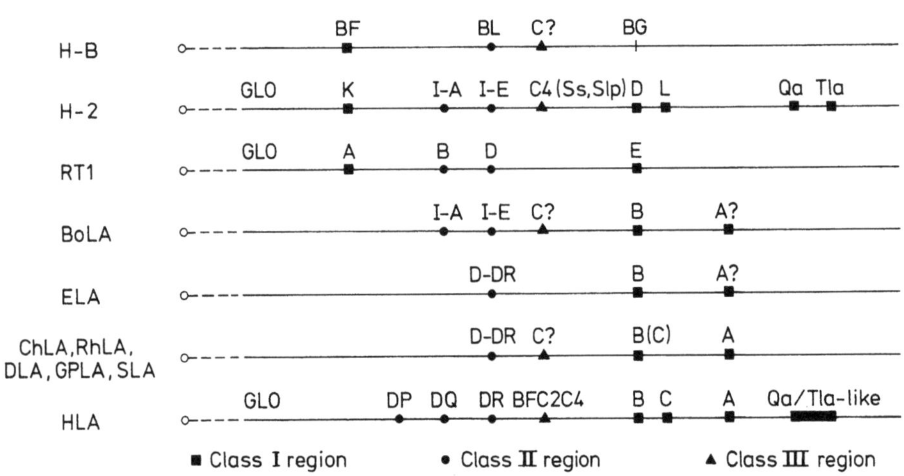

Fig. 3. Organization of MHC in various species

Table 1. Number of class II genes in man and mouse

Class II gene	Man	Mouse
Alpha	6	2
Beta	7	4–6

Class II Gene Expression in Various Species

Whereas the human/mouse model for class II antigens has been elaborated in great detail, fewer data have been accumulated for other species. At least two types of class II molecule have been defined in several species [7, 22]. Xenoimmune and alloimmune cross-reactive mouse sera were widely used in these studies. Immunochemical detection of hamster class II molecules was achieved by alloimmune anti-Ia^k mouse antibodies [62]. Two distinct groups of rat [7, 93] and bovine [33] Ia antigens were detected by A^k- and E^k-specific alloantibodies.

Certainly, antibodies obtained in the combination A.TH anti-A.TL (two congeneic mouse strains which differ only for class II antigens) have been used most often for these pioneer surveys or expeditions into the universe of class II molecules along their evolutionary paths. This antibody probe could hit a target even on *Drosophila* cells [73]. Surprisingly, whereas in most cases the anti-E^k antibodies from A.TH anti-A.TL sera (or the respective monoclonal antibodies) became the prominent (but certainly not exclusive) reagent for the interspecies class II cross-reactions [54], on *Drosophila* cells anti-A^s antibodies (A.TL anti-A.TH) were positive.

The human/mouse model and data from other species show that class II antigens are not (or only very weakly) expressed on resting T cells. Only about 5% of human or murine resting T cells (or human peripheral blood T lymphocytes) express class II antigens. A rather different situation was found in dogs [23, 25], where virtually all resting T cells express a similar amount of class II antigens to B cells. However, in man, class II antigen expression can be detected on peripheral T cells after stimulation (in vitro or in vivo). Therefore it was questioned whether the presence of class II molecules on dog "resting" T cells is due to an unusual state of stimulation (infections?). This was found not to be so, because peripheral T cells of SPF dogs express class II antigens too. These findings show that the "differential" tissue distribution of class I and class II antigens was not a principal "must" in their evolutionary history. A similar situation was found in swine [86]. The canine class II antigens were detected by xenoimmune (anti-human) or alloimmune (mouse) cross-reactive anti-class II sera. From the various mouse antibodies that recognized dog class II antigens, only some xenoimmune and anti-E or anti-E+A monoclonal antibodies detected class II antigens on resting canine T lymphocytes, whereas several anti-A monoclonal antibodies did not react with canine T cells [25].

Another deviation from expectations is that of the cat, the only species in which the mixed lymphocyte culture was not positive among unrelated individuals [68]. Possibly the dog is a species in which the difference in class II expression on T vs B cells is not as important as it appears in man and mouse, and the cat a species with such a low class II expression that more sensitive techniques are needed.

Class II Gene Polymorphism in Various Species

In the human/mouse model, class II antigen polymorphism is extensive. A similar situation is indicated for other species, including the Syrian hamster, where difficulties are reported in establishing class I polymorphism. For class II antigens, an unexpectedly low extent of polymorphism was found in rats. However, unless much more extensive population studies are performed it will be difficult to conclude how much of this information is really representative for the species (and would allow speculations about the biological significance of the observed extent of intraspecies polymorphism), or are due to some kind of stratification of the "population sample" and/or insufficient discriminative power of the techniques used.

Homology of DNA and Protein Sequences

The class II molecules have been well characterized by biochemical methods mainly in mouse and man, but also in primates [31], rat [8], cattle [33, 49], hamster [82], and guinea pig [27].

The class II molecules are heterodimers, composed of two chains, α and β. The α chains range in molecular weight from 30 to 35 kd and the β chains from 26 to 29 kd. By using alloantisera or monoclonal antibodies, it has been shown that there are two (mouse, rat, hamster, cattle, primates) or three (man) types of class II molecule.

The mouse A (Aα Aβ) and E (Eα Eβ) molecules are homologous to human DQ and DR molecules respectively. The structural similarity is based on the following observations: (a) Both DQ and A heavy chains are lower in molecular weight than are DR and E heavy chains.The DQ and A light chains are generally more basic in charge than the DR and E light chains. (b) The N-terminal amino acid sequence of the DR and DQ heavy chains show homology to the sequence of the E and A heavy chains respectively [12, 77].

Amino acid sequences deduced from cloned DNA have complemented protein sequencing and other structural studies. Each chain is composed of four domains: a polymorphic terminal domain (α1, β1) without homology with immunoglobulin, a second (α2, β2), relatively conserved domain, having a striking homology with immunoglobulin, a hydrophobic (transmembrane) region, and a C-terminal hydrophilic region.

The first domains of human and murine heavy chains (α1) are all glycosylated at a homologous residue (residue 78) and are homologous: DQα1 is most homologous to Aα1, and DR α1 most homologous to Eα1.

Long et al. [52] have published data on nucleotide sequence homologies between human and murine class II β genes (Table 2). The nucleotide sequence homology is greater between DR and E or between DQ and A β genes than intraspecies homologies between β genes of different subregions. This may suggest that the gene duplication which generated the DR/E and DQ/A β genes had taken place before separation of these two species.

It is interesting that DQβ cytoplasmic domain lacks a stretch of eight amino acids present in the other light chains, which corresponds to a single exon in murine Aβ and Eβ chains [48].

Table 2. Nucleotide sequence homologies between human and murine class II β genes. The nucleotide sequences are compared separately for each exon encoding the first, second, and third domains. The numbers represent the homology between two sequences expressed as a percentage. References and data were published by Long et al. [52]

	β chain domain											
	First				Second				Third			
	Man		Mouse		Man		Mouse		Man		Mouse	
	DR	DQ	E	A	DR	DQ	E	A	DR	DQ	E	A
DR		75	79	72		74	83	71		78	87	75
DQ			68	79			74	83			75	86
E				74				70				70
DP	76	77	67	72	77	79	77	76	68	71	71	70

One difference between man and mouse is the existence of a third family of class II antigens DP, in the human system. There are data [52] showing the preferential hybridization of the DPβ cDNA to the second murine Eβ gene. However, a comparison of nucleotide sequences shows that the DPβ gene is neither E-like nor A-like. At the nucleotide level the DPβ gene is not more closely related to the DQβ gene than to the DRβgene (Table 2). At present it is difficult to guess whether a murine counterpart to the DP antigen exists but remains undetected or whether it was lost during evolution. It is also possible, that the DP genes were generated by gene duplications after the mouse/man divergence.

There are several similarities between class I, class II, β2-microglobulin, and immunoglobulin genes. All these genes exhibit a precise correlation between exon-intron organization and the protein domains. The DNA sequences of the exons encoding the closest membrane domains (α3 of the class I, α2 and β2 of the class II) and for the β2-microglobulin are homologous to the exon sequences encoding immunoglobulin constant regions. A low level of homology has also been observed between the class I α1 and the class II β1 domains [47]. The class II heavy chain genes and β2-microglobulin have a similar genomic structure, whereas the class II light chain genes are more similar to class I heavy chain genes [34]. Although class I and II antigens serve different functions, their structural similarity makes it likely that their modes of action at the molecular level are similar. One can ask a question: Is it possible to find an antibody reacting with a determinant carried by class I and class II molecules? At present, there are no data available to answer this question. Monomorphic monoclonal class I-specific antibodies can inhibit class II-restricted proliferative responses [81] and cocap class II antigens [58]. These results suggest some insufficiently understood relationship between class II and class I antigens at the cell membrane.

Class II Interspecies Cross-reactions Detected by Antibodies

A. Xenoimmune Antibodies

Class II molecules in different species are highly homologous, but they exert sufficient interspecies variations to become a strong immunogen. Therefore, xenoimmune sera are expected to react (a) with all class II products of the species from which the antigen was used for immunization (monomorphic pattern of reactivity), (b) only with a part of the class II products but carried by all individuals of the donor species (monomorphic pattern of reactivity, region-specific antibodies), or (c) only with allele-specific antigenic determinants (polymorphic pattern of reactivity, which may or may not be region-specific). An extreme example of the latter would be antiprivate xenoimmune antibodies, i.e., antibodies directed against determinants of one class II molecule.

Obviously, most of the xenoimmune sera are mixtures of all these kinds of antibody. The recipients were usually rabbits, immunized by various forms of antigen (whole cells, isolated cell membranes, or soluble preparations in various degree of purity including highly purified light and heavy chain material). The main aim of such immunization was to obtain a large quantity of a strong serum for biochemical study on human class II molecules to replace weak alloimmune human sera.

The specificity of xenoimmune rabbit anti-Ia^k serum antibodies was directed against common parts of murine class II molecules because cells of some third-party strains absorbed all activity; donor haplotype-specific antibodies could not be detected [60]. Similar results were obtained with rabbit anti-human class II sera (Klareskog et al. 1978). However, in another study, six of 31 rabbit anti-human class II sera showed preferential activity with cells bearing the donor-specific class II antigens [78]. These types of broad xenoimmune serum also reacted with class II antigens of third-party species and allowed only one conclusion, that class II molecules of various species broadly cross-react. Only monoclonal antibodies allowed the examination of more specific questions.

Are Xenogeneic Monoclonal Antibodies Directed Against Monomorphic or Polymorphic Class II Determinants?

The distinction between polymorphic (allotypic) and monomorphic (isotypic) determinants, and the antibodies directed against them, is operational. A monomorphic antibody reacts with all cells tested. However, it was not always clear whether the binding to comparable cell suspensions of various haplotypes was always the same. Absorption experiments, variations in titer, or dissociation rate constants might show a hidden preference of a "monomorphic" antibody to certain polymorphic determinants. A polymorphic monoclonal antibody recognizes antigenic determinants carried only by certain cells from the test panel.

So far, 199 monoclonal antibodies directed against human class II antigens have been registered by Colombani et al. [20, 21] and Colombani and Lepage [19]. Of the 125 mouse anti-human monoclonal antibodies, 82 reacted as monomorphic and 39 as polymorphic; of four rat anti-human antbodies, two reacted as monomorphic and two as polymorphic. The remaining monoclonal antibodies were either allogeneic (see later) or the combination of immunization was unknown. Among the polymorphic antibodies, only about 10% recognized a single DR specificity (as defined by human antibodies). The majority of the polymorphic monoclonal antibodies recognized public or broad specificities, as for example DRw52 and DRw53. Some of these broad specificities had already been defined by alloimmune human sera, others defined "new" public determinants [3, 11]. Among the broadly reactive monoclonal antibodies, some are particularly interesting, as they point to a relationship between human and mouse class II determinants. Some of them react with all cells except those which are DR7-homozygous. They were usually produced by BALB/c (H-2^d) mice. The most straightforward interpretation of these results is that class II products of H-2^d haplotype express a determinant identical with or similar to DR7. In the rat an "all except DR7" (SFR P 1.1) as well as a DR7-specific (SFR 16-DR7) monoclonal antibody was produced [69].

Along with the polymorphism of DR molecules, the polymorphism of DQ and DP molecules had also become well established. Part of the data published about monoclonal antibodies against human class II antigens were analyzed for their specificity against the distinct human class II region products. In Table 3 data on 66 monoclonal antibodies of mouse origin are summarized. As to the monoclonal antibodies reacting only with a single type of class II molecule, 28 are monomorphic: 27 antibodies recognize DR, one reacts with DP and none with DQ molecules. However, of the 24 polymorphic monoclonal antibodies, 17 recognize DR and seven (nearly 30%) recognize DQ molecules. Although the immunogen was presented in a variety of forms and the assignment of the specificities of monoclonal antibodies to human class II regions is rather an indication than a final conclusion, the results show an apparently pronounced immunogenicity of polymorphic DQ determinants as compared with the monomorphic DQ determinants.

Table 3. Molecular specificity of 66 mouse monoclonal antibodies directed against human class II molecules. References for these monoclonal antibodies can be found in Colombani et al. [20, 21] and Colombani and Lepage [19]. Molecular specificity of monoclonal antibodies was studied during the First International Workshop on Monoclonal Antibodies to Human MHC Class II Antigens (Edinburgh 1983) [80] and during the Ninth Histocompatibility Workshop [11]

Molecular assignment	Reaction pattern	Monoclonal antibodies	
		Identity	*n*
DR	monomorphic	D1.11; D1.12; D1.17; D4.22; FMC.4; FMC.14; FMC.15; L1.1.6; L203; L227; L243; NE4; Q2/70; SG157; Tu34; Tu35; Tu36; Tu37; W1691.13.17; 1.35; 1.41; 2.06; 2E11; 307; 406; 7B2; IVG1	27
	polymorphic	AB8.25; D4.90; D7.69; DA6.164; E13.11; E15.4; FMC.2; HU30; MAJA7.3; MCS7; Q2/80; Q5/13; S3; 16.23; 21R5; I-1; I-LR2	17
DQ	monomorphic		0
	polymorphic	Genox3.53; HU18; HU23; S1; Tu22; 5F6; 17.15	7
DP	monomorphic	IB4	1
	polymorphic		0
DR+DQ	monomorphic	TDR31.1	1
	polymorphic	BT3/4; SDR1	2
DR+DP	monomorphic	BT2.9; Da6.147; Tu39; Tu43	4
	polymorphic	SG520, I-LR1	2
DP+DQ	monomorphic		0
	polymorphic	SG171	1
DR+DQ+DP	monomorphic	AA3.83; DA6.121; DA6.231	3
	polymorphic	SG465	1

Shaw et al. [74] analyzed 52 monoclonal antibodies on a panel of 17 HLA-deletion mutants derived from a single-parent cell line. The mutant cell lines varied in expression of class II molecules owing to deletion of various HLA subregions. Twenty-two monoclonal antibodies reacted only with DR or DQ or DP molecules expressed by the given cell line, 18 reacted with DR and DP, and one reacted with DR, DQ, and DP molecules. These results and those summarized in Table 3 show that xenogeneic monoclonal antibodies can detect class II molecule determinants shared by several subregion products. Similar results have been obtained with rat anti-mouse monoclonal antibodies [4].

We have no clear explanation concerning the rules that regulate the outcome of MHC xenoimmunization and its dissection by monoclonal antibodies. Nor is it clear whether and to what extent the diversity of xenoimmune monoclonal antibodies reflects the influence of the MHC genotype of the immunized animal due to partial sharing of structures with the immunogen. Thus, the relationship of allo and xeno repertoire of murine B cells for class II antigen remains unclear.

Can Xenogeneic Monoclonal Antibodies Detect MHC Polymorphism in Third-Party Species?

There are examples of monoclonal antibodies that detect polymorphism in third-party species; here we shall only summarize data obtained with xenogeneic anti-human monoclonal antibodies tested against bovine lymphocytes.

Brodsky et al. [15] examined nine mouse anti-human class II specific monoclonal antibodies for binding activity to lymphocytes from five breeds of cattle. Two showed essentially monomorphic binding to cattle (and human) class II molecules, and one was polymorphic in both species. In the study of Chardon et al. [18], neither of the two polymorphic anti-human class II monoclonal antibodies reacted with bovine animals, but all four monomorphic anti-human class II monoclonals reacted with all animals tested. Spooner and Ferrone [79] examined eight anti-human monoclonal antibodies which, among various species, recognized only cattle B lymphocytes. One was monomorphic, seven reacted with between 11 and 23 of the 27 samples tested. The polymorphic reaction pattern did not correlate with any defined BoLA class II antigens. However, it was noteworthy that the two anti-human antibodies which recognized distinct and spatially distant monomorphic determinants on human class II molecules displayed a similar reactivity pattern on bovine cells. Two other antibodies that cross-inhibited one another in inhibition binding assays with human B cells showed a different reactivity pattern on the panel of bovine lymphocytes.

In general, bovine MHC antigens cross-react much more with HLA antigens than do antigens from other nonprimate species [15, 79]. It was hypothesized that the close association between cattle and humans arising from domestication had, by virtue of common pathogens, selected for similar histocompatibility antigens and might explain a shared susceptibility to some pathogens [15].

Can Xenogeneic Monoclonal Antibodies detect MHC Polymorphism in the Immunized Species Itself?

Phylogenetically distant species share not only a general homology for the MHC molecules but also some aspects – albeit not well understood – of intraspecies polymorphism. Hence, xenogeneic monoclonal antibodies might detect some kind of polymorphism when tested on a panel of targets of the immunized species itself. This was found for class I antibodies: B10 (H-2^b) mice immunized with human cells produced (variable per individual mouse) H-2K- or H-2D-specific (private or public) antibodies [36]. Serum antibodies against polymorphic mouse class II determinants were induced by immunization of A.TH mice with lymphocytes of chicken, frog, and fish [76].

Some xenogeneic class II specific monoclonal antibodies produce the same phenomenon. McMaster and Williams [57] examined four BALB/c anti-rat class II monoclonal antibodies against a panel of mouse spleen cells and found a polymorphic reaction pattern which mapped the mouse target structure(s) in the I-A subregion. Falk et al. [26] prepared an A.TH anti-human class II monoclonal antibody which also reacted on mouse cells. While monomorphic on human cells, the antibody detected the Ia.7 specificity on mouse cells. However, on E^k molecules, this anti-human monoclonal antibody detected an epitope related to, but not identical with, that defined by Ia.7-specific allogeneic monoclonal antibodies. We have screened 56 mouse anti-human class II monoclonal antibodies for their lymphocytotoxic reactivity on mouse spleen cells. A polymorphic anti-class II reactivity on mouse cells was found in 15 of these xenogeneic monoclonal antibodies, of which ten were polymorphic and five monomorphic on human cells [Pla, unpublished data].

Hence, xenogeneic anti-MHC monoclonal antibodies can detect polymorphism in the immunized species itself (and in third-party species), whereas the reaction pattern on the cell donor species is monomorphic or polymorphic. The factors that regulate all these aspects of the fine specificity of xenogeneic monoclonal antibodies remain unclear. Probably, most variations are due to complex cross-reactions among the multiple epitopes of class II molecules of various regions and species. Moreover, the MHC haplotype of the immunized strain, the form of the immunogen, and immune-response genes will be involved in the regulation of the specificity of xenoimmune class II antibodies.

B. Alloimmune Class II-Specific Antibodies Detect Polymorphism Across Species Barriers

Alloimmune MHC-specific antibodies are directed against determinants that are polymorphic for the given species. In general, it is believed that most of the polymorphism developed after speciation by mechanism(s) and to extents that might be rather various for individual immunogenetic systems (compare, e.g., hemoglobin, serum protein, blood group, immunoglobulin, and MHC polymorphism). Alloimmune reagents to blood groups or Ig allotypes often do not recognize polymorphism across species barriers. The intriguing observation that alloimmune MHC antibodies frequently recognize polymorphic determinants of widely separated species is now well documented for MHC class I and class II antigens (see [36] and this review). The reactivity of alloimmune MHC antibodies across species barriers is of interest, because (a) such antibodies point to determinants that are shared by widely separated species, or (b) they point to polymorphic determinants that are not identical but express sufficient resemblance to be detected as cross-reactive target structures. The intriguing fact is that such alloimmune antibodies detect polymorphism in various species. Intraspecies polymorphism developed after speciation from a rather limited pool of genetic material – and thus with a restricted number of allelic variants – that was available at the beginning of the species. Because we do not known how large (and polymorphic) the original "founder" population was, we also do not know how much was "inherited" from ancestors and how much of the polymorphism emerged after speciation. For the human HLA-B locus alone, probably the most polymorphic locus in mammals, more than 50 alleles are known, and possibly many more exist in the total of the human species. Other genes (of comparable size), although examined on a great number of individuals from various ethnic groups, appear to be much less polymorphic. Only the number of variants, and not their frequency for a given population, illustrates the biologically significant and real extent of polymorphism for a given gene. Clearly, the explanation of the specificity of the cross-reactions of alloimmune MHC-specific antibodies is related to our understanding of the origins of MHC polymorphism in general and for every species separately.

Several other facets of interest appear in the studies of class II cross-reactions. The class II molecules are coded by a multigene family and therefore the interspecies homology (cross-reactions) for individual loci is of interest. Moreover, the mouse alloimmune anti-class II antibodies might present a special situation. Some mice (H-$2^{b,f,q,s}$) do not express E molecules (E^o). Therefore the cross-reactions of anti-E antibodies produced by E nonexpressing mice is of special interest. In fact, such alloimmune antibodies might be seen as analogous to xenoimmune antibodies. Class II antigens are important as foreign antigen-presenting structures. This function of the class II molecules is dependent on their structure, including the polymorphic determinants. Therefore it is important to examine which and how many of these functionally active determinants are shared among individuals of various species.

The ability of some alloimmune mouse class II-specific antibodies to react with human [38] and rat [72] cells was first shown in 1977. At that time biochemical studies had begun to illustrate that homologous class II molecules can be detected in several species, and a rabbit anti-human DR serum reacted with Ia-like antigen molecules from monkey, rat, mouse, guinea pig, cow, pig, and chicken lymphocytes [45]. After these initial findings, the interspecies cross-reactions of class II antigens were elaborated in various directions.

Mouse Alloimmune Class II Antibodies Cross-react with Human Cells

In 1979, three laboratories reported detailed studies on cross-reactions of alloimmune H-2 class II specific antibodies on human cells [24, 37, 53]. The potent anti-Ia^k antibodies obtained in the combination A.TH anti-A.TL (Table 4) dominated these studies. The same combination was later explored by series of monoclonal antibodies [64, 65]. Supported by panel studies, absorption experiments, sequential immunoprecipitation, direct binding assays on various cell subpopulations and comparison of sera from various other donor-recipient combinations, the following conclusions were tentatively offered:

1. E and DR are homologous.
2. A might be expected to be homologous to a second human class II region product. Subsequently, DQ was found to be homologous with A.
3. The reaction pattern of A.TH anti-A.TL antibodies on human cells is nonpolymorphic because cells from all individuals tested could be lysed.
4. Anti-E antibodies (namely anti-Ia.7) are responsible for the (strong) cytotoxic action of mouse alloimmune antibodies on human B cells.

Table 4. H-2 haplotypes of inbred mouse strains often used in work on class II interspecies cross-reactions. For various reasons, there is no expression of the E molecule on the cell surface for strains with E^b, E^f, E^q, and E^s (E^0 strains). The E^k molecule expresses public specificity Ia.7; the same determinant is present of all E cell surface molecules. This means that Ia.7 is a monomorphic public class II determinant which can be detected only by sera raised in E^0 strains. (These comments do not consider the situation in a heterozygous F1 individual)

Strain	H-2 regions				H-2 molecules			
	K	I-A	I-E	D	K	A	E	D
A. TH	s	s	s	d	K^s	A^s	E^0	D^d
A. TL	s	k	k	d	K^s	A^k	E^k	D^d

The first and second of these conclusions are fully confirmed (see sequence homology data), but the others have to be modified (see below). The reason for the situation being in fact more complex than it appeared at the beginning of these cross-reaction studies is the simple fact that A and E molecules (and DR and DQ molecules) express cross-reactive determinants by virtue of homology (and thus common origin); therefore, in principle, anti-E might cross-react with DQ and anti-A with DR molecules (monoclonal antibodies were isolated which recognize both E and A determinants). A second reason for oversimplification was the highly heterogeneous anti-E antibody population in the A.TH anti-A.TL sera. The E^k molecules express several determinants ("clusters of antigenic factors") as shown by epitope mapping by a series of monoclonal antibodies [63, 70]. Therefore, a polyvalent (serum pool) antibody population (although restricted exclusively against the E^k molecule) might have reacted with all human cells tested, although exceptions and differences between human cells in titer and affinity were noticed. Monoclonal antibodies (and to some extent sera of individual mice) partially illustrated this complex situation (see below).

Nevertheless, the anti-E^k antibodies are a predominant cross-reactive antibody population in A.TH anti-A.TL sera, and a number of interesting observations was made with these sera:

1. The anti-E antibodies broadly cross-react with class II antigens of widely different mammalian and submammalian vertebrates, such as chicken and frog. To confirm these findings, mouse (A.TH) immune sera were raised against chicken, frog, and fish lymphocytes and tested for reactivity on mouse lymphocytes. (Antixeno- cross-react with alloantigens!) The reactivity of these sera on B10.S(9R) i.e., A^s, E^k cells, located the gene encoding the cross-reactive determinant to the I-E region. From these studies, the origin of the primordial I-E gene has been traced back at least to fish [76].

2. In binding assay with isolated class II human molecules, the A.TH anti-A.TL serum reacted poorly with a class II preparation from DR7-homozygous cells [87]. This was proved by the proportion of reactive molecules. The sequential binding data on the DR7-homozygous cell preparation suggested the presence of two distinct types of DR7 molecule, one reacting and the other not reacting with the mouse serum. The alternative possibility, low affinity of A.TH anti-A.TL (anti-E^k) antibodies to DR7 molecules in general, would point to an exceptional

behavior of the DR7 molecules as the only polymorph poorly recognized by hyperimmune A.TH anti-A.TL serum antibodies. This would indicate some special feature(s) for DR7. DR7 was found associated with a rare feature of benign persistent polyclonal B-cell lymphocytosis [30], and the DR7 epitope, as defined by alloreactive antibodies, was mapped in an area on the DR molecule separate from the area where DR1, 2, and 3 were mapped [32, 85].

3. A.TH anti-A.TL sera were used to detect class II antigens in various species. These antibodies were used for the initial steps to identify class II molecules in rat [71, 72, 75], hamster [62], cattle [33], and dog [25].

4. A.TH anti-A.TL sera have the ability to eliminate subpopulations of human adherent cells and thus inhibit primary human MLRs, induction of cytotoxic lymphocytes and proliferative response to concanavalin A and purified protein derivate (PPD) [83, 91].

The Polymorphic Reaction Pattern of A.TH Anti-A.TL (Anti-Ia^k) Antibodies on Human Cells

Whereas most initial reports indicate that strong A.TH anti-A.TL antisera (pooled from a number of hyperimmunized mice) can lyse B cells (but not T cells) from all individuals tested, it was also noticed that the sera exhibit some variations in titer and binding affinity. These variations were most prominent when sera from individual mice (and not serum pools) were examined [37, 39]. Sera from individual mice lysed, in a titer higher that 1 : 10, only some of the ten human B cells tested. Therefore nine sera from individual mice were tested during an HLA workshop in four laboratories on a large panel of DR-typed B peripheral blood lymphocytes [89]. One serum was found to react significantly more weakly with DR5- and/or DR7-positive cells. Six other sera showed the same tendency. Although these results did not allow many conclusions to be drawn about the exact specificity of the serum antibodies, they showed that A.TH anti-A.TL antibodies do not exhibit a monomorphic reaction pattern on human cells due to cross-reaction with a conserved (Ia.7-like) determinant on all DR molecules.

A series of studies with monoclonal antibodies isolated from the combination A.TH anti-A.TL partially dissected the complex nature of these cross-reactions.

Pierres et al. [63, 64] produced an extensive series of 35 monoclonal antibodies from the combination A.TH anti-A.TL. These monoclonal antibodies were first characterized for specificity and epitope cluster mapping (by cross-inhibition experiments) on mouse cells. When nine of these monoclonal antibodies were tested on human cells [65] two E- and one A-specific antibody exerted a monomorphic cross-reactivity pattern on 50 human cells. However, differences between human cells in their ability to bind these monoclonal antibodies were observed. Strongly reacting human cells absorbed all reactivities against the mouse (Ia^k) cells. All monoclonal antibodies precipitated human class II molecules. The same monoclonal antibodies were also positive against rat, cow, rabbit, and hamster cells; only one (E) was positive on pig cells, and only one (A) was positive on guinea pig cells. Cross-inhibition experiments showed that the multiple cross-reactive epitope cluster specificity of the monoclonal antibodies on mouse and human cells does not always correspond. In other words, monoclonal antibodies that exhibited complete cross-inhibition on mouse (Ia^k) cells were not competitive on human cells. This indicates that monoclonal antibodies – although mutually cross-inhibiting – detect distinct determinants of the public Ia.7 specificity. These first results on mouse/human cross-reactions detected by monoclonal antibodies (a) confirmed that alloimmune class II specific mouse antibodies detect distinct epitopes on human class II molecules and (b) showed that not only E- but also A-specific antibodies cross-react [65]. When 30 monoclonal antibodies were examined on an extensive panel of human B cells, ten were found nonreactive (!), four monomorphic, and 16 polymorphic [66]. Thus (c) it was conclusively shown that A.TH anti-A.TL antibodies can exert a polymorphic reaction pattern on human cells. Again, E-, A-, and E+A-specific antibodies were found to be cross-reactive. The fine allospecificity of the antibodies on mouse cells was not predictive for the cross-reactivity pattern in human cells. The polymorphic reaction pattern on human cells did not correspond to any well-defined class II antigens. Eight polymorphic monoclonal antibodies detected supertypic and eight detected subtypic HLA-DR associated determinants. One monoclonal antibody (A+E-specific) was further characterized [67]. On murine cells the monoclonal antibody 40.B had the specificity $A^{k,b,d}+E^{k,d}$; on human cells it strongly correlated with MT1 +MT2 (DQw1 + DRw52), but did not bind, or bound only very weakly, to MT3 (DRw53, DR4,7,DRw9) cells. The fine specificity of monoclonal antibodies remained an intriguing problem. Two E-specific monoclonal antibodies were examined in detail for affinity by measuring the dissociation rate constant of labeled Fab fragments on a series of human lymphoblastoid cell lines. One antibody was found nonpolymorphic. The other showed high-avidity binding pattern only to cells with DR1, and low-avidity binding was observed to cells with all other DR types. The same phenomenon was observed by immunoprecipitation, as the polymorphic antibody precipitated a large amount of class II molecules only from DR1-positive cells [5].

One of the important conclusions of Pierres' work was that not only E-specific but also A-specific antibodies cross-react with human class II molecules. If that is so, cross-reactions of A antibodies with human DQ molecules would be expected. However, nature did not bless us with a situation that simple Hurley et al. [35] examined the molecules precipitated by A-specific monoclonal antibody (anti-$A^{k,b,t,q}$ from an A.TH anti-A.TL immunization) and found by sequencing that the precipitated molecules are DR and not DQ. Moreover, the antibody exerted a monomorphic reaction pattern on human cells. Hence, an A-specific aloimmune anti-public monoclonal antibody recognizes a monomorphic determinant on human DR molecules.

Another anti-A monoclonal antibody gave analogous results. In the combination (H-2^k × H-2^d)F_1 anti-H-2^b, an anti-A^b (anti-private) monoclonal antibody was isolated. The antibody reacted (strongly) only with A^b cells and was negative even on A^{bm12} mutant cells (the A^{bm12} mutant molecule differs from A^b only by three nucleotide substitutions at the β chain). Weak cross-reactions were observed with A^s target cells. With few exceptions, the reactivity of this monoclonal antibody on a panel of 66 human B cells correlated with the presence of HLA-DR2. In high antibody dilutions, only a fraction of DR2 cells was lysed. This suggests that a "short" or subtypic split of DR2 is detected by this anti-A^b private antibody. Among the many examples of cross-reactions exerted by alloimmune anti-Ia antibodies, this appears to be "most private" for both mouse and man and indicates the hidden and unpredictable potentials for mouse/human class II cross-reactions as detected by monoclonal antibodies [96].

However, another anti-A monoclonal antibody provides strong evidence for cross-reaction of mouse A antibodies with DQ molecules. From the alloimmunization A.TH anti-A.TL a broad public A^k (anti-Ia.17-like) monoclonal antibody was isolated which was able to precipitate human class II polypeptide chains (30 and 35 kd). Preclearance with anti-E^k serum (anti-Ia.7) antibodies did not remove the molecule precipitable by this monoclonal antibody, and vice versa. The reaction pattern on human cells was evidently monomorphic, since B peripheral blood lymphocytes from all 46 individuals tested were lysed. The monoclonal antibody also reacted with rat, guinea pig, rabbit, and dog lymphocytes [98].

The following scenario for A.TH anti-A.TL cross-reactions with human class II antigens appears probable. In the combination A.TH anti-A.TL, A-, E-, and A+E specific antibodies are induced. Any of them (and without a possible prediction on the basis of their reaction pattern on the mouse panel) might cross-react with DR or DQ molecules respectively, and possibly also cross-react with DR+DQ (and possibly also DP) determinants. However, in the A.TH anti-A.TL serum pool, E antibodies that recognize DR determinants predominate, and therefore the serum antibody pool appears to cross-react with DR molecules [87].

However, the E antibodies in A.TH anti-A.TL sera represent a special situation, because A.TH cells do not express E molecules. Because E is homologous to DR, the anti-E antibodies resemble xenoimmune "anti-DR" antibodies. This might be the reason why E antibodies in serum pools dominate the interspecies cross-reactions. Lunney et al. [54] analyzed this presumption by using monoclonal antibodies. Anti-E monoclonal antibodies isolated from the A.TH anti-A.TL combination were of four types: (a) anti-E^k private, (b) anti-E^k public polymorphic, (c) anti-E^k + A^k public polymorphic, and (d) anti-E^k public "monomorphic", i.e., reacting with all strains that express E molecules (anti-Ia.7). The species cross-reactivity was expected to be due to the latter type of E^k antibody; however, this expectation was not confirmed. Of 17 E-specific monoclonal antibodies, ten were cytotoxic on pig cells. Eight of them were of the anti-E public polymorphic type (non-Ia.7), and only two of the I-E public "monomorphic" type (Ia.7-like). A similar distribution of reactivities was also found for human cells (Table 5). However, a new aspect emerged from these detailed studies. There are three (at least) epitope clusters recognized on E (and DR) molecules desig-

Table 5. Relationship between determinant specificity and epitope specificity of A.TH anti-A.TL (anti-E^k) monoclonal antibodies for reactions on pig and human cells

MoAb	Reaction pattern on mouse cells	Specificity	Epitope cluster[a]	Cross-reactions	
				Pig	Man
E^k	private	Ia.22			
E^k	public	various	III(12)[a]	most	most
E^k+A^k	public	various			
E^k	public monomorphic	Ia.7[b]	II (2)	all	all
			I (6)	none	some

[a] Figures in parentheses are number of monoclonal antibodies tested
[b] Positive on all strains that express E molecules

nated I, II, and III [70]. Most monoclonal antibodies which exerted cross-reaction on pig (and human) cells were those specific for epitope cluster III, which is detected by the polymorphic type of public E antibody. Thus the species cross-reactions correlated better with the epitope cluster specificity of E^k antibodies (cluster III and II) than with I-E public monomorphic (i.e., Ia.7-like) specificity. The complex nature of these relationships is depicted in Table 5. The mapping and sequencing of the E (and DR) epitope cluster III might provide an explanation of some E/DR cross-reactions.

As shown in Fig. 2 and Table 2, there is a higher heterogeneity in the human class II molecular pool than in its mouse counterpart. Therefore it seemed of interest to examine the structural heterogeneity of human class II molecules by A.TH anti-A.TL antibodies. Class II molecules precipitated by 11 monoclonal antibodies (six E, two A, and three E+A) were heterogenous. All 11 monoclonal antibodies precipitated DR-like (29–32 kd) molecules. However, two E, two A, and one E+A monoclonal antibodies recognized a broader family of human class II molecules, including DQ-like (28–30 kd) molecules. These results did not allow to conclude whether the various molecules (26, 28, 29, 30, and 32 kd) are coded by different genes. The results indicate that A.TH anti-A.TL monoclonal antibodies might provide a powerful tool to dissect the heterogeneity of the human class II pool [1, 2, 6].

As shown by the extensive data referred to above, most experiments on mouse/human cross-reactions were performed with anti-Ia^k antibodies from the A.TH anti-A.TL immunization. These sera were found mostly positive in the initial studies. The anti-Ia^s sera from the opposite combination A.TL anti-A.TH were found negative [37, 53] or weakly positive [24]. Uemura and Yano [88] obtained A.TL anti-A.TH (anti-A^s) serum antibodies positive with antigen-presenting cells and able to block the PPD-specific proliferative response of human peripheral blood lymphocytes by eliminating antigen-presenting cells. These variable results might be due to differences between the strength of the antibodies in various serum pools, or to the high expression of human class II molecules on antigen-presenting cells.

In general, only a limited number of donor/recipient combinations of mouse strain for class II antibodies was examined for cross-reactions on human cells [24, 37, 53, 90]. Gasser et al. [28] produced a rat monoclonal antibody (by fusion with mouse myeloma cells) directed against rat class II antigens. This rat alloimmune monoclonal antibody also reacted with most mouse strains and B cells of all (14) human donors tested.

Anti-DR Serum Antibodies Cross-react with Mouse Class II (E) Molecules

Of 14 human alloreactive anti-DR sera (anti-DR1,2,3,4,5,w6,7), 12 reacted positively with mouse B cells. Tests on H-2 congeneic and recombinant strains and blocking studies with E antibodies tentatively mapped the target molecules to the I-E region. These antibodies were too weak for immunoprecipitation, and mouse spleen cells were unable to absorb activity against human B cells, indicating that only some of the antibodies were cross-reactive with the mouse class II molecules. An apparent cross-reactivity between certain DR and mouse Ia antigens was not ascertained. The serum with a broadest reactivity on mouse cells contained anti-DR7 antibodies [90].

Class II Interspecies Cross-Reactions Detected by T Cell Receptors

Xenoreactive Anti-Class II T Cells

A high frequency of T cells responds to allogeneic MHC antigens. This response comprises a bias by restricting the killer function to class I antigens and the helper function to class II antigens. This dichotomy in the association between T cell function and the class of the MHC molecules (and the respective markers of the responding T cells) is recognized and also operates across species barriers. The separation is known not to be absolute, but for the assays used, dominated the overall response. Therefore, human cytotoxic lymphocytes are generated to mouse class I antigens (and vice versa) [50, 89], whereas a proliferative response can be measured against xenogeneic class II antigens [51, 84].

Class II antigens stimulate T cells in the primary allogeneic MLR and restimulate specifically a proliferative response in secondary primed lymphocyte test (PLT) MLR. Lindahl and Bach [51] studied the response of human lymphocytes to mouse cells in PLT. Human lymphocytes recognized, by a strong secondary response, only those lymphocytes that had the I-A region structure of the original stimulator cells. Thus, human T cell receptors specifically recognized private murine A antigens. Analogous results were obtained by Boylston and Anderson [13] and Carnaud et al. [17]. Swain et al. [84] examined the specificity of the induction of interleukin-2 (IL-2) production in the human anti-mouse combination, which appeared to be specific for stimulator A^b molecule. Interestingly, A^b and A^{bm12} mutant cells restimulated equally well, but the A^k molecule could not restimulate. Experiments with cells from four human donors gave similar results.

In variance with the specificity of the human anti-mouse secondary proliferative responses, in the mouse anti-human secondary and tertiary xenogeneic MLR, class II-positive cells from whichever of six human blood donors could be recognized equally well by primed mouse cells [100]. The proliferative response was blocked by monoclonal anti-DR antibodies. Thus, the murine T cells recognized a shared determinant(s) of DR antigens. The suggested determinants were coined as common part(s) of DR antigens. However, it is not clear whether the shared common DR determinant(s) are species-specific or represent "long" public determinants (e.g., DRw52,53). These problems will probably be examined at the clonal level.

Alloreactive Anti-Class II T Cells

Martinis and Bach [55, 56] sensitized human lymphocytes with a pool of 20 allogeneic stimulator cells. Xenogeneic monkey, dog, and cattle (but not mouse) cells induced significant restimulation. Lymphocytes from rhesus monkeys restimulated human cells specifically for LK1 (Dw3). These results indicate the allospecific T cell receptors (class II specific) recognize alloantigens from widely separated species. However, in comparison with serological data (see this review), little is known about the interspecies cross-reactivity of alloimmune anti-class II T cell receptors.

Self-Class II-Restricted T Cells

Yamamoto and Yano [97] examined the specificity of interspecies sharing of antigen-presenting determinants. Two human cell donors were selected with class II antigens on antigen-presenting cells known to cross-react with anti-A^s and E^k antibodies [59, 88]. Individual A was E^{k+}, A^{k-}, and E^k antibodies blocked antigen presentation by syngeneic cells; individual B was A^{s+}, E^{k-}, and A^s-specific antibodies blocked antigen presentation by syngeneic cells. The cross-reactions were examined in both directions. PPD-specific T cells from individuals A and B were not stimulated by PPD-pulsed A^sE^k [B10.S(9R)] cells. On the contrary, B10.S(9R) T cells primed to PPD were stimulated by PPD-pulsed human A and B cells. In other terms, human antigen-presenting cells express a nonpolymorphic (?) determinant suitable for triggering of mouse PPD-specific T cells. However, the class II specificity on the human cells was not examined in detail. Murine antigen-presenting cells lack a determinant suitable for triggering of human PPD-specific cells, although they share a cross-reactive determinant recognized by antibodies.

Waters et al. [92] found at the clonal level that human cells can stimulate an I-E-restricted murine T-cell clone. A CB6F1 murine T cell hybridoma exhibited E-restricted response (IL-2 secretion) to keyhole limpet haemocyanin (KLH). Cells from ten of 30 humans presented KLH (but elicited no response in absence of KLH). The ability to present KLH segregated in families with the HLA haplotype and correlated significantly with the presence of MT3 (DRw53, i.e., DR4,7,w9). There was also a significant correlation with a determinant detected on the human cells by an E^k (anti-Ia.22)-specific monoclonal antibody. The monoclonal anti-E antibody inhibited IL-2 production by blocking of KLH presentation by murine and all human cells. However, although the ability of human cells to present KLH correlated strongly with MT3 and/or with the presence of an E-like determinant (Ia.22) for neither of them was the correlation perfect. These results at the clonal T-cell level clearly show that E-restricted murine T cells can recognize foreign antigen (KLH) presentation by a related polymorphic human class II determinant. The data conclusively show that polymorphic MHC molecules in widely separated species share determinants of the same function. Such finding(s) support the view, that MHC polymorphism might have been developed by the action of common (interspecies) selective forces.

Discussion Without Conclusion: Significance and Perspectives of Interspecies Class II Cross-Reactions

The MHC appears to be the most polymorphic genetic system. In several species the linkage group is analogous and the gene products exert a high degree of homology. Therefore, xenoimmune sera cross-react with MHC molecules of various distant species. Strong sera are useful for isolation of the respective molecules or separation of subsets of lymphocytes. The specificity of most (xenoimmune) sera is monomorphic or broad. However, the registers of monoclonal antibodies show that antibodies of restricted specificity can also be found. We could not find data to guide us to produce antibodies of predicted or desired specificity.

Biochemical studies show that E/DR and A/DQ are homologous. Much more complicated and uncertain are conclusions about the fine specificity of individual cross-reacting antibodies. Certainly, anti-E antibodies recognize DR molecules. However, sharing of determinants among the subsets of class II molecules appears to be extensive, and therefore the fine specificity of cross-reaction is very complex. Whether this high degree of determinant sharing among the various subsets of class II molecules will refute or reinforce the usefulness of species cross-reactions in further work depends on more experience and also on the aim of certain experiments. In general, class II molecules appear more cross-reactive than class I molecules. However, we might be biased by the special circumstances under which A.TH anti-A.TL antibodies are induced (the recipient strain does not express E molecules).

The study on interspecies class II cross-reactions pointed to several interesting findings and problems, most of which have been already discussed in this review. New and barely explored questions are introduced by the finding that not only antibodies, but also T cell receptors, recognize determinants across species barriers in class II-restricted foreign antigen recognition. The function of class II molecules is to present foreign antigens to T helper cells. The responder T cells must share MHC determinants with the antigen-presenting cells in order to be able to recognize the foreign antigen. The restriction is a requirement for identical or almost identical structures between the responder and antigen-presenting cells. In many systems only syngeneic (autologous) molecules are able to fulfill this requirement; in terms of the human situation, this means sharing of identical class II molecules between the donor of responder and the donor of antigen-presenting cells. Recent data show, surprisingly, that some class II molecules express such a high degree of homology across widely distant species barriers that they are recognized by xenogeneic (responder) T cells. Antibodies "easily" cross-react (in spite of their specificity) with structures that sufficiently "resemble" the immunogen, but T cell receptors involved in MHC-restricted recognition of nominal (foreign) antigens appeared to behave much more specifically. In most experimental systems, identity in MHC molecules is required between responder and antigen-presenting cells. Do mouse and human class II molecules really share identical determinants (as indicated by shared restriction elements), or is cross-species antigen presentation permitted by such a high degree of homology (not identity, but resemblance) that the T cell receptor is somehow blinded? The need for a conclusive answer to this basic question in immunology is a sufficient reason to continue with the analysis of the interspecies comparative aspects of MHC antigens. Evolutionary aspects of sharing of functionally unique and important molecules provide new perspectives for the understanding of the biological role of MHC polymorphism.

The intriguing and unique nature of MHC cross-reactions has already emerged from serological studies. Beside the extreme polymorphism of MHC genes and the structural homology across widely distant species barriers stands the unique feature of extensive interspecies cross-reactions exerted by alloimmune antibodies. There are almost no similar data in other polymorphic systems. Immunoglobulin molecules are also homologous, but alloreactive anti-immunoglobulin antibodies only exceptionally detect polymorphism (allotypes) in widely distant species [61]. For alloimmune MHC antibodies, recognition of polymorphism in distant species is not regular (?), but at least frequent. This was first found for class I alloimmune antibodies and appears even more frequent for class II antibodies. The explanation of this serological phenomenon is unclear and closely related to the inherent problem about how polymorphism in individual species developed. Alloantibodies are directed against intraspecies antigenic variations; in other words, they detect variations that are unique for the given species; see the extensive tables of the WHO-HLA nomenclature committee, which still show only a part of the HLA iceberg. Compare these extensive HLA tables with the even more extensive H-2 antigen charts. Do these charts identify shared determinants or determinants of sufficient resemblance which are recognized, sometimes in very specific manner – by antibodies and T cell receptors – across species barriers?

There are various theories about the origin of MHC polymorphism. Bodmer [9] proposed that individuals of various species share a quasi-complete set of homologous genes, and that if two identical genes are derepressed, their products can be recognized by alloimmune antibodies. Klein [43, 44] proposed an alternative explanation: Whereas Bodmer's model started with the assumption that the situation for the MHC is analogous to that in other immunogenetic systems, Klein proposes a special situation. According to his view, the development of MHC polymorphism is different from that of other polymorphic systems. Because the MHC genes were extensively polymorphic in the preceding species, the new species will "inherit" a great part of the original polymorphism. This means that the polymorphism flows along with evolution, and the same, or slightly modified, molecule(s) or allele(s) spread along the evolutinary tree (Fig. 4).

We presume that the major part of MHC polymorphism develops after speciation from the rather restricted genetic pool inherited by the new species. This is illustrated in Fig. 4. The difference between the various proposals might be only numerical, but if the founders of a new species inherited not much more than 2–10 alleles, then the existence of more than 100 at later stages of the species evolution says that most (if not all) polymorphism of distant species is divergent. If so, how can alloimmune antibodies (and self-restricted T cell receptors) recognize polymorphism across species barriers?

Two possibilities are apparent. In the first, the allelic forms are only minor variations on a given theme which nevertheless retains sufficient homology for alloan-

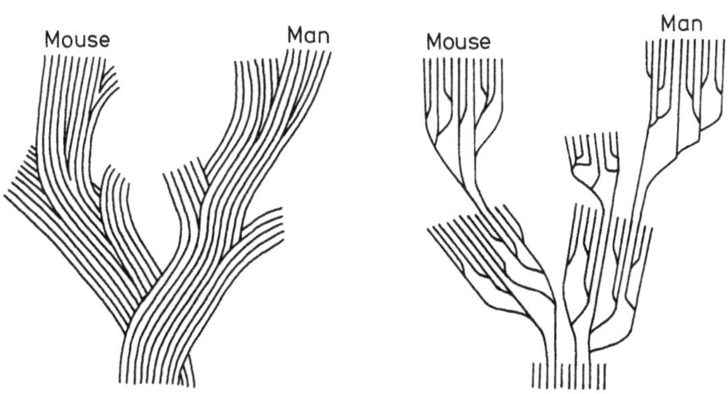

Fig. 4. Two hypotheses of MHC gene evolution. *Left:* MHC alleles evolve independently of speciation from heterogeneous gene pools (Klein [43, 44]. *Right:* The generation of alleles appears after speciation using rather limited gene pools. (In the figure, the extreme situation – one homozygous breeding pair – is presented.)

tibodies raised against analogous variations in other species to recognize them by virtue of cross-reactions. A chance component is involved which regulates the extent of these variations and stratification. This would expose the polymorphism of MHC as comparable with some of the masterpieces of Johan Sebastian Bach's variations on a theme. Another possibility is that for some common reasons, such as continuous exposure to certain pathogens, various species developed and retained by selection (from the enormous pool of possibilities) identical or almost identical determinants: they are good for the same functional role(s). This might appear as innocent or unconscious mutual plagiarism, similar to e.g., that of Braque and Picasso (E/DR sharing of determinants). We can hardly imagine how this might happen.

Some possibilities of the mechanism have been discussed in previous reviews [14, 36]. Certainly some polymorphism develops by mutation. Schematically, a point mutation will produce one public and one private allodeterminant. The anti-public antibody will gain a broad chance to detect homologous determinants in various species. Subsequent mutations at the same residue position and at other positions will create a number of polymorphic determinants. Antibodies against some of them will cross-react across species barriers. Other knowledge emerges from the new information coming from molecular biology. Recent data indicate that MHC polymorphism may arise by gene-conversion-like events between nonallelic MHC genes. This involves the transfer of a DNA segment from one gene to another gene (of the same related class) on the same chromosome. For class I antigens this was illustrated by the origin of some K^b mutants from a common donor gene reservoir. Possibly, some (nonexpressed or expressed) MHC genes are transferred during evolution from one species to another without many variations. However, such (hidden) donor genes might become the "donors" of homologous stretches of DNA. If the same event has happened in various species, cross-reactive determinants will also be found in distant species. While this possibility appears as a general scenario, little is yet known about the actual mechanism, origin, and extent of gene-conversion-like events. For both alternatives and probably other mechanisms of generation of diversity [16], the possibility appears that some determinants in various species are maintained and/or selected for functional reasons. This possibility is now strongly supported by the finding that determinants of shared function have been detected in mouse and man by functional assays [92, 97, 99]. Foreign antigen presentation involves specific determinants of MHC molecules. If so, and if at least for a limited array, the vital enemies of mouse, cattle, and man were identical or homologous, then selective forces will lead to the occurrence of these – albeit cross-reactive – determinants in various species.

This review shows that the phenomenon of MHC class II interspecies cross-reactions provides some facts, exposes a very complex situation, and is sometimes the subject of wild speculations. In fact, though, we derive pleasure from the continued existence of facets of MHC which are difficult to understand.

References

1. Accolla RS, Pierres M (1983) Structural heterogeneity of the human Ia molecular pool as detected by cross-reacting mouse monoclonal antibodies. J Immunol 130:283–288
2. Accolla RS, Birnbaum D, Pierres M (1983) The importance of cross-reactions between species: mouse allo-anti-Ia monoclonal antibodies as a powerful tool to define human Ia subsets. Hum Immunol 8:75–82
3. Beckman I (1984) Monoclonal antibodies to HLA-DR antigens. Immunol Today 5:29–32
4. Bhattacharya A, Dorf ME, Springer A (1981) A shared alloantigenic determinant on Ia antigens encoded by the I-A and I-E subregions: evidence for gene duplication. J Immunol 127:2488–2495
5. Birnbaum D, Dosseto M, Bourge F, Pierres M, Kourilsky FM (1982) A cross-reactive mouse anti-IE^k monoclonal antibody detects an HLA-DR polymorphism linked to HLA-DR1. Mol Immunol 19:755–764
6. Birnbaum D, Rohner C, Dubreuil P, Bourge F, Pierres M, Goridis C (1983) Mouse monoclonal anti-Ia antibodies recognize cross-reacting determinants expressed on distinct subsets of human Ia-like cell-surface molecules. Mol Immunol 20:511–520
7. Blankenhorn EP, Cecka JM, Frelinger J, Götze D, Hood L (1980) Structure of Ia antigens from the rat. Mouse alloantisera demonstrate at least two distinct molecular species. Eur J Immunol 10:145–151
8. Blankenhorn EP, Symington FW, Cramer V (1983) Biochemical characterization of Ia antigens encoded by the RT1.B and RT1.D loci in the rat MHC. Immunogenetics 17:475–484
9. Bodmer WF (1973) A new genetic model for allelism at histocompatibility and other complex loci: polymorphism for control of gene expression. Transplant Proc 5:1471–1475
10. Bodmer JG, Bodmer WF (1984) Histocompatibility 1984. Immunol Today 5:251–254
11. Bodmer JG, Kennedy L, Aizawa M, Dawkins R, Lepage V, Mazzilli MC, Richiardi P (1984) HLA-D region monoclonal antibodies. In: Albert ED, Baur MP, Mayr WR (eds) Histocompatibility testing 1984. Springer, Berlin Heidelberg New York Tokyo, pp 217–236
12. Bono MR, Strominger J (1982) Direct evidence of homology between human DC-1 antigen and murine I-A molecules. Nature 299:836–838
13. Boylston AW, Anderson RL (1978) Human-mouse mixed lymphocyte cultures. Immunology 35:455–461
14. Brodsky FM, Parham P (1982) Evolution of HLA antigenic determinants: species cross-reactions of monoclonal antibodies. Immunogenetics 15:151–166
15. Brodsky FM, Stone WH, Parham P (1981) Of cows and men: a comparative study of histocompatibility antigens. Hum Immunol 3:143–152
16. Burnside SS, Hunt P, Ozato K, Sears DW (1984) A molecular hybrid of the H-2D^d and H-2L^d genes expressed in the dm1 mutant. Proc Natl Acad Sci USA 81:5204–5208
17. Carnaud C, Fadai-Ghotbi M, Lesavre P, Bach JF (1977) Education of human lymphocytes against mouse cells: specific recognition of H-2. Eur J Immunol 7:81–85
18. Chardon P, Kalil J, Leveziel H, Colombani J, Vaiman M (1983) Monoclonal antibodies to HLA recognize monomorphic and polymorphic epitope on BoLA. Tissue Antigens 22:62–71
19. Colombani J, Lepage V (1984) HLA monoclonal antibody registry: third listing. Tissue Antigens 24:209–214
20. Colombani J, Dausset J, Lepage V, Degos L, Kalil J, Fellous M (1982) HLA monoclonal antibody registry: a proposal. Tissue Antigens 20:161–171
21. Colombani J, Lepage V, Kalil J (1983) HLA monoclonal antibody registry: second listing. Tissue Antigens 22:97–106
22. Crone M, Jensenius J, Koch C (1981) Evidence for two populations of B-L (Ia-like) molecules encoded by the chicken MHC. Immunogenetics 13:381–391

23. Deeg HJ, Wulff JC, Derese S, Sale GE, Braum M, Brown MA, Springmeyer SC, Martin PJ, Storb R (1982) Unusual distribution of Ia-like antigens on canine lymphocytes. Immunogenetics 16:445–457
24. Delovitch TL, Falk JA (1979) Evidence for structural homology between murine and human Ia antigens. Immunogenetics 8:405–418
25. Doveren RFC, Buurman WA, Schutte B, Greenewegen G, Van Der Linden CJ (1985) Class II antigens on canine T lymphocytes. Tissue Antigens 25:255–265
26. Falk JA, Addis JBL, Letarte M (1983) Species cross-reactive Ia determinants: detection with a monoclonal antibody to human Ia of murine Ia.7 epitope. Hum Immunol 7:79–88
27. Fuge Abruzzini LNK, Schwartz BD (1982) Tentative assignment of alleles for guinea pig Ia antigens. 1. Ia.3,5 and Ia.4,5 share structural homology expected for alleles. J Immunol 128:2682–2690
28. Gasser DL, Winters BA, Haas JB, McKearn TJ, Kennett RH (1979) Monoclonal antibody directed to a B-cell antigen present in rats, mice and humans. Proc Natl Acad Sci USA 76:4636–4640
29. Gill TJ, Cramer DV, Kunz HW, Misra DN (1983) Structure and function of the major histocompatibility complex of the rat. J Immunogenet 10:261–273
30. Gordon DS, Jones BM, Browning SW, Spira TJ, Lawrence DN (1982) Persistent polyclonal lymphocytosis of B lymphocytes. N Engl J Med 307:232–236
31. Goyert SM, Silver J (1981) Isolation of I-A subregion-like molecules from subhuman primates and man. Nature 294:266–268
32. Grumet FC, Charron DJ, Fendly BM, Levyr R, Ness DB (1980) HLA-DR epitope region definition by use of monoclonal antibody probes. J Immunol 125:2785–2789
33. Hoang-Xuan M, Charron D, Zilber MT, Levy D (1982) Biochemical characterization of class II bovine major histocompatibility complex antigens using cross-species reactive antibodies. Immunogenetics 15:621–624
34. Hood L, Steinmetz M, Malissen B (1983) Genes of the major histocompatibility complex of the mouse. Annu Rev Immunol 1:529–568
35. Hurley CK, Pierres M, Capra JD (1982) A murine anti-IA^k monoclonal antibody recognizes human DR (IE-like) antigens. Hum Immunol 6:199–205
36. Ivanyi P (1981) Interspecies MHS relationships studied by serological and cellular cross-reactions. In: Reisfeld RA, Ferrone SS (eds) Current trends in histocompatibility, vol 1. Plenum, New York, pp 133–181
37. Ivanyi P, van Mourik P (1979) Murine anti-H-$2I^k$ sera exhibit a strong cytotoxic effect on human B lymphocytes. Immunogenetics 9:591–596
38. Ivanyi P, Gyody E, Gyorffy G, Pavljukova H, Ivaskova E, Petranyi G (1977) Cytotoxic effect of anti-H-2 and anti-Ia antisera on human B and T cells. Scand J Immunol 6:431–437
39. Ivanyi P, van den Berg-Loonen EM, de Greeve P (1978) Individual mice of one inbred strain produce anti-H-2 and anti-HLA antibodies of different specificities. Tissue Antigens 12:32–38
40. Ivaskova E, Dausset J, Ivanyi P (1972) Cytotoxic reactions of anti-H-2 sera with human lymphocytes. Folia Biol (Praha) 18:194–197
41. Ivaskova E, Ivanyi P, Mickova M, Demant P (1975) Cross-reactions between the major histocompatibility system of man and mice (HL-A and H-2): Cytotoxic action of anti-H-2 sera on lymphocytes. Tissue Antigens 6:286–311
42. Klareskog L, Tragardh L, Lindblom JB, Peterson PA (1978) Reactivity of a rabbit antiserum against highly purified HLA-DR antigens. Scand J Immunol 7:199–208
43. Klein J (1980) Generation of diversity at MHC loci: implications for T cell receptor repertoires. In: Fougereau M, Dausset J (eds) Immunology 80. Academic, London, pp 239–253 (Progress in immunology IV, vol 1)
44. Klein J (1982) Evolution and function of the major histocompatibility complex. In: Parham P, Strominger J (eds) Receptors and recognition. Histocompatibility antigens. Chapman and Hall, London, pp 221–240
45. Kvist S, Ostberg D, Petersen PA (1978) Reactions and cross-reactions of a rabbit anti-H-2 antigen serum. Scand J Immunol 7:265–276
46. Lafuse WP, David CS (1984) Ia antigens. Genes, molecules, and function. Transplantation 38:443–453

47. Larhammar D, Schenning L, Gustafsson K, Wiman K, Claesson L, Rask L, Peterson PA (1982) Complete amino acid sequence of a HLA-DR antigen-like β chain as predicted from the nucleotide sequence: Similarities with immunoglobulins and HLA-A, -B, and -C antigens. Proc Natl Acad Sci USA 79:3687–3691
48. Larhammar D, Hammerling U, Denaro M, Lund T, Flavell RA, Rask L, Peterson PA (1983) Structure of the murine immune response I-Aβ locus: sequence of the I-Aβ gene an adjacent β-chain second domain exon. Cell 34:179–188
49. Letesson JJ, Coppet, Lostrie-Trussart N, Depelchina A (1983) Bovine "Ia-like" antigen detected by a xenogeneic monoclonal antibody. Anim Blood Groups Biochem Genet 14:239–240
50. Lindahl KF, Bach FH (1975) Human lympocytes recognize mouse alloantigens. Nature 254:607–609
51. Lindahl KF, Bach FH (1976) Genetic and cellular aspects of xenogeneic mixed leukocyte culture reaction. J Exp Med 144:305–318
52. Long EO, Gorski J, Mach B (1984) Structural relationship of the SB β-chain gene to HLA-D region genes and murine I-region genes. Nature 310:233–235
53. Lunney JK, Mann DL, Sachs DH (1979) Sharing of Ia antigens between species. III. Ia specificities shared between mice and human beings. Scand J Immunol 10:403–413
54. Lunney JK, Osborne BA, Sharrow SO, Devaux C, Pierres M, Sachs DH (1983) Sharing of Ia antigens between species. IV. Interspecies cross-reactivity of monoclonal antibodies directed against polymorphic mouse Ia determinants. J Immunol 130:2786–2793
55. Martinis J, Bach FH (1977a) Human LD antigens are present on xenogeneic cells. Nature 266:540–542
56. Martinis J, Bach FH (1977b) LD sharing between species. Transplant Proc 9:1235–1237
57. McMaster WR, Williams AF (1979) Identification of Ia glycoproteins in rat thymus and purification from rat spleen. Eur J Immunol 9:426–433
58. Neppert J, Mueller-Eckhardt C (1984) Monoclonal mouse antibodies to human MHC class I antigens cocap class II antigens. Tissue Antigens 24:187–189
59. Okubo Y, Kusama S, Yamashita Y, Kitazawa K, Nagasaka M, Yano A (1983) Serological cross-reactivity of murine A.TH anti-A.TL antibody (anti-IE^k antibody) with Ia-like molecules of human antigen-presenting cells. Cell Immunol 76:1–9
60. Parish CR, McKenzie IFC (1978) A detailed serological analysis of xenogeneic anti-Ia serum. Immunogenetics 6:183–196
61. Parsons M, Herzenberg LA (1981) Monoclonal mouse anti-allotype antibody reacts with certain human and other vertebrate immunoglobulins: genetic and phylogenetic findings. Immunogenetics 12:207–219
62. Phillips JT, Duncan WR, Klein J, Wayne-Streilein J (1979) Immunochemical detection of hamster class II MHC homologues by murine anti-Ia^k sera. Immunogenetics 9:477–486
63. Pierres M, Kourilsky FM, Rebouah JP, Dosseto M, Caillol D (1980) Distinct epitopes on I^k gene products identified by monoclonal antibodies. Eur J Immunol 10:950–957
64. Pierres M, Devaux C, Dosseto M, Marchetto S (1981) Clonal analysis of B and T cell responses to Ia antigens. I. Topology of epitope regions on IA^k and IE^k molecules analyzed with 35 monoclonal antibodies. Immunogenetics 14:481–495
65. Pierres M, Rebouah JP, Kourilsky FM, Dosseto M, Mercier P, Mawas C, Malissen B (1981) Cross-reactions between mouse Ia and human HLA-D/DR antigens analyzed with monoclonal alloantibodies. J Immunol 126:2424–2429
66. Pierres M, Mercier P, Madsen M, Mawas C, Kristensen T (1982) Monoclonal mouse anti-IA^k and anti-IE^k antibodies cross-reacting with HLA-DR supertypic and subtypic determinants rather than classical dR allelic specificities. Tissue Antigens 19:289–300
67. Pierres M, Lafuse WP, Dosseto M, Devaux C, Birnbaum DZ, David CS (1982) Molecular specificity of a monoclonal anti-I^k alloantibody identifying a highly conserved determinant on mouse IA, IE, and human DR antigens. Tissue Antigens 20:208–220

68. Pollack MS, Mastrota F, Chin-Louise J, Mooney S, Hayes A (1982) Preliminary studies of the feline histocompatibility system. Immunogenetics 16:339–347
69. Radka SF, Amos DB, Quackenbush LJ, Cresswell P (1984) HLA-DR7-specific monoclonal antibodies and a chimpanzee anti-DR7 serum detect different epitopes on the same molecule. Immunogenetics 19:63–70
70. Rebai N, Malissen B, Pierres M, Accolla RS, Corte G, Mawas C (1983) Distinct HLA-DR epitopes and distinct families of HLA-DR molecules defined by 15 monoclonal antibodies (mAb) either anti-DR or allo-anti-Ia^k cross-reacting with human DR molecule. I. Cross-inhibition studies of mAb cell surface fixation and differential binding of mAb to detergent solubilized HLA molecules immobilized to a solid phase by a first mAb. Eur J Immunol 13:106–111
71. Rozing J, Vaessen LMB, Ewijk van W, Lameijer LDF (1979) Cross-reactivity between mouse Ia antigens and rat Ia-like antigens as determined by monoclonal anti-mouse Ia.A^k antibodies. Transplant Proc 11:1574–15576
72. Sachs DH, Humphrey GW, Lunney JK (1977) Sharing of Ia antigens between species. I. Detection of Ia specificities shared by rats and mice. J Exp Med 146:381–393
73. Shalev A, Pla M, Ginsburger-Vogel T, Echalier G, Logdberg L, Bjorck L, Colombani J, Segal S (1983) Evidence for beta-2-microglobulin-like and H-2-like antigenic determinants in *Drosophila.* J Immunol 130:297–302
74. Shaw S, Ziegler A, Demars R (1985) Specificity of monoclonal antidoes directed against human and murine class II histocompatibility antigens as analysed by binding to HLA-deletion mutant cell lines. Hum Immunol 12:191–212
75. Shinohara N, Lunney JK, Sachs DH (1978) Sharing of Ia antigens between species. II. Molecular localization of shared Ia determinants implies the existence of more than one I sublocus of the rat MHC. J Immunol 121:637–640
76. Shinohara N, Sachs DH, Nonaka N, Yamamoto H (1981) Phylogenetic tracing of Ia genes. Nature 292:362–363
77. Silver J, Walker LE, Reisfeld RA, Pellegrino MA, Ferrone S (1979) Structural studies of murine I-E and human DR antigens. Mol Immunol 16:37–42
78. Solheim BG, Fuks A, Smith L, Strominger JL, Thorsby E (1978) Possible detection of HLA-DR alloantigenic specificities in man with unabsorbed rabbit antisera. Scand J Immunol 8:15–20
79. Spooner RL, Ferrone S (1984) Cross reaction of monoclonal antibodies to human MHC class I and class II products with bovine lymphocyte subpopulations. Tissue Antigens 24:270–277
80. Steel CM (1984) Human MHC class II antigens: genetics, structure and function. Dis Markers 2
81. Sterkers G, Henin Y, Kalil J, Bagot M, Levy JP (1983) Influence of HLA class I and class II-specific monoclonal antibodies on DR-restricted lymphoproliferative responses. J Immunol 131:2735–2740
82. Sung E, Duncan WR, Streilen JW, Jones PP (1982) Detection of two distinct class II α:β:Ii complexes in the Syrian hamster. Immunogenetics 16:425–433
83. Suzuki T, Ochiai T, Taniguchi M, Shinohara N (1983) The ability of interspecies cross-reactive anti-Ia murine alloantibodies to eliminate a subpopulation of human adherent cells responsible for induction of alloimmunity. Transplantation 35:368–373
84. Swain SL, Dutton RW, Schwab R, Yamamoto J (1983) Xenogeneic human anti-mouse T cell subsets responsible for allospecific and major histocompatibility complex restricted responses. J Exp Med 157:720–729
85. Taylor CG, Grumet FC (1982) HLA-DR antigen grouping by use of monoclonal antibody probes: expansion of known groups, and mechanism of cytotoxicity blocking. J Immunol 128:1489–1490
86. Thistlewaite JR, Pennington DR, Lunney JK, Sachs DH (1983) Immunological characterization of MHC recombinant swine. Transplantation 35:394–400
87. Tosi R, Tanigaki N, Sorrentino R, van Mourik P, Ivanyi P (1982) Human Ia molecules carrying DC1 or BR4X7 determinants are not homologous to murine IE molecules. Immunogenetics 16:187–199
88. Uemura K, Yano A (1982) Serological cross-reactivity of murine allo-anti-Ia^s antibody with the molecule on human antigen-presenting cells. Immunol Lett 5:293–299

89. van Mourik P, Petranyi G, Gyodi E, Lindblom B, Holmlund G, Kastelan A, van den Rijden HJ, Ivanyi P (1983) Allo-immune anti-Ia^k sera of individual mice detect HLA-DR associated polymorphism on human B cells. Tissue Antigens 22:134–141
90. Vaughan HA, Sandrim MS, McKenzie IFC, Tait BD, Ting A (1981) Cross-reactions of Ia antigens between mouse and man. Hum Immunol 2:113–123
91. Watanabe M, Suzuki T, Taniguchi M, Shinohara N (1983) Monoclonal anti-Ia murine alloantibodies crossreactive with the Ia homologous of other mammalian species including humans. J Immunol 36:712–718
92. Waters SJ, Winchester RJ, Nagase F, Thorbecke GJ, Bona CA (1984) Antigen presentation by murine and human cells to a murine T-cell hybridoma: demonstration of a restriction element associated with a major histocompatibility complex class II determinant(s) shared by both species. Proc Natl Acad Sci USA 81:7559–7563
93. Wettstein PJ, Frelinger JG, Hood L (1981) Serological and biochemical characterization of rat (RT1) class I molecules with restricted mouse anti-Ia sera. Immunogenetics 13:93–107
94. White PC, New MI, Dupont B (1984a) HLA linked congenital adrenal hyperplasia results from a defective gene encoding a cytochrome P-450 specific for steroid 21-hydroxylation. Proc Natl Acad Sci USA 81:7507–7509
95. White PC, Chaplin DD, Weis JH, Dupont B, New ML, Seidman JG (1984b) Two steroid 21-hydroxylase genes are located in the murine S region. Nature 312:465–467
96. Wong DM, Skelly RR, Walsh WD, Ahmed A, Mittal KK (1985) An anti-I-A murine monoclonal antibody which cross-reacts with HLA-DR2. Hum Immunol 12:37–45
97. Yamamoto M, Yano A (1984) Serological and biological cross-reactivity of class II antigens between mice and humans in antigen-specific T-cell proliferative responses. Cell Immunol 87:659–673
98. Yamamoto K, Kumagai Y, Hiramatsu K, Okumura K, Tada T (1983) I-A homologous antigen on human lymphocytes detected by a monoclonal antibody. Immunogenetics 17:101–108
99. Yano Y, Yabu K, Yuji K, Yamashita K, Aosai F (1984) Interspecies cross-reactivity of class II antigens of MHC determined by syngeneic, allogeneic, and xenogeneic B and T cells. Immunobiology 168:154–166
100. Yoshizawa K, Yano A (1984) Mouse T lymphocytes proliferative responses specific for human MHC products in mouse anti-human xenogeneic MLR. J Immunol 132:2820–2829

Differences Between Ethnic Groups

Human Class II Antigen in Different Ethnic Groups *

K. Tsuji, K. Sato, Y. Nose, H. Inoko, T. Nakatsuji, A. Ando, and N. Ikewaki

Table of Contents

Introduction

The history and the development of HLA-ology over the past 35 years can be roughly classified into four stages, as shown in Table 1. The fourth stage, from 1981 up to date, may be called one of revision. After the Ninth International Histocompatibility Workshop [1], biochemical and molecular genetic analyses of the genes and gene products associated with the class II D region revealed the existence of at least three subregions, DR, DQ, and DP, each of which consists of a noncovalently associated α and β chain [10].

This chapter, deals with HLA class II antigens from populations in various parts of the world, including Asia, Oceania, and Japan, and the complexity of HLA-Dw4 regions in Japanese.

* This work was supported in part by the Ministry of Welfare and Health and a grant from Tokai University

Table 1. A history of HLA and its development

Stage	Time	International workshop (chairman)	Remarks	Methodology and application
I Period of discovery	1951 ~ 1960		Discovery of HLA antigen by J. Dausset, R. Payne, J. J. van Rood	Leukoagglutination Cytotoxicity Complement fixation
II Period of growth	1961 ~ 1970	1st, 1964 (D. B. Amos) 2nd, 1965 (J. J. van Rood) 3rd, 1967 (R. Ceppellini) 4th, 1970 (P. I. Terasaki)	Establishment of HLA typing Clinical application: Kidney transplantation (Hamburger, Terasaki) Disease association (Amiel et al.) Immune response (Levine, Marsh, et al.)	Microlymphocytotoxicity HLA typing: SD, LD
III Period of development	1971 ~ 1980	5th, 1972 (J. Dausset) 6th, 1975 (F. Kissmeyer-Nielsen) 7th, 1977 (W. Bodmer) 8th, 1980 (P. I. Terasaki)	Regional workshops held Nobel prize received (G. Snell, J. Dausset, B. Benacerraf)	PLT Monoclonal antibodies 2D gel
IV Period of revision	1981 ~	9th, 1984 (E. D. Albert, W. Mayr) 10th, 1987 (B. Dupont)	Biochemical and molecular approach DNA analysis for genetics, disease association and transplantation	Biochemical technique with monoclonal antibodies DNA typing Southern hybridization etc.

HLA Class II Antigens in Different Ethnic Groups

HLA-DR Antigens in Various Populations

It is a challenging and very interesting task in population genetics to search for the origin of different populations. There have been many studies of genetic polymorphism, using blood group, serum protein, enzymes, and HLA antigens in various population groups [2–4, 7, 11, 20, 23, 34, 35, 43].

This study concentrated on HLA-DR antigens of different ethnic groups from the data of the Eighth International Histocompatibility Workshop [38], the First and Second Asia and Oceania Histocompatibility Workshop [36, 39], the data of the Japanese region in the Ninth International Workshop [42], and many individual papers. Gene frequencies in different populations worldwide are shown in Table 2. Genetic distance was computed by the formula of Cavalli-Sforza and Edwards [6].

A dendrogram computed by Nei's method [28] is shown in Fig. 1. A group of Mexicans with the same data (numbers 50 and 51 in the figure) was used as a control. Furthermore, groups 43, 44, and 45 were Australian Caucasian, 47 and 48 were American and North American Caucasians respectively, and 34 and 35 were Japanese. The data from Australian Caucasian group 43 came from the Second Asia and Oceania Histocompatibility Workshop, those of groups 44 and 45 from the Eighth International Histocompatibility Workshop. They were clustered in one group. American Caucasian group 47 North American Caucasian group 48 were also included in one cluster, as were the Japanese groups 34 (Ninth International Histocompatibility Workshop) and 35 (Eighth International Histocompatibility Workshop). Five general clusters were observed (Fig. 1): Caucasians; Blacks; Chinese; Micronesians/Melanesians; and American Indians/Japanese.

Caucasian group included Scandinavians, French, Germans, Mexicans, English, Spanish, Italians, Hindu Indians, Ashkenazi Jews, North Africans, Dutch, Austrians, Swiss, North Americans, Australians, and Canadians. However, Mexicans and Scandinavians were clustered at a genetic distance of 0.1136. This should be reexamined.

In the black group, Negroids, American blacks, and African blacks were clustered at a genetic distance of 0.1418. It is interesting that gypsies, Hungarians, and Yugoslavians were clustered close to the black group at a genetic distance of less than 0.1887. However, this needs further analysis.

South Africans, North Indians, Asian Indians, and non-Ashkenazi Jews were clustered with the Caucasian group at a genetic distance of 0.1949–0.2620.

In the third group, Filipinos and Chinese from Thai and Singapore, and China were clustered at a genetic distance of 0.2527.

In the fourth group, Micronesians and Melanesians, New Zealand Maoris, and Cook Islanders were clustered at a genetic distance of 0.2703, Czechoslovakians and Iranians at 0.1582, and Australian aborigines and Pima Indians at 0.2299. At a genetic distance of 0.2976, Czechoslovakians/Iranians and Australian aborigines/Iranians were clustered. However, at a genetic distance of 0.2885, the Chinese and Micronesian/Melanesian groups were not clustered.

In the fifth group (North American Indians and Japanese) the two Japanese groups (columns 34 and 35 in Fig. 1), at a genetic distance of 0.1207, American Indians and North American Indian, at 0.1693, and Balinese and Tenganans, at

Table 2. Gene frequencies in different populations worldwide

	1	2	3	4	5	6	7	8	9	10	11	12	13	14	15	16	17	18	19	20
	Scand	English	N-african	South-african	Spanish	other Cau	NEG	BL-african	German	Dutch	French	Austria	Swiss	Eur Ca	Hungarian	Gipsy	Hungarian	Italian	Czech	Yugoslav
	*	*	#	*	*	*	*	*	*	*	*	*	*	*	#	#	*	*	*	*
n	313	221	38	13	181	145	323	138	336	73	438	56	87	2499	118	176	105	455	133	70
DR1:	.0662	.0687	.0705	.1231	.0571	.0529	.0492	.0258	.0487	.1089	.0767	.1033	.0900	.0689	.0978	.0829	.0567	.0884	.0151	.0362
DR2:	.1191	.0978	.1754	.2665	.1621	.1253	.1544	.1072	.1462	.1699	.1282	.1657	.1421	.1346	.1123	.2132	.2503	.1219	.0662	.2069
DR3:	.0972	.1705	.1815	.1681	.1078	.0939	.1729	.2063	.0989	.1163	.1072	.1236	.0967	.1078	.1123	.1913	.2069	.0862	.0346	.1380
DR4	.1392	.1491	.1550	.0802	.0835	.1017	.0492	.0635	.0742	.1322	.1179	.0939	.1225	.0961	.1317	.0614	.0640	.0635	.0346	.0587
DR5:	.0492	.1000	.1078	.0802	.1174	.1288	.1328	.0950	.0694	.1089	.0884	.1550	.1028	.1028	.1265	.0890	.0487	.1988	.0582	.1462
DR6:	.0146	.0025	.0550	.0000	.0166	.0279	.0524	.0635	.0212	.0070	.0243	.0550	.0413	.0217	.0840	.0202	.0192	.0346	.0192	.0217
DR7:	.1168	.1129	.1185	.1231	.2101	.1134	.0978	.0716	.1253	.1322	.1123	.1340	.1491	.1248	.1265	.0403	.0640	.1305	.1033	.1134
DR8:	.0424	.0161	.0000	.0000	.0197	.0388	.0555	.0481	.0227	.0419	.0419	.0362	.0177	.0274	.0136	.0983	.0243	.0243	.0040	.0146
DR9:	.0161	.0090	.0000	.0000	.0197	.0141	.0269	.0258	.0243	.0000	.0070	.0090	.0233	.0111	.0000	.0085	.0000	.0055	.0116	.0000
7J:	.0000	.0000	.0000	.0000	.0000	.0000	.0000	.0000	.0000	.0000	.0000	.0000	.0000	.0000	.0000	.0000	.0000	.0000	.0000	.0000
DR10:	.0000	.0025	.0000	.0393	.0111	.0070	.0187	.0294	.0090	.0000	.0035	.0000	.0116	.0070	.0000	.0000	.0050	.0202	.0000	.0000
DR b1:	.3392	.2739	.1334	.1195	.1949	.2962	.1902	.2637	.3600	.1826	.2925	.1242	.2030	.2979	.1953	.1948	.2588	.2261	.6533	.2643

* Data from [3]. # Data from *Tissue Antigens* or Second Asia and Oceania Histocompatibility Workshop Conference (see individual reference)
References: Column 3 [16]; 15, 16 [15]; 23 [44]; 24 [37]; 25 [27]; 27 [13, 17]; 28 [9]; 29 [8]; 30 [21];32 [19]; 33 [22]; 34 [42];36, 37 [5]; 38–40 [13, 17]; 41 [14, 17]; 42 [33]; 43 [36]; 53–55 [12]; 57 [31]

Table 2 (continued)

	21	22	23	24	25	26	27	28	29	30	31	32	33	34	35	36	37	38	39	40
	Jewish Ashken	non Ashk	Iranian	N-Indian	HINDU Ind	Asian Ind	Thai	Thai-Chi	Sing-Chi	CHI-1	Chinese	CHI-2	Filipino	Japanese	Japan	Bali	Tenganau	PNG-C	PNG-H	Aust Abor
	*	*	#	#	#	*	#	#	#	#	*	#	#	#	*	#	#	#	#	#
n	133	61	49	109	138	32	28	49	37	140	31	48	36	541	884	51	175	31	32	35
DR1:	.0824	.0694	.0630	.0566	.0445	.0646	.0362	.0000	.0136	.0150	.0161	.0000	.0141	.0630	.0630	.0197	.0055	.0161	.0000	.0330
DR2:	.0906	.0694	.0970	.2158	.1925	.3152	.0939	.1938	.1456	.1720	.1772	.1963	.3130	.1521	.2000	.3583	.3872	.2597	.4414	.0497
DR3:	.0699	.0689	.0310	.1168	.0673	.0481	.0362	.0202	.0846	.0740	.1022	.0868	.0721	.0035	.0161	.0398	.0497	.0000	.0000	.0000
DR4:	.1288	.0857	.0310	.1598	.0873	.0481	.1340	.0835	.1456	.1190	.1969	.1462	.1669	.2430	.2345	.0000	.0000	.0840	.2293	.0840
DR5:	.2196	.1894	.0200	.1168	.0753	.0813	.0742	.0513	.0274	.0590	.0161	.0868	.0721	.0524	.0217	.2332	.1963	.3277	.0000	.0161
DR6:	.0227	.0305	.0100	.1276	.0294	.0320	.0182	.0305	.0000	.0000	.0000	.0759	.0141	.0721	.0466	.2457	.2713	.0161	.0481	.0000
DR7:	.1462	.1106	.0410	.1168	.2063	.0813	.1981	.1515	.0136	.0370	.0497	.1219	.0721	.0030	.0050	.1033	.0835	.0000	.0000	.0000
DR8:	.0269	.0000	.0000	.0000	.0481	.0156	.0742	.0202	.0413	.0680	.0161	.0646	.0571	.1185	.0651	.0000	.0000	.1022	.0156	.1574
DR9:	.0192	.0305	.0000	.0146	.0182	.0156	.0550	.0619	.1456	.1230	.1202	.1963	.0571	.1485	.1225	.0000	.0000	.0497	.0000	.0000
7J:	.0000	.0000	.0000	.0000	.0000	.0000	.0000	.0000	.0000	.0000	.0000	.0000	.0000	.0000	.0000	.0000	.0000	.0000	.0000	.0000
DR10:	.0075	.0382	.0000	.0141	.0182	.0481	.0000	.0000	.0136	.0040	.0161	.0000	.0000	.0045	.0060	.0000	.0000	.0000	.0000	.0000
DR bl:	.1862	.3075	.7070	.0611	.2129	.2500	.2800	.3872	.3691	.3290	.2892	.0254	.1614	.1394	.2194	.0000	.0065	.1443	.2655	.6597

Table 2 (continued)

	41	42	43	44	45	46	47	48	49	50	51	52	53	54	55	56	57	58
	New Zealand	Cook Islan	Aust Cau	Australian	AAC	Canad	American	Nor Am Ca	BL-American	Mexican	MEX	North Am Ind	PIMA Indian	Hopi	Navajo	Am Indian	Venezuelan	South Am Ind
	#	#	#	*	*	*	*	*	*	*	*	*	#	#	#	*	#	*
n	68	43	167	154	167	99	979	1145	168	88	88	25	113	90	93	67	32	42
DR1:	.0020	.0095	.0878	.0846	.0878	.1067	.1078	.1056	.0710	.0408	.0408	.0408	.0131	.0455	.0217	.0151	.0815	.0000
DR2:	.0035	.0212	.1282	.1174	.1282	.1294	.1415	.1357	.1870	.0770	.0770	.1754	.0737	.3675	.1022	.2672	.0986	.3277
DR3:	.0846	.0630	.1736	.1742	.1736	.1236	.1208	.1179	.1515	.0829	.0835	.0202	.0315	.1633	.3359	.0305	.0481	.0362
DR4:	.2424	.1729	.1699	.1784	.1699	.1532	.1515	.1473	.0424	.1538	.1538	.3675	.0829	.0513	.1901	.2775	.2295	.2286
DR5:	.2044	.0619	.0780	.0775	.0780	.0791	.0989	.1022	.1586	.1473	.1473	.0408	.1123	.3668	.3122	.0151	.1522	.0000
DR6:	.1089	.0630	.0429	.0466	.0429	.0413	.0372	.0377	.0455	.0289	.0289	.0000	.0000	.0000	.0000	.0382	.0986	.0614
DR7:	.0146	.0212	.1456	.1473	.1456	.1833	.1214	.1259	.1168	.1208	.1208	.0619	.0000	.0055	.0055	.0227	.1708	.0000
DR8:	.1340	.0372	.0182	.0197	.0182	.0151	.0299	.0269	.0646	.0408	.0408	.1515	.0310	.0000	.0000	.2082	.0986	.2444
DR9:	.0603	.1299	.0151	.0166	.0151	.0310	.0126	.0151	.0243	.0055	.0055	.0000	.0000	.0000	.0000	.0075	.0000	.0121
7J:	.0000	.0000	.0000	.0000	.0000	.0000	.0000	.0000	.0000	.0000	.0000	.0000	.0000	.0000	.0000	.0000	.0000	.0000
DR10:	.0000	.0000	.0060	.0035	.0060	.0100	.0035	.0060	.0009	.0055	.0055	.0835	.0000	.0000	.0000	.0382	.0000	.0121
DR b1:	.1454	.4201	.1346	.1342	.1346	.1272	.1750	.1796	.1374	.2966	.2960	.0584	.6555	.0000	.0323	.0797	.0221	.0777

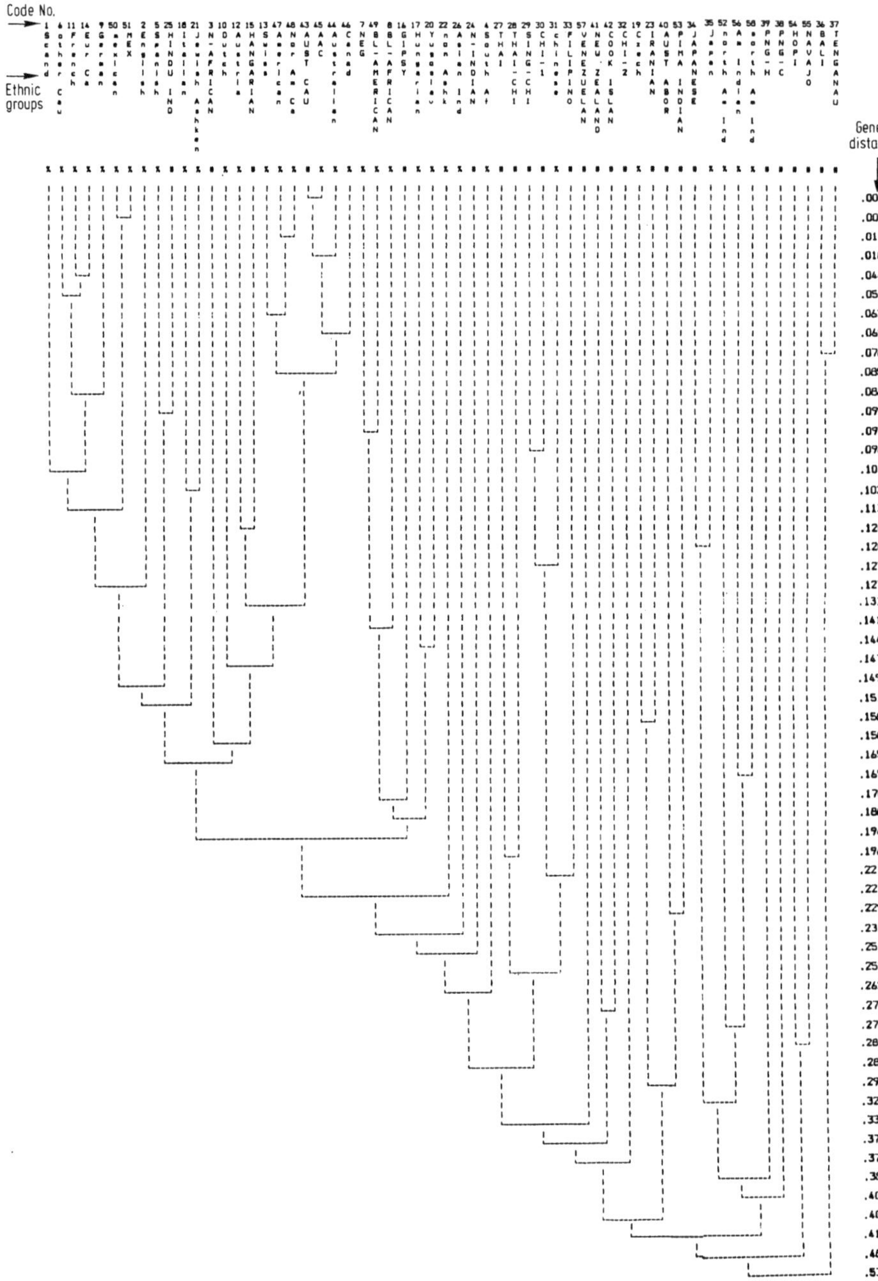

Fig. 1. Dendrogram of HLA-DR antigens on a worldwide scale

0.0787, were shown to be in one cluster. Furthermore, Japanese and American Indians were clustered at a genetic distance of 0.3284. Also, both highlanders and coastal dwellers of Papua New Guinea were clustered to the Japanese and the American Indian group at a genetic distance of 0.4050. Hopi and Navajo Indians were clustered at a genetic distance of 0.2815.

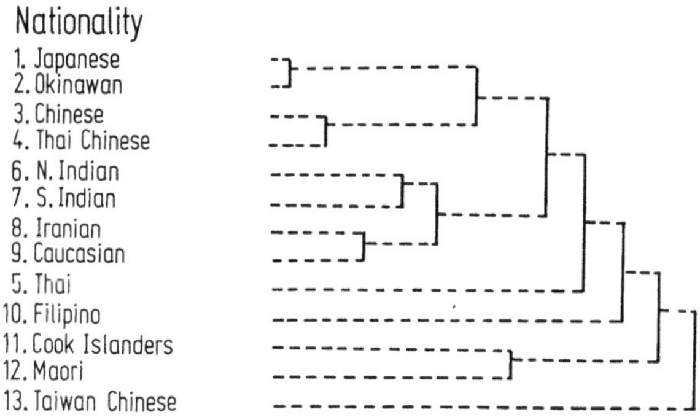

Fig. 2. Dendrogram of HLA-A, B, C antigens in Asia-Oceania populations

It is still obscure where the Japanese originated from, and several theories can be proposed. They may have come from Siberia, China, Korea, or Micronesia, or they could have been present originally on the Japanese islands. Due to the link found with American Indians, it may be that a common ancestor of North Scandinavian, e.g., Icelandic, origin migrated separately into Central Europe, China, Siberia, Japan, and North then South America. Another possibility is the origin in South America of a race that migrated north. A close relationship between Japanese and American Indians was observed from our dendrogram analysis. However, in our recent study of the Mongolian population using human immunoglobulin allotype, similarity between the Japanese and Siberian populations was observed [25, 26]. Therefore, from these recent studies it may be considered that the Japanese have a common origin with both American Indians and Siberians, but there is no clear explanation for the existence of the HLA antigenic cline. However, we observed that HLA-DRw9 antigen frequency was high in Japanese, Chinese, Micronesians, and Melanesians, and lowest in American Indians, Australian aborigines, Balinese, Iranians, Africans, and Caucasians.

We have not yet confirmed this using the Ninth International Histocompatibility Workshop data; more studies are necessary. Because this is the first attempt to make dendrograms of HLA-DR antigens on a worldwide scale, further consideration will be needed. A great similarity was noticed between the clusters found in this study and the dendrogram from the HLA-ABC antigen in the first Asia and Oceania Workshop population study [44] (Fig. 2).

Gene Frequencies of HLA-DR Antigens and DRw9 Antigen Cline in Japanese

Gene frequencies of HLA-DR antigens of Japanese from seven different localities in Japan are shown in Table 3. The gene frequencies of DRw9 antigens decreased from Okinawa (0.2631) to Hokkaido (0.0426). It was observed that the gene frequency cline of DRw9 antigen was statistically significant ($F < 0.05$; Table 4, Fig. 3).

No other cline of HLA-DR antigen was observed. We preliminarily observed in 1976 that there was a tendency for HLA-A2 to decline and HLA-A9 to increase in frequency from north to south [44], but further investigation did not confirm this finding. Also, a strong association between IDDM and HLA-DRw9 in Japanese was shown [41]. Gene frequency of HLA-DRw9 was mapped on a world map (Fig. 4). Interestingly, DRw9 in the Asian and Oceanian population, espe-

Table 3. Gene frequencies of HLA-DRw9 antigens of Japanese in seven different localities in Japan

	68 SAPPORO	69 TOKYO	70 NAGOYA	71 OSAKA	72 EHIME	73 KYUSYU	74 NAHA
n	52	224	30	93	19	65	35
DR1:	.0703	.0619	.0689	.0721	.0540	.0310	.0737
DR2:	.2100	.1438	.1633	.1766	.0540	.1777	.0289
DR3:	.0000	.0040	.0000	.0000	.0000	.0075	.0000
DR4:	.2327	.2437	.1633	.2031	.3115	.1777	.3450
DR5:	.0499	.0646	.0513	.0382	.0269	.0075	.0000
DR6:	.0000	.0813	.0000	.0000	.0000	.0233	.0000
DR7:	.1629	.0020	.0000	.0000	.0000	.0000	.0000
DR8:	.0000	.0105	.0868	.1140	.2050	.0884	.1214
DR9:	.0426	.1340	.1438	.1444	.2050	.0716	.2631
7J:	.0208	.0000	.0000	.0000	.0000	.0000	.0000
DR10:	.0000	.0000	.0000	.0217	.0269	.0000	.0000
DR bl:	.2109	.2542	.3225	.2298	.1168	.4153	.1679

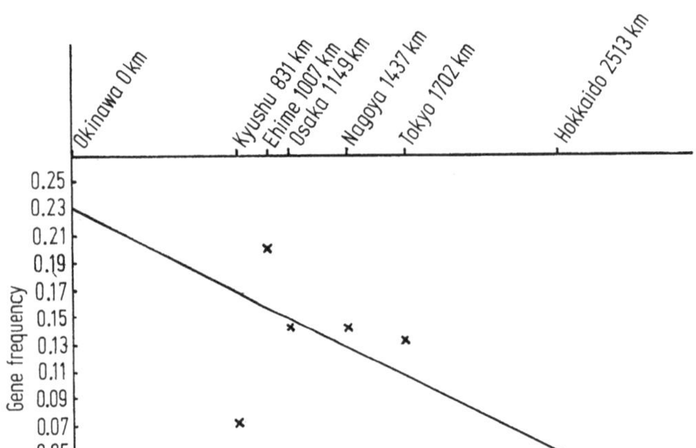

Fig. 3. DRw9 antigen frequency cline in Japanese

cially in Japanese, increased, whereas there was a very low incidence in other Caucasians, blacks, American Indians, and Australian aborigines.

The relationship between HLA antigen frequency, natural selection, immune response, and disease susceptibility should be investigated in the different ethnic groups as well as on a worldwide scale. Furthermore, studies of HLA antigen and/or genetic markers in the pan-Pacific, South Pacific, and northern parts of the world will be necessary.

Table 4. Statistical analysis of DRw9 antigen frequency in Japan

Locality (city)	*Y* (observed)	*Y* (estimated)	*T* value
Okinawa (Naha)	23.31	23.37	0.805
Kyushu (Fukuoka)	7.17	17.29	−5.941
Ehime (Matsuyama)	20.50	16.00	0.905
Osaka (Osaka)	14.44	14.97	−0.097
Nagoya (Hamamatsu)	14.38	12.86	0.279
Tokyo (Tokyo, Isehara)	13.40	10.93	0.479
Hokkaido (Sapporo)	4.26	5.00	−0.196

$\hat{Y}i = 23.38 - 0.007\,Xi$
Xi distance
less 5% significance
Y = gene frequency × 1000

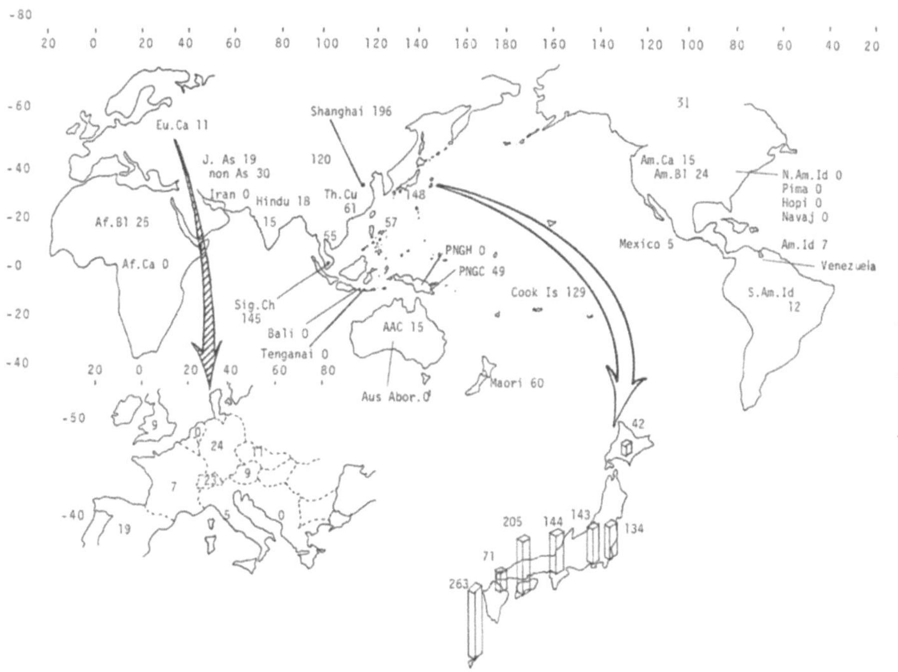

Fig. 4. Geographic distribution of HLA-DRw9 (g.f. × 1000) *J.As, non As,* Ashkenazi and non-Ashkenazi Jews; *AAC,* Australian Caucasians; *PNGH, PNGC,* Papua New Guinea highlanders, coastal dwellers *Sing. Ch., Th. Ch.,* Singapore and Thai Chinese

Complexity of DR4-Associated D Antigens

There have been many investigations concerning the complexity of HLA-D/DR antigens. We have already found that DR2 was associated with D2J [40], DR6 with DEn, and DRw9 with DKT.

Table 5. HLA-DR-associated D antigens in Japanese and Caucasians

HLA-D specificity	Japanese [29] (n=42) Antigen frequency (%)	Caucasian [32] (n=116) Antigen frequency (%)
Dw15 (=DYT)	40.5	3
DB3	16.7	9
DKT2	16.7	0
Dw4	9.5	44
LD40	0	18
Dw10	0	16

DR4-Associated D Antigens in Japanese and Caucasians

HLA-DR4 associated D antigens in Japanese [29] and Caucasians [32] are compared in Table 5. In Japanese, Dw15 had the highest frequency, followed by DKT2 and DB3 with the lowest, and in Caucasians the order was Dw4; LD40; Dw10; DB3 and DYT. However, no other population was tested.

PLT Clones Detecting HLA-Dw15 and Dw4 Antigen Determinant

PLT clones were established as described elsewhere [18]. KN(HLA-Dw1, Dw15, DR1, DR4, DQ1, DRw53, DPw2, DPw4) and OS(HLA-Dw1, Dw4, DR1, DR4, DQ1, DRw53, DPw2, DPw4) were used as stimulator and responder cells respectively. More detailed data were presented at the Ninth International Workshop [30]. Four Dw15-specific PLT clones, C-4, C-11, C-14, and C-17 and one Dw4-specific PLT clone, 1-3, were obtained. The relationship of HLA-D determinant and two PLT clones, C-11 and 1-3, are shown in Fig. 5. The results indicate that the response of the clones is very specific to Dw15 or Dw4.

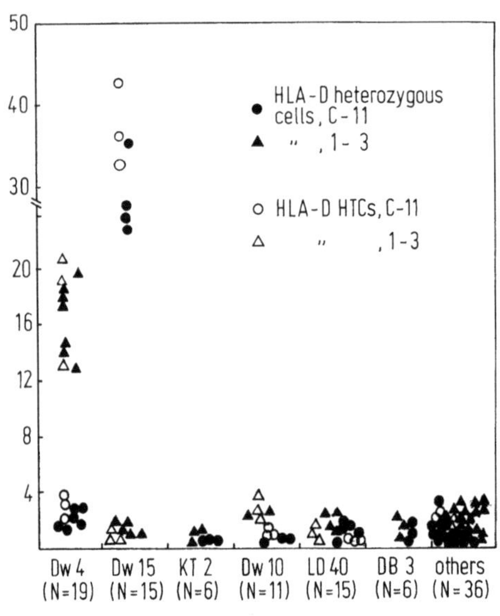

Fig. 5. PLT clones specific for Dw15(C-11) and Dw4(1-3)

Table 6. New DRYT alloantisera specific for Dw15

Cell no.	DR	DQ	D			DR4					DRw53					DQw3		TA10				DRYT			
			w15	KT2	w4																				
501	4, w13, w52, w53	w1	+			4	8	8	6	8	8	8	6	8	6	1	6	1	1	1	1	8	4	4	8
502	2, 4, w53	w1	+			4	8	6	4	8	8	8	8	8	8	4	1	1	1	1	1	6	6	6	8
601	2, 4, w53	w1	+			4	8	8	6	8	6	8	8	8	8	1	1	1	1	1	1	8	4	6	8
204	4, –, w53	–	+			4	8	6	4	8	6	1	4	6	8	1	4	1	1	1	1	8	4	8	8
270	2,4, w53	w1	+			6	6	6	1	6	8	8	4	8	8	4	1	4	1	1	1	6	1	8	8
002	4, –, w53	–	+			8	8	8	6	8	8	2	8	8	8	1	1	1	4	1	1	8	6	1	6
082	1, 4, w53	w1	+			6	8	1	1	6	8	1	8	8	8	1	1	1	1	1	1	4	4	1	6
511	2, 4, w53	w1	+			4	6	4	4	6	8	6	6	8	6	1	1	1	1	1	1	4	6	6	8
512	4, w13, w52, w53	w1	+			1	8	6	1	6	8	1	6	8	8	1	1	1	1	1	1	4	1	4	8
611	2, 4, w53	w1	+			4	2	6	4	6	6	4	6	6	4	1	1	1	1	1	1	6	1	4	6
219	4, –, w52, w53	w1, w3	+			4	8	6	6	6	8	6	8	8	8	6	6	1	1	1	1	8	6	8	8
274	4, w9, w53	w1, w3	+			8	6	4	4	6	4	8	6	8	8	6	8	1	1	4	1	8	8	8	8
258	4, w9, w53	w1, w3	+			4	6	4	4	8	8	8	8	8	8	8	8	1	1	1	1	8	8	8	8
701	4, w9, w53	w3		+		6	6	6	2	4	6	2	6	6	4	6	6	1	1	1	1	1	1	1	1
711	1, 4, w53	w1, w3		+		6	6	6	6	6	8	6	4	8	6	6	6	4	1	1	1	4	1	1	1
801	4, w13, w52, w53	w1, w3		+		6	8	6	4	8	8	4	6	8	6	8	4	1	1	1	1	1	1	6	1
811	4, w14, w52, w53	w1, w3		+		4	8	6	4	6	8	8	8	6	6	4	4	1	1	1	1	1	1	1	1
280	4, –, w52, w53	w3		+		4	4	4	4	8	6	1	4	8	6	8	8	1	1	1	1	1	1	1	4
226	4, –, w52, w53	w1, w3		+		8	6	6	1	8	8	8	8	8	8	8	8	4	1	1	1	4	1	1	1
034	4, –, w53	w1, w3		+		6	8	8	4	8	8	1	6	8	6	6	6	1	1	1	1	1	1	1	1
261	4, –, w53	w3			+	6	8	8	8	8	6	6	4	6	1	8	8	8	4	6	4	4	1	1	1
009	1, 4, w53	w3			+	6	8	8	8	8	8	8	1	8	8	8	8	8	8	8	8	4	1	1	1

Scores
8: >80% cell lysis
6: 50%–79% cell lysis
4: 30%–49% cell lysis
2: 20%–29% cell lysis
1: 0%–19% cell lysis

New DRYT Alloantisera Specific for Dw15

Positive panel cells of 13 Dw15, seven DKT2 and two Dw4 were tested for DR typing using the Eighth Japanese Workshop antisera. Table 6 shows the relationship between DR4-associated D antigens and DR4, DRw53, DQ3, TA10, and DRYT. A high correlation between Dw15 and DRYT was found, and DRYT did not react with any other DR antigens. DRYT antisera react only with the Dw15 antigen. Dw10, Dw13, and Dw14 were not tested. DKT2 could be completely identified by DR4, DRw53, and DQ3, and Dw4 by DR4, DRw53, DQ3, and TA10. However, DQ3 also reacted with DR5, DRw9, and DRNJ2, and TA10 with DR5 and DRNJ2 [24].

It was suggested that the DR4-associated D region is encoded by DR(DR4, DRYT, DRw53) and DQ(DQ3, TA10) antigens. Using DR and DQ antisera, it was found that Dw15 is comprised of DR4, DRw53, and DYT. By using DRYT antisera, Dw15 antigen can be selectively recognized, so DRYT is a specific antigen of Dw15. It is still unclear whether the MLR gene is single or compound. Also, the mechanism of MLR is as yet unsolved, and must be analyzed using biochemical, molecular, PLT clone, and monoclonal antibody techniques.

Summary

An attempt was made at making dendrograms using HLA-DR antigens on a world-wide scale. Five clusters of ethnic groups were observed.

A geographical distribution of HLA-DRw9 antigen was drawn and an antigenic cline was found in Japan.

The complexity of HLA-DR4-associated D antigen in Japanese was studied. PLT clones detected HLA-Dw15 and Dw4 antigen and new DRYT alloantisera specific for the Dw15 specificity.

Further studies on a worldwide scale into HLA-D complexity will be necessary.

Acknowledgments. We would like to thank Professor T. Takahashi for the computer program, Y. Yamashita for computer analysis, Mrs Nadia El Borai for correcting the English, and A. Oki for typing the manuscript.

References

1. Albert ED, Baur MP, Mayr WR (eds) (1984) Histocompatibility testing 1984. Springer, Berlin Heidelberg New York Tokyo
2. Amos DB, Pool P, Grier J (1980) HLA-A, HLA-B, HLA-C, and HLA-DR. In: Am. Soc. for Microbiology (ed) Manual of clinical immunology, 2nd edn. Washington, pp 978–986
3. Baur MP, Danilov JA (1980) Population analysis of HLA-A, B, C, DR and other genetic markers. In: Terasaki PI (ed) Histocompatibility testing 1980. UCLA Tissue Typing Laboratory, Los Angeles, pp 955–993
4. Bodmer W, Bodmer JG (1978) Evolution and function of the HLA system. Br Med Bull 34:309–316
5. Breguet G, Wolnizer CM, Doran T, Bashir H, Jeannet M, Benzonana G, Ney R, Adiputra N, Scherz R, Blake NM (1982) HLA antigens in Bali (Indonesia) with a special reference to an isolated community. Tissue Antigens 20:229–238

6. Cavalli-Sforza LL, Edwards AWF (1967) Phylogenetic analysis; model and estimation procedures. Am J Hum Genet 19:233–257
7. Cavalli-Sforza LL, Bodmer WF (1971) The genetics of human populations. Freeman, San Francisco
8. Chan SH, Wee GB (1981) HLA and nasopharyngeal cancer in Singapore Chinese. Proceedings of the Second Asia and Oceania Histocompatibility Workshop Conference 1981, pp 495–496
9. Chandanayingong C, Chiewsilp P (1981) HLA antigens in Thais. Proceedings of the Second Asia and Oceania Histocompatibility Workshop Conference 1981, pp 276–287
10. Crumpton MJ, Bodmer JG, Bodmer WF, Heyes JM, Lindsay J, Rudd CE (1984) Biochemistry of class II antigens: workshop report. In: Albert ED, Baur MP, Mayr WR (eds) Histocompatibility testing 1984. Springer, Berlin Heidelberg New York Tokyo, p 29
11. Dausset J, Svejgaard A (eds) (1977) HLA and disease. Munksgaard, Copenhagen
12. Ensroth AF, Mann DL, Johnson AH, Knowler WC, Pettitt DJ, Bennett PH (1983) HLA-A and B lymphocyte alloantigens in Gila River Indians. Tissue Antigens 21:198–207
13. Fong R, Dagger J, Locke H (1981) Analysis of HLA-ABC and DR antigens in New Zealand Maoris. Proceedings of the Second Asia and Oceania Histocompatibility Workshop Conference, pp 261–271
14. Fong R, Dagger J, Locke H (1981) Analysis of HLA-ABC and DR antigens in New Zealand Maoris. Proceedings of the Second Asia and Oceania Histocompatibility Workshop Conference, pp 272–274
15. Gyodi E, Tausxik T, Petranyi GY, Kotrasz A, Palffy GY, Takacs I, Nemak P, Hollan SR (1981) The HLA antigen distribution in the Gipsy population in Hungary. Tissue Antigens 18:1–12
16. Herait P, Tursz T, Guillard MY, Hanna K, Lipinski M, Micheau C, Sancho-Garnier H, Schwaab G, Cachin Y, Degos L, deThe G (1983) HLA-A, -B, and -DR antigens in North African patients with nasopharyngeal carcinoma. Tissue Antigens 22:335–341
17. Honeyman M, Bashir H (1981) Cellular typing. Proceedings of the Second Asia and Histocompatibility Workshop Conference, pp 231–260
18. Inouye H, Hank JA, Chardonnens X, Segall M, Alter BJ, Bach FH (1980) Cloned primed lymhocyte test reagents in the dissection of HLA-D. J Exp Med 152:143s
19. Jaraquemada D, Alonso A, Awad J, D'Amaron J, Olliver W, Doyle P, Ikoye RC, Williams E, Restenstein H et al. (1984) HLA polymorphisms in a Shanghai Chinese population. Tissue Antigens 23:23–32
20. Kostyu D, Dawson D, Ciftan E, Stewart A, Lewis D, Parc F, Laigrat J, McCollum M, Amos DB (1984) HLA in two islands of French Polynesia. Tissue Antigens 23:217–228
21. Lee TD, Zhao T, Chi Z, Wong H, Shen M, Rodey G (1983) HLA-A, -B, and HLA-DR phenotypes in mainland Chinese patients with diabetes mellitus. Tissue Antigens 22:92–95
22. Lingao LL, Chavez C (1981) HLA antigens in the Philippines. Proceedings of the Second Asia and Oceania Histocompatibility Workshop Conference, pp 288–289
23. MacArthur RH, Connell JH (1966) The biology of populations. Wiley, New York
24. Maeda H (1984) Mouse monoclonal antibody detects a new polymorphic Ia determinant other than HLA-DR antigen: a possible allele of DC-1. Tissue Antigens 23:163
25. Matsumoto H, Miyazaki T, Ishida N, Katayama K (1982) Mongoloid populations from the viewpoint of Gm patterns. Jpn J Hum Genet 27:271
26. Matsumoto H, Miyazaki T, Rychkov YG, Zhukova OV, Lebedeva IA, Kondik VM, Udima IG, Spitzin VA, Batsuur J, Shnader YV, Tsuji K, Takahashi T, Nakao Y (1984) Studies of the human immunoglobin allotypes in five populations in the USSR. Jpn J Hum Genet 29:10
27. Mittal KK, Naik S, Sansonetti N, Cowherd R, Kuman R, Wong DM (1982) The HLA antigens in Indian Hindus. Tissue Antigens 20:223–226
28. Newberger A, Jatum E (1975) In: Nei M (ed) Molecular population genetics and evolution. North-Holland, Amsterdam, pp 199–201 (Frontiers in biology, vol 40)

29. Nose Y, Sato K, Nakagawa M, Kondho K, Inouye H, Tsuji K (1982) HLA-D clusters associated with DR4 in the Japanese population. Hum Immunol 5:199–203
30. Nose Y, Sukegawa T, Tsuchida F, Nakatsuji T, Tsuji K (1984) PLT analysis of D region complexity by cloned cells: a new non-DP antigen. In: Albert ED, Baur MP, Mayr WR (eds) Histocompatibility testing 1984. Springer, Berlin Heidelberg New York Tokyo, pp 475–477
31. Ottenhoff THM, Gonzales NM, deVries RRP, Convit J, van Rood JJ (1984) Association of HLA specificity LB-E12(MB1, DC1, MT1) with lepromatous leprosy in a Venezuelan population. Tissue Antigens 24:25–29
32. Reinsmoen NL, Bach FH (1982) Five HLA-D clusters associated with HLA-DR4. Hum Immunol 4:249–258
33. Roberts MW, Minnee KE, Woodfield DG (1981) HLA antigens in the Cook Islands. Proceedings of the Second Asia and Oceania Histocompatibility Workshop Conference, pp 261–271
34. Ryder LP, Andersen E, Svejgaard A (1978) An HLA map of Europe. Hum Hered 28:171–200
35. Serjeantson SW, Kirk RL, Ranford P, Beauchamp M (1983) HLA antigens and non-HLA chromosome 6 markers in Micronesians from Nauru. Tissue Antigens 22:49–58
36. Simons MJ, Tait BD (eds) (1981) Proceedings of the Second Asia and Oceania Histocompatibility Workshop Conference
37. Singh SPN, Mehra NK, Dingley HB, Pande JN, Vaidya MC (1983) HLA-A, -B, -C, and -DR antigen profile in pulmonary tuberculosis in North India. Tissue Antigens 21:380–384
38. Terasaki PI (ed) Histocompatibility testing 1980. UCLA Tissue Typing Laboratory, Los Angeles
39. Tsuji K, Komori K (eds) (1979) Proceedings of the First Asia and Oceania Histocompatibility Workshop and Conference, Japan HLA Association
40. Tsuji K, Nose Y, Komori K, Tajika R, Nakagawa M, Inouye H, Yamamura M (1979) Probable existence of four subloci in the HLA-DR (or D) region. Transplant Proc 11:1792–1795
41. Tsuji K, Nakagawa M, Sato K, Kondo K, Nose Y, Inouye H, Nakazawa M, Hirata M (1982) HLA specificities associated with insulin-dependent diabetes mellitus in Japan. In: Mimura G, Baba S, Goto Y, Köbberling J (eds) Clinico-genetic genesis of diabetes mellitus. Excerpta Medica, Amsterdam, pp 114–124 (Int. Congress Series 597)
42. Tsuji K et al. (1984) Collecting data in Japan region. Ninth International Histocompatibility Workshop and Conference, Munich-Vienna, May 1984
43. Troup GM, Schanfield MS, Singaraju CH, Harvey RL, Jameson J, Capper J, Baker B (1982) Study of HLA alloantigens of the Navajo Indians of North America. Tissue Antigens 20:339–351
44. Yasuda N, Komori K, Tsuji K (1979) Workshop report in genetics. In: Tsuji K, Komori K (eds) Proceedings of the First Asia and Oceania Histocompatibility Workshop and Conference, Japan HLA Association, p 113

Serological Definition

Serology of HLA Class II Antigens: Methodological Aspects *

P. Richiardi and E. S. Curtoni

Table of Contents

Serological Methods for the Study of HLA Class II Antigens

Lymphocytotoxicity

Most of HLA class II serology is essentially based on a complement-dependent lymphocytotoxicity reaction. The principle of this reaction is as follows: cytotoxic antibodies are incubated with a purified suspension of living lymphocytes in the

* Supported by CNR, Centro per l'Immunogenetica e Istocompatibilitá, by Progetto Finalizzato Tecnologie Biomediche, and by Ministero Pubblica Istruzione

presence of complement. Attachment of the antibodies to the antigens on the cell surface specifically activates the complement. The final result will be an irreversible lesion of the cell membrane, allowing the extracellular fluids to enter the cell. The results of the reaction are evaluated by counting the percentage of living and dead cells. If the cells are alive, it means that the complement has not been activated, therefore the reaction is negative. In contrast, dead cells indicate a positive reaction.

The complement-dependent lymphocytotoxicity techniques are generally micromethods, using very small amounts of reagents, and are all derived from the original technique described by Terasaki and McClelland [47]. The technique most widely used is the cytotoxicity test by dye exclusion, performed in Falcon microtest tissue culture plates with a purified suspension of class II-antigen-bearing lymphocytes (see below): to better distinguish living from dead cells, a stain such as eosin Y or trypan blue is used, which is excluded from the living lymphocytes (which when examined with a phase contrast inverted microscope appear small and nonstained), but enters into the dead ones (which appear larger and stained).

The main advantage of this technique is that it employs very small amounts of reagents and very few target cells (1 μl antiserum and 3000 lymphocytes per reaction), thus allowing extended population studies of random individuals as well as family studies including children and patients. Moreover, when technical conditions are accurately standardized it has very good reproducibility.

Disadvantages that may hamper the use of this technique are as follows:

1. Conditions for complement activation are not always present. In fact, the antigen density must be sufficiently high to allow the attachment of two IgG molecules close enough to trigger complement-dependent lysis. Moreover, not all antibody subclasses are able to fix complement: this constitutes a problem when using monoclonal antibodies (MoAbs).
2. Cell suspensions to be tested must have a viability greater than 80%.
3. Positive reactions with less than 20%–30% killed cells are difficult to detect. For this reason, class II-positive cell-enriched suspensions must be used.

This problem can be overcome by the two-colour fluorescence test described by van Rood et al. [51], which can make use of total lymphocyte suspensions and not necessarily of purified suspensions of class II-bearing lymphocyte subpopulations. The cells are previously incubated with fluorescein-conjugated anti-immunoglobulin; after the reaction with class II antiserum in the presence of complement, killed cells are stained by addition of ethidium bromide, which enters dead cells and stains the nuclei with a red fluorescence. It is thus possible to distinguish dead from living cells by the ethidium bromide, and B cells, T cells, and monocytes by the anti-immunoglobulin: B lymphocytes develop distinct green fluorescent caps, monocytes do not form caps but show fluorescent spots on the surface, and T lymphocytes are not stained by green fluorescence. According to van Rood et al., the main advantages of this test compared with the above-mentioned cytotoxicity test on purified class II-bearing lymphocyte suspensions is that it takes a shorter time and that one can ascertain whether the fraction of the cells killed are B cells and monocytes.

The sensitivity of the cytotoxicity tests may depend on several parameters, the most important of which seem to be incubation time, temperature, cell storage, and complement. If the incubation time is prolonged, the sensitivity is increased. A prolonged incubation of cells and antiserum allows the fixation of low-avidity antibodies; if the incubation time of complement is prolonged, the action of complement may be stronger. Class II antisera are often rather weak; therefore, they are more easily detected using a "long incubation" technique. A temperature increase is generally proportional to an increase of the reaction speed. Also, the storage of test cells increases the reaction sensitivity. In our laboratory, DR sera were tested against class II-bearing lymphocytes immediately after cell separation and 16 h later, after storage overnight at 15 °C; of all the positive reactions, about 20% were present only with stored cells. The reactions positive only with stored cells correlated with DR antigens. It seems therefore that weak class II antibodies may be detected only on stored lymphocytes.

Complement Fixation

As known, immune complexes formed on a cell membrane by class II antigens and anti-class II antibodies usually activate the complement sequence. This phenomenon can be seen using either a cytotoxicity technique (as described above) or a complement fixation technique [32]. This latter method is less sensitive, but can also be used on nonviable cells or on subcellular extracts. The principle of the method is to evaluate the amount of complement fixed by antigen-antibody complexes. The reference hemolytic system used to detect the complement consists of sheep erythrocytes sensitized by an anti-sheep erythrocyte antibody. The method can be qualitative (giving only a positive or negative result of the reaction, according to the absence or presence of residual hemolytic activity) or semiquantitative (in which case the tests are made at various dilutions of antigens and antibodies).

Beyond the relatively low sensitivity already mentioned, another disadvantage is anticomplementarity which can be observed in several sera when they are tested pure or at low dilution. Tests should therefore be performed with serum diluted at least 1:5.

Radioimmunoassay

The radioimmunoassay technique [45] is based on a direct binding assay based on the double antibody technique. It measures the extent of binding obtained by incubating the labeled human class II antigen preparation (obtained from solubilized cell membranes) with antiserum and recovering the immune complex with an anti-IgG antiserum. The reaction can be performed in a small test tube, using about 5 μl antiserum and 10000–20000 cpm labeled class II preparation. The reaction volume and ionic strength of the reaction mixture can influence the reaction remarkably. After incubation, the immune complexes are precipitated with an anti-Ig antiserum or with *Staphylococcus aureus* protein A. The immune precipitates are washed and the radioactivity is determined by a gamma-ray counter.

This method allows class II molecules to be isolated and therefore makes it possible to distinguish different class II molecules against which a single antiserum can react and to perform structural studies on the isolated molecules.

Indirect Immunofluorescence

Indirect immunofluorescence has the advantage that noncytotoxic antisera may be used. It can be useful mainly with MoAbs, which are often unable to induce cytotoxicity. After incubation with anti-class II antibody, the cells are washed with cold phosphate-buffered saline added with bovine serum albumin (PBS+BSA), then the supernatants are removed and the cells are resuspended in fluorescent anti-Ig diluted in PBS+BSA. After a further incubation the cells are accurately washed and then transferred to a reading plate (Hamax). The reaction can be evaluated on an inverted fluorescence microscope equipped with an epi-illuminator.

A disadvantage of this method is that it cannot be considered a microtechnique; in fact, it makes use of relatively high amounts of cells (50 000) and serum (20 μl). Reactions can be performed on Seromat-Greiner plates (60 wells, each of 200 μl capacity; see Richiardi et al. [43]).

ELISA

The ELISA technique [30] is based on an unlabeled antibody-enzyme method consisting of incubating the cells first with the mouse anti-class II MoAb under study, then with an anti-mouse Ig xenoantiserum. Subsequently a soluble complex peroxidase-antiperoxidase is added; the antiperoxidase is a mouse MoAb, which will be bound by the anti-mouse Ig already present. Finally, the cells are incubated with a substrate solution for the peroxidase reaction.

The advantages of this technique, generally used to study MoAbs, are (1) the possibility of detecting noncytotoxic antibodies, (2) that it requires a rather small amount of antiserum and cells, and (3) that the cells do not need to be alive, so that they can be stored long before they are used.

Class II-Positive Target Cells

Polymorphism of HLA class II antigens in man has until recently been studied mainly by serological methods, using the lymphocytotoxicity technique. This requires the selection of appropriate target cells, since class II antigens exhibit a restricted expression on subpopulations of lymphoid cells. Moreover, there is a differential expression of class II antigens coded by different loci and a differential expression depending both on the maturation stage of the target cells and on different pharmacological or immunological stimuli to which they may be exposed. Thus, target cells obtained with the same technical procedures from various donors can exhibit a quite variable reactivity with the same serological reagents. The following target cells have been more often employed for selection and characterization of class II antibodies.

Peripheral Blood Mononuclear Cells. These include T lymphocytes, B lymphocytes, monocytes, and the so called null cells, which form a distinct cell population with a larger mean size than either T or B lymphocytes and do not express the E receptor [22]. They have also been variously referred to as "third lymphocyte population" [24], "unclassified lymphoid cells" [27], and "L cells" [28].

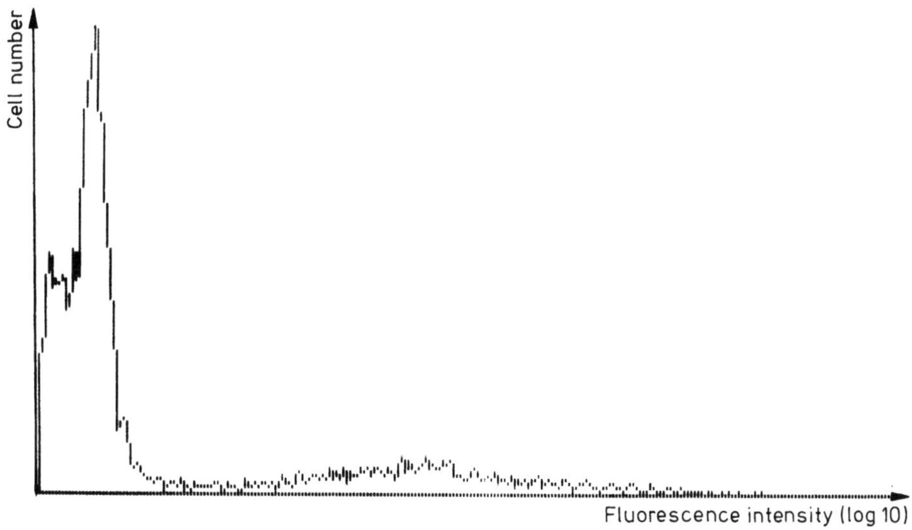

Fig. 1. Cytofluorometric analysis of DR antigen expression on peripheral blood mononuclear cells using an anti-DR MoAb

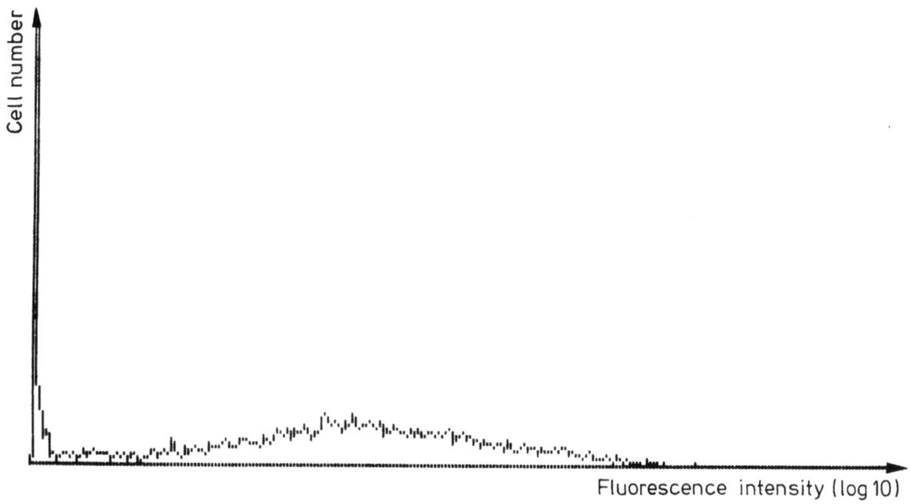

Fig. 2. Cytofluorometric analysis of DR antigen expression on E− peripheral blood mononuclear cells using an anti-DR MoAb

Expression of Ia antigens is quite variable on the above subpopulations. Figure 1 shows the cytofluorometric analysis of reactivity of an anti-DR monomorphic MoAb with peripheral blood mononuclear cells: it ranges from completely negative to strongly positive and it can be seen that the strongly positive cells are only a minority.

Analyzing the reactivity of anti-class II monomorphic reagents (murine MoAbs or xenoantisera) against purified lymphoid subpopulations, it appears that peripheral blood T cells do not express class II antigens, which are restricted to cells not rosetting (E−) with sheep red blood cells (SRBC). Even among E−

subpopulations, however, there is a wide range of reactivity (see Fig. 2) that can be represented (oversimplified) as follows:

Class II antigens	
Monocytes	+
B lymphocytes	+
Null cells	–

The various technical procedures that have been used to purify class II-positive peripheral lymphoid cells and the results obtained will be discussed in the following paragraphs. Since HLA class II serology has been performed mainly on peripheral blood cells and using the cytotoxicity technique, it is obvious that purification of positive target cells is one of the central problems whose solution is essential to class II typing.

Cultured B Lymphoid Lines. These express class II antigens and have been advantageously used. Many anti-class II antibodies (both alloantisera and MoAbs) have been screened and selected against a panel of lymphoid lines [18, 23], yielding results comparable to those obtained with peripheral B lymphocytes.

The advantages of using cultured lines as target cells are that they homogeneously express class II antigens at high density [50] and are always available. Moreover, high amounts of cells can be produced, thus making biochemical studies possible. Particularly useful have been the Epstein-Barr virus (EBV)-induced lymphoid lines produced from genetically homozygous individuals. Some disadvantages may be the following:

1. Though it is theoretically possible to produce EBV-induced lymphoid lines from any individual, in practice only a few lines are available and commonly used, because of the time-consuming and expensive procedures necessary for the production and conservation of these cellular reagents. Therefore any serological analysis of HLA class II polymorphism performed using lymphoid lines is bound to be limited to a small panel and generally does not include population and family analysis. A panel of EBV-transformed lymphoid lines proposed by Dausset and coworkers during the Ninth International Histocompatibility Workshop (1984, personal communication), including 12 lines fully typed for all HLA antigens, is now available.

2. Lymphoid lines express 5–6 times more class II antigens than peripheral B lymphocytes [50]. It is thus possible that antisera that show a positive reaction against cultured cells become negative when tested against peripheral blood cells. Therefore the reagents selected against lymphoid lines should always be tested and characterized against peripheral blood cells before being used as typing antisera.

3. Some lymphoid lines are particularly sensitive to the lytic action of rabbit complement used for the cytotoxicity technique. Thus a careful selection of complement, by previous testing against the target cell lines, is required.

Lymphocytes from Patients with Chronic Lymphocytic Leukemia. These cells are a convenient source of B cells for screening anti-Ia antibodies since the majority of patients with chronic lymphocytic leukemia (CLL) have more than 90% surface immunoglobulin (SIg)-positive cells in the peripheral blood mononuclear cells. The advantages of using these cells are the high yield of lymphocytes and the avoidance of the time-consuming procedures involved in the separation of enriched B cell suspensions from normal blood. The disadvantage is that the results are not always reproducible and that many sera selected as positive against CLL cells may appear negative when tested against normal B-enriched cells [3]. For those sera that are reactive both with CLL and normal cells, however, the results generally appear to be comparable [23, 31]. There is one important exception: some sera have been reported which, though positive with normal B cells, do not react with CLL cells. It is now clear that peripheral blood cells in B-CLL are heterogeneous with respect to MHC class II: while they all express DR antigens, only a small proportion express DQ antigens [26]. In contrast, DR and DQ are equally present on normal peripheral blood B cells. It is therefore likely that the above reported alloantisera (positive with normal B cells but negative with CLL cells) recognize a DQ allospecificity.

Spleen and Lymph Node Lymphocytes. These target cells are used for class II typing of necrokidney donors. For these individuals, typing of HLA class II antigens on peripheral B lymphocytes is often impossible because of their frequent lack of reactivity with even strong HLA alloantisera [35], probably a result of steroid treatment. In contrast both spleen and lymph node B cells normally express HLA class II antigens and can usually be class II-typed without difficulties. According to Goldman (personal communication), spleen and lymph node B cells can be clearly typed in more than 75% of cases; moreover, lymph node cells give the best B cell-enriched suspensions for DR typing and provide the best source of cells for pretransplant cross-match purposes. For this reason, the Eurotransplant tissue typing working committee suggested urging surgical teams, whenever possible, to obtain some lymph nodes in addition to the spleen. Following this policy, the Turin transplantation unit generally performs DR typing of the cadaver kidney donor, prior to the choice of the recipient, on lymph node B-enriched cells. Among 78 necrokidney donors, lymph node cells could not be typed at all in ten cases (12.8%), mostly because they were not reactive; four donors showed poor DR typing and six poor DQ typing. Altogether 70% of the donors could be typed without problems for both DR and DQ antigens.

Methods of Obtaining Class II-Positive Mononuclear Cells from Peripheral Blood

As mentioned above, class II-antigen-bearing leukocytes are only a minority of peripheral blood mononuclear cells. DR structures are present mainly on B lymphocytes and monocytes, while DQ can be found on B lymphocytes and on a minority of monocytes [37]. The class II-typing techniques adopted by most laboratories make use of cell suspensions enriched with leukocytes possessing at their surface a significant number of class II molecules. Therefore several methods have been proposed to purify from peripheral lymphocytes subpopulations enriched with class II-bearing cells.

E Rosette Method

The E rosette technique is based on the principle that T lymphocytes have a surface receptor (E receptor) able to bind SRBC. When lymphocytes are incubated at 4 °C with SRBC, rosettes are formed which include one T cell and several

SRBC. The ability to form rosettes is increased if SRBC are pretreated with 2-aminoethilisothiouroniumbromide (AET) [39] or with neuraminidase [29]. The rosettes can easily be separated from the residual free lymphocytes by centrifugation on density gradient. The remaining suspension is composed of E− cells: these include B lymphocytes, monocytes, and null cells. Of these, only B lymphocytes and monocytes express DR antigens in a quantity allowing strong and reproducible reactivity with anti-class II antibodies using the lymphocytotoxicity technique. The relative proportion of the three cell populations may vary considerably in cell suspensions, both from healthy donors and from patients of some diseases; therefore in several cases the suspension obtained by E rosette depletion is not sufficiently enriched with class II-bearing cells to allow reliable class II typing (see next paragraph).

Nylon Wool Method

It was demonstrated several years ago [25] that if lymphocytes are incubated with nylon fibers, non-T cells adhere to the fibers and a pure T population can be obtained. It has further been shown [49] that a non-T population which adheres to nylon fibers can be eluted without damaging the cells. The best way of obtaining adherence of cells to fibers seems to be to pack nylon into small columns (as common drinking straws) and to incubate cells in fibers maintained at 37 °C and wetted (with McCoy's solution + 5% foetal calf serum). After incubation the nonadherent cells (T and null lymphocytes) are collected by allowing McCoy's medium to drop through the column. The cells adherent to the nylon may be eluted by repeatedly squeezing the straw; these are mainly B lymphocytes and monocytes. The yield of B lymphocytes is generally around 30% of the B cells present in the blood [52]. The proportion of Ig-bearing cells in the adherent fraction varies between 50% and 80%. The efficiency of this technique for preparing cells for Ia serology is considered by some authors higher than the E rosette method [4, 33, 34], while others [53] obtain more satisfactory typing on E rosette-depleted lymphocytes. In our laboratory the nylon wool method, which allows removal of T and null cells, both class II-negative, gives better results (see next paragraph), particularly in typing individuals such as dialysis patients in whom the E rosette method often does not allow sufficient purification of the class II-bearing cells.

Plastic Plate Incubation

A useful modification of the above-mentioned method of nylon wool adherence is adherence to plastic surfaces. If a lymphocyte suspension (depleted from E-rosetting lymphocytes) is incubated in a plastic Petri dish at 37 °C, monocytes and B cells adhere to the dish. The nonadherent cells may be removed by gentle washing, a more vigorous washing allows recovery of B cells while monocytes, which are the most adherent to plastic, may be recovered either by incubation and subsequent washing in McCoy's medium + 1% alcohol solution (5 parts ethanol, 1 part benzyl alcohol) [13], or mechanically with the help of a rubber policeman.

Since both adherent populations express DR but only B cells express DQ (see next paragraph), this method has the advantage of providing two cell populations that can be used together for DR typing or separated for DQ typing, sera screening, or other serological analysis.

MoAb Rosetting Method

This technique makes use of a mouse monomorphic MoAb specific for DR antigens. The antibody-coated cells form rosettes with bovine erythrocytes [44] or alternatively with Sepharose-4β beads [19], coupled with anti-mouse Ig, and can be purified by density gradient centrifugation. For this technique it is recommended to use defibrinated and not heparinized blood, because platelets present in the latter adhere to leukocytes, resulting in cell clumping and some nonspecific rosette formation. Of the cells obtained with this method, 70%–80% show SIg. The cell suspension reacts strongly with DR antisera, and it has been observed that this suspension, being composed solely of class II-positive cells, may show positive reactions with some antisera which contain weak extra antibodies undetectable when the sera are tested with target cells obtained with other methods. The method has, however, proved to be useful in separating blood from which it is difficult to purify B cells (cord blood, patients undergoing therapy with particular drugs, previously frozen lymphocytes, etc.).

Characterization of Lymphocyte Subsets Present in B Enriched Suspensions and Determination of Class II-Positive Cells

As stated above, B cell-enriched suspensions prepared from peripheral blood mononuclear cells include a heterogeneous population of cells that express class II antigens differently (see Fig. 2). The techniques more widely used to purify B lymphocytes are the depletion of T cells by E rosetting and the adherence of B cells to nylon wool. Neither procedure is standardized, and their reproducibility is rather poor. The final suspension may thus be contaminated by a variable amount of non-B cells. Differences among individuals and between categories of patients, according to the variety of diseases, make it necessary to use a system of monitoring each cell preparation for component purity and for the presence of class II-positive target cells. Exact evaluation of the contaminant cells is essential for correct interpretation of serological reaction patterns. This may be achieved by checking the cell preparations for the presence of specific surface markers and differentiation antigens recognized by MoAbs (see Table 1). The ad-

Table 1. Markers characterizing mononuclear cell subpopulation

	T cells	Monocytes	B cells	Null cells
Adherence	−	++	+	−
E receptor (SRBC rosettes)	+	−	−	−
MoAb OKT11	+	−	−	−
SIg	−	(+)	+	(+)
MoAb B1	−	−	+	−
MoAb OKM1	−	+	−	+
Anti-DR MoAbs	−	+	+	(−)
Anti-DQ MoAbs	−	+/− [a]	+	−
Size (μm)	6.76	9.02	6.42	7.16

Data form El-Awar et al. [22], Crepaldi et al. [15], Guy et al. [25], Chen et al. [12]
[a] Two monocyte populations are present, one DQ+ and one DQ−

Table 2. Peripheral blood mononuclear cell subpopulations present in enriched suspensions

Technique:	T cells	Monocytes	B cells	Null cells
E rosetting	–	+	+	+
Nylon wool adherence	+ (mainly OKT8+)	+	+	–

vantage of using complement-fixing MoAbs is that characterization of cell subpopulations can be achieved using the complement-dependent lymphocytotoxicity technique. This allows to test every cell suspension to be studied for class II antigens in a simple way, using a small amount of target cells and reagents. Moreover, El-Awar et al. [22] succeeded in discriminating between different lymphoid cell subpopulations from peripheral blood, on the basis of their size as measured by a Coulter counter. The cell subpopulations that can be found in B-enriched suspensions obtained with the two procedures mentioned above are indicated in Table 2. It thus appears that the nylon adherence technique yields cell suspensions that have less of the nonadherent null cell component than suspensions obtained after removal of E rosettes. The class II-negative component detectable in the nylon adherent suspensions is mainly represented by a heterogeneous, preferentially OKT8-positive, T cell subpopulation. T lymphocytes in the nylon-adherent cells are more frequent among uremic patients (65% of nylon-adherent cell suspensions from uremic patients contain more than 40% T cells, vs. 33% of suspensions from healthy donors [15]). On the other hand, no T cells are detectable in B-enriched suspensions obtained with the E rosette technique, with which the class II-negative cells are mainly null cells. The proportion of null cells in E− suspensions is variable. Among 244 samples prepared from healthy donors, El-Awar et al. [22] found only eight (3.2%) not containing null cells: these showed strong reactivity with anti-DR alloantisera. In contrast, 21 samples that contained no B cells at all never reacted strongly with anti-DR alloantisera. Altogether, El-Awar et al. found 36% of suspensions reacting strongly with the control anti-class II xenoantisera and with anti-DR alloantisera (and showing less than 30% null cells), 48% of cell suspensions with intermediate reactions (30% –80% null cell contamination) and 8% of practically unreactive samples (more than 80% null cells). It must be noted that in these experiments monocytes had been eliminated with thrombin. It thus appears that simple SRBC rosette depletion can yield highly pure B lymphocytes only in a minority of samples, especially when the samples are from dialysis patients.

The above results are reflected in the quality of typing for class II antigens. We have examined the results of class II typing concerning both dialysis patients and normal individuals, in relation to the percentage of "B cells" (cells positive with MoAb B1) present in the cell suspensions (Table 3). It appears that an acceptable DR typing can be obtained independently of B cell enrichment, though while all B1+ samples can be satisfactorily typed, this is not always true for B1− samples. In contrast, DQ typing significantly depends on the presence of B1+ cells. It must be noted that monocytes were present in these cell suspensions and are responsible for the positive reactions with anti-DR alloantisera when B cells are absent or few. B1+ suspensions are seldom (25%) obtained from dialyzed patients when

Table 3. Correlation between presence of B lymphocytes in the target cell suspensions and reactivity of anti-DR and anti-DQ antibodies, in complement-dependent cytotoxicity assay

	++	+−	−+	−−	X^2	r
B1/DR[a]	29	0	64	27	n.s.	
B1/DQw1[b]	14	3	10	25	13.32	0.51
B1/Tu22[c]	23	7	5	91	67.53	0.73

Note: A reaction with a monoclonal antibody is considered positive when more than 40% of the cells in the sample are killed. DR and DQ typing are considered positive when the mean percentage of cells killed by all antisera specific for an antigen present on the cells is higher than 40%

[a] DR typing; [b] DQw1 typing; [c] Anti-DQ MoAb

using the E rosetting technique: this explains why class II typing of uremic patients is so frequently troublesome, especially for DQ specificities. The difficulty can be in part overcome using B-enriched suspensions obtained with the nylon technique, in which case we obtain more than 80% B1+ cell samples, but it should be remembered that remarkable T cell contamination is frequently found (see above).

A surprisingly high percentage of B1-positive samples (70%) was obtained from patients with HBsAg+ chronic active hepatitis using the E rosetting cell depletion technique. In this case, 90% of the cell suspensions could easily be typed for DR and DQ specificities. These findings can be explained by the hypothesis that the viral infection increases the amount of circulating B lymphocytes.

Reactivity of Anti-Class II Antibodies with Different Mononuclear Cell Subpopulations; Characterization of Antibody Specificity

It is obvious from the above data that different reactivities of anti-class II antibodies must be expected, depending upon the target cells.

Two main consequences can be envisaged and have indeed been demonstrated:

1. Anti-DR antibodies may show a different reactivity (ranging from negative to strongly positive) against different B cell-enriched suspensions from the same individual, depending on the relative amounts of B cells, monocytes, and null cells. When pure B cells are tested, standardized typing alloantisera may show many extra-reactions due to the presence in the sera of weak extra antibodies that do not generally react with the usually prepared cell suspensions.

In a screening of 350 alloantisera negative against total peripheral blood lymphocytes, we found a significantly higher percentage of positive reactions with the purified B lymphocytes than with the standard E rosette-depleted cell suspensions. Moreover, the mean strength of the positive reactions was 70% of killed cells in the first case and 40% in the second case.

2. The majority of circulating monocytes do not express DQ specificities [26, 37]. Therefore anti-DQ antibodies are able to react only against the cell suspensions that contain a sufficient amount of B cells (more than 40% of cells positive

with MoAb B1). This explains why a significant correlation has been found between reactivity with MoAb B1 and liability of DQ typing (Table 3).

A practical consequence of the differential expression of DR and DQ antigens on B cells and monocytes is that in some cases it allows definition of the specificity of anti-class II alloantisera. As a matter of fact the specificity of anti-class II antibodies is usually defined through population studies and significant correlation with known class II specificities in 2×2 contingency tables. Since DR and DQ antigens show very strong linkage disequilibrium, it is often impossible to discriminate between anti-DR and anti-DQ antibodies with the same distribution in the population.

Serologic reactions specific for DQ antigens can be better identified through the following characteristics:

1. Expression on B cells but not on monocyte-enriched suspensions
2. Inhibition of cytotoxicity by anti-DQ MoAbs but not by anti-DR MoAbs [36].

We have thus been able to characterize some apparently anti-DR5 alloantisera which, probably recognize a DQ new specificity in linkage disequilibrium with DR5 (Richiardi et al., paper in preparation). Among 11 alloantisera used for DR5 typing, three (GEG 503, TORP 718, PA 125) were identified whose reactivity was significantly correlated with the positive reaction of the cell suspensions with MoAb B1. These three alloantisera very often did not show a clear segregation with HLA in families, in the sense that they were positive only with some of the DR5+ members. This pattern excluded the possibility that they might recognize a specificity subtypic to DR5. When tested against separated monocytes and B lymphocytes from DR5+ individuals, they showed a positive reaction only against B cells. In contrast, the remaining eight anti-DR5 alloantisera showed a similar reactivity against B cells and monocytes. Furthermore, the reactivity of the former antisera was not blocked by a non-complement-fixing anti-DR MoAb, while the contrary was true for the latter eight anti-DR5 antisera. Altogether, these data indicate that the above three antisera recognize a DQ specificity.

Differentiation of Anti-Class II from Antibodies with Other Specificity

If a serum reacts only with B (or, better, non-T) cells and is negative when tested against T lymphocytes, this is not sufficient evidence that it is anti-class II. There are antibodies specific for several antigens other than HLA class II antigens that react only with B lymphocytes.

Anti-HLA-A, B, C. Antibodies have been described that are specific for HLA-A, B, or C antigens, but cytotoxic only for B cells [14, 42].This is due to the fact that B cells express on the cell surface three times more A, B, C antigens than T cells. Therefore the density of the target antigen on T cells might not be enough to trigger complement-dependent cytotoxicity. These antibodies can be differentiated from anti-class II antibodies by studying the serum after extensive absorption with platelets, since platelets may absorb only anti-A, B, C, not anti-class II. If the serum is investigated for a pretransplant cross-match there may not be enough time for platelet absorption with classical methods. In this case, quick absorptions can be performed directly in Terasaki plates [10]. Another efficient method is to test serum against B cells coated by a turkey anti-human-B2-microglobulin (anti-B2M) serum (which is not cytotoxic in the presence of rabbit complement). Such cells can no longer react with antibodies directed against B2M-associated structures, such as HLA class I antigens, while they are still able to react with anti-class II antibodies. This test, named "bb test" [5], is very quick and efficient in differentiating anti-class II from anti-A, B, C and is used routinely in our kidney transplantation department for pretransplant cross-match procedures.

Anti-Lewis. The presence of Lewis antigens on lymphocytes has long been demonstrated. Lymphocytotoxic sera specific for these antigens have been found [20]; some of them react only with B lymphocytes [17, 38]. The Lewis antigens may have a different structure according to the ABO blood group of an individual, therefore some sera react with either Le(a) or Le(b), while others react only with cells whose phenotype is A1+ Le(b+), and yet others only with B+ Le(b+). Their specificity can be identified only by testing the serum with a panel typed for ABO and Lewis.

Screening of Anti-Class II Antibodies

The major source of anti-Ia antibodies have up to now been sera from pluriparous women or from immunized individuals. Recently also polymorphic monoclonal antibodies have been produced that recognize known and new allospecificities [6]. In the alloantisera the proportion of sera reacting with B lymphocytes is smaller among sera devoid of anti-HLA-A, B antibodies (20%) than among sera that also contain anti-class I antibodies (50%) [9]. Of all the B cell-positive antisera, around 20% correlate with known class II antigens. Since many sera contain both anti-class II and anti-class I antibodies one major problem is to eliminate reactivity of the unwanted anti-class I antibodies. As mentioned above, this has been obtained in two ways:

1. Absorbing anti-A, B, C with platelets, that express class I but not class II molecules.
2. Masking class I antigens on the cell surface with non cytotoxic anti-B2-microglobulin antibodies (bb test).

Absorptions are performed with pools of platelets from at least 200 individuals, from which all class II-positive leukocytes have been accurately removed by differential centrifugation. A large pool of platelets assures that all HLA-A, B, C specifificities are represented, even those with a very low frequency. Most anti-class I antibodies can be eliminated from alloantisera after absorption with 30 $\times 10^9$ platelets/ml serum. In a few cases larger amounts are needed. Obviously, when the specificity of anti-A, B, C antibodies present is known and specific platelets are available, absorptions can be performed with lower doses. Failure to completely absorb anti-A, B, C antibodies might be due to the presence of antibodies directed against class I specificities that are not well expressed on platelets, such as HLA-C antigens (which disappear upon conservation), B8, B12, etc. [2, 16]. Absorptions can also be performed with identical results using lyophilized platelets [40].

Not all anti-class II sera show a constant pattern when they are absorbed with different pools. In our experience, among 35 sera of known specificity absorbed with two different platelet pools, 23 maintained the same reactivity, while in the remaining 12 the reaction patterns were different [7, 8]. The platelet absorption is therefore a critical step in serum manipulation which needs rigid standardization both of the technical procedure and of the criteria of platelet selection. In this respect, lyophilized platelets that assure indefinite conservation of very large pools may prove to be very useful.

Storage of antisera is again critical [1]. A remarkable loss of activity can be seen in some sera upon storage at −30 °C; anti-DR reagents should thus be stored in the deep freeze (−70 °C).

The bb test has been explained above. It is a way of "purifying" anti-class II activity in a serum without platelet absorption. A comparison between the reactivity of unabsorbed sera in the "bb test" and of absorbed sera against nonpretreated cells demonstrates that the "bb test" shows a larger number of positive results. In a study of 318 sera with the two techniques [9], we showed that 53% of the sera were positive with the bb test, while 20% reacted with nonpretreated B cells after platelet absorption. All the sera reacting against B lymphocytes after platelet absorption were also positive with the bb test, while 99 sera showed a positive reaction against B cells only with the bb test. It is worthwhile to note that platelet-absorbed sera also displayed more frequent positive reactions against anti-B2M-pretreated lymphocytes. The reactivity of some of the antibodies positive only with the bb test was significantly correlated with known DR specificities, confirming the report by Ceppellini et al. [11] that anti-B2M-pretreated cells show an increased reactivity with anti-class II antibodies. On the other hand, these investigators could not exclude the possibility that the bb test may also reveal non-HLA antibodies. We too observed that some sera, whose reactivity in the bb test is not correlated to known class II antigens, are able to react with T lymphocytes only after pretreatment with anti-B2M, thus supporting the hypothesis that non-HLA lymphocytotoxic antibodies may be revealed by the bb test.

Relevance of Complement in HLA Class II Serology

Differences between pools of rabbit complement are a major source of variability in HLA typing results. To check the extent of variability due to complement in DR serology, we compared three pools of complement that had been standardized for A, B, C typing. The pools had been checked against total peripheral blood lymphocytes for absence of spontaneous cytotoxicity after long incubation (2 h) and titrated with known anti-A and B antisera. The three complement pools gave identical results. When tested against B cells, one of the three showed a clear, albeit low, spontaneous cytotoxicity and had to be discarded. Titrated in conjunction with three different DR antisera, the remaining two showed the same strength. It therefore seems that complement is no more a source of variability for DR than for A, B, C serology. However, rabbit complement pools not showing spontaneous cytotoxicity must be selected by direct testing against B cell-enriched suspensions [7, 16].

Serological Analysis of Anti-Class II Antibodies

Classical serological analysis of anti-HLA antibodies includes the following steps.

Population and Family Studies. These allow assessment of whether the reactivity of antibody is correlated with a known HLA specificity and whether it segregates with a HLA haplotype in families.

Problems that can be encountered in HLA class II serology concerning this step have been exhaustively discussed above and refer mainly to differential expression of HLA antigens on different peripheral blood mononuclear target cells.

Absorption and Elution Experiments. These aim at analysis of the different antibody populations that can be present in alloantisera. Procedures for elimination of anti-class I antibodies have already been discussed. We are now left with the problems of dissecting various anti-class II antibodies. Absorptions must be performed with class II-positive cells: therefore, lymphoid lines with an appropriate class II phenotype are the ideal material. If peripheral blood cells are employed, it is convenient to use total, unseparated leukocytes where a larger amount of class II-positive cells can be found. The main problem is to select absorbing cells with the appropriate phenotype: very often, antibodies against more than one antigen, belonging to a common haplotype, coexist in alloantisera. Separation of these antibody populations can be achieved only using cells from the rare individuals not carrying both specificities. Alternatively, DQ-negative CLL B cells or monocytes could be used, but these should be purified from the DQ-positive subpopulations.

Identification of the Target Molecules. Classical serology of HLA-A, B, C antigens has achieved this goal by means of the lysostrip technique (for a review see [41]). In brief, incubation of lymphocytes with the anti-HLA antibody plus a second anti-IgG antibody at 37 °C induces "capping" of the relevant target molecule, with the consequent abrogation of reactivity (detected by lymphocytotoxicity) with all the antibodies recognizing antigenic epitopes carried by that molecule. In contrast antibodies directed against epitopes carried by different molecules are still able to react. It was by using this technique that it was possible to demonstrate that HLA-B and C antigens controlled by genes in high linkage disequilibrium are carried by different molecules.

For some unknown reason it is generally difficult or impossible to induce lysostrip of class II molecules. Positive results have been claimed by Duquesnoy et al. [21], who succeeded in obtaining a separate lysostrip of DR1 and DQw1 molecules, though they report that they "experienced considerable difficulties with the lysostrip procedures. In most cases lysostripping was either incomplete or the cells showed an unusually high background in subsequent lymphocytotoxicity testing." Anyhow, all those who have succeeded in inducing lysostrip of Ia molecules have used F(ab')2 fragments of anti Ig as the second antibody [21] (P. Stastny, personal communication).

For the analysis of human class II molecules a different approach proved particularly useful [45, 48]. The procedure involves isolation of class II antigens from class II-typed lymphoid cell lines on the basis of physicochemical properties, radioiodination of the labeled antigens, and subsequent analysis of the reactivity to alloantisera by molecular binding assay. A sequential binding assay can indicate whether two antisera which may bind different proportions of class II molecules in a preparation do recognize separate subsets of molecules. In this case, prior binding with one antiserum and elimination of the reacting molecules does not affect the reaction of the second antiserum. If this also holds true in the reciprocal experiment, it is demonstrated that the two tested antisera recognize antigenic epitopes carried by different subsets of class II molecules. This approach has an obvious limitation in the fact that class II alloantisera are usually complex mixtures of antibodies produced against the associated allelic products of loci in linkage disequilibrium. Since these are the components that one wishes to separate immunospecifically by means of antisera, this is a closed circle that can be broken only by the use of antibodies that, in a given antigen combination, only react with one component.

With this approach Tanigaki et al. [46] were able to demonstrate quite convincingly that alloantigenic determinants are localized on three molecular subsets, which they called DR, DC, and BR. Allelic specificities at each of these loci are in strong linkage disequilibrium. It has now been demonstrated definitively by biochemical analysis of the class II molecules and by analysis of the gene sequence that DR and BR are different molecules coded by the DR region (they possess the same alpha chain but different beta chains), while DC molecules are coded by the DQ region.

References

1. d'Apice AJF, Tait BD, Lambert G (1977) Inhibition of B cell cytotoxicity by aggregated IgG and immune complexes. Tissue Antigens 10:373–378
2. Aster RH, Szarkowski N, Liedert M, Duquesnoy RJ (1977) Expression of HLA-B12, HLA-B8, w4 and w6 on platelets. Transplant Proc 9:1695–1696
3. Baricordi O, Belvedere M, Fagiolo U, Neri TM, Trabace S, Savi M (1978) Screening for B cell specific antisera. Results from region Italy. Haematologica (Pavia) 63:125–131
4. Belvedere M, Diotallevi P, Savina C (1977) Purificazione di linfociti B dal sangue periferico: studio di vari aspetti delle tecniche relative. Riv Emoter Immunoematol 24:25–37
5. Bernoco D, Bernoco M, Ceppellini R, Poulik MD, van Leeuwen A, van Rood JJ (1976) B cell antigens of the HLA system: a simple serotyping technique based on non-cytotoxic anti-B2-microglobulin reagents. Tissue Antigens 8:253–260
6. Bodmer J, Kennedy L, Aizawa M, Dawkins R, Lepage V, Mazzilli MC, Richiardi P (1984) HLA-D region monoclonal antibodies. In: Albert ED, Baur MP, Mayr WR (eds) Histocompatibility Testing 1984. Springer, Berlin Heidelberg New York Tokyo, pp 217–236
7. Borelli I, Diotallevi P, Neri TM, Olivetti E, Savi M, Curtoni ES (1978) Studio immunogenetico delle strutture HLA-DR. I. Importanza di alcune variabili delle tecniche sierologiche. Riv Emoter Immunoematol 25:18–36
8. Borelli I, Cornaglia M, Olivetti E, Curtoni ES (1979) HLA-DR typing: some relevant difficulties. Transplant Proc 11:1319–1332
9. Borelli I, Amoroso A, Richiardi P, Durtoni ES (1982) Evaluation of different technical approaches for the research of human anti-Ia alloantisera. Tissue Antigens 19:380–387
10. Cecchi V, Belvedere M, Luciani G, Curtoni ES (1977) A new HLA antigen apparently not controlled by the known HLA loci. J Immunogenet 4:7–14
11. Ceppellini R, Garotta G, Malavasi F, Trucco M (1981) Modulation of expression of HLA components at the cell surface induced by anti-B2M reagents. Tissue Antigens 17:28–36

12. Chen Y-X, Evans RL, Pollack MS, Lanier LL, Phillips JH, Rousso C, Warner NL, Brodsky FM (1984) Characterization and expression of the HLA-DC antigens defined by anti-Leu 10. Hum Immunol 10:221–235
13. Cicciarelli JC, Bernoco D, Terasaki PI, Shirahama S (1978) Studies of HLA-A, B, C, and D antigens on monocytes. Transplant Proc 10:863–865
14. Coxe-Gililand R, Cross DE (1980) A comparison of the sensitivities of T and B lymphocytes to HLA-A, B, C antibodies. In: Terasaki P (ed) Histocompatibility Testing 1980. UCLA University Press, Los Angeles, p 927
15. Crepaldi T, Richiardi P, Borelli I, Malavasi F, Carbonara AO (1982) Characterization by monoclonal antibodies of lymphocyte subsets present in B-enriched suspensions. Tissue Antigens 20:282–288
16. Curtoni ES, Borelli I, Carbonara AO, Diotallevi P, Olivetti E, Neri TM, Savi M (1979) Serologic and genetic aspects of HLA-DR antigen study. Transplant Proc 11:1317–1318
17. Curtoni ES, Borelli I, Cornaglia M, Olivetti E, Peyretti F (1980) Antibodies for other blood systems present in Workshop DR sera and interaction with anti-DR antibodies. In: Terasaki P (ed) Histocompatibility Testing 1980. UCLA University Press, Los Angeles, p 900
18. Curtoni ES, Pellegrino MA, Indiveri F, Borelli I, Ferrone S (1981) Persistence of cytotoxic antibodies to HLA-A, B, C antigens and to Ia-like antigens in parous women. J Immunogenet 8:281–285
19. de Kretser TA, Bodmer JG, Bodmer WF (1980) The separation of cell populations using monoclonal antibodies attached to Sepharose. Tissue Antigens 16:317–325
20. Dorf ME, Eguro SY, Cabrera G, Yunis EJ, Swanson J, Amos DB (1972) Detection of cytotoxic non-HLA antisera. I. Relationship to anti-Le(a). Vox Sang 22:447–456
21. Duquesnoy RJ, Marrari M, Annen K (1980) Association of the B-cell alloantigen MB1 with HLA-DRw1 and DRw2. Transplant Proc 12:138–140
22. El-Awar N, Terasaki PI, Perdue S, Cicciarelli J, Mickey MR (1980) Discrimination of T, B, and null lymphocytes by electronic sizing. Tissue Antigens 15:346–360
23. Ferrone S, Pellegrino MA, van Rood JJ, van Leeuwen A (1977) Functional properties of anti-B cell antigen alloantisera. Transplant Proc 9:675–678
24. Froland SS, Natvig J (1974) Identification of three different human lymphocyte populations by surface markers. Transplant Rev 16:114
25. Greaves MF, Brown G (1974) Purification of human T and B lymphocytes. J Immunol 112:420–423
26. Guy K, Ritchie AWS, van Heyningen V, Dewar AE (1983) Further serological characterization of the heterogeneity of expression of human MHC class II antigens: chronic lymphocytic leukemia cells and monocytes differentially express DR and DC antigens. Dis Markers 1:249–262
27. Hayward A, Greaves MF (1977) Human T and B lymphocytes populations in blood. Recent Adv Clin Immunol 1:149–167
28. Horwitz DA, Bakke A (1984) An Fc receptor-bearing third population of human mononuclear cells with cytotoxic and regulatory function. Immunology Today 5:148–153
29. Kovithavongs T, Shivji S, Dossetor JB (1978) Human K cells do not have Ia antigens. Transplant Proc 10:839–843
30. Lansdorf PM, Oosterhof F, Astaldi GC, Zeijlemaker WP (1982) Detection of HLA antigens on blood platelets and lymphocytes by means of monoclonal antibodies in an ELISA technique. Tissue Antigens 19:11–19
31. Lawler SD, Dewar PJ, Mrazek I, Jones EK, Hockley AB (1978) Antisera with Ia specificity selected by lymphocytes from patients with chronic lymphocytic leukemia. Vox Sang 34:200–207
32. Lepage V, Gaudy Y, Terrier E, Dausset J, Colombani J (1981) Screening and use of high titered anti-HLA-DR sera in PHA blasts complement fixation and B-lymphocytotoxicity techniques. Tissue Antigens 17:37–42
33. Lowry RP, Person AE, Goguen JE, Carpenter CB, Garovoy MR (1978) Technical modification for antibody-dependent cell-mediated cytotoxicity versus separated T and B lymphocytes: T- and B- cell separation by nylon wool columns. Transplant Proc 10:833–837

34. Lowry RP, Goguen J, Carpenter CB, Strom TB, Garovoy MR (1979) Improved B cell typing for HLA-DR using nylon wool column enriched B lymphocyte preparations. Tissue Antigens 14:325–330
35. Madsen M (1979) False negative HLA-DR assignment of necrokidney donors. A glucocorticoid effect? Tissue Antigens 14:353–358
36. Nunez G, Latimer MJ, Ball EJ, Myers LK, Stastny P (1984) Serologic detection of new polymorphisms on DQ molecules distinct from the DQw1, 2, and 3 specificities. In: Albert ED, Baur MP, Mayr WR (eds) Histocompatibility testing 1984. Springer, Berlin Heidelberg New York Tokyo, pp 421–422
37. Nunez G, Giles RC, Ball EJ, Hurley CK, Capra JD, Stastny P (1984) Expression of HLA-DR, MB, MT, and SB antigens on human mononuclear cells: identification of two phenotypically distinct monocyte populations. J Immunol 133:1300–1306
38. Park MS, Oriol P, Terasaki PI, Nakata S (1980) Lewis-related specificities of the 8th Workshop. In: Terasaki P (ed) Histocompatibility testing 1980. UCLA University Press, Los Angeles, p 929
39. Pellegrino MA, Ferrone S, Dierichard MP, Reisfeld RA (1975) Enhancement of sheep red blood cell human lymphocyte rosette formation by the sulphhydryl compound 2-amino ethylisothiouronium bromide. Clin Immunol Immunopathol 3:324–327
40. Prou O, Kaplan C, Muller JY (1980) Freeze-dried platelets for HLA alloantibodies absorption. Tissue Antigens 16:105–107
41. Richiardi P (1982) Lysostrip, F(ab)2 blocking. In: Solheim B, Ferrone S (eds) HLA typing: methodology and clinical aspects. CRC Press, Boca Raton, p 39
42. Richiardi P, Diotallevi P, Matejc T, Carbonara AO, Curtoni ES (1977) HLA antibodies cytotoxic only for B lymphocytes. Tissue Antigens 10:323–329
43. Richiardi P, Crepaldi T, Carbonara AO (1984) Reactivity of monoclonal anti-T Workshop reagents in immunofluorescence and cytotoxicity techniques. In: Bernard A, Boumsell L, Dausset J, Milstein C, Schlossmann SF (eds) Leukocyte typing. Springer, Berlin Heidelberg New York Tokyo, pp 231–236
44. Stocker JW, Garotta G, Hausmann B, Trucco M, Ceppellini R (1979) Separation of human cells bearing HLA-DR antigens using a monoclonal antibody rosetting method. Tissue Antigens 13:212–222
45. Tanigaki N, Tosi R (1982) Assessment of the specificity of human Ia alloantisera and alloantigens by the use of radioiodinated human Ia antigens. Tissue Antigens 20:1–21
46. Tanigaki N, Tosi R, Duquesnoy R, Ferrara GB (1983) Three Ia species with different structures and alloantigenic determinants in an HLA-homozygous cell line. J Exp Med 157:231–247
47. Terasaki PI, McClelland JD (1964) Microdroplet assay of human serum cytotoxins. Nature 204:998
48. Tosi RM, Tanigaki N, Centis D, Ferrara GB, Pressmann DJ (1978) Immunological dissection of human Ia molecules. J Exp Med 148:1592–1611
49. Trizio D, Cudkowicz G (1974) Separation of T and B lymphocytes by nylon wool columns. Evaluation of efficacy by functional assays in vivo. J Immunol 113:1093–1097
50. Trucco M, De Petris S, Garotta G, Ceppellini R (1980) Quantitative analysis of cell surface HLA structures by means of monoclonal antibodies. Hum Immunol 1:233–243
51. van Rood JJ, Van Leeuwen A, Ploem JS (1976) Simultaneous detection of two cell populations by two-colour fluorescence and application to the recognition of B-cell determinants. Nature 262:795–797
52. Werner C, Klouda P, Correa MC, Vassalli P, Jeannet M (1977) Isolation of B and T lymphocytes by nylon fiber columns. Tissue Antigens 9:227–229
53. Wong DM, Mittal KK (1981) HLA-DR typing: a comparison between nylon wool adherence and T cell rosetting in the isolation of B cells. J Immunol Methods 46:177–186

Alloantisera Against Human Class II Antigens: Definition and Methodology *

G. M. T. Schreuder and A. van Leeuwen

Table of Contents

* This work was in part supported by the Dutch Foundation for Medical Research (FUNGO), which is subsidized by the Dutch Organization for the Advancement of Pure Research (ZWO) and the J. A. Cohen Institute for Radiopathology and Radiation Protection (IRS)

Introduction

Alloantisera have been and still are the major source of reagents for the recognition of antigenic determinants on class II molecules. The importance of these determinants in immunological processes is clearly recognized, but still poorly understood. Class II determinants are also extensively studied by cellular techniques using homozygous typing cells (HTCs) and primed lymphocyte typing (PLT) reagents. Careful comparison between serological and cellular studies has led to a better understanding of the relations between the serologically defined HLA-DR and DQ specificities and the cellularly defined HLA-D specificities. Recently the addition of monoclonal antibodies that can be used in serological, cellular, and especially biochemical assays has added much to the unravelling of the relationships between the class II determinants.

The Ninth International Histocompatibility Workshop and Conference (9WS) presented an excellent opportunity to put together the presently acquired knowledge concerning major histocompatibility complex (MHC) and in particular class II determinants. One of the lessons that could be learned was that the definitions based upon the conventional alloantisera are needed as a reference to which other data can be compared. However, these definitions are still incomplete and will certainly be extended in future.

HLA-DR and DQ Nomenclature

The designation of the HLA-DR locus alleles did not change after the Eighth International Histocompatibility Workshop. The alleles are still numbered DR1-w10 (Table 1). Provisional designations for HLA-DR5 and DRw6 subgroups were added [1]: DRw11 (previously LB5) and DRw12 (previously LB5x8 or DR5 short) are splits of DR5, while DRw13 (previously 6.6, 6.1, 6Z) and DRw14 (previously 6.3, 6.9, 6X, 901) are splits of DRw6. Two other specificities, originally defined as cross-reacting specificities, have also been given HLA-DR numbers: DRw52 (previously mT2) and DRw53 (previously MT3).

Another group of serologically defined specificities is coded for by genes of the DQ locus. At present three alleles can be recognised: DQw1, DQw2, and DQw3. Most previously used equivalent designations are given in Table 1.

Another group of specificities which are encoded in the HLA-D region are designated as DP (previously SB). The six alleles (DPw1-w6, Table 1) can at present be defined only by cellular techniques. Serological recognition of DP specificities is possible by the use of alloantisera [2]. Such sera are rare, and will not be discussed here.

Table 1. 1984 WHO nomenclature of HLA-DR and DQ specificities with the previously used equivalents

Present	Previous
DR1	
DR2	
DR3	
DR4	
DR5	
DRw6	
DR7	
DRw8	
DRw9	
DRw10	
DRw11 (5)	LB5
DRw12 (5)	LB5 × 8, DR5 short, 8wDRw13, 8wDRw17
DRw13 (w6)	6.6, 6.1, 6Z
DRw14 (w6)	6.9, 6.3, 6X, 901
DRw52	MT2
DRw53	MT3
DQw1	DC1, MT1, MB1, LB-E12
DQw2	MB2, DC3, Te24, LB-E17
DQw3	MB3, MT4, DC4, TB21
DPw1	SB1, PL3A
DPw2	SB2
DPw3	SB3
DPw4	SB4, PL3B
DPw5	SB5
DPw6	SB6

HLA-DR in Relation to HLA-D

It should be kept in mind that the original definition of HLA-DR specificities was based on the specificities defined by cellular studies with homozygous typing cells (HTCs) [3]. When results from cellular and serological studies performed during the 9WS were compared, HLA-DR typings could be predicted by the HLA-D typings without exception, indicating a very close relationship between HLA-D and HLA-DR [4].

HLA-DR1

DR1 can be defined without any great problems. Monospecific alloantisera are available. Several anti-DR1 sera show cross-reactivity towards DRw10. DR1 is strongly associated with Dw1.

HLA-DR2

The DR2 specificity can be readily defined, but heterogeneity has been reported [5–7]. DR2 is associated with a number of HTC-defined specificities. The most common DR2 is associated with Dw2 and Dw12, whereas DR2 short (as defined

Table 2. HLA-DR2: DR, DQ serum patterns and D relationships

HLA-DR specificity	Groups of antisera					
	DR2	DR2 short (9w555)	DQw1	DQw3	TA10	HLA-D specificity
DR2	+	+	+	−	−	Dw2, Dw12
DR2 short	+	−	+	−	−	'FJO'
DR2 short	+	−	−	+	+	DB9
DR2 short	+	−	?	?	?	AZH

?: not known

by 9WS serum 9w555, CCB1000 from W. E. Braun) is associated with DB9, FJO [8], and AZH [9]. Association of DR2 with DW9 has been reported [10], but not confirmed. Table 2 summarizes the possible relations between DR2, other class II determinants, and HLA-D. For TA10 definition see below.

HLA-DR3

DR3 is a well-defined specificity which is strongly associated with Dw3.

HLA-DR4

The DR4 specificity is heterogeneous. Two DR4 subgroups (LB4 and LB10) were described by our group [11]. Dw4-positive cells typed as LB4, and Dw10-positive cells typed as LB10. Subdivisions into DR4.1, 4.2, and 4.3 resulted from the 9WS analysis [12], but were hampered by the weak reactivity of some sera.

The DR4 heterogeneity is also reflected by the large number of HTC-defined specificities that associate with it, including Dw4, Dw13 (DB3), Dw14 (LD40), Dw15 (DYT), and DKT2. Table 3 summarizes the three serologically defined patterns and their possible association with HLA-D [12, 13] together with other class II specificities (see below). The patterns are partly based on observations with HTCs.

The double gene dose expression on a homozygous cell may cause positive reactions with sera that do not recognize that specificity on a heterozygous cell. Therefore Dw10 cells may all be DR4.3.

Table 3. HLA-DR4: DR, DQ serum patterns and D relationships

HLA-DR specificity	Groups of antisera						
	DR4 (4.1+ 4.2+4.3)	4.1+ 4.2	4.1	LB14	DQw3	TA10	HLA-D specificity
DR4.1 (LB4)	+	+	+	+	+	+/−	Dw4
	+	+	+	+	+	−	Dw14
	+	+	+	+	−	−	Dw15
DR4.2 (LB10)	+	+	−	−	+	+/−	Dw13
DR4.3 (LB10)	+	−/+	−	−	+	−/+	Dw10

+/−: most cells positive; −/+: most cells negative

Table 4. HLA-DR5, DRw6, and DRw8: DR, DQ serum patterns and D relations

HLA-DR, DQ specificity	DR serum groups								DQ serum groups					
	w52	w11	5+ w13	5+w8 +w13	w14	3+w6	w8	DR5+ TA10	TA10	DQw3	2+w6	DQw1	DQw2	HLA-D specifictiy
DR5														
DRw11, DQw3	+	+	+	+	–	–	–	+	+	+	–	–	–	Dw5
DRw11, DQw1	+	+	+	+	–	–/+	–	+	–	–	–	+	–	Dw5?
DRw11, DQ–	+	+	+	+	–	–	–	+	–	–	–	–	–	?
DRw12, DQw3	+	–	+	+	–	–/+	–	+	+	+	–	–	–	DB6
DRw12, DQ–	+	–	+	+	–	–	–	+	–	–	–	–	–	?
DRw6														
DRw13, DQw1	+	–	+	+	–	+/–	–	–	–	–	+	+	–	Dw18, Dw19 (Dw6)
DRw13, DQw3	+	–	+	+	–	+	–	+	+	+	–	–	–	HAG
DRw13, DQ–	+	–	+	+	–	+/–	–	–	–	–	–	–	–	?
DRw14, DQw1	+	–	–	–	+	+/–	–	–	–	–	+	+	–	Dw9
DRw14, DQw3	+	–	–	–	+	+	–	+	+	+	–	–	–	Dw16
DRw8, DQ–	+	–	–	+	–	–	+	–	–	–	–	–	–	Dw8
DRw8, DQw1	+	–	–	+	–	–	+	–	–	–	–	+	–	DB7 (8.2)
DRw8, DQw3	+	–	–	+	–	–	+	+	+	+	–	–	–	DB7 (8.2)

+/–: most cells positive; –/+: most cells negative

HLA-DR5

Two subgroups of DR5 were described by us as LB5 (now DRw11) and LB5x8 (now DRw12) [11]. The DRw11 specificity can be easily defined with monospecific antisera, and is associated with Dw5. The DRw12 specificity is difficult to define and has been confused with some DRw6 variants [14]. As yet no monospecific DRw12 antisera are available. So-called long DR5 sera recognize DRw12, but also DRw11, and contain DQ-related antibodies. Other DR sera react with DR5 – but also with DRw13 (w6) – and often DRw8-positive cells.

DRw12 was originally defined as LB5x8 with HTC Herluf (from A. Svejgaard). Serological typing of 9WS HTCs showed that HTC BM16 (from G. B. Ferrara) also typed as DRw12 [13]. Both HTCs have been provisionally designated as DB6 [15].

DR5-related serum patterns are summarized in Table 4.

HLA-DRw6

The definition of DRw6 has been greatly complicated by the lack of monospecific antisera. The Seventh Workshop indicated the use of DR2 + w6 sera [16]. During the Eighth Workshop the DRw6 definition was predominantly based on DR3 + w6 sera, which led to an underestimation of DRw6 [17]. Moreover, heterogeneity was reported which included selective reactivity of DR5 + w6 + w8 sera [14, 18].

Analysis of the 9WS family data and HTCs enabled a more precise definition of DRw6 through the consideration of two subgroups, DRw13 and DRw14 [19]. This was facilitated by the availability of two monospecific anti-DRw14 sera, one of which had been described as recognizing a Dw9-associated DR specificity called 901 [20]. In Table 4 groups of sera are shown that enable the recognition of DRw6 subgroups, even in the presence of DR5. The DRw6 definition is also complicated by the fact that both DR5 and DRw6 (sub)types can occur in conjunction with different DQ specificities (see below).

DRw13 is associated with Dw6. Although alloantisera are not (yet) able to define the two cellularly defined subgroups of Dw6 (Dw18 and Dw19) [21], monoclonal antibodies may do so [22]. DRw13 is also associated with an HTC-defined specificity, HAG (HTC 9w1802 from P. Wernet). The serological distinction between the DRw12-DB6 and DRw13-D"HAG" is very difficult and predominantly based on the reactivity of DR3 + w6 sera. Here again, monoclonal antibodies may enable a more reliable definition [19, 22].

DRw14 is associated with Dw9 and Dw16.

Table 5 summarizes the present and previously used nomenclature for DRw6-related specificities.

Table 5. Present and previous nomenclature used for DRw6 specificities [19]

Present	Previous
DRw13, associated with DQw1	DRw6.1, 6.6, 8w6Y, 6Z, LB6.6
DRw13, associated with DQw3	DRw6.2, 6Y, LB6.2
DRw14, associated with DQw1	DRw6.3, 6.9, 6X, LB6.9, IaLad9, FT19, KD5, 901.
DRw14, associated with DQw3	DRw6.2, 6A, LB6.2

HLA-DR7

The DR7 specificity is well defined by serology. It is associated with Dw7, Dw11, and Dw17.

HLA-DRw8

The DRw8 specificity can be reasonably well defined, although monospecific anti-DRw8 sera are still rare. Other sera helpful for DRw8 recognition also react with DR5 (and DRw6). Reaction patterns of such sera are summarized in Table 4 in relation to DR5 and DRw6. DRw8 is associated with Dw8, DB7 (Dw8.2), and possibly other D specificities [23].

HLA-DRw9

The DRw9 specificity is reasonably well defined. Few monospecific sera are available at present. Most DRw9 antisera show also reactivity towards DR4- and/or DR7-positive cells. DRw9 is associated with DB5 [24].

HLA-DRw10

The DRw10 specificity is quite well defined. Several monospecific antisera are now available. A number of antisera with broader reactivity can also be helpful for DRw10 definition: DR1+w10 and DR1+w9+w10 [25].

DRw10 has been reported to associate with HTC SHY [26].

HLA-DR-Blank

A possible DR-blank specificity has been reported as DR"Br" [27]. As yet no DR antisera react with it. We have observed it in a family typed for the 9WS.

Surprisingly, the HTC BON (M. Thomsen, personal communication) appears to type for this specificity.

Two other specificities have been added to the DR series which were originally defined by so-called broadly reacting antisera. Their antigenic determinants are expressed both on DR and on other molecules coded for in the DR region [28, 29].

HLA-DRw52

DRw52 is present on all DR3-, DR5 (DRw11 and DRw12)-, DRw6 (DRw13 and DRw14)-, and DRw8-positive cells. Many alloantisera are available to type for DRw52. It probably comprises several antigenic determinants [28], which is also demonstrated by a monoclonal antibody that reacts with all DR3-, 5-, and w6-positive cells but not with DRw8 [30].

Anti-DRw52 sera can be very helpful for the definition of DR3, DR5, DRw6, and DRw8 specificities.

HLA-DRw53

Similarly, DRw53 is present on all DR4-, DR7-, and DRw9-positive cells. Very few good DRw53 antisera are available. Some sera show incomplete reactivity toward DR4, 7, or w9, but react strongly with the other DRw53-included specificities. Some DR4, 7, and w9 cells have been reported that do not react with any DRw53 antisera [31]. This could be due to technical factors, but it is also possible that DRw53 determinants are absent on some cells [29]. Other sera recognize DRw53 completely but contain additional antibodies toward DQw2, DQw3, DR5, and/or DR3.

Earlier reports also included DRw10 in DRw53 [32]. This was probably due to difficulties in DRw9 and DRw10 recognition.

HLA-DQ and Its Relation to DR

Substantial biochemical evidence has accumulated to prove that the so-called DC, MB, MT, LB-E, or DS specificities reside on molecules that are different from DR [29, 33] and are products of the DQ locus.

The position of the DQ locus in the D region is still unclear. Biochemists prefer to locate it between the DR and DP loci, but several reported B:DQ recombinations would suggest a site between DR and B [34, 35].

The DQ antisera were originally described as broadly reacting DR sera. Such observations were based on two phenomena: (a) many alloantisera are mixtures of DR and DQ antibodies; (b) the strong associations between DR and DQ specificities depend on the population studied.

When two loci are tightly linked, their association will be stable in a certain population. In a purely Caucasoid population, DR-DQ associations are very strong and make it almost impossible to discover, for example, an anti-DR2 antibody in a DQw1 serum or an anti-DR3 antibody in a DQw2 serum. When several antisera for each specificity are used, it is possible to discover occasional exceptional DR-DQ combinations.

The expression of DQ molecules appears to be restricted to peripheral blood B lymphocytes and a small subpopulation of monocytes [36]. Differential expression of DR and DQ has also been observed on hematopoietic progenitor cells [37] and on certain leukemic blast cells [38].

At present, three DQ specificities can be recognized.

HLA-DQw1

The DQw1 specificity is strongly associated with DR1, DR2, DRw6 (DRw13 and DRw14), and DRw10, but can also be found in association with DR3, DRw11 (DR5), DRw8, and DR"Br" (DR-blank).

Many anti-DQw1 allosera also contain anti-DR2 antibodies thus, complicating the observation of DR2-positive, DQw1-negative cells. Similarly, additional DR1 (+w10) antibodies can be found in DQw1 sera. Other sera appear as short anti-DQw1 sera. For example, DR2+w6 sera, originally used for the DRw6 definition, do not react with cells that carry DRw6 in combination with DQw3 (Table 4).

HLA-DQw2

DQw2 is strongly associated with DR3 and to a lesser extend with DR7. Occasional DRw9-DQw2 combinations have been reported [39]. Many DQw2 alloantisera contain additional antibodies to DR7 (and to DRw9). Also, anti-DR3 antibodies can often be observed in anti-DQw2 sera. Such sera accounted for the slightly different definitions of MB2, Te24 and LB-E17.

HLA-DQw3, LB-E13, and TA10

The DQw3 specificity is associated with DR4, DR5 (DRw11 and DRw12), DR7, and DRw9. Occasional combinations of DQw3 with DR2, DR3, DRw6 (DRw13 and DRw14), and DRw8 have also been reported [40, 13]. Recently, a family where DR-blank segregated with DQw3 was also observed [M. de Haan, personal communication].

Most anti-DQw3 alloantisera contain additional anti-DR4, -DR5 and/or -DRw53 antibodies and thus complicate DQw3 definition. DQw3 is probably heterogeneous.

The LB-E13 specificity appears to be included in DQw3, but is absent on DR7-DQw3 and on most DRw9-positive cells [11]. LB-E13 may account for a short DQw3 pattern observed on DRw9 cells [41].

TA10 is another DQ-related specificity which is probably included in DQw3 [42]. It was first described by a monoclonal antibody, but can also be recognized with alloantisera [43]. Almost all DR5-DQw3-positive cells are TA10-positive (Table 4), but only some DR4-DQw3-positive cells are also TA10-positive (Table 3). Many so-called long DR5 sera also react with TA10. Such sera may have caused the definition of triplets with DR4 and DR5 and with DRw8 and DR5 in the past.

The TA10 specificity is related to the 8wDRw13 specificity as defined by serum 8w719 in the Eighth Histocompatibility Workshop [44]. Ferrara suggested that this serum could recognize a product of a locus different from DR. However the 8wDRw13 designation was also used for the present DRw12 specificity, thus complicating the definitions.

HLA-DQ-Blank

Sometimes DR specificities are observed without serologically detectable DQ specificities. It is not yet known whether DQ products are really absent, or whether we have to await the discovery of antisera that will detect this DQ-blank.

Examples of DQ-blank associations are DRw8 and some DR4. Careful analysis of DR-DQ segregation in families that were typed in our laboratory, but also of the 9WS family data, showed that almost all DR specificities can occasionally occur in association with DQ-blank.

Figure 1 summarizes DQ-DR combinations as observed in local and 9WS data analysis without consideration of ethnic origin. The length of the horizontal lines indicates whether combinations were observed frequently or only occasionally. The LB-E13 and TA10 specificities are shown as variants of DQw3.

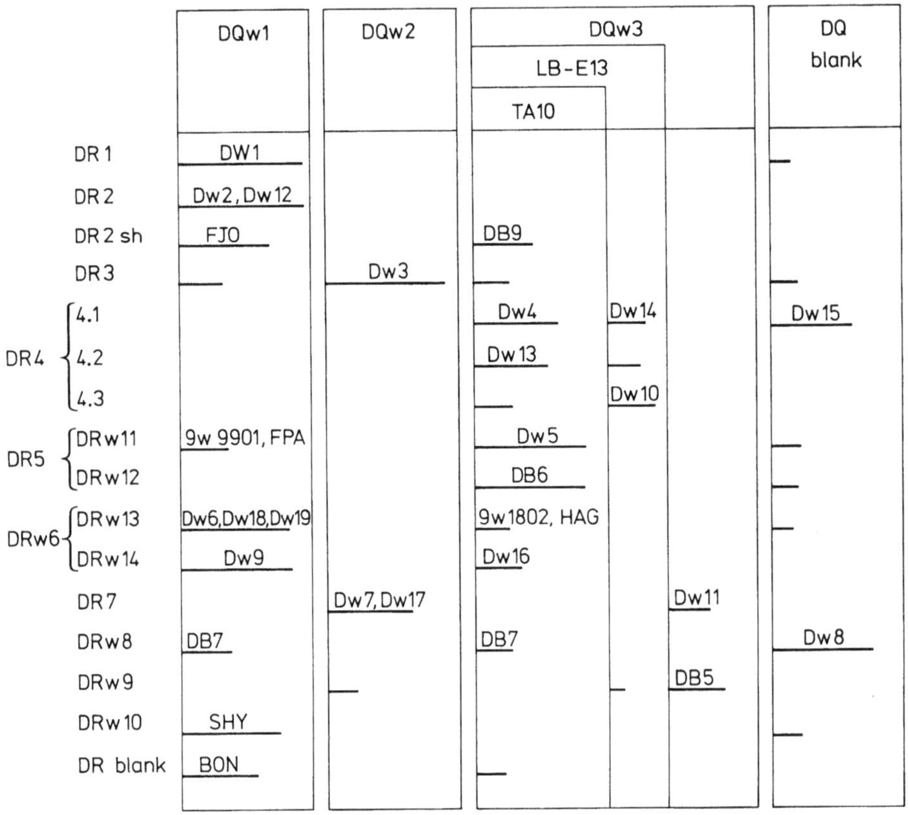

Fig. 1. HLA-DR, DQ associations and their relation to HLA-D

MC1, Te23, LB14

This specificity has been described as a DR1- and DR4-associated specificity [45, 46]. In our laboratory the designation LB14 has been used for what is probably the same specificity and can be recognized with two local alloantisera. It is present on almost all DR1- and DRw10- and on some DRw9-positive cells. Furthermore, all DR4-LB4 (DR4.1) cells carry this specificity, whereas DR4-LB10 (DR4.2 and 4.3) cells are LB14-negative. LB14 does not correlate with DQw1-w3. It is not yet known whether LB14 is a DR-like or a DQ-like specificity.

HLA-DR and DQ in Relation with HLA-D

Many of the above-mentioned DR-DQ combinations can be observed on HTCs [13]. Conversely, all of the DR-typed individuals who typed with these HTCs carried the equivalent DR-DQ combination [4]. This demonstrates a very close relationship of HLA-D and DR-DQ combinations.

In Fig. 1 HLA-D specificities are indicated with their HLA-DR and DQ associations. The less well defined specificities, provisionally designated as DB, are also shown. Some single HTCs represented exceptional DR-DQ combinations. They are shown by their 9WS number and local name. Some HTC specificities have been reported but not yet included in histocompatibility workshops. Where their DR-DQ assocations are known they are represented by their local name in Fig. 1.

DR2 short–DQw3 HTCs type for DB9. HTC FJO may also belong to this cluster [47], but is DR2 short–DQw1-positive.

The DR4-positive HLA-D specificities show a variety of DR4- and DQw3-related subtypes. As shown in Table 3, the associations within one HLA-D group are not homogeneous. Figure 1 summarizes their most likely associations.

Of the group of Dw5 HTCs, one (9w9901-FPA) was DRw11, DQw1, whereas all others were DRw11, DQw3.

In the DRw14-Dw9 HTC cluster, another exception was found: HTC 9w1902-DJ appeared to be DR3, DRw14, DQw1, DQw2.

HTCs that are DR7-positive can be divided into Dw7 and Dw17 (both DQw2-positive) and Dw11 (DQw3-positive). One Dw11 HTC, (9w1105-SM11), appeared as DQw2, DQw3-positive.

The majority of DRw8 HTCs are Dw8, DRw8, DQ-blank. A less well defined group of DB7 (Dw8.2) HTCs was typed as either DRw8, DQw1 or DRw8, DQw3.

Some Serological Considerations

Alloantisera reactive to B cells can be used very effectively to define HLA-DR, DQ, and other new specificities. However, alloantisera have to be considered as mixtures of antibody populations. Careful screening methods are required to select reagents that monospecifically recognize a certain DR or DQ specificity.

Sera that appear as short may prove to recognize splits. However, care should be taken that such sera show strong positive vs clearly negative reactions that segregate in families.

Broadly reacting sera may prove to be good anti-DQ reagents, but will almost always contain additional DR antibodies.

Another problem in the search for B cell antibodies is the presence of HLA-A, B, and/or C antibodies. Most HLA-A and B antibodies can be absorbed by platelets, but antibodies towards HLA-C and some B groups (e.g., B8 and B12) are very difficult to remove because of their variable expression on platelets [48, 49].

Platelet-absorbed sera should be retested for the presence of HLA-A, B, or C antibodies, even when they no longer react with T cells. The expression of HLA-ABC antigens is much stronger on B cells than on T cells [50], and B cell reactions can therefore still be caused by HLA-A, B, or C antibodies.

Especially with regard to DQ typing, the ratio of B cells to monocytes in the cell suspension is of importance. False-negative assignment of DQ is possible when predominantly monocytes are used [36].

A great number of cell separation and typing methods are in use for DR, DQ typing and have been published in detail. We will now present a selection of earlier published methods.

Detection of Anti-B Cell Antibodies by the Two-Color Fluorescence Test [51]

Heparinized blood is diluted with one volume of phosphate buffered saline (PBS) and this suspension is carefully layered upon Ficoll-Isopaque or Lymphoprep (sg 1.077). The tubes are spun for 15 min at 1000 *g* (2400 rpm), and the mononuclear cells are harvested from the interface and washed twice in PBS containing 1% bovine serum albumin (PBS+BSA 1%). From 4 to 6×10^6 cells suspended in 0.5 ml PBS+BSA 1% are incubated with one drop (0.025 ml) goat anti-human immunoglobulin FITC conjugate diluted 1:2 or 1:3 (Central Blood Transfusion Laboratory, Amsterdam) for 5 min in a 37 °C waterbath. After washing twice with PBS+BSA 1%, the cells are suspended in tissue culture medium with 20% heat-inactivated fetal calf serum (FCS) and the count is adjusted to 12000/µl. Do not use too much heparin, since this increases the background. Blood drawn on the day before testing: it is better to isolate and freeze lymphocytes than to leave the blood overnight. Make sure that the anti-immunoglobulin is not toxic by itself. It is often necessary to screen several batches. The incubation temperature of the trays should not exceed 22 °C, and the trays should be kept in darkness during incubation. PBS+BSA 1% should be made up freshly each time, since bacterial contaminations will interfere with the assay. Use plastic or siliconized glass tubes to avoid loss of B cells, which tend to adhere to glass.

Next, 0.5 µl platelet-absorbed anti-B cell serum (see below for absorption method) is incubated in a glass Hamax tray (Hamax AS, N1501, Moss, Norway) under paraffin oil with 0.5 µl mononuclear cell suspension (6000 cells) for 60 min at 20 °C. Then 2.5 µl fresh rabbit serum is added to provide an excess of complement factors and the mixture is incubated for 2 h at 20 °C. Finally, 0.5 µl of a 1:70 dilution of a stock solution of ethidium bromide (Sigma Chemical Co., 100 µg/ml dissolved in saline with EDTA 5%) is added.

The reading is done with an inverted Leitz or Zeiss microscope with an epi-iluminator (filter combination: excitation filters LB455-SP490; barrier filter LP520). The test will simultaneously detect antibodies reacting with B cells (HLA-DR and others), T cells, and, with some training, monocytes. Trays can be left overnight at 4 °C in darkness.

Detection of Anti-B Cell Antibodies by the Long, B Cell-Enriched (LB) Lymphocytotoxicity Test [3]

Lymphocytes are obtained from heparinized blood by Ficoll-Isopaque separation. The yield of B cells is often increased by physical exercise (e.g., cycling or running upstairs) before the blood sample is taken. The separated lymphocytes are washed three times in PBS+BSA 1%, counted, and resuspended in tissue culture medium with 25% heat-inactivated (FCS 2000 cells/µl).

To this suspension an equal volume of papainized or AET-treated sheep red blood cells (SRBC) is added and the mixture is spun at 200 *g* for 5 min and then gently mixed by manual tilting. In preparing a B cell enriched suspension, plastic or siliconized glass tubes are preferable to increase the final yield.

Preparation of SRBC with Papain

Washed (three to five times) SRBC at 5% concentration in PBS (pH 7.2) are mixed with an equal volume of 0.25% papain solution. [The papain (Sigma) is kept as a stock solution of 25 mg/ml.] An additional volume of Na_2HPO_4 solution (36 g/l in water) is added, together with two volumes of 9.2% L-cysteine in PBS. The treated SRBC are then incubated for 10 min at 37 °C and washed three times in PBS. For preparing rosettes, it is recommended to use 0.8% papainized SRBC.

Preparation of SRBC with AET

Washed (three to five times) SRBC are incubated for 15 min at 37 °C with 10 ml freshly prepared AET solution [AET (Sigma) 0.14 *M* in sterile distilled water, pH adjusted to 9.0 using 10 *N* NaOH]. The treated SRBC are washed at least four times with PBS. A 1% suspension of the AET-treated SRBC is made in tissue culture medium containing 40% heat-inactivated FCS and can be stored at 4 °C for a week. It is generally not necessary to wash the SRBC before preparing the rosettes.

The lymphocyte/SRBC mixture is then centrifuged over a Ficoll-Isopaque gradient and the B cell-enriched suspension at the interface is harvested. The rosetted T cells sediment to the bottom. The B cell-enriched suspension is washed three times in siliconized glassware in PBS + BSA 1% and resuspended at 2000–3000 cells/μl in tissue culture medium with 20% heat-inactivated FCS.

The LB Lymphocytotoxicity Test Proper

One microliter of the B cell-enriched suspension is incubated with 1 μl of the platelet-absorbed serum for 1 h at 20 °C, then 5 μl of fresh rabbit serum is added and the total mixture further incubated for 2 h at 20 °C. Dead cells are stained by the addition of 3 μl 5% eosin in water, and the reaction is stopped by the addition of 8 μl 40% formalin (pH 7.2).

The remaining T cells can be used for HLA-A, B, C typing. The SRBC in the pellet are lysed by incubating for 15 min at 0 °C with ammonium chloride buffer (8.3 g NH_4Cl, 1 g $KHCO_3$, and 1 ml 0.1 *M* EDTA per liter). After lysis of the erythrocytes, the lymphocytes are washed twice. Adjust the cell concentration to 2000 cells/μl in tissue culture medium and perform the cytotoxicity test.

Absorption of Antisera Containing Anti-HLA-DR Antibodies to Remove Anti-HLA-A, B, and C Antibodies

Selection of Donors

If the specificity of the antibody in the serum is known, a pool of platelets should be obtained from donors who carry the corresponding antigens.

Care should be taken that if two antibodies are present, one in a high titer and one in a low titer, proportionally more platelets from donors carrying the antigens against which the high-titered antibody is directed should be present in the pool. One should keep in mind that HLA-B8 and B12 antigens, as well as C locus antigens, are often poorly expressed on platelets. Such antibodies will be difficult to absorb. If the specificity of the serum is not known, then a pool from donors with as many different HLA-A, B, C antigens as possible is collected. Isolated platelets should have been stored before use for at least 4 weeks at 4 °C in PBS containing 0.1% sodium azide. Prior to absorption they should be washed four times in PBS. It should always be checked whether leukocytes are still present.

If more than 1/μl leukocytes are present, they should first be removed by differential centrifugation.

Absorption Technique

One volume of serum and one volume of packed platelets are incubated for 30 min at 20 °C after carefully mixing the platelets and the serum. To avoid dilution of the antisera to be absorbed, all PBS in which the platelets are suspended should be removed by centrifugation before the serum is added. During incubation, the platelets are resuspended by shaking. At least three absorptions are necessary.

If possible, use polystyrene round-bottom tubes which can be centrifuged in an angle-head centrifuge for 10 min at 15000 rpm, making it much easier to remove the absorbed serum from the platelet sediment. After absorption, sera should be checked against T cells for any residual anti-HLA-A, B, or C activity.

Freezing of Lymphocytes

The following media are used for freezing: medium A, 25% FCS in RPMI 1640, medium B. 25% FCS and 20% DMSO in RPMI 1640. In the preparation of medium B, the DMSO should be added to the RPMI + 25% FCS at the last possible moment and the tube placed immediately in ice.

A suspension of the lymphocytes is made in cold medium A at a maximum concentration of 20×10^6/ml, and placed in melting ice. An equal volume of cold medium B is slowly added. When the ampules are filled and sealed, they are placed in a vertical position in a polystyrene foam box of room temperature. The box with the ampules should be placed immediately in a −70 °C Revco for up to 24 h. The ampules can then be stored in liquid nitrogen. The ampules can also be frozen in a controlled manner, using a machine which cools the cells at the rate of 1°–1.5 °C/min down to −30 °C, with a careful compensation at the critical point of crystallization (around −18 °C), and thereafter at 7 °C/min down to the temperature of liquid nitrogen.

Thawing of Frozen Lymphocytes

Tubes are prepared with FCS and RPMI. The ampules are transported in liquid nitrogen to the laboratory, placed in a waterbath at 37 °C, and thawed quickly. The cell suspension is then transferred to a plastic or siliconized glass tube. An equal volume of FCS is added dropwise to the tube, with thorough mixing between drops, and the tube is spun for 5 min at 400 *g* (1700 rpm). The pellet is suspended in 1.5 ml RPMI + 20% FCS and left for 30 min at 37 °C (waterbath). In this way the cells will recover best from the thawing procedure. After another spinning for 5 min at 400 *g* and one more washing in RPMI + 10% FCS, the suspension is ready for use.

References

1. Bodmer WF, Albert E, Bodmer JG, Dausset J, Kissmeyer-Nielsen F, Mayr W, Payne R, van Rood JJ, Trnka Z, Walford RL (1984) Nomenclature for factors of the HLA system 1984. Immunogenetics 20:593–601
2. van Leeuwen A, Termijtelen A, Shaw S, van Rood JJ (1982) Recognition of a polymorphic monocyte antigen in HLA. A systematic approach to recognize yet undefined gene products. Nature 298:565–567
3. van Rood JJ, van Leeuwen A, Keuning JJ, Blussé van Oud Alblas A (1975) The serological recognition of the human MLC determinants using a modified cytotoxicity technique. Tissue Antigens 5:73–79
4. Doxiadis I, Grosse-Wilde H, Valentine-Thon E (1984) Segregation analysis (HTCs). In: Albert ED, Baur MP, Mayr WR (eds) Histocompatibility testing 1984. Springer, Berlin Heidelberg New York Tokyo, pp 265–269
5. Richiardi P, Belvedere M, Borelli I, De Marchi M, Curtoni ES (1978) Split of HLA-DRw2 into subtypic specificities closely correlated to two HLA-D products. Immunogenetics 7:57
6. Mervart H, Kalovsky E, Moore BPL (1983) Splits of the HLA-DR2 antigen. Tissue Antigens 22:29–31
7. Batchelor JR, Hors J, Dodi IA, Bétuel H, Borelli I (1984) Antigen report: HLA-DR2. In: Albert ED, Baur MP, Mayr WR (eds) Histocompatibility testing 1984. Springer, Berlin Heidelberg New York Tokyo, pp 186–187
8. Reinsmoen NL, Layrisse Z, Bétuel H, Freidel AC, Bach FH (1984) A study of HLA-DR2 associated HLA-Dw/LD specificities. Hum Immunol 11:105–115
9. Cohen N, Amar A, Brautbar C (1984) Definition of a new DR2 short associated HLA-D specificity with the Ninth Histocompatibility Workshop reagents. Tissue Antigens 24:184–186
10. Suciu-Foca N, Rohowsky C, McKiernan P, Godfrey M, Susinno E, Broell J, Hardy M (1979) Association of Dw9 with DRw2. Transplant Proc 11:1799–1803
11. Schreuder GMT, van Leeuwen A, Termijtelen A, Parlevliet J, D'Amaro J, van Rood JJ (1982) Cell membrane polymorphisms in the HLA-D/DR region. Hum Immunol 4:301–302
12. Williamson J, Tait B, Richiardi P, Awad J, Fauchet R, Curtoni S, Festenstein H, Dawkins RL (1984) Antigen report: HLA-DR4. In: Albert ED, Baur MP, Mayr WR (eds) Histocompatibility testing 1984. Springer, Berlin Heidelberg New York Tokyo, pp 188–189
13. Schreuder GMT, Doxiadis I, Parlevliet J, Grosse-Wilde H (1984) HLA-DR, DQ, LB, and TA10 specificities of Ninth Workshop homozygous typing cells. In: Albert ED, Baur MP, Mayr WR (eds) Histocompatibility testing 1984. Springer, Berlin Heidelberg New York Tokyo, pp 243–248
14. Schreuder GMT, Parlevliet J, Termijtelen A, van Rood JJ (1983) Reanalysis of the HLA-DRw6 complex. Tissue Antigens 21:62–74
15. Grosse-Wilde H, Doxiadis I, Brandt H (1984) Definition of HLA-D with HTC. In: Albert ED, Baur MP, Mayr WR (eds) Histocompatibility testing 1984. Springer, Berlin Heidelberg New York Tokyo, pp 249–264
16. Bodmer JG, Pickbourne P, Richards S (1978) Joint report: Ia serology. In: Bodmer WF et al. (eds) Histocompatibility testing 1977. Munksgaard, Copenhagen, pp 35–84
17. Terasaki PI, Park MS, Bernoco D, Opelz G, Mickey MR (1980) Overview of the 1980 International Histocompatibility Workshop. In: Terasaki PI (ed) Histocompatibility testing 1980. UCLA Tissue Typing Laboratory, Los Angeles, pp 1–17
18. Awad J, Jaraquemada D, Festenstein H (1982) Serological analogue of HLA-Dw9. Tissue Antigens 19:233–237
19. Schreuder GMT, Kennedy LJ, Gebuhrer L, Awad J, Bétuel H, Degos L, Jeannet M (1984) Antigen report: HLA-DRw6 and its subgroups HLA-DRw13 and HLA-DRw14. In: Albert ED, Baur MP, Mayr WR (eds) Histocompatibility testing 1984. Springer, Berlin Heidelberg New York Tokyo, pp 192–197
20. Bétuel H, Gebuhrer L, Lambert J, Freidel AC, Farre A (1983) A possible new HLA-DR allele. Hum Immunol 8:227–237

21. Termijtelen A, Schreuder GMT, Mickelson EM, van Rood JJ (1984) Ninth International Histocompatibility preworkshop testing of Dw6 HTCs. Two subtypes of Dw6. Tissue Antigens 24:10–17
22. Bodmer J, Kennedy L, Aizawa M, Dawkins R, Lepage V, Mazilli MC, Richiardi P (1984) D region monoclonal antibodies. In: Albert ED, Baur MP, Mayr WR (eds) Histocompatibility testing 1984. Springer, Berlin Heidelberg New York Tokyo, pp 217–236
23. Mickelson EM, Nisperos B, Layrisse Z, Kim SJ, Thomas ED, Hansen JA (1983) Analysis of the HLA-DRw8 haplotype: recognition by HTC typing of three distinct antigen complexes in Caucasians, native Americans, and Orientals. Immunogenetics 17:399–410
24. Mickelson EM, Nisperos B, Thomas ED, Hansen JA (1982) Definition of LD "4 × 7": a unique HLA-D specificity defined by two homozygous typing cells. Hum Immunol 4:79–86
25. Fauchet R, van Leeuwen A, Yunis ED, Schreuder GMT (1984) Antigen report: HLA-DRw10. In: Albert ED, Baur MP, Mayr WR (eds) Histocompatibility testing 1984. Springer, Berlin Heidelberg New York Tokyo, pp 201–202
26. Amar A, Mickelson E, Hansen JA, Shalev Y, Brautbar C (1984) HLA-D "SHY": a new lymphocyte defined specificity associated with HLA-DRw10. Hum Immunol 11:143–149
27. Laundy GJ, Lewis L (1984) HLA-DR'Br', a new MT1-related specificity. Ninth Workshop Newsletter VII
28. Tanigaki N, Tosi R, Sagawa K, Minowada J, Ferrara GB (1983) The distribution of DR5, MT2, and MB3 specificities on human Ia subsets. Immunogenetics 17:371–386
29. Tanigaki N, Tosi R, Duquesnoy RJ, Ferrara GB (1983) Three Ia species with different structures and alloantigenic determinants in an HLA-homozygous cell line. J Exp Med 157:231–247
30. Koning F, Schreuder GMT, Giphart M, Bruning H (1984) A mouse monoclonal antibody detecting a DR-related MT2-like specificity: serology and biochemistry. Hum Immunol 9:221–230
31. Lepage M, Grumet C, Busson M, Colombani J, Ness D, Degos L (1984) Antigen report: HLA-DRw53. In: Albert ED, Baur MP, Mayr WR (eds) Histocompatibility testing 1984. Springer, Berlin Heidelberg New York Tokyo, pp 203–204
32. Nakata S, Park MS, Omori K (1980) Joint report MT3. In: Terasaki PI (ed) Histocompatibility testing 1980. UCLA Tissue Typing Laboratory, Los Angeles, p 569
33. Tosi R, Tanigaki N, Centis D, Ferrara GB, Pressman D (1978) Immunological dissection of human Ia molecules. J Exp Med 148:1592–1611
34. van Leeuwen A, Festenstein H, D'Amaro J, Navarette C, Awad J, van Rood JJ (1980) A new B cell locus defined by a recombinant family. In: Terasaki PI (ed) Histocompatibility testing 1980. UCLA Tissue Typing Laboratory, Los Angeles, p 853
35. Suciu-Foca N, Godfrey M, Rohowsky C, McKiernan P, Susinno E, Broell J (1979) Evidence that HLA-D is different from DR and that two different HLA loci code for B-cell antigens. Transplant Proc 11:1781–1787
36. Nunez G, Giles RC, Ball EJ, Hurley CK, Capra JD, Stastny P (1984) Expression of HLA-DR, MB, MT, and SB antigens on human mononuclear cells: identification of two phenotypically distinct monocyte populations. J Immunol 133:1300–1306
37. Falkenburg JHF, Jansen J, van der Vaart-Duinkerken N, Veenhof WFJ, Blotkamp J, Goselink HM, Parlevliet J, van Rood JJ (1984) Polymorphic and monomorphic HLA-DR determinants on human hematopoietic progenitor cells. Blood 63:1125–1132
38. Newman RA, Delia D, Greaves MF, Navarette C, Fainboim L, Festenstein H (1983) Differential expression of HLA-DR and DR-linked determinants on human leukemias and lymphoid cells. Eur J Immunol 13:172–176
39. Marrari M, Duquesnoy RJ (1984) Antigen report: HLA-DQw2. In: Albert ED, Baur MP, Mayr WR (eds) Histocompatibility testing 1984. Springer, Berlin Heidelberg New York Tokyo, pp 207–209
40. Oudshoorn M, Schreuder GMT, Campbell E, Du Toit ED (1984) Segregation of MB and DR: "exceptions to the rule". In: Albert ED, Baur MP, Mayr WR (eds) Histocompatibility testing 1984. Springer, Berlin Heidelberg New York Tokyo, pp 419–420

41. Duquesnoy RJ, Marrari M (1984) Antigen report: HLA-DQw3. In: Albert ED, Baur MP, Mayr WR (eds) Histocompatibility testing 1984. Springer, Berlin Heidelberg New York Tokyo, pp 209–211
42. Maeda H (1984) Mouse monoclonal antibody detects a new polymorphic Ia determinant other than HLA-DR antigen: a possible allele of DC-1. Tissue Antigens 23:163–170
43. Bétuel H, Gebuhrer L, Schreuder GMT, Goldmann SF, Arnaiz-Villena A, Layrisse Z (1984) Antigen report: HLA-DR5 and its subtypes HLA-DRw11 and HLA-DRw12. In: Albert ED, Baur MP, Mayr WR (eds) Histocompatibility testing 1984. Springer, Berlin Heidelberg New York Tokyo, pp 190–192
44. Ferrara GB, Longo A, Zappacosta S, Biagnini A, Mennucci M (1980) 8w DRw13. In: Terasaki PI (ed) Histocompatibility testing 1980. UCLA Tissue Typing Laboratory, Los Angeles, pp 546–547
45. Park MS, Terasaki PI (1980) Second DR locus. In: Terasaki PI (ed) Histocompatibility testing 1980. UCLA Tissue Typing Laboratory, Los Angeles, pp 578–582
46. Duquesnoy RJ, Marrari M, Hackbarth S, Zeevi A (1984) Serological and cellular definition of a new HLA-DR associated determinant, MC1 and its association with rheumatoid arthritis. Hum Immunol 10:165–176
47. Ollier W, Doxiadis I, Jaraquemada D, Okoye R, Grosse-Wilde H, Festenstein H (1984) First level testing of HLA-D "blank" HTC. In: Albert ED, Baur MP, Mayr WR (eds) Histocompatibility testing 1984. Springer, Berlin Heidelberg New York Toyko, pp 281–285
48. Thorsby E, Helgesen A, Gjemdal T (1972) Repeated platelet transfusions from HLA-A compatible unrelated and sibling donors. Tissue Antigens 2:397–404
49. Aster RH, Szatkowski N, Liebert M, Duquesnoy RJ (1977) Expression of HLA-B12, HLA-B8, w4, and w6 on platelets. Transplant Proc 9(4):1695–1696
50. Richiardi P, Diotallevi P, Matejč T, Carbonara AO, Curtoni ES (1977) HLA antibodies cytotoxic only for B lymphocytes. Tissue Antigens 10:323–329
51. van Rood JJ, van Leeuwen A, Ploem JS (1976) Simultaneous detection of two cell populations by two colour fluorescence and application to the recognition of B cell determinants. Nature 262:795–797

Monoclonal Antibodies Against HLA Class II Antigens *

J. Colombani and V. Lepage

Table of Contents

Introduction

It is now clear that monoclonal antibodies (MoAb) represent invaluable reagents for the study and analysis of HLA molecules and specificities. This is especially true for HLA class II products because of the complexity of the HLA-D region. MoAb are used conjointly with classical serology and cellular immunology techniques, as well as biochemical and molecular biology methods.

We present here a review of class II MoAb as presently known, attempting to discover any general properties of the MoAb and to describe their present contribution to our understanding of the HLA-D region. The comparison of allospe-

* This work was supported by contracts from INSERM, the Caisse Régionale d'Assurance Maladie de l'Ile de France, and the Fondation pour la Recherche Médicale

cificities seen by allosera and MoAb seems particularly useful for the description of HLA polymorphism. Examples will be given concerning the description of a new specificity (MC1-LE) associated with HLA-DR1 and 4 and the study of the HLA-DRw6 specificity. In addition MoAb are essential for studies of the expression, molecular structure, and functions of class II molecules.

Distribution of Polymorphic/Monomorphic, Class I/Class II MoAb

In order to keep track of the HLA MoAb available, we started a registry in 1982 [21]. By December 1984 a fourth list of the HLA MoAb registry was in progress [20]. A total of 393 HLA MoAb are currently listed. They include 127 class I MoAb and 266 class II MoAb (Table 1). The reason for preponderance of class II MoAb is that more research is devoted to HLA class II products; all class II MoAb produced (polymorphic or monomorphic) are studied and eventually published, since they provide new information, but only polymorphic HLA class I MoAb are published. It seems very likely that many hybridomas producing monomorphic class I MoAb are no longer being developed, maintained, and published. The numbers of polymorphic MoAb in both groups support this explanation: 88 of a total of 127 in class I vs 107 of 266 in class II. It is clear that the difference is mainly due to an excess of monomorphic class II MoAb.

At present, the majority of fusions for the production of HLA MoAb are made after immunization with human lymphoid cell lines derived from B lymphocytes. It seems that such immunization equally favors the production of hybridomas secreting class I and class II MoAb. The observed difference is thus the result of a selection by the laboratories producing MoAb.

The classical distinction between polymorphic (allotypic) and monomorphic (isotypic) MoAb is operational. A MoAb is said to be polymorphic when it does not react with certain cells from the test panel. It is said to be monomorphic when it reacts with all cells. The number of donors in the panel and its composition are thus critical. A panel of at least 20–30 donors representing all HLA class II specificities seems to be the minimum for an effective analysis. Homozygous cells are

Table 1. Distribution of 266 HLA class II MoAb by specificity

Polymorphic	
13	Recognizing a single DR specificity (DR1, 2, 4, 5, w6, 7, w8)
13	Recognizing DRw52 or 53
27	Recognizing DQw1 or DQw3
38	HLA class II polymorphism correlated with several HLA-DR and/or DQ specificities
16	HLA class II polymorphism not correlated with known allospecificities [a]
107	
Monomorphic	
86	Recognizing defined class II molecules or chains (DR and/or DQ and/or DP)
73	Molecular specificity not known [a]
159	

Details in [8, 9, 19–22, 93]

[a] Uncertainties may be due to insufficient study

important for the detection of certain broadly reactive MoAb which would seem monomorphic if tested against heterozygous cells.

A simple interpretation would assume that each MoAb is specific for a class II molecule and chain. A polymorphic MoAb would recognize a determinant located at a variable site; a monomorphic MoAB would recognize a framework determinant.

It is now recognized that HLA-D region products comprise two (or maybe three) DR molecules, one (or maybe two) DQ molecule, and one (or maybe two) DP molecule. Each molecule is composed of a beta chain (highly variable) and an alpha chain. The DR alpha chain is invariable, whereas the DQ alpha chain is variable. A polymorphic MoAb would thus recognize a variable determinant located on a beta chain or an a DQ alpha chain, but a monomorphic MoAb would recognize a framework determinant located on the DR alpha chain or on the most conserved part of any chain, i.e., the domain close to the cell membrane.

Some MoAb will probably follow this simple model, but there are certainly many exceptions. At least one polymorphic MoAb, I-LR1 [71, 72] recognizes a variable determinant shared by HLA-DPw2,3 and DR5 molecules. This is an example of interlocus cross-reaction, comparable to that observed for class I polymorphic MoAb (e.g., HLA-A2,B17 [67]). Monomorphic MoAb show a high degree of interlocus cross-reactivity (see discussion on molecular specificity below).

Specificity of Polymorphic MoAb

Among the 107 polymorphic MoAb, only 13 recognize narrow DR specificities. The majority recognize broad specificities: HLA-DRw52 ($n=10$), DRw53 ($n=3$), DQw1 ($n=20$), DQw3 ($n=7$) (Tables 1, 2). Not a single DQw2 MoAb has been described: this observation will be discussed later. According to the results of the Ninth International Histocompatibility Workshop [9], it is clear that MoAb alone would not suffice to accomplish safe HLA class II tissue typing. Several specificities are not yet defined by MoAb. In the case of classical DR specificities, usually only a single MoAb is available. Nevertheless, MoAb used in conjunction with allosera would contribute substantially to the typing. Several good or fairly good reagents are now available. Most MoAb presented in Table 3 were evaluated during the Ninth Workshop in relatively difficult conditions. Even then, most correlation coefficients were higher than 0.70. HLA-DQw1 and w3 reagents were good or excellent.

MoAb SFR3-DR5 is excellent provided that a suitable complement for the lymphocytotoxicity technique is selected. SFR3-DR5 and SFR16-DR7 were both produced in the rat, which could thus be particularly capable of recognizing HLA polymorphic determinants [86, 87].

A new specificity TA10, related to HLA-DQw3, seems to be defined by two MoAb, HU23 (9w909) [56] and A10-83 (9w790), highly correlated with one another ($r=0.89$). TA10 appears to be a split of DQw3 more closely related to DR5 than to DR4.

Table 2. HLA class II polymorphic MoAB recognizing (or correlated with) a single classical allospecificity

DR1:	62-74 [52] HPA49.11.10 (9w963) H4O-242.3 [7]
DR2:	NDS-1538 [35] HU30 [55] (9w906)
DR4:	FMC2 [103] NFDL.M1 (Dover 1984, personal communication)
DR5:	SFR3-DR5 [86] (9w960)
DRw6:	S2 [50]
DR7:	SFR16-DR7M and SFR16-DR7G [87] 17.3.3 (9w949)
DRw8:	HU46 (9w921)
DRw52:	JMSDR8.1.1 (9w947) ILR-2 [72] E15.4 [99] E13.11 [99] 7.3.19.1 [59] D4.90 [69] R3 [50] MCS7 [96] CHE64 (9w953) VR71319.1 (9w930)
DRw53:	109d6 [78], X.2.7 (9w941), PL3 [44]
DQw1:	Genox 3.53 [11, 12] 77.34 [33] SH1 (9w901) JMSDR4.1.1 (9w945) SH2 (9w927) JAF77.3410 (9w943) FU1 (9w914) FU4 (9w903) NFB.14.12 (9w964) IIB3 (Koning 1984, personal communication) SDR1 [26] 5F6 [58] S3/4 [102] F5C9 [92] MRC-OX3 [65, 66] S1 [50] R1 [50] HU11 (9w913), HU28 (9w907) GAP.D1 (9w962)
DQw3:	FU2 (9w908) TER.M (9w968) TA10 [64] (9w790) IVD12 [37] HU18 [56] (9w915) HU23 [56] (9w909) HU48 (9w923)

For MoAb studied during the Ninth International Histocompatibility Workshop, the workshop number is indicated with the prefix 9w [9]

Table 3. A selection of MoAb potentially usuable for tissue typing

HLA specificity	MoAb		*r*
DR1	HPA49.11.10	(9w963)	0.54 (w, a)
DR2	HU30	(9w906)	0.74 (w)
DR4	NFDL.M1 (c)		1 (l)
DR5	SFR3-DR5	(9w960)	0.96 (l, b)
DRw6	S2		0.68 (b)
DR7	SFR16.DR7M		1 (l)
	17.3.3	(9w949)	0.64 (w)
DRw8	HU46	(9w921)	0.50 (w, d)
DRw52	JMSDR8.1.1	(9w947)	0.87 (w)
	CHE64.2	(9w953)	0.74 (w)
DRw53	109d6		0.77 (l)
	X.2.7	(9w941)	0.50 (w)
DQw1	SH1	(9w901)	0.82 (w)
	SH2	(9w927)	0.80 (w)
	JMSDR4.1.1	(9w945)	0.78 (w)
DQw3	HU18	(9w915)	0.97 (w)
	HU48	(9w923)	0.90 (w)
	17.15	(9w969)	0.97 (w)

The best MoAb were selected from the analysis made during the Ninth International Histocompatibility Workshop. Correlation coefficients (*r*) are in most cases from the Workshop (w). *l*, Correlation coefficient obtained in local laboratory in which the McAb was produced; *a*, reacted also with DQw1; *b*, practically nonreactive during Ninth Workshop, probably because a selected rabbit complement is necessary to obtain good results in the lymphocytotoxicity microtechnique; *c*, non-complement-fixing MoAb; *d*, +Dw15

Technical Problems Concerning the Use of MoAb for HLA Class II Tissue Typing

The use of MoAb in serological techniques raises specific problems which were reviewed by J. Bodmer et al. [9].

Carry-over from one well to the next in the typing tray is a major problem with high-titered MoAb. Several solutions to the problem have been proposed. A "no-touch" technique is difficult to use routinely and is probably not absolutely safe. Another solution, though not very convenient, would be to put several wells containing only diluent between the wells containing the MoAb. The simplest solution is obviously to dilute the MoAb at an optimal concentration; however, this would lead to other problems, such as loss of reactivity during conservation and variation in sensitivity of the lymphocytotoxicity technique between laboratories. The latter problem could be solved by each laboratory finding the appropriate dilution of the MoAb with the local technique and complement.

Loss of reactivity during conservation seems to be a problem with certain MoAb, especially after dilution. There is no simple explanation or solution, but the following proposals can be made: Conservation at +4 °C in sterile conditions seems better than multiple freezing and thawing. For dilution, a high protein concentration (at least 20% final concentration) is necessary. Normal human serum inhibits MoAb activity and should be avoided. Fetal calf serum or bovine serum albumin are satisfactory protein sources.

It has been suggested that MoAb stick to the plastic in the typing tray. This could be avoided by coating the surface of the trays with protein (for instance bovine serum albumin) before adding the MoAb.

Selection of rabbit complement for use of MoAb in the lymphocytotoxicity technique is a major problem. Reactivity and specificity of certain MoAb are dependent on the complement batch used. At present, only empirical selection of the right batch seems possible.

The choice of the best target for use with MoAb has to be discussed. It has been observed that several complement-fixing MoAb can be nonreactive with peripheral blood B lymphocytes in the lymphocytotoxicity technique, but clearly reactive with B blasts (lymphoid cell lines) (SFR3-DR5) [86] or phytohemagglutinin (PHA) blasts, as observed with several MoAb from our laboratory. A likely explanation for this phenomenon is the higher number of reactive sites on B or T blasts than on resting B lymphocytes, a sufficient number of sites being necessary to induce the killing of the target. In addition, the choice of panel for identification of the MoAb specificity is critical. For instance, certain MoAb can behave as monomorphic antibodies when tested on a panel of B lymphoid cell lines, and as polymorphic antibodies on other targets (B lymphocytes from normal blood, chronic lymphocytic leukemias, or acute lymphoblastic leukemias).

It is probably difficult to contemplate the use of B blasts for routine typing. On the other hand, the use of PHA blasts is possible either with lymphocytotoxicity or complement fixation microtechniques.

For several years we have been using the complement fixation microtechnique on PHA blasts for HLA class II typing [18]. This technique is well adapted to the use of HLA class II MoAb. PHA blast have also the advantage of a good expression of HLA-DQ as well as HLA-DR specificities. Complement fixation on PHA blasts would thus be a good candidate for HLA class II typing with MoAb.

However, the ideal technique to replace lymphocytotoxicity would be a complement-independent technique. Several techniques using enzyme-labeled antibodies have been proposed, but so far they have been unable to replace the lymphocytotoxicity technique, probably because they cannot be used for large scale typing and/or because they use too many target cells (more than 100000 per test).

Such a technique would be convenient for non-complement-fixing MoAb. It has been proposed that non-complement-fixing MoAb could be used in a lymphocytotoxicity technique assisted by adjunction of anti-mouse immunoglobulin antibodies [36].

Technical problems are particularly important when polymorphic MoAb are being used for HLA typing, but are also significant when using monomorphic MoAb.

Recognition of Two or More Classical Specificities by Polymorphic MoAb

Several polymorphic MoAb are correlated with two or three classical specificities. They can be useful as typing reagents in the same way as bispecific allosera.

Table 4. HLA class II polymorphic MoAb correlated with several classical allospecificities

DR1+4:	AC1.59 [69] 21R5 [32] CC-C1 20 (Dejelo 1984, personal communication) HU43 (9w918) Y62C10 (9w928) XI.21.4 (Mazzilli 1983, personal communication)
DR3+w6:	16.23 [51] (9w929) CHE41 (Colombani 1983, personal communication)
Other bispecific:	DRw6+8: S3 [50] DR7+Dw15: 17.3.3 (9w949) DRw8+Dw15: HU46 (9w921)
DPw2+w3+DR5:	I-LR1 [47, 71, 72]
Broadly reactive:	DR3+7+w9: 26.1 [92] DR3+4+7: IIIE3 [45, 46] (Edinburgh 195) DR1+3+4: PD3 and IB6 (Koning 1984, personal communication) DR1+3+4: IVGI [45] (Edinburgh 197) DR3+5+w6+7+w8: PL2 [43] DQw3+DRw53: 17.15 (9w969) [42] Negative on DR5 cells: Q2/80 [85] Negative on DRw8 cells: IVF7 (Edinburgh 196) DR2+DRw52: D7.69.6 (Edinburgh 176)
Reactive with all cells except homozygous DR7:	Q5/6 [85] DA6.164 [94] 50D6A (Edinburgh 199) MHM4 [69] (Edinburgh 201) AB8.25 (Edinburgh 177) I-2 [72] (9w944) HU26 (9w904)
Reactive with all cells except Homozygous DR3 and DR7	AC.BM50 (Edinburgh 168) 33.1 [70] Leu 10 [17] (Edinburgh 133) SFR.P1.1 (Edinburgh 175) BL12 (Betuel 1982, personal communication) (9w951) MCLB.8 [12] BT3/4 [23] (Edinburgh 170) 21R5 (Edinburgh 200)

For MoAb studied during the Ninth International Histocompatibility Workshop, the workshop number is indicated with the prefix 9w [9]. Workshop numbers are also given for MoAb studied during the Edinburgh Workshop [93]

Moreover, they can recognize potentially interesting new specificities. When allosera detect such a specificity, it is difficult to exclude an artifact due to a mixture of antibodies. In contrast, when a MoAb, by definition monospecific, detects the same specificity, it confirms the existence of a new determinant shared by several allospecificities previously considered as unrelated. Examples of such observations (DR1+4 and DR3+w6) will be described in detail below. However, it is quite possible that several bispecific or broadly reactive MoAb in Table 4 recognize other new specificities, the molecular localization of which is not presently known.

Several broadly reactive MoAb have been described as positive on all cells except cells homozygous for the HLA-DR7 haplotype ("all except DR7" specificity). The first MoAb described could have been considered as a mere oddity, but now that many similar if not identical MoAb have been described independently, it is clear that the phenomenon corresponds to a property of HLA class II molecules and to the way in which they are seen by the immunized mouse (Table 4). During the Ninth International Histocompatibility Workshop the specificity of these MoAb was more precisely defined, and they were recognized as nonreactive with DR7 and DRw9 cells [9]. During the Edinburgh Workshop [93], it was also recognized that certain MoAb were nonreactive with DR7 and DR3 cells [49].

These MoAb react with a determinant common to all HLA-DR and/or DQ allotypes but absent in all class II molecules coded by the HLA-DR7 haplotype (and possibly the haplotypes DR3 and DRw9). It has been suggested that such a specificity would be the consequence of a tolerance of the immunized mouse (in most cases Balb/c, H-2^d) for DR7-associated molecules resulting from antigenic similarities between class II molecules coded by the human HLA-DR7 haplotype and the murine H-2^d haplotype [8, 13]. This hypothesis could perhaps account for the absence of HLA-DQw2 MoAb, since this specificity is strongly associated with HLA-DR3 and DR7. However, other observations should be considered. Surprisingly, the molecular specificity of these MoAb is not always the same. In most cases they recognize the DR molecule, but at least one MoAb (Leu 10) is specific for the DQ molecule, and another (MHM4) could be DP-specific. The tolerance hypothesis should take into account a MoAb (17.3.3, 9w949) correlated with DR7 ($r = 0.64$). This MoAb is a mouse anti-murine Ia antibody. Another mouse MoAb (26.1, Edinburg 145) [92] was correlated with DR3,7,w9. In the rat an "all except DR3 and DR7" MoAb has been produced (SFR. P1.1, Edinburgh 175) as well as a DR7 McAb (SFR16-DR7) [87]. This curious observation requires further investigation. For instance, it would be interesting to compare the structure of class II molecules or genes from H-2^d and HLA-DR7 haplotypes. It would also be interesting to study the specificity of anti-class II antibodies produced by homozygous DR7 individuals. According to the above hypothesis, these antibodies should resemble the MoAb.

When discussing the way the immunized mouse recognizes HLA class II molecules, the following observation should be mentioned. The majority of HLA-DR MoAb are monomorphic, while the majority of HLA-DQ MoAb are polymorphic (Table 5); in other words, the mouse recognizes more polymorphism on

Table 5. Prevalence of monomorphic HLA-DR and polymorphic HLA-DQ MoAb

Specificity	Monoclonal antibodies		
	Monomorphic	Polymorphic	Total
HLA-DR	58	13	71
HLA-DQ	4	27	31
Total	62	40	102
$\chi^2 = 42.83$			
$p = 10^{-7}$			

Only MoAb for which the molecular specificity was clearly established were included. For this reason DRw52, w53 and broadly reactive MoAb, as well as monomorphic MoAb recognizing two or three class II molecules, were excluded

DQ than on DR. This is what could be expected when considering the mouse response against murine Ia molecules. In this allogeneic situation, more polymorphism is seen on I-A-coded molecules (DQ equivalent) than on I-E-coded molecules (DR equivalent). This interpretation would also suggest that there is no basic difference between allo- and xenoimmunization against products of the major histocompatibility complex [54]. It can also be noted that the DQ molecule is polymorphic on both chains, while the DR molecule is polymorphic only on the beta chain.

Contribution of MoAb to the Analysis of HLA-DRw6-Related Specificities

One example of the way in which MoAb can contribute to the analysis of HLA class II polymorphism is given by Johnson et al. [51] and Johnson and Wank [50]. Six MoAb were produced in three fusions: 16.23 (immunizing cell JuSo, HLA-DR2,3); R1 and R3 (immunizing cell Rebma, DRw6,6, 16.23-negative); S1, S2, and S3 (immunizing cell Sch, DRw6,6, 16.23-positive). Analysis of the allospecificity of the MoAb and of their molecular specificity led to the conclusion that three clusters of specificities could be used to define DRw6 haplotypes:

1. DQw1 (defined by R1 and S1 MoAb, $r=0.66$ and 0.60 respectively)
2. 16.23 and S2, probably carried by a DRw52 molecule recognized by MoAb R3 ($r=0.71$). 16.23 was correlated to DR3 ($r=0.80$) and DR3+w6. S2 was correlated to DRw6 ($r=0.68$). A specificity correlated to DR3+w6 has been described by allosera [28, 48].
3. S3 was correlated to DRw6+w8 ($r=0.56$), independent from DQw1 and DRw52 and possibly carried by a DR molecule.

Molecules	DQw1	DRw 52	DR
Epitopes and MoAb	R1, S1 [a]	R3, CHE64 [b]	S3? [e]
		16.23, CHE41 [c]	
		S2 [d]	

[a] Public epitope common to DR1,2,w6 and w8 haplotypes
[b] Public epitope common to DR3,5,w6 and w8 haplotypes
[c] Epitope restricted to DR3 and w6 haplotypes
[d] Epitope restricted to DRw6 haplotype
[e] Epitope restricted to DRw6 and w8 haplotypes

The model should be adapted to take into account the DRw6 splits, DRw13/14.

Fig. 1. A provisional model for the epitopes defined by monoclonal antibodies, carried by class II molecules coded by DRw6 haplotypes

In our laboratory a fusion was made after immunization against the lymphoid cell line Chevallier (DR3,7, DRw52, DQw2). Among the MoAb produced, CHE41 was correlated to DR3+w6 ($r=0.69$) and CHE64 (9w953) was correlated to DRw52 ($r=0.72$). Three allosera were highly correlated to CHE41, confirming that the DR3+w6 specificity is recognized by both MoAb and allosera. Our

MoAb have not yet been directly compared to those of Johnson and colleagues, but it is likely that CHE41 is similar to 16.23, and CHE64 to R3. A very preliminary model of the epitopes related to DRw6, summarizing these results, is given in Fig. 1.

The model emphasizes the fact that DRw6 is recognized indirectly. The DRw6 haplotype is marked by determinants carried by DQw1 and especially DRw52 molecules. The DRw6 molecule would be relatively devoid of specific determinants. In other words, DRw6 would be non- or poorly immunogenic. This would fit with the observation that in several cells the DRw6 beta chain was absent or weakly expressed [43].

It should be mentioned that the four fusions which produced these MoAb were made after a single immunizing injection, and that most MoAb were IgM. This would suggest that polymorphic MoAb are more frequent after a primary immunization, and would fit with the suggestion by Parham et al. [80] that low-affinity MoAb are polymorphic, while high-affinity MoAb are monomorphic.

Recognition by Several MoAb of a New HLA Class II Specificity Associated with DR1+4

A new HLA class II specificity (MC1) present on HLA-DR1 and/or DR4 cells has been described by Duquesnoy et al. [29]. A Te23 specificity similar or related to MC1 has been reported [81], and we ourselves have also described a similar specificity (LE) [62]. In all instances, alloimmune sera were used. Absorption-elution experiments demonstrated that the allosera were not a mixture of anti-DR1 and anti-DR4 antibodies. To date six MoAb have been reported (Table 4), all of which correlate to various degrees with DR1+4+w9. Three of these MoAb (Y62C10, XI-21-4, and HU23) were compared during the Ninth International Histocompatibility Workshop and formed a cluster; the correlation coefficients between them were 0.50, 0,52, and 0.69. They had a negative association with DRw52, thus suggesting a possible allelic relationship with DRw52 [9].

No direct comparison has yet been made between the MoAb and the allosera. Nevertheless, it is likely that at least some sera and some MoAb will be correlated. If such is the case, the MoAb will be very useful in determining the precise definition of the new specificity. They demonstrate the existence of an epitope shared by class II molecules and coded by DR1 and DR4 haplotypes. This specificity is also recognized by alloreactive T cell clones [29] and by HLA-restricted anti-influenza T cell clones [31]. It is not yet known if the specificity is carried by a DR or DR-like molecule [62] or by a non-DR molecule [29]. MoAb will be used for immunoprecipitation and biochemical identification of the molecule.

Difficulty in Ascertaining the Molecular Specificity of Monomorphic HLA Class II MoAb

While polymorphic MoAb contribute to the analysis of HLA polymorphism, monomorphic MoAb are used for structural or functional studies. A precise definition of the molecular specificity of the MoAb is thus needed. Molecular specificity can be studied by serological methods using B lymphoid cell lines carrying various mutations affecting the HLA region. Mutant cell lines will then lack one or several HLA products, – class I, DR, DQ, DP – in various associations. By comparing the reactivity of a MoAb with a panel of mutant cell lines, it is generally possible to determine which HLA product is recognized [27, 91]. It is also possible to use monocytes, the majority of which do not express DQ molecules [38], or certain leukemia cells, also DQ-negative in the same way [77]. Capping techniques can also be used.

Biochemical methods involve sequential immunoprecipitation with reference MoAb and/or immunoprecipitation followed by analysis of the precipated molecules by two-dimensional polyacrylamide gel electrophoresis. Western blotting can also be used.

Table 6. Molecular specificity of 86 monomorphic HLA class II MoAb

DR molecule ($n=58$):	Three examples: HC2.2 (DR alpha) [60] DA6.147 (DR alpha) [94] SG171 (DR-monomorphic + recognizes DQ on DR7 haplotype) [40]
DQ molecules ($n=4$):	HAK-75 [101] B2 (Crepaldi 1984, personal communication) Tu22 [82] L2 (DQ alpha) (Fermand 1984, personal communication)
DR + DQ + DP molecules ($n=10$):	DA6.121 and DA6.231 (DR beta + DQ + DP?) [94] SG465 (DQ + DP? monomorphic + recognize DR on DR3 haplotype) [40] CR3.43 (Edinburgh 148) NFG2 (Edinburgh 172) HIG78 (Edinburgh 158) AA3.84 (Edinburgh 178) TAL-1B5 and TAL-3C3 (alpha chain from several class II molecules) [1] SG520 (recognizes different molecules depending on the haplotype tested: on DR1 and DR4, DR and DP; on DR3, DR and DQ: on DR5, DR; on DR7, DQ) [40]
DR + DP molecules ($n=14$):	2.06 and 1.35 [14] BT2.9 (Edinburgh 169) DAG-147 (DR alpha chain + DP) [94] HIG48 (Edinburgh 157) NFG1 (Edinburgh 171) XD5.H7 (Edinburgh 173) LC12/3 (Edinburgh 184) LC12/9 (Edinburgh 185) 506.AF (Edinburgh 187) YD1/63HLK Tu39 Tu43 ACP53 (Edinburgh 161)

Many data were obtained during the Edinburgh Workshop [93]
These molecular specificities should be considered as provisional; they could be modified by further studies. In addition to these monomorphic MoAb, three polymorphic MoAb were used for studies on DP molecules: I-LR1 (DPw2, 3 + DR5) [71, 72], B7/21 (recognizing FA antigen) [100], and MHM4 (Edinburgh 201) [68]

A complete study (which is rarely performed) should involve several methods applied to several targets. A molecular specificity defined by one technique does not exclude another specificity when another technique is used, for instance, a cross-reactivity with a second molecule observed in a serological test and not seen by less sensitive immunoprecipitation methods.

More importantly, it is clear that certain molecular cross-reactions are dependent on the haplotype studied. Classical examples of this phenomenon are given by Goyert and Silver [40]. Three MoAb, SG171, SG465, and SG520, recognize one or two class II molecules in different associations depending on the target cell used (Table 6). SG171 and SG465 are monomorphic for one molecule (DR and DQ respectively) and recognize a certain allotype from another molecule, thus they are polymorphic for the other molecule. SG520 is polymorphic for DR, DQ, and probably DP, but reacts with all targets, since in all cases it recognizes one or two molecules. There is no basic difference between SG520, which is operationally monomorphic, and I-LRI (DPw2,3+DR5), which is clearly polymorphic.

Thus it seems reasonable to conclude that definition of the molecular specificity of a MoAb is always provisional and cannot be generalized from a single experiment on a given target. In addition to original publication, many data in Table 6 were obtained during the Edinburgh Workshop [93]. These data are based mainly on reactivity of the MoAb with loss-mutant cell lines [90]. As already mentioned, a majority of monomorphic MoAb recognize DR molecules and a minority recognize DQ molecules. Relatively few MoAb recognize DR+DQ+DP or DR+DP.

Exclusively DP-specific MoAb are very rare. B7/21 [4, 100] and MHM4 [68] have this specificity. MHM4 was described as recognizing the "all except DR7" specificity.

Only molecular cross-reactivity could be expected in view of the structural homology between the various alpha and beta chains, especially for their domain close to the cellular membrane. It is likely that cross-reacting allosera do exist, but they would be difficult to analyze due to technical problems. In the mouse, cross-reactivity between I-A and I-E subregion products has been demonstrated with allosera [6, 63] and allogeneic MoAb [83, 95].

Importance of MoAb in Studies on Tissue Distribution and Function of HLA Class II Specificities

MoAb have already proved invaluable tools for studying the tissue distribution of class II molecules. An ideal protocol should use a large battery of monomorphic and polymorphic MoAb covering all class II molecules and specificities (DR, DRw52,53, DQ, and if possible DP). Several individual donors should be tested for each target in order to take into account the possible variations in molecular specificity from one HLA haplotype to another.

Several observations will be of importance to the understanding of the biological functions of class II molecules. For instance, DR molecules and DRw52 specificities have been found on all hematopoietic progenitor cells [34, 88], whereas DQw1 determinant could not be demonstrated on these cells. Differential expression of DR and DQ molecules was also observed on leukemic cells. DR is expressed on non-T acute lymphoblastic leukemias, on B chronic lymphocytic leukemias, and on acute myeloblastic leukemias. DQw1 specificity has been found on B chronic lymphocytic leukemias, but not on certain non-T acute lymphoblastic leukemias [77].

Variable expression of DR, DQ, and DP molecules has been reported on mature cells. DR molecule is expressed on B lymphocytes, monocytes, macrophages, and activated T cells. DQ molecule is found on B lymphocytes, activated T cells, and 15% of monocytes [79]. It has been shown that these DR+, DQ+ monocytes presented certain antigens [38]. The relative roles of DR and DQ in antigen presentation deserve further study. DP molecule is expressed on monocytes [79] and B lymphocytes [91].

Aberrant expression of DR has been observed during certain pathological processes, for instance on thyrocytes in Graves' disease [41], on melanoma cells [84], and on bile duct epithelium in primary biliary cirrhosis [5].

It is clear that further studies on these "experiments of nature" will provide informations on the biological role of class II molecules.

Importance of MoAb in Structural Studies on Class II Molecules

The first evidence of a second HLA class II molecule (DC1) was produced by biochemical studies performed with allosera [97]. However, it was only the systematic use of MoAb which enabled extensive structural studies on class II molecules (for review, see [89]). The three-chain structure (alpha, beta, invariant) of the DR molecule was established and the existence of a second DR beta chain demonstrated. The structure of the DC(DQ) molecule was then further investigated, particularly with the use of MoAb Genox 3.53, SG171, and BT3/4 [10, 23]. The DP(SB) molecule was then characterized with MoAb I-LRI [71, 72] and BT7/21 (FA) [4, 100]. The existence in man of hybrid class II molecules produced by transcomplementation was demonstrated with MoAb Genox 3.53, 2.06, SG171 [16].

A biochemically defined polymorphism of class II molecules is currently being described. Class II molecules immunoprecipitated by MoAb (or possibly by allosera) are analyzed by bi-dimensional polyacrylamide gel electrophoresis (2D-PAGE). Electrophoretic patterns are observed which are allele-specific. Initial studies showed a correlation between biochemically and serologically defined polymorphisms of the DR molecule [14, 15]. It then became apparent that biochemical studies showed a heterogeneity among serologically homogeneous specificities. The DR4 specificity was thus split into several biochemically defined subtypes [74]. Very often, these subtypes correlated with the HLA-Dw specificities defined by cellular immunology methods. DR2 specificity was split by biochemical analysis [75] in the same way. The same biochemical heterogeneity is demonstrated for HLA-DQ specificities [40].

In our laboratory, in collaboration with D. Charron, we analyzed the molecular heterogeneity of HLA-DRw6 antigens using 2D-PAGE in 15 unrelated individuals and in four informative families [43]. Assignment of DRw6 was done with Ninth Workshop sera, recognizing DRw6 in association with other DR specificities, and with DQw1 and DRw52 sera. In most cells, a DR beta chain corresponding to the DRw6 haplotype was present. Four different molecular species were identified from the 2D-PAGE profile of the DR beta chain. The molecular subtypes defined correlated only partially with DRw52 sera, and did not correlate with DQw1 sera. Preliminary results suggested that allosera and/or MoAb could be found which recognized certain molecular subtypes. In several cells, the DR beta chain associated with the DRw6 haplotypes was absent or only weakly detected, suggesting a quantitative polymorphism.

This example illustrate an approach currently developed in our laboratory, namely the biochemical definition of subtypes in a serological specificity, followed by the systematic search for serological reagents corresponding to the subtypes. This approach would thus take advantage of both the high analytical power of the biochemical method and the efficiency of the serological techniques, which are well adapted to large-scale studies.

Use of MoAb in Studies on the Role of Class II Molecules in Immunological Recognition by T Cells

MoAb are extensively used in blocking experiments in which class II molecules are recognized by T lymphocytes. Needless to say, the molecular specificity of the MoAb used should be well defined in order to enable correct evaluation of the results.

Such experiments have thus confirmed the role of HLA-DR and DP molecules as stimulators of proliferative allogeneic T lymphocytes [82]. In these experiments, a class I MoAb (w6/32) was unexpectedly able to block the proliferative response of anti-DR and anti-DP T lymphocytes. The blocking effect seemed to affect the responding rather than the stimulating cells. This unexplained observation was confirmed with another class I MoAb (M18) [53].

Corte et al. [25] reported that unlike DR MoAb, DQw1 MoAb (BT3/4) had no effect on the proliferation of T cells in response to alloantigens or soluble antigens. However, DQw1 MoAb inhibited the generation of allogeneic cytolytic T lymphocytes. These results suggested different functions for DR and DQ molecules.

Other blocking experiments confirmed that DR molecules can serve as targets for cytolytic T lymphocytes generated during the allogeneic response [3, 61]. Such experiments have also confirmed the role of class II molecules in antigen presentation to proliferative T lymphocytes [30, 73].

In recent experiments a battery of class II MoAb was used to inhibit several proliferative T cell clones specific for influenza virus [31], varidase, or diphtheria toxoid [98]. In each case, clones showed a distinct inhibition pattern according to the clone specificity. Moreover, a certain heterogeneity was apparent between clones with the same specificity. These results suggest that the associative recognition of foreign antigen + class II self molecules by T lymphocytes is molecule-specific (molecular restriction), and epitope-specific (epitope restriction). Such experimental protocols using a battery of MoAb should contribute to the analysis of the fine specificity of T cell clones.

Conclusions

It is clear that at the present time, several MoAb can be used as typing reagents. However, in order to obtain satisfactory results from the use of MoAb, certain precautions are necessary with regard to the appropriate dilution of the MoAb, its conservation, and the selection of complement for the lymphocytotoxicity technique. HLA-DQw1,3 and DRw52,53 are among the specificities which can be defined by MoAb.

The contribution of MoAb to the solution of serological problems is already important: for instance, MC1-LE specificity, DR3+w6 specificity, analysis of DRw6, TA10 as a split of DQw3. Other polymorphic MoAb will contribute to the analysis of HLA class II polymorphism, together with classical serology using allosera. It is interesting to note that MoAb serology and classical (allosera) serology are developing simultaneously. One can thus expect fruitful interactions from them, in contrast to what happened with class I, where classical serology was almost complete before the first MoAb appeared.

A future field of research will be the systematic comparison of polymorphisms as seen by allosera, MoAb, cellular immunology methods (HLA-Dw), and biochemical techniques: 2D-PAGE for the gene product, and restriction fragment length polymorphism for the gene itself.

Summary

An inventory of all HLA class II MoAb known in December 1984 has been made; 266 are listed, of which 107 are polymorphic and 159 monomorphic. A few polymorphic MoAb recognize DR1, 2, 4, 5, w6, 7, w8 specificities; many MoAb recognize DRw52, w53, DQw1,3 specificities, none recognizes DQw2. Several MoAb recognize specificities associated with DR1+4, DR3+w6: both of these specificities are also detected by allosera and are thus new classical specificities. Among broadly reactive MoAb, several react with all cells except homozygous DR7 (and DRw9 or DR3) cells. Several MoAb can be used as typing reagents. However certain technical problems remain to be solved: preservation of MoAb in the typing trays, reproducibility of lymphocytotoxicity results with different batches of complement and/or dilution of MoAb.

It is important, though sometimes difficult, to establish a satisfactory definition of the molecular specificity of MoAb. Several aparently monomorphic MoAb recognize one, two, or three different class II molecules (DR, DQ, DP), depending on the HLA haplotype of the target cell. Such cross-reactions between alleles and molecules reflect structural homologies between DR, DQ, and DP alpha and beta chains.

MoAb are essential for the study of tissue distribution, structure, and functions of class II molecules. They are invaluable tools for future studies on HLA polymorphism.

Acknowledgments. We thank all our colleagues for helpful discussions and suggestions, particularly M. Colombani, M. Pla, A. Haziot, and P. Loiseau. We also thank D. Charron for suggestions concerning biochemical studies, E. May for reviewing the manuscript, and P. Lacombe for expert secretarial assistance.

References

1. Adams TE, Bodmer JG, Bodmer WF (1983) Production and characterization of monoclonal antibodies recognizing the alpha-chain subunits of human Ia alloantigens. Immunology 50:613–624
2. Albert ED, Baur MP, Mayr WR (eds) (1984) Histocompatibility testing 1984. Springer, Berlin Heidelberg New York Tokyo
3. Anichini A, Bach FH (1984) HLA-Dw/LD directed cytotoxic T cell clones. Hum Immunol 10:153–164
4. Austin P, Trowsdale J, Rudd C, Bodmer W, Feldmann M, Lamb J (1985) Functional expression of HLA-DP genes transfected into mouse fibroblasts. Nature 313:61–64
5. Ballardini G, Bianchi F, Doniach D, Mizakian R, Pisi E, Bottazo GF (1984) Aberrant expression of HLA-DR antigens on bileduct epithelium in primary biliary cirrhosis: relevance to pathogenesis. Lancet 3:1009–1013
6. Birnbaum D, Pla M, Colombani M, Colombani J (1982) Serological cross-reactivity between products of separate I region. Immunogenetics 15:71–77
7. Birnbaum D, Dosseto M, Bourge F, Pierres M, Kourilsky FM (1982) A cross-reactive mouse anti-I-E^k monoclonal antibody detects an HLA-DR polymorphism linked to HLA-DR1. Mol Immunol 19:755–764
8. Bodmer JG, Bodmer WF (1984) Monoclonal antibodies to HLA determinants. Br Med Bull 40:267–275
9. Bodmer J, Kennedy L, Aizawa M, Dawkins R, Lepage V, Mazzili MC, Richiardi P (1984) HLA-D region monoclonal antibodies. In: Albert ED, Baur MP, Mayr WR (eds) Histocompatibility testing 1984. Springer, Berlin Heidelberg New York Tokyo, pp 217–236
10. Bono MR, Strominger JL (1982) Direct evidence of homology between human DC-1 antigen and murine I-A molecules. Nature 299:836–837
11. Brodsky PM, Parham P, Barnstable CJ, Crumpton MJ, Bodmer WF (1979) Monoclonal antibodies for analysis of the HLA system. Immun Rev 47:3–61
12. Brodsky FM, Stone WH, Parham P (1981) Of cows and men: a comparative study of histocompatibility antigens. Hum Immunol 3:143–152
13. Charron DJ (1984) Serology with 100 monoclonal antibodies to MHC class II antigens: an overview of workshop presentations. Dis Markers 2:145–149
14. Charron DJ, McDevitt HO (1979) Analysis of HLA-D region associated molecules with monoclonal antibody. Proc Natl Acad Sci USA 76:6567–6571
15. Charron DJ, McDevitt HO (1980) Characterization of HLA-D region antigens by two-dimensional gel electrophoresis. Molecular genotyping. J Exp Med 152:18s–36s
16. Charron DJ, Lotteau V, Turmel P (1984) Hybrid HLA-DC antigens provide molecular evidence for gene trans-complementation. Nature 312:157–159
17. Chen YX, Evans RL, Pollack MS, Lanier LL, Phillips JH, Rousso C, Warner NL, Brodsky FM (1984) Characterization and expression of the HLA-D antigens defined by anti-Leu 10. Hum Immunol 10:221–236
18. Colombani J (1982) Complement fixation tests in HLA typing. In HLA typing: methodology and clinical aspects, vol II. In: Ferrone S, Solheim BG (eds) CRC Press, Boca Raton, pp 1–9
19. Colombani J, Lepage V (1984) HLA monoclonal antibody registry: third listing. Tissue Antigens 24:209–214
20. Colombani J, Lepage V (1985) HLA monoclonal antibody registry: 4th listing (in preparation)
21. Colombani J, Dausset J, Lepage V, Degos L, Kalil J, Fellous M (1982) HLA monoclonal antibody registry. A proposal. Tissue Antigens 20:161–171
22. Colombani J, Lepage V, Kalil J (1983) HLA monoclonal antibody registry: second listing. Tissue Antigens 22:97–106
23. Corte G, Calabi F, Damiani G, Bargellesi A, Tosi R, Sorrentino R (1981) Human Ia molecules carrying DC1 determinants differ in both alpha- and beta-subunits from Ia molecules carrying DR determinants. Nature 292:357–360
24. Corte G, Damiani G, Calabi F, Fabbi M, Bargellesi A (1981) Analysis of HLA-DR polymorphism by two-dimensional peptide mapping. Proc Natl Acad Sci USA 78:534–538

25. Corte G, Moretta A, Cosulich ME, Ramarli D, Bargellesi A (1982) A monoclonal anti-DC1 antibody selectively inhibits the generation of effector T cells mediating specific cytolytic activity. J Exp Med 156:1539–1544
26. De Kretser TA, Crumpton MJ, Bodmer JG, Bodmer WF (1982) Two dimensional gel analysis of the polypeptides precipitated by a polymorphic HLA-DR1,2 and w6 monoclonal antibody: evidence for a third locus. Eur J Immunol 12:600–606
27. De Mars R (1984) Mutations that dissect the D-region of a human B-lymphoblastoid cell line. Dis Markers 2:175–182
28. Duquesnoy R (1980) Definition of three subdivisions of HLA-DRw6. In: Terasaki PI (ed) Histocompatibility testing 1980. UCLA Tissue Typing Laboratory, Los Angeles, pp 817–818
29. Duquesnoy RJ, Marrari M, Hackbarth S, Zeevi A (1984) Serological and cellular definition of a new HLA-DR associated determinant, MC1, and its association with rheumatoid arthritis. Hum Immunol 10:165–176
30. Eckels DD, Lamb JR, Lake P, Woody JN, Johnson AH, Hartzman RJ (1982) Antigen specific human T-lymphocyte clone. Genetic restriction of influenza virus-specific responses to HLA-D region genes. Hum Immunol 4:313–324
31. Eckels DD, Sell TW, Bronson SR, Johnson AH, Hartzman RJ, Lamb JR (1984) Human helper T-cell clones that recognize different influenza hemagglutinin determinants are restricted by different HLA-D region epitopes. Immunogenetics 19:409–423
32. Falk JA, Addis JBL, Letarte M (1983) Species cross-reactive Ia determinants: Detection with a monoclonal antibody to human Ia of a murine Ia.7 epitope. Hum Immunol 7:79–88
33. Falk JA, Cannon M, Nakouda A, Lewis W, Letarte M, Falk RE (1983) Monoclonal antibody to MT1 inhibits antibody production (abstract). American Association Clinical Histocompatibility testing, Ninth Conference 1983
34. Falkenburg JHF, Jansen J, Van Der Vaart-Dunkerken N, Veenhot WFJ, Blotkamp J, Goselink HM, Parlevilet J, Van Rood JJ (1984) Polymorphic and monomorphic HLA-DR determinants on human hematopoietic progenitor cells. Blood 63:1125–1132
35. Fuggle SV, Kirkley J, Ting A, Morris PJ (1983) A monoclonal antibody recognizing HLA-DR2 on malignant and activated cells. Immunogenetics 18:415–428
36. Fuller TC, Phelan D, Gebel H, Rodey G (1982) Antigenic specificity of antibody reactive in the antiglobulin augmented lymphocytotoxicity test. Transplantation 34:24–29
37. Giles RC, Nunez G, Hurley CK, Nunez-Roldan A, Winchester R, Stastny P, Capra D (1983) Structural analysis of a human I-A homologue using a monoclonal antibody that recognizes an MB3-like specificity. J Exp Med 157:1461–1470
38. Gonwa TA, Picker LJ, Raff HV, Goyert SM, Silver J, Stobo JD (1983) Antigen-presenting capabilities of human monocytes correlates with their expression of HLA-DS an Ia determinant distinct from HLA-DR. J Immunol 130:706–711
39. Goyert SM, Silver J (1981) Isolation of I-A subregion-like molecules from subhuman primates and man. Nature 294:266–267
40. Goyert SM, Silver J (1983) Further characterization of HLA-DS molecules: implications for studies assessing the role of human Ia molecules in cell interactions and disease susceptibility. Proc Natl Acad Sci 80:5719–5723
41. Hanafusa T, Chiovato L, Doniach D, Borell RP, Russel RCG, Bottazzo GF (1983) Aberrant expression of HLA-DR antigen on thyrocytes in Graves' Disease: relevance for autoimmunity. Lancet 2:1111–1115
42. Hansen JA, Martin PJ, Kamoun M, Nisperos B, Thomas ED (1981) A supertypic HLA-DR specificity (DR4 + 5) defined by murine monoclonal antibody. Hum Immunol 2:103–112
43. Haziot A, Lepage V, Degos L, Charron DJ (1984) Molecular dissection of DRw6. In: Albert ED, Baur MP, Mayr WR (eds) Histocompatibility testing 1984. Springer, Berlin Heidelberg New York Tokyo, pp 522–526
44. Horibe K, Knowles RW, Pollack MS, Dupont B (1983) Two monoclonal antibodies which recognize polymorphic determinants related to HLA-DR7 antigens (abstract). American Association Clinical Histocompatibility testing, Ninth Conference 1983

45. Hurley CK, Nunez G, Winchester R, Finn OJ, Levy R, Capra JD (1982) The human HLA-DR antigens are encoded by multiple beta-chain loci. J Immunol 129:2103–2108
46. Hurley CK, Shaw S, Nadler L, Schlossman S, Capra JD (1982) Alpha and beta chains of SB and DR antigens are structurally distinct. J Exp Med 156:1557–1562
47. Hurley CK, Giles RC, Nunez G, DeMars R, Nadler L, Winchester R, Stastny P, Capra JD (1984) Molecular localization of human class II MT2 and MT3 determinants. J Exp Med 160:472–493
48. Jeannet M (1980) Joint report on DRw6. In: Terasaki PI (ed) Histocompatibility testing 1980. UCLA Tissue Typing Laboratory, Los Angeles, pp 524–525
49. Johnson JP (1984) Monoclonal antibodies against human MHC class II antigens: analysis of binding to HLA-D/DR homozygous cells, melanoma cell lines, and isolated Ia antigens. Dis Markers 2:255–262
50. Johnson JP, Wank R (1984) Monoclonal antibodies to polymorphic epitopes on Ia antigens: three independent groups of determinants expressed on DRw6 homozygous cells. Eur J Immunol 14:739–743
51. Johnson JP, Meo T, Riethmuller G, Schendel DJ, Wank R (1982) Direct demonstration of an HLA-DR allotypic determinant on the low molecular weight (beta) subunit using a mouse monoclonal antibody specific for DR3. J Exp Med 156:104–111
52. Kalil J, Fellous M (1982) Monoclonal antibodies to HLA-DR antigens. In: Ferrone S, David C (eds) Murine Ia and human DR, CRC Press, Boca Raton, pp 55–80
53. Kalil J, Wollman EE (1983) Role of class I and class II antigens in the allogenic stimulation. Class I and class II recognition in allogenic stimulation. Blocking of MLR by monoclonal antibodies and F(ab′)2 fragments. Cell Immunol 79:367–373
54. Kalil J, Lepage V, Fellous M, Colombani J (1982) Anticorps monoclonaux anti-HLA. Bull Inst Pasteur 80:97–126
55. Kasahara M, Ogasawara K, Ikeda H, Tsugoyo O, Ishikawa N, Takenouchi T, Wakisaka A, Kikuchi Y, Aizawa M (1983) A monoclonal antibody that detects a polymorphic determinant, common to HLA-DR1 and 2. Tissue Antigens 21:105–113
56. Kasahara M, Takenouchi T, Ogasawara K, Ikeda H, Okuyama T, Ishikawa N, Moriuchi J, Wakisaka A, Kikuchi Y, Aizawa M, Kaneko T, Kashiwagi N, Nishimura Y, Sasazuki T (1983) Serological dissection of HLA-D specificities by the use of monoclonal antibodies. Immunogenetics 17:485–495
57. Kasahara M, Takenouchi T, Ikeda H, Ogasawara K, Okuyama T, Ishikawa N, Wakisaka A, Kikuchi Y, Aizawa M (1983) Serologic dissection of HLA-D specificities by the use of monoclonal antibodies. II. Distinction between HLA-Dw2 and HLA-Dw12. Immunogenetics 18:525–536
58. Koide Y, Awashima F, Yoshida TO, Takenouchi T, Wakisaka A, Moriuchi J, Aizawa M (1982) The role of three distinct Ia-like antigen molecules in human T cell proliferative responses. Effect of monoclonal anti-Ia-like antibodies. J Immunol 129:1061–1069
59. Koning F, Schreuder I, Giphart M, Bruning H (1984) A mouse monoclonal antibody detecting a DR-related MT2-like specificity: serology and biochemistry. Hum Immunol 9:221–230
60. Korman AJ, Knudsen PJ, Kaufman JF, Strominger JL (1982) cDNA clones for the heavy chain of HLA-DR antigen obtained after immunopurification of polysomes by monoclonal antibody. Proc Natl Acad Sci 79:1844–1848
61. Krensky AM, Clayberger C, Reiss CS, Strominger JL, Burakoff SJ (1982) Specificity of OKT4+ cytotoxic T lymphocyte clones. J Immunol 129:2001–2003
62. Lepage V, Alcalay D, Douay C, Mallet C, Loiseau P, Degos L, Colombani M, Colombani J (1985) Evidence for a new HLA class II determinant present on cells from HLA-DR1 and/or -DR4 individuals. Tissue Antigens 25:96–102
63. Lowry PA, Murphy DB (1981) Serological cross-reactivity between products of different Ia loci. Immunogenetics 14:189–201
64. Maeda H (1984) Mouse monoclonal antibody detects a new polymorphic Ia determinant other than HLA-DR antigen: a possible allele of DC-1. Tissue Antigens 23:163–170

65. McMaster WR, Williams AF (1979) Monoclonal antibodies to Ia antigens from rat thymus: cross reactions with mouse and human and use in purification of rat Ia glycoproteins. Immunol Rev 47:117–137
66. McMaster WR, Winearls BC, Parham P (1979) A monoclonal mouse anti-rat Ia antibody which cross react with a human HLA-DRw determinant. Tissue Antigens 14:453–458
67. McMichael AJ, Parham P, Rust N, Brodsky F (1980) A monoclonal antibody that recognizes an antigenic determinant shared by HLA-A2 and B17. Hum Immunol 1:121–129
68. Makgoba MW, Hildreth JEK, McMichael AJ (1983) Identification of a human Ia antigen that is different from HLA-DR and DC antigens. Immunogenetics 17:623–636
69. Malavasi F, Fabbi M, Milanese C, Richiardi P, Ferrero E, Bergui L, Dellabona P, Carbonara AO (1983) Production and characterization of murine monoclonal antibodies against human B cell surface determinants. XXX Col. Protides. Biol. Fluids. Pergamon, Oxford
70. Marti GE, Kuo MC, Shaw S, Chang CC, De Mars R, Sogn JA, Coligan JE, Kindt TJ (1983) A novel HLA-D/DR-like antigen specific for human B lymphoid cells: biochemical evidence for similarity to but nonidentity with known HLA-D/DR antigens. J Exp Med 158:1924–1937
71. Nadler LM, Stashenko P, Hardy R, Pesando JM, Yunis EJ, Schlossman SF (1981) Monoclonal antibodies defining serologically distinct HLA-D/DR related Ia like antigens in man. Hum Immunol 1:77–80
72. Nadler LM, Stashenko P, Hardy R, Tomaselli KJ, Yunis EJ, Schlossman SF, Pesando JM (1981) Monoclonal antibody identifies a new Ia-like (p29,34) polymorphic system linked to the HLA-D/DR region. Nature 290:591–593
73. Ng AG, Zhang YH, Russo C, Ferrone S (1982) Immunochemical and functional analysis of Ia-like antigens on human monocytes macrophage with monoclonal antibodies. Cell Immunol 66:78–87
74. Nepom BS, Nepom GT, Mickelson E, Antonelli P, Hansen JA (1983) Electrophoretic analysis of human HLA-DR antigens from HLA-DR4 homozygous cell lines: correlation between beta chain diversity and HLA-D. Proc Natl Acad Sci 80:6962–6966
75. Nepom GT, Nepom BS, Wilson ME, Mickelson E, Antonelli P, Hansen JA (1984) Multiple Ia-like molecules characterize HLA-DR2 associated haplotypes which differ in HLA-D. Hum Immunol 10:143–152
76. Neppert J, Mueller-Eckhardt C (1984) Monoclonal mouse antibodies to human MHC class I antigen cocap class II antigens. Tissue Antigens 24:187–189
77. Newman RA, Delia D, Greaves MF, Navarrete C, Fainboim L, Festenstein H (1983) Differential expression of HLA-DR and DR-linked determinants on human leukemias and lymphoid cells. Eur J Immunol 13:172–176
78. Nunez-Roldan A, Szer I, Toguchi T, Cuttner J, Winchester R (1982) Association of certain Ia allotypes with the occurence of chronic lymphocytic leukemia. Recognition by a monoclona anti-Ia reagent of a susceptibility determinant not in the DR series. J Exp Med 156:1872–1877
79. Nunez G, Giles RC, Ball EJ, Hurley CK, Capra JD, Stastny P (1984) Expression of HLA-DR, MB, MT, and SB antigens on human mononuclear cells: identification of two-phenotypically distinct monocytes populations. J Immunol 133:1300–1306
80. Parham P, Androlewicz MJ, Brodsky FM, Holmes NJ, Ways JP (1982) Monoclonal antibodies, purification, fragmentation and application to structural and functional studies of class I MHC antigens. J Immunol Methods 53:133–174
81. Park MS, Terasaki PI (1980) Second DR locus. In: Terasaki P (ed) Histocompatibility testing 1980. UCLA Tissue Typing Laboratory, Los Angeles, pp 578–582
82. Pawelec GP, Shaw S, Ziegler A, Muller C, Wernet P (1982) Differential inhibition of HLA-D or SB-directed secondary lymphoproliferative responses with monoclonal antibodies detecting human Ia-like determinants. J Immunol 129:1070–1075
83. Pierres M, Mercier P, Madsen M, Mawas C, Kristensen T (1982) Monoclonal mouse anti-I-A^k and anti-I-E^k antibodies cross reacting with HLA-DR supertypic and subtypic determinants rather than classical DR allelic specificities. Tissue Antigens 19:289–300

84. Pollack MS, Chin-Louie J, Moshief RD (1984) Functional characteristics and differential expression of class II DR, DS, and SB antigens on human melanoma cell lines. Hum Immunol 9:75–87
85. Quaranta V, Pellegrino MA, Ferrone S (1981) Serologic and immunochemical characterization of the specificity of four monoclonal antibodies to distinct antigenic determinants expressed on subpopulations of human Ia-like antigens. J Immunol 126:548–552
86. Radka SF, Machamer C, Cresswell P, Kostyu DD, Ward FE, Amos DB (1983) SFR3-DR5, a monoclonal antibody with HLA-DR5 specificity. J Immunol 130:1863–1866
87. Radka SF, Amos DB, Quackenbush LJ, Cresswell P (1984) HLA-DR7 specific monoclonal antibodies and a chimpanzee anti-DR7 serum detect different epitopes on the same molecule. Immunogenetics 19:63–76
88. Robinson J, Sieff C, Delia C, Edwards PAW, Greaves MF (1981) Expression of cell-surface HLA-DR, HLA-A,B,C and glycophorin during erythroid differentiation. Nature 289:68–71
89. Shackelford DA, Kaufman JF, Korman AJ, Strominger JL (1982) HLA-DR antigens: structure, separation of subpopulations, gene cloning, and functions. Immunol Rev 66:133–187
90. Shaw S, DeMars R (1984) Binding specificity of anti-human Ia monoclonal antibodies analysed with HLA-deletion mutant cell lines: patterns of binding to products of two different HLA haplotypes and of three subregions of a single haplotype. Dis Markers 2:183–195
91. Shaw S, DeMars R, Schlossman SF, Smith PL, Lampson LA, Nadler LM (1982) Serological identification of the human secondary B cell antigens. J Exp Med 156:731–743
92. Sparrow RL, McKenzie IFG (1983) Human "Ia" antigen populations defined by monoclonal antibodies. J Immunogenet 10:179–190
93. Steel CM (ed) (1984) Human MHC class II antigens: genetics, structure, and function. Wiley, Chichester
94. Steel CM, Vanheyningen V, Guy K, Cohen BB, Deane DL (1982) Influence of monoclonal anti-Ia-like antibodies on activation of human lymphocytes. Immunology 47:597–604
95. Symington FW, Sprent J (1981) A monoclonal antibody detecting an Ia specificity mapping in the I-A or I-E subregion. Immunogenetics 14:53–61
96. Tanigaki N, Tosi R, Sagawa K, Minowada J, Ferrara GB (1983) The distribution of DR5, MT2, and MB3 specificities on human Ia subsets. Immunogenetics 17:371–386
97. Tosi R, Tanigaki N, Centis D, Ferrara GB, Pressman D (1978) Immunological dissection of human Ia molecules. J Exp Med 148:1592–1611
98. Triebel F, Missenard-Leblond V, Conty MC, Charron D, Debre P (1984) Differential inhibition of human antigen specific T cell clone proliferative responses by distinct monoclonal anti-HLA-DR antibodies. J Immunol 132:1773–1778
99. Trucco MM, Garotta G, Stocker JW, Ceppellini R (1979) Murine monoclonal antibodies against HLA structures. Immunol Rev 47:219–252
100. Watson AJ, DeMars R, Trowbridge IS, Bach FH (1983) Detection of a novel human class II HLA antigen. Nature 304:358–360
101. Yamamoto K, Kumagai Y, Hiramatsu K, Okumura K, Tada T (1983) I-A homologous antigen on human lymphocytes detected by a monoclonal antibody. Immunogenetics 17:101–108
102. Yasukawa M, Zarling JM (1984) Human cytotoxic T cell clones directed against herpes simplex virus infected cells. I. Lysis restricted by HLA class II MB and DR antigens. J Immunol 133:422–427
103. Zola H, Bradley J, Macardle P, McEvoy R, Thomas M (1980) A hybridoma antibody which reacts with human cells carrying the DRw4 tissue type. Evidence for heterogeneity of DRw4. Transplantation 29:72–73

Preparation, Characterization, and Utilization of Monoclonal Antibodies to the Gene Products of the HLA-D Region, with Special Emphasis on Those to Polymorphic Determinants *

M. Igarashi, L. Imberti, M. Maio, M. Tsujisaki, F. Perosa, K. Sakaguchi, P.G. Natali, and S. Ferrone

Table of Contents

* This work was supported by the National Institute of Health Grants AI21384 and CA38469, by a grant-in-aid from the American Heart Association, Westchester/Putnam Chapter, and by a grant from the Cancer Research Institute, New York, NY. M.T. was supported by a fellowship from the National Kidney Foundation

Introduction

The hybridoma technology has been applied successfully by a large number of investigators to develop anti-HLA class II monoclonal antibodies (for reviews, see [10, 12, 59, 90]). A large number of these reagents have been analyzed in two recent international workshops [4, 117].

In this chapter we will first review the approaches used to develop and characterize anti-HLA class II monoclonal antibodies, then describe the specificity of the antibodies thus far published, and finally discuss the application of anti-HLA class II monoclonal antibodies, with emphasis on investigations which have been facilitated by the availability of these reagents. We will not attempt a comprehensive review of the extensive available literature, but will mainly focus on our own studies. Where appropriate, the work by others will be mentioned to discuss our own results.

Development of Anti-HLA Class II Monoclonal Antibodies

Immunogens

Cultured B lymphoid cells have been the most common immunogens utilized. Antigens partially purified from cultured B lymphoid cells, activated T cells, and melanoma cells have also been utilized. It is of interest that the latter two types of immunogens have generated antibodies to HLA-DQ antigens and to HLA-DR allospecificities more frequently than immunization with cultured B lymphoid cells. These findings suggest that the immunogenicity of HLA class II antigens expressed by activated T cells and by melanoma cells may be different from that of their counterparts expressed by cultured B lymphoid cells. In view of the structural homology and serological cross-reactivity of HLA class II antigens with their counterparts in other animal species [31], it is not surprising that immunization with murine and rat lymphoid cells has yielded antibodies cross-reacting with HLA class II antigens.

Immunization Schedule

Various immunization schedules have been utilized. Although no systematic comparison has been made of various immunization schedules, the available information and our own experience suggest that this variable does not play a major role in determining the specificity of the antibodies developed, but influences the Ig class and subclass of the antibodies.

Animals Immunized

BALB/c mice have been most frequently used for immunization. To broaden the specificity of monoclonal antibodies, it may be useful to continue to use other strains of mice, since the differential cross-reactivity of anti-H-2 class II antibodies with various HLA class II alloantigens (for review see Pla and Ivanyi, Cross-reactions of Class II Histocompatibility Antigens of Various Species, this volume) suggests that the antibody repertoire of various murine strains may be different and that HLA class II antigens may differ in their immunogenicity in various murine strains.

Screening Procedures

Screening of hybridoma supernatants to identify anti-HLA class II antibodies has relied on their differential reactivity with B and T lymphoid cells in serological assays. The latter include binding assays, conventional cytotoxicity, and antiglobulin assays. Blocking assays with $F(ab')_2$ fragments of conventional anti-HLA xenoantibodies and sodium dodecyl sulfate – polyacrylamide gel electrophoresis of antigens immunoprecipitated by the monoclonal antibodies have provided additional serological and immunochemical evidence about their reactivity with the gene products of the HLA-D region. Binding assays with HLA deletion mutant cell lines [112] and two-dimensional gel electrophoresis of antigens purified with monoclonal antibodies (Fig. 1) have been useful approaches to characterize their reactivity with HLA-DR, DQ, and/or DP antigens. Testing in serological and immunochemical assays with homozygous HLA cells has provided

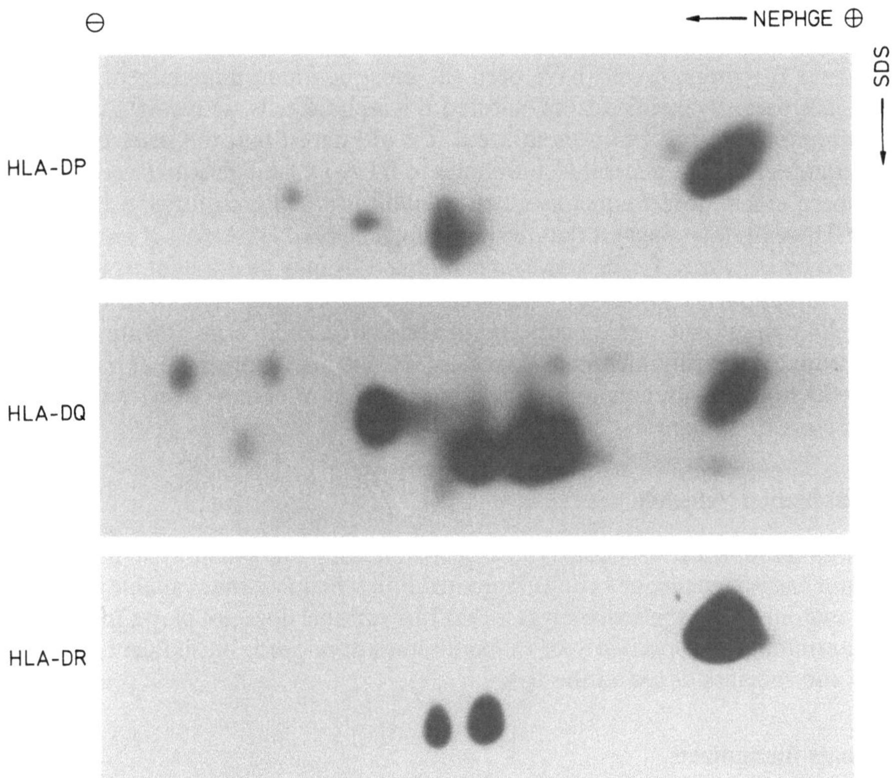

Fig. 1. Two-dimensional gel electrophoresis [nonequilibrium pH-gradient gel electrophoresis (*NEPHGE*) according to O'Farrell et al. [93] in the first dimension, sodium dodecyl sulfate polyacrylamide slab gel electrophoresis (*SDS*) according to Laemmli [65] in the second dimension] of antigens immunoprecipitated by the anti-HLA-DP MoAb B7/27 (*top panel*), by the anti-HLA-DQ MoAb anti-Leu 10 (*middle panel*), and by the anti-HLA-DR MoAb Q2/70 (*bottom panel*) from biosynthetically labeled cultured B lymphoid cells. Gels were fluorographed as described by Bonner and Laskey [11]

valuable information about the distribution of the determinants recognized by monoclonal antibodies on HLA class II allospecificities. Serological assays with HLA typed cells have identified antibodies to conventional HLA class II allospecificities. Binding assays with isolated subunits of HLA class II antigens and Western blotting analysis have characterized the reactivity of the antibodies with the subunits of HLA class II antigens.

Specificity of Anti-HLA Class II Monoclonal Antibodies

Monoclonal Antibodies to Monomorphic Determinants

Antibodies recognizing monomorphic determinants restricted to the gene products of the HLA-DR, DQ, and DP loci have been the exception and not the rule. It is noteworthy that the determinants restricted to the gene products of HLA-DR are mainly expressed by fully processed forms of the antigens, i.e., glycosylated α and β chain complex which is not associated with γ chain. The large majority of the antibodies recognize determinants expressed on HLA-DR and DP antigens or react strongly with these two antigens and weakly with HLA-DQ antigens. It has been reported in the literature [21, 39] and has also been our own experience that the distribution of monomorphic determinants on the gene products of the various loci may vary in cells with different phenotypes, thus adding to the complexity of the analysis of the specificity of monoclonal antibodies. The expression of determinants recognized by monoclonal antibodies on the gene products of the three loci of the HLA-D region may also vary during the biosynthesis of these antigens. For instance, the determinant recognized by the MoAb I2 is expressed on early biosynthetic products of HLA-DR, DP, and DQ antigens; as the processing of the antigens proceeds, the determinant becomes restricted to HLA-DR and DP antigens. In our own experience, monoclonal antibodies with high affinity for monomorphic determinants shared by HLA-DR, DQ, and DP antigens have not been very frequent. We have identified only two antibodies with such a specificity, Q5/13 and 26.163.

The distribution of monomorphic determinants recognized by monoclonal antibodies on conventional serologically defined HLA-DR allospecificities may display various types of heterogeneity: some monoclonal antibodies, like Genox 3.32 [12], Q5/6 [102], D7.69 [73], AB8.25/5, AC.BM.50, DA6.164, and 50D6A [15] react with all but one or two HLA-DR allospecificities. It is of interest that the HLA-DR7 allospecificity is the most frequently nonreactive alloantigen with this group of monoclonal antibodies. Other monoclonal antibodies recognize determinants with a heterogeneous distribution on HLA class II allospecificities which are indistinguishable with conventional alloantisera. Thus the determinants recognized by the MoAb Q2/80 [52] is differentially expressed on HLA-DR4 allospecificities which are indistinguishable with alloantisera, but are structurally different and are associated with different cellularly defined HLA-D allospecificities. Furthermore, the MoAb Q2/80, Q5/6, and Q5/13 display a differential titer in the cytotoxic assay with homozygous HLA-DR2 antigens bearing cells which express different HLA-D allospecificities (Table 1). These results suggest that monoclonal antibodies can enhance the discriminatory power of serological assays to an extent similar to that of cell-mediated immunity assays.

Table 1. Differential reactivity of monoclonal antibodies to monomorphic determinants of HLA class II antigens with homozygous HLA-DR2 positive lymphoid cells which express different HLA-D allospecificities

MoAb	DR2/DW2	DR2/DW9	DR2/LD14
Q5/13	80	80	320
Q5/6	20	320	320
Q2/80	20	20	320

Results expressed as reciprocal of titer in the cytotoxic test

Monoclonal Antibodies to HLA Class II Allospecificities

Among the antibodies recognizing conventional allotypic specificities, only a slightly higher number of antibodies to HLA-DR allospecificities than to HLA-DQ allospecificities have been described (Tables 2–4). Anti-HLA-DQw1 antibodies have been reported most frequently. It is of interest that, as observed with conventional alloantisera, antibodies to certain allospecificities have been developed utilizing immunogens which lack this specificity or express only a cross-reacting specificity. For instance, the anti-HLA-DR7 MoAb 62.74 was developed utilizing an immunogen with the phenotype HLA-DR3, w6 [58]. It should also be noted that some monoclonal antibodies (e.g., AC1.59 and D7.69) acquire specificity only when they are used at an appropriate dilution [73]. Monoclonal antibodies to polymorphic determinants, like those to monomorphic determinants, have identified heterogeneity in allospecificities which are indistinguishable with conventional antisera. The MoAb 16.23 recognizes a subset of the HLA-DR3 allospecificity [56]. The MoAb AC1.59 displays differential reactivity with HLA-DR4 allospecificities which are indistinguishable with conventional antisera, but are associated with different HLA-D specificities [20]. The MoAb NDS 15.38 identifies a determinant expressed on HLA-DR2 antigens synthesized by B lymphoid cells in long-term culture, by B lymphocytes from patients with chronic lymphocytic leukemia, and by activated T lymphocytes, but not by resting B lymphocytes [34]. A similar, although not identical, reactivity pattern has been described for the MoAb DA6.147 to a monomorphic determinant of HLA class II antigens [41].

Reactivity of Monoclonal Antibodies with Isolated Subunits of HLA Class II Antigens

Reactivity with the isolated subunits of HLA class II antigens has been determined for a limited number of monoclonal antibodies to monomorphic and polymorphic determinants. Antibodies to HLA-DR allospecificities have been found to react with the β subunit [56], as one would have predicted from the available information about the structural polymorphism of the two subunits of HLA-DR antigens [113]. The large majority of monoclonal antibodies recognizing monomorphic determinants expressed on HLA-DR and DP antigens or on HLA-DR, DQ, and DP antigens have been found to react with the β subunit or with the complex of the α and β subunit [14, 17, 103]. We are aware of only two monoclo-

Table 2. Monoclonal antibodies to HLA-DR allospecificities

Monoclonal antibody	Immunogen	Schedule of immunization	Strain	Myeloma	Specificity[a]	Ig subclass	Ref.
62.74	B-LCL: Raji (DR3,w6)	–	Lewis rat	–	DR1	G2ak	[58]
H40-242.3	Lymphoid cells from A.TL mice ($K^sI^kD^d$)	–	A.TH ($K^sI^sD^d$) mouse	X63-Ag8.653	DR1	G2ak	[9]
NDS 15.38	B-LCL: GIR_2 (DR2,7)	1×10^7 cells ip; 1.8×10^7 cells iv after 6 weeks; fusion: 5 days later	BALB/c mouse	P3-NS1/1Ag4.1	DR2 (on malignant activated cells)	–	[34]
AB8.25	PBL	2×10^7 cells iv single injection	BALB/c mouse	X63-Ag8.653	DR2 (DR2, DR5)	M	[73]
16.23	Melanoma cell line: Mel JuSo	Single injection	BALB/c mouse	–	DR3	–	[56]
FMC2	B-LCL: RPMI 8866 (DR2,4)	7×10^7 cells ip; 1×10^7 cells ip after 4 weeks; fusion: 5 days later	–	P3-NS1/1 Ag4.1	DR4 (short)	–	[131]
SFR16-DR7M }	Glycoproteins from B-LCL: P Bur (DR7,–)	20 µg glycoproteins (footpath)	KGH rat	Sp2/0-Ag14	DR7	M	[107]
SFR16-DR7G }					DR7	G2a	
12.7G3	Mouse splenocytes: BXSB	1×10^8 irradiated splenocytes + 4 mg aluminum ip; 1×10^8 iv after 2 weeks; fusion: 3 days later	(CBBC)F1 mouse	Sp2/0	DR2	–	[130]
7.3.19.1	B-LCL: ALA1 (DR3,3)	1×10^7 cells ip; 3×10^7 cells iv after 3 weeks; fusion: 3 days later	BALB/c mouse	Sp2/0	DRw52	G2b	[64]

Table 2 (continued)

Monoclonal antibody	Immunogen	Schedule of immunization	Strain	Myeloma	Specificity[a]	Ig subclass	Ref.
H10-81.10, H39-91.1	Splenocytes, thymocytes, or ConA-activated spleen cells from A.TL ($K^sI^kD^d$) mice	–	A.TH (K I D) mouse	NS1-1Ag4.1 or X63.Ag8.653	DRw52	G2ak	[100]
E.13.11	B-LCL: Daudi (DRw6, DQw1)	2,5–3,5 × 10^7 cells ip; 2,5–3,5 × 10^7 cells iv after 10 days; fusion: 3 days later	–	P3-X63-Ag8	DRw52	–	[123]
SFR3-DR5	Detergent-solubilized membranes from B-LCL: JK (DR4,w6)	10 µg of membranes (in CFA); 10 µg of membranes (in CFA) after 2 weeks; fusion: 3 days later	KGH rat	SP-2/0-Ag14	DR5	G2b	[106]
PL3	B-LCL: PLH (DR7)	1 × 10^7 cells ip biweekly, 3 times; fusion: 3 days after last injection	BALB/c mouse	Sp2/0-Ag14	DRw53	G3	[49]

B-LCL, human B-lymphoblastoid cell line; PBL, periphered blood lymphocytes

[a] According to the nomenclature of the Ninth International Histocompatibility Workshop

Table 3. Monoclonal antibodies to HLA-DQ allospecificities

Monoclonal antibody	Immunogen	Schedule of immunization	Strain	Myeloma	Specificity[a]	Ig subclass	Ref.
PLM12 PLM2	B-LCL: EBV-Sh (DR2,w6)	1×10^7 cells ip; 1×10^7 cells iv after 4 weeks; fusion: 3 days later	BALB/c mouse	X63-Ag8.653	DQw3 DQ(DR5, DR6.2)	G2a	[72]
BT 3/4	E-rosetting cells from a secondary MLC	1×10^7 cells ip every 10 days (3 times); fusion: 4 days later	BALB/c mouse	P3/X63-Ag8-U1	DQw1	G1	[19]
T10	B-LCL: KCCL 1448 (DR5, w9)	1×10^7 cells ip; 1×10^7 cells ip after 3 weeks; fusion: 3 days later	BALB/c mouse	X63Ag8.653	DQw1	M	[71]
Genox 3.53	Glycoproteins from B-LCL: Bristol-8 (DR2)	30 µg glycoproteins (in CFA) sc; 30 µg glycoproteins in ICFA) sc after 7 weeks; 30 µg glycoproteins iv; fusion: 6 days later	C3H mouse	P3-NS1/1Ag4.1	DQw1 (DR1, 2, w6)	G1	[12]
MRC.0X3	Glycoproteins from rat thymocytes	–	BALB/c mouse	P3-NS1/1Ag4.1	DQw1	–	[77]
SDR1	B-LCL: MST(DR2)	–	–	–	DQw1	G1	[25]
5F6	B-LCL	–	BALB/c mouse	P3-X63-Ag8	DQw1	G2a	[63]
HU-18	B-LCL: ISH (DR4,-/DRw52/ DQw3)	3×10^7 cells ip; 3×10^7 cells iv after 3 weeks; fusion: 3 days later	BALB/c mouse	X63-Ag8.653	DQw3	G2b	[62]
IVD 12	B-LCL: PRIESS (DR4,4)	1×10^7 cells ip every week (for 3 weeks); 1×10^7 cells iv after 33 days; fusion: 3 days later	BALB/c mouse	Sp2/0-Ag-14	DQw3(DR4,5)	G1k	[37]
SG 171	B-LCL: GM3163(DR7)+ GM3107(DR2)+ GM3158 (M)	–	BALB/c mouse	–	DS7	–	[38]

B-LCL, human B lymphoblastoid cell line
[a] According to the nomenclature of the Ninth International Histocompatibility Workshop

Table 4. Monoclonal antibodies recognizing determinants shared by allospecificities encoded by the HLA-DR, DQ, and DP loci

Monoclonal antibody	Immunogen	Schedule of immunization	Strain	Myeloma	Specificity[a]	Ig subclass	Ref.
I-LR2	Burkitt's lymphoma cells	5×10^6 cells ip; 5×10^6 cells iv after 4 weeks; fusion: 4 days later	BALB/c mouse	P3/NS1/1-Ag4-1	DRw52 (DR3, 5, w6)	–	[81]
E15.4	B-LCL: Daudi (DRw6/DQw1)	2.5–3.5×10^7 cells ip; 2.5–3.5×10^7 cells iv after 3 days; fusion: 3 days later	–	P3-X63-Ag8	DRw52 (DR3,5,w6)	–	[123]
MCLB.8	–	–	–	–	DR1,2,4,w6,w8	–	[13]
MC-26.1	B-LCL: Raji (DR3,w6)	1×10^8 cells ip; 5×10^7 cells iv after 2 weeks; fusion: 3 days later	CBA/H mouse	NS-1	DRw53(DQw3) (DR7,w9) (DR4,5)	G2ak	[119]
17.15	B-LCL: PHU(DR3,4)	1×10^7 cells ip; 1×10^7 cells ip after 10 days; fusion: 3 days later	BALB/c mouse	MOPC21 NS1/1	DRw53(DQw3)	–	[44]
HU-30	B-LCL: Shi-C3 (DR2,-/DQw1, DRw52,DRw3)	3×10^7 cells ip; 3×10^7 cells iv after 3 weeks; fusion: 3 days later	BALB/c mouse	X63-Ag8.653	DR1,2	G2	[61]
AC1.59	B-LCL: IBW4(DR1)	2×10^7 cells iv single injection	BALB/c mouse	X63-Ag8/653	DR1,4(short) w6,w8	M	[20]
H40-164.3 H40-315.7 H8-15.9 H39-352.4	Splenocytes, thymocytes, or ConA-activated spleen cells from A.TL ($K^sI^sD^d$) mice	–	A.TH($K^sI^sD^d$) mouse	NS1-Ag.4.1 or X63-Ag.8.653	DR1,2,3,w6,w8, w9,w10 DR1,2,w6(short) w9,w10 DR1,2,3,w6(short) w9,w10 DR1,2,w6(short) w9,w10	G2ak	[100]

I-LR1	Burkitt's lymphoma cells	1×10^6 cells ip; 5×10^6 cells iv after 4 weeks; fusion: 4 days later	BALB/c mouse	P3-NS1/1-Ag-1	DPw2,w3,DR5	–	[111]
D4.90	B-LCL: Daudi (DRw6,DQw1)	2×10^7 cells iv single injection	BALB/c mouse	X63-Ag8/653	DR3, DRw52	M	[73]
Anti-Leu10	Purified B cells (non-E-rosette forming lymphocytes) from human tonsil	–	BALB/c mouse	P3/NS1/1-Ag4-1	DQw1,w3,DRw10	–	[16]
33.1	B-LCL: TRAL (DR2,2, w52/DQw1/DPw4)		BALB/c mouse	P3-X63-Ag-U1	DQw1,w3	G1k	[75]
IIIE3	B-LCL: XNEW (DR3/DRw10)	1×10^7 cell ip every week for 3 weeks; 1×10^7 cells iv after 33 days; fusion: 3 days later	BALB/c mouse	SP2/0-Ag14	DRw52,w53	G1k	[51]
109d6	Hairy cell leukemia cells (DR4,5)	–	BALB/c mouse	Sp/20	DRw10,w52	G2a	[121]

B-LCL, human B lymphoblastoid cell line; PBL, human peripheral blood lymphocytes
[a] According to the nomenclature of the Ninth International Histocompatibility Workshop

nal antibodies, DA6.147 [41] and TAL-1B5 [2], reacting with the α chain, and one, VIC-Y1 [105], reacting with the γ chain. One antibody, L227 [32], has been found to recognize a determinant shared by the β and γ chains. The higher frequency of antibodies reacting with the β chain than with the α chain may reflect the low immunogenicity of the latter subunit, as suggested by its conserved primary amino acid sequence through phylogenetic evolution. The low frequency of antibodies to the γ chain may reflect its low immunogenicity and/or the lack of detection of antibodies to intracytoplasmic components, such as the γ chains, by assays with viable cells which are the most widely used to screen hybridoma supernatants.

Applications of Anti-HLA Class II Monoclonal Antibodies

In this section we will discuss investigations which have been facilitated by anti-HLA class II monoclonal antibodies.

Analysis of the Distribution of HLA Class II Antigens in Normal and Malignant Tissues

Immunohistochemical staining of surgically removed tissues with monoclonal antibodies (Figs. 2 and 3) has shown that HLA class II antigens have a broader tissue distribution than originally suggested (for review see [78]), as they are expressed by cells not directly associated with the immune system, may display variability in their expression among different donors, and may be induced by a number of stimuli [6, 23, 43, 83, 86, 89, 125]. This may be exemplified by summarizing the information about the distribution of HLA class II antigens in the kidney, an organ extensively investigated because of the influence of HLA-DR matching on graft survival (see A. Ting, The Role of HLA Class II Antigens in Clinical Transplantation, this volume) and because of the occasional association between hyperacute and accelerated rejection and anti HLA-DR antibodies. HLA class II antigens are expressed by glomeruli, intertubular capillaries and veins, and interstitial dendritic cells, but are not detected on the endothelia of the majority of large vessels [28, 33, 42, 83]. Expression of HLA class II antigens on tubules varies among individual kidneys, ranging from strong to very weak or undetectable. The intensity of the staining is also influenced by the specificity of the antibodies used. This latter variability may reflect heterogeneity in the distribution of monomorphic determinants of HLA class II antigens and/or differences in the affinity of the antibodies. The expression of HLA class II antigens on tubular cells is considerably increased in transplanted kidneys which show acute cellular rejection [42]. This phenomenon may reflect induction of HLA class II antigens on renal tubular cells by immune interferon produced by infiltrating activated T cells, or may be a consequence of tubular regeneration following rejection or ischemic damage.

Recently, analysis of surgically removed tissues with monoclonal antibodies to the gene products of the HLA-D region has shown differences in their ontogeny and in their tissue distribution in adults; HLA-DR and DP antigens have a broader distribution than HLA-DQ antigens [67, 87, 89]. The latter have a tissue

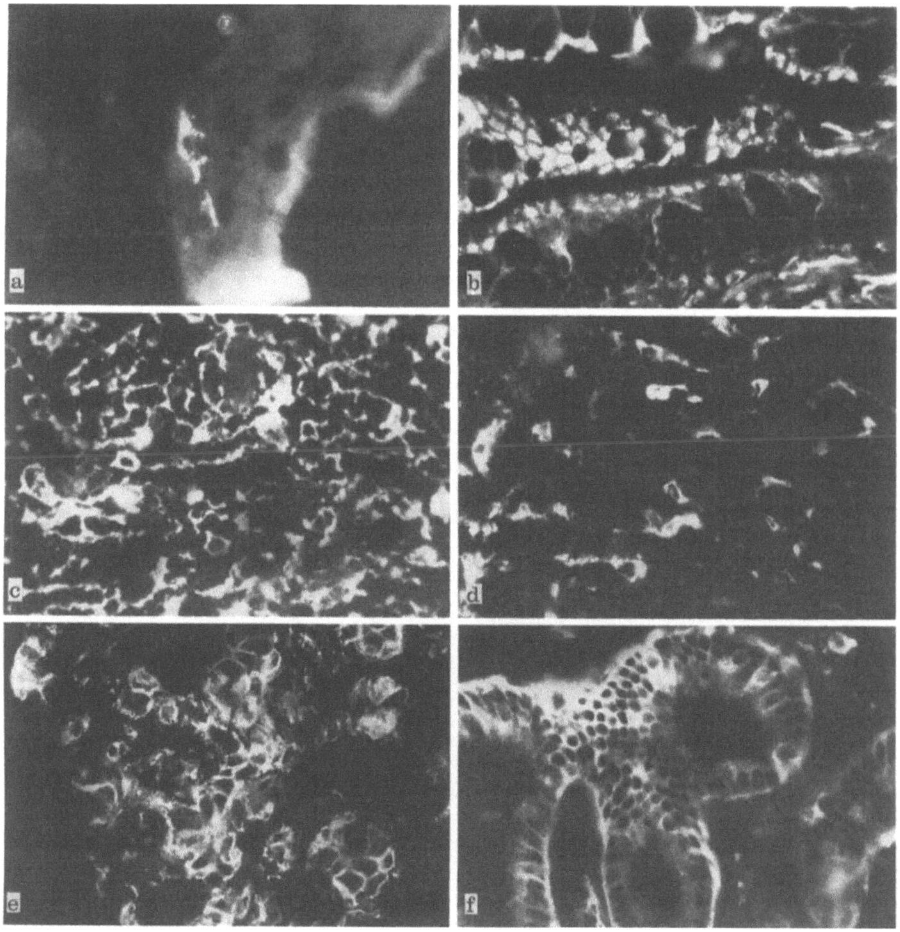

Fig. 2. Indirect immunofluorescence staining of 4-μm cryostat sections of fetal skin (**a**), jejunum (**b**), and thymus (**c**) with the anti-HLA-DR + DQ + DP MoAb Q5/13, of liver (**d**), and parotid (**e**) with the anti-HLA-DQ MoAb anti-Leu 10, and of endometrium (**f**) with the anti-HLA-DP MoAb I-LR1. **a,** × 1000, **b–f,** × 650

distribution different from that of their murine counterparts, since I-A antigens are expressed in epithelia of small intestine and colon, but are not detectable in acinar cells of parotid and in Kupffer cells [84].

In view of the potential role of HLA class II antigens in the interaction of tumor cells with the host's immune system, it is noteworthy that in agreement with studies performed with cell lines in long-term culture [14, 45, 70, 92, 101, 126, 129], analysis of surgically removed tissues has shown that malignant transformation of cells may be associated with the appearance of HLA class II antigens [22, 82, 85, 118, 120, 128]. The frequency of the phenomenon is different in various types of malignancies, being greatest in melanoma. Of the three types of HLA class II antigens analyzed, HLA-DR antigens are the most frequently found in malignancies of lymphoid [5, 30, 76] and nonlymphoid [89] origin. In our own studies, no malignant lesion has been found to express either HLA-DQ or DP

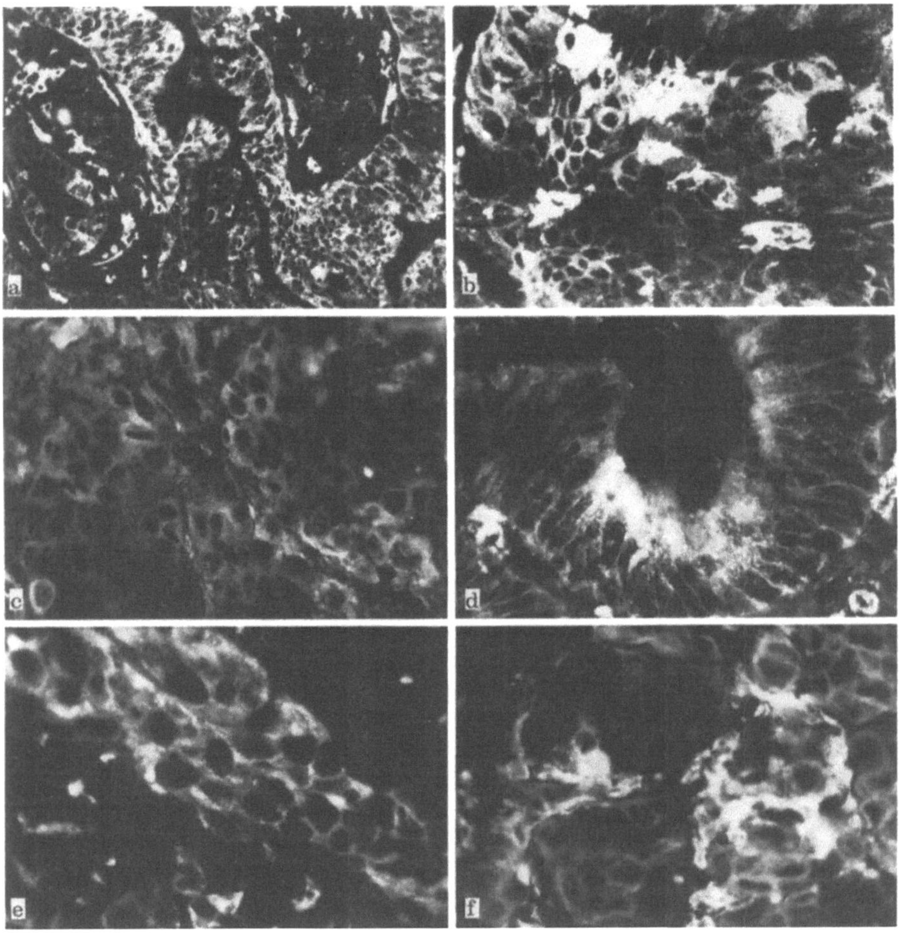

Fig. 3. Indirect immunofluorescence staining of 4-μm cryostat sections of metatastic melanoma (**a**) and epidermoid skin carcinoma (**b**) with the anti-HLA-DP MoAb I-LR1, of thyroid follicular carcinoma (**c**) and endometrial carcinoma (**d**) with the anti-HLA-DR MoAb PTF29, and of a rectal adenocarcinoma (**e**) and a metastatic melanoma (**f**) with the anti-HLA-DQ MoAb anti-Leu 10. **a–f,** ×650

antigens without HLA-DR antigens, while several lesions can express only HLA-DR antigens. The differential expression of HLA-DR and HLA-DQ antigens has been found not only in lesions from different patients, but also among autologous lesions removed from different anatomic sites from a given patient [88, 89]. Representative results are shown in Table 5. The mechanism(s) underlying these phenomena is not known. The differential susceptibility of the gene products of the HLA-D region to induction by interferons may play a role in this regard [7, 18, 35, 36, 50, 124]. Furthermore, no information is available about the relationship between HLA class II phenotype and the clinical course of the disease. It will be of interest to determine whether the differential expression of these antigens affects the biology of malignant cells.

Table 5. Heterogeneous expression of the gene products of the HLA-D region in multiple metastases removed from patients with melanoma

Patient		HLA-DR	HLA-DQ	HLA class I	β–μ	HMW-MAA
T.A.	M1	2+ cyt.	–	2+	1+	2+
	M2	Isolated cells	–	trace	var.	trace
	M3	Isolated cells	–	2+	var.	1+
Z.C.	M1	1+	–	2+ var.	–	1+
	M2	1+ var.	–	1+	1+	2+
	M3	–	–	–	–	1+
	M4	–	–	–	–	2+
C.O.	M1	2+ var.	2+	1+	1+ var.	1+ var.
	M2	1+ var.	1+ var.	2+	2+	1+ var.

Frozen sections of surgically removed lesions were stained with monoclonal antibodies in indirect immunofluorescence. The staining was classified as: 2+ = bright and homogeneous staining; 1+ = dull and homogeneous staining; var. = variable staining; trace = barely detectable staining; cyt. = cytoplasmic staining
HMW-MAA, high-molecular-weight melanoma-associated antigen

Development of Double-Determinant Immunoassays to Measure HLA Class II Antigens

Double-determinant immunoassays developed with monoclonal antibodies have been applied to detect and quantitate HLA class II antigens [46, 109]. Thus far, the studies have been performed only with antibodies to monomorphic determinants. The results have confirmed early observations that HLA class II antigens, like HLA class I antigens [97], are present in serum [53, 127], and have shown that the level of HLA class II antigens, like that of HLA class I antigens, may be increased in pathological conditions (such as various types of leukemia). The results obtained with monoclonal antibodies to a limited number of HLA class I allospecificities [Russo et al., in preparation] suggest that a major application of the double-determinant immunoassay will be typing for HLA class II antigens, once antibodies with the appropriate specificity become available, because of the technical difficulties of HLA-DR typing utilizing the lymphocytotoxic test.

Development of Anti-idiotypes to Anti-HLA Class II Monoclonal Antibodies

The high degree of homogeneity and the availability in large amounts of anti-HLA class II monoclonal antibodies has facilitated the development of anti-idiotype antibodies. These reagents have been developed in rabbits and in mice utilizing antibodies to monomorphic determinants of HLA class II antigens as immunogens [98, 99, 104]. In agreement with results in the murine system [26, 27, 40, 95], both syngeneic and xenogeneic anti-idiotypic antibodies define a limited number of idiotopes, some of which are associated with the antigen binding site. Whether these recurrent idiotopes are also expressed on antibodies directed to different antigenic systems is not known. On the other hand, idiotopes recognized by conventional antisera elicited in rabbits and BALB/c mice with the anti-HLA-A2, A28 MoAb CR11-351 have been found also on the anti-HLA class II MoAb

127, CR10-343, CR11-462, CR12-230, Q2/47, Q5/6, and Q5/13 [110; unpublished observations]. Sharing of idiotopes among antibodies to different antigenic structures has already been described in other antigenic systems [57, 60, 68, 94]. This phenomenon may reflect the random occurrence of idiotypic determinants on antibodies to unrelated specificities or the involvement of related IgV-gene families in the diversification of corresponding B cell precursors. In view of the cross-reactivity between human and murine class II histocompatibility antigens (for review, see Pla and Ivanyi, Cross-reactions of Class II Histocompatibility Antigens of Various Species, this volume), it is also noteworthy that anti-HLA class II antibodies appear to share idiotopes with anti-murine class II histocompatibility antigen antibodies. Dr. S. L. Epstein at the National Cancer Institute, Bethesda, Maryland, found that our anti-HLA class II MoAb Q2/70, Q2/80, Q5/13, and CR11-462 cross-reacted in a binding assay with anti-idiotype antibodies elicited in pigs and rabbits with the anti-murine Ia7 MoAb 14-4-4S.

Topography of Determinants Recognized by Anti-HLA Class II Monoclonal Antibodies

Utilizing cross-inhibition binding assays, the spatial relationship among determinants recognized by a number of monoclonal antibodies has been analyzed. According to the information in the literature [1, 108] [Russo et al., in preparation], as well as to our own results, the determinants recognized by the monoclonal antibodies appear to be restricted to limited areas on the HLA class II-bearing molecules. These results are in agreement with the differences in the amino acid sequence in restricted areas between human and murine class II histocompatibility antigens. Interesting observations have been made in the course of the mapping of antigenic determinants on HLA class II molecules. The spatial relationship among monomorphic determinants, as well as between monomorphic and polymorphic determinants may vary on different allospecificities [8; unpublished observations]. This finding, in conjunction with the differential reactivity of populations of HLA class II antigen cells with monoclonal antibodies to monomorphic determinants [3, 9, 74] (Table 6), suggests that the polymorphism of HLA class II antigens is more extensive than anticipated. Tosi et al. [122] have reported that binding of one monoclonal antibody to HLA class II antigens can enhance the binding of antibodies to distinct determinants. Two mechanisms have been suggested to account for this phenomenon [48]. In one, binding of the first antibody induces a conformational change in the antigen which increases its affinity for the combining site of the second antibody. In the other, the binding of the first antibody arranges the antigens in pairs, with a subsequent increase in the rate of association of the second antibody. Some monoclonal antibodies to HLA class II antigens have been found unexpectedly to inhibit the binding of monoclonal antibodies to HLA class I antigens [Russo et al., in preparation]. Although there is homology in the sequence of the second domain of the two subunits of HLA class II antigens with the third domain of the heavy chain of HLA class I antigens and with β_2 microglobulin [66], this blocking is not likely to reflect binding of anti-HLA class II monoclonal antibodies with HLA class I antigens. Recently published serological and immunochemical results suggest that this phenomenon may reflect an association between HLA class II and class I antigens following reaction with monoclonal antibodies. Neppert and Mueller-Eckhardt [91] have

Table 6. Heterogeneity in the expression of monomorphic determinants of HLA class II antigens by leukemic cells

Cells	Percent of cells stained by monoclonal antibodies		
Type Donor	Q2/80	Q5/6	Q5/13
CLL			
AB	71	15	10
SZ	ND	88	8
RE	50	10	15
HO	15	64	57
B-lymphoma			
EC	70	0	73
Null-ALL			
NO	0	78	56
NU	3	72	60

CLL, chronic lymphocytic leukemia; ALL, acute lymphoblastic leukemia; ND, not done

reported that anti-HLA class I monoclonal antibodies can cocap HLA class II antigens on B lymphocytes. Adams et al. [2] have reported that anti-HLA class II monoclonal antibodies coprecipitate a protein with the approximate molecular weight of 43K which appears to be the heavy chain of HLA class I antigens. Redistribution of HLA class I antigens induced by anti-HLA class II monoclonal antibodies has to be taken into account when interpreting the blocking of T cell cytotoxicity by anti-HLA class II monoclonal antibodies.

Phylogenetic Evolution of Determinants Defined by Anti-HLA Class II Monoclonal Antibodies

The restricted reactivity of monoclonal antibodies has greatly facilitated the characterization of the phylogenetic evolution of antigenic determinants of HLA class II antigens. In agreement with previous results with conventional allo- and xeno-antisera (for review see Pla and Ivanyi, Cross-reactions of Class II Histocompatibility Antigens of Various Species, this volume) a number of monoclonal antibodies has been found to cross-react with class II histocompatibility antigens in other animal species [24, 47, 54, 69, 96] [Crepaldi et al., in preparation). The extent of cross-reactivity varies from antibody to antibody. Some of our monoclonal antibodies, like Q5/13, cross-react with lymphocytes from a variety of mammalian species and even from some nonmammalian vertebrates. The mechanism(s) underlying the immunogenicity of highly conserved determinants have recently been dicussed by Jemmerson et al. [55], who investigated the immunogenicity of an evolutionarily conserved region of mammalian cytochrome c in rabbits.

It is of interest that monoclonal antibodies to monomorphic determinants of HLA class II antigens may recognize determinants which are polymorphic in other animal species [29, 116]. Furthermore, the cross-reactivity of monoclonal antibodies recognizing determinants expressed by HLA-DR antigens appears to be more extensive than that of those restricted to HLA-DQ antigens. The latter finding is in agreement with the higher cross-reactivity of anti-murine I-E^k than anti-murine I-A^k monoclonal antibodies with their human counterparts [100]. Results from these studies have both theoretical and practical implications. Information about the phylogenetic evolution of HLA class II antigens, when correlated with changes in the function of the immune system, may contribute to our understanding of the structure-function relationship of HLA class II antigens. Furthermore, identification of anti-HLA class II monoclonal antibodies cross-reacting with xenogeneic class II histocompatibility antigens provides reagents to characterize the gene products of the immune response region in animal species in which alloantisera and/or monoclonal antibodies are not available.

Role of Determinants Defined by Anti-HLA Class II Monoclonal Antibodies in Cell-Cell Interactions

Monoclonal antibodies have facilitated the utilization of blocking assays to analyze the role of the gene products of the HLA-DR, DQ, and DP loci and of distinct determinants on each molecule in cell-cell interactions. The conclusions from these experiments have to be interpreted with caution, since monoclonal antibodies claimed to be specific for the gene products of one locus have been subsequently shown to cross-react with the gene products of other loci. Monomorphic determinants of both HLA-DR and DQ antigens can function as targets of cytotoxic T cells [114, 115]. Some, but not all, monoclonal antibodies to monomorphic determinants of HLA-DR and DQ antigens have been found to inhibit the proliferation of T cells stimulated with mitogens, with soluble antigens, with allogeneic cells, with autologous non-T cells, and with autologous phytohemagglutinin-activated T cells. Polymorphic determinants of HLA-DQ antigens differ from monomorphic determinants of HLA-DR and DQ antigens in their involvement in the sequence of events which lead to proliferation of T cells activated by a variety of stimuli. Anti-HLA-DQw1 monoclonal antibodies do not affect proliferation of T cells stimulated with alloantigens or soluble antigens, but inhibit the generation of effector T cells mediating specific cytolytic activity. Anti-HLA class II monoclonal antibodies appear to regulate T cell proliferation through different mechanisms. Some inhibit production of interleukin-2 by T cells [79], others induce suppressor cells that inhibit T cell proliferation [80]. Finally, destruction of cells via an antibody-dependent cell-mediated cytotoxicity phenomenon cannot be excluded, since the inhibitory activity of the whole immunoglobulin may be lost when $F(ab')_2$ fragments are used [80].

Conclusions

The available information indicates that anti-HLA-DR antibodies are found with a markedly higher frequency than anti-HLA-DQ and anti-HLA-DP antibodies among hybridomas generated with splenocytes from mice immunized with HLA class II antigens. At present it is not known whether this finding reflects the higher expression of HLA-DR antigens than of HLA-DQ and DP antigens or differential immunogenicity of the gene products of the HLA-D region, or both. The low frequency of anti-HLA-DP specific antibodies is a surprising and unexpected finding, since analogues of HLA-DP antigens have not been detected in mice, while HLA-DR and DP antigens display a high degree of homology in their primary amino acid sequence with the murine I-E and I-A antigens. Monomorphic and polymorphic determinants expressed by the three types of HLA class II antigens differ in their immunogenicity: anti-HLA-DR monoclonal antibodies to monomorphic determinants are markedly more frequent than those to polymorphic determinants, while this difference is less pronounced among anti-HLA-DQ monoclonal antibodies. The majority of monoclonal antibodies to polymorphic determinants have low affinity and therefore have not been very useful for the immunochemical characterization of the corresponding specificities.

It has been a general experience that the development of monoclonal antibodies to polymorphic determinants of HLA class II antigens has been less frequent than anticipated, although a variety of immunogens have been utilized. It is not known wheter this reflects low immunogenicity of polymorphic determinants, their low representation in the antibody repertoire of the murine immune system, or both. Furthermore, it would appear that purification of antigens is associated with a marked reduction in their immunogenicity, especially that of polymorphic determinants. Whether the utilization of synthetic peptides can overcome these limitations is not known at present, although the immunization of rabbits with synthetic peptides has met with limited success.

Monoclonal antibodies have detected a high degree of cross-reactivity among the products of the HLA-DR, DQ, and DP loci, especially among the incompletely processed forms. The cross-reactivity is markedly higher than that detected among the gene products of the HLA-A, B, and C loci. The findings are in agreement with the high degree of homology in the primary amino acid sequence of HLA-DR, DQ, and DP antigens, and are consistent with the derivation of HLA-DR, DQ, and DP antigens by gene duplication. Furthermore, these findings suggest that maturation of HLA class II antigens is associated with changes in their antigenic profile.

The availability of monoclonal antibodies has greatly facilitated the analysis of the tissue distribution of HLA class II antigens. There is general agreement that these antigens are not restricted to cells directly associated with the immune system and that the expression of these antigens can be induced by a variety of stimuli. The functional significance of these findings remains to be determined. The detailed characterization of the tissue distribution of the gene products of the HLA-D region provides an explanation for findings such as the association between kidney hyperacute rejection and anti-HLA class II cytotoxic antibodies.

The exquisite specificity of monoclonal antibodies has sharpened the discriminatory power of serological assays. Various types of heterogeneity have been identified which could not be detected with conventional antisera. Among them is the heterogeneous distribution of monomorphic determinants on populations of cells. This finding has both theoretical and practical implications: it shows that the polymorphism of HLA class II antigens is more extensive than anticipated on the basis of studies with conventional antisera, and useful markers can be provided to isolate subpopulations of HLA class II antigen cells. Characterization of the functional properties of the cell subsets in conjunction with analysis of the effect of anti-HLA class II monoclonal antibodies on immunological phenomena will contribute to our understanding of the structure-function relationship of

HLA class II antigens. Furthermore, monoclonal antibodies have detected heterogeneity within HLA-DR allospecificities which are indistinguishable with conventional alloantisera but display structural polymorphism and are associated with different HLA-D allospecificities. These reagents will allow application of serological techniques to define the biological and clinical significance of the structural heterogeneity of HLA-DR allospecificities.

An area which has greatly benefited from the availability of monoclonal antibodies is the development of anti-idiotype antibodies. Conventional antisera to idiotypes of monoclonal antibodies to monomorphic determinants of HLA class II antigens have been described, and monoclonal antibodies are being prepared. The latter reagents may facilitate the development of new approaches to modulate the immune response in patients with abnormalities of their immune system. The results of these investigations will contribute to our understanding of the role of HLA class II antigens in immunopathological conditions and will help to assess the impact of monoclonal antibodies on clinical applications of HLA class II antigens.

Acknowledgments. The authors wish to acknowledge the excellent secretarial assistance of Mrs. Edwina L. Jones and Mrs. Vicky Temponi.

References

1. Accolla RS, Corte G, Tosi R (1984) Classification of anti-class II monoclonal antibodies based on epitope and molecular assignment. Dis Markers 2:39–45
2. Adams TE, Bodmer JG, Bodmer WF (1983) Production and characterization of monoclonal antibodies recognizing the α-chain subunits of human Ia alloantigens. Immunology 50:613–624
3. Addis JBL, Tisch R, Falk JA, Letarte M (1982) The analysis with monoclonal antibodies of the heterogeneity of Ia glycoproteins on chronic lymphocytic leukemia cells. J Immunol 129:2033–2039
4. Albert ED, Baur MP, Mayr WR (eds) (1984) Histocompatibility testing 1984. Springer, Berlin Heidelberg New York Tokyo
5. Al-Katib A, Koziner B (1984) Leu-10 (HLA-DC/DS) antigen distribution in human leukaemic disorders as detected by a monoclonal antibody: correlation with HLA-DR expression. Br J Haematol 57:373–382
6. Ballardini G, Mirakian R, Bianchi FB, Pisi E, Doniach D, Bottazzo GF (1984) Aberrant expression of HLA-DR antigens on bileduct epithelium in primary biliary cirrhosis: relevance to pathogenesis. Lancet II:1009–1013
7. Basham T, Smith W, Lanier L, Morhenn V, Merigan T (1984) Regulation of expression of class II major histocompatibility antigens on human peripheral blood monocytes and Langerhans cells by interferon. Hum Immunol 10:83–93
8. Beckman IGR, Bradley J, Zola H (1984) Delineation of serologically distinct monomorphic determinants of human MHC class II antigens: evidence of heterogeneity in their topographical distribution. Dis Markers 2:101–105
9. Birnbaum D, Dosseto M, Bourgue F, Pierres M, Kourilsky FM (1982) A cross-reactive mouse anti-I-E^k monoclonal antibody detects an HLA-DR polymorphism linked to HLA-DR1. Mol Immunol 19:755–764
10. Bodmer JG, Bodmer WF (1984) Monoclonal antibodies to HLA determinants. Br Med Bull 40:267–275
11. Bonner WM, Laskey RA (1974) A film detection method for tritium-labelled proteins and nucleic acid in polyacrylamide gels. Eur J Biochem 46:83–84
12. Brodsky FM, Parham P, Barnstable CJ, Crumpton MJ, Bodmer WF (1979) Monoclonal antibodies for analysis of the HLA system. Immunol Rev 47:3–61

13. Brodsky FM, Stone WH, Parham P (1981) Of cows and men: a comparative study of histocompatibility antigens. Hum Immunol 3:143–152
14. Carrel S, Gros N, Heumann D, Mach JP (1979) Expression of "Ia-like" antigens on cells from a human endometrial carcinoma cell line, END-1. Transplantation 27:431–433
15. Charron DJ (1984) Serology with 100 monoclonal antibodies to MHC class II antigens: an overview of workshop presentation. Dis Markers 2:145–149
16. Chen Y-K, Evans RL, Pollack MS, Lanier LL, Phillips JH, Rousso C, Warner NL, Brodsky FM (1984) Characterization and expression of the HLA-DC antigens defined by Anti-Leu 10. Hum Immunol 10:221–235
17. Cohen B, Deaned D, Moxley M (1984) Analysis of antibody specificity by western blotting. Dis Markers 2:135–144
18. Collins T, Korman AJ, Wake CT, Boss JM, Kappes DJ, Fiers W, Ault KA, Gimbrone MA Jr, Strominger JL, Pober JS (1984) Immune interferon activates multiple class II major histocompatibility complex genes and the associated invariant chain gene in human endothelial cells and dermal fibroblasts. Proc Natl Acad Sci USA 81:4917–4921
19. Corte G, Calabi F, Damiani G, Bargellesi A, Tosi R, Sorrentino R (1981) Human Ia molecules carrying DC1 determinants differ in both α- and β-subunits from Ia molecules carrying DR determinants. Nature 292:357–360
20. Crepaldi T, Richiardi P, Malavasi F, Carbonara AO, Igarashi M, Ferrone S (1985) The monoclonal antibody AC1.59 define a new polymorphic determinant on HLA-DR molecules. Tissue Antigens 26:25–34
21. Crumpton MJ, Bodmer JG, Bodmer WF, Heyes JM, Lindsay J, Rudd CE (1984) Biochemistry of class II antigens: workshop report. In: Albert ED, Baur MP, Mayr WR (eds) Histocompatibility testing 1984. Springer, Berlin Heidelberg New York Tokyo, pp 29–37
22. Daar AS, Fuggle SV, Ting A, Fabre JW (1982) Anomalous expression of HLA-DR antigens on human colorectal cancer cells. J Immunol 129:447–449
23. Daar AS, Fuggle SV, Fabre JW, Ting A, Morris PJ (1984) The detailed distribution of MHC class II antigens in normal human organs. Transplantation 38:293–298
24. Deeg HJ, Wulff JC, De Rose S, Sale GE, Braun M, Brown MA, Springmeyer SC, Martin PJ, Storb R (1982) Unusual distribution of Ia-like antigens on canine lymphocytes. Immunogenetics 16:445–457
25. De Kretser TA, Crumpton MJ, Bodmer JG, Bodmer WF (1982) Two-dimensional gel analysis of the polypeptides precipitated by a polymorphic HLA-DR1,2,w6 monoclonal antibody: evidence for a third locus. Eur J Immunol 12:600–606
26. Devaux C, Pierres M (1982) Clonal analysis of B and T cell responses to Ia antigens. III. Characterization of 12 xenogeneic anti-idiotypic antisera to A.TH-derived anti-I-A^k and anti-I-E^k monoclonal antibodies. J Immunol 128:751–757
27. Epstein SL, Ozato K, Bluestone JA, Sachs DH (1981) Idiotypes of anti-Ia antibodies I. Expression of the 14-4-4S idiotype in humoral immune responses. J Exp Med 154:397–410
28. Evans PR, Trickett LP, Smith JL, Maciver AG, Tate D, Slapak M (1984) Variable expression of HLA-DR antigens in the human kidney. Dis Markers 2:251–253
29. Falk JA, Addis JBL, Letarte M (1983) Species cross-reactive Ia determinants: detection with a monoclonal antibody to human Ia of a murine Ia.7 epitope. Hum Immunol 7:79–88
30. Faille A, Turmel P, Charron DJ (1984) Differential expression of HLA-DR and HLA-DC/DS molecules in a patient with hairy cell leukemia: restoration of HLA-DC/DS expression by (12-0-tetradeconayl phorbol-13-acetate), 5 azacytidine, and sodium butyrate. Blood 64:33–37
31. Ferrone S, David CS (eds) (1982) Ia antigens. Vol II. Man and other species. CRC Press, Boca Raton, Florida
32. Finn OJ, Stackhouse CJ, Metzgar RS (1983) Human Ia beta chains and the invariant chain share a common antigenic determinant. J Exp Med 158:1344–1349
33. Fuggle SV, Errasti P, Daar AS, Fabre JW, Ting A, Morris PJ (1983) Localization of MHC (HLA-ABC and DR) antigens in 46 kidneys. Differences in staining of tubules between kidneys. Transplantation 35:383–390

34. Fuggle SV, Kirkley J, Ting A, Morris PJ (1983) A monoclonal antibody recognizing HLA-DR2 on malignant and activated cells. Immunogenetics 18:415–428
35. Giacomini P, Aguzzi A, Pestka S, Fisher PB, Ferrone S (1984) Modulation by recombinant DNA leukocyte (α) and fibroblast (β) interferons of the expression and shedding of HLA- and tumor-associated antigens by human melanoma cells. J Immunol 133:1649–1655
36. Giacomini P, Aguzzi A, Ferrone S (1985) Differential susceptibility to modulation by recombinant immune interferon of HLA-DR and DQ antigens synthesized by melanoma cells Colo 38. J Invest Dermatol (submitted)
37. Giles RC, Nunez G, Hurley CK, Nunez-Roldan A, Winchester R, Stastny P, Capra JD (1983) Structural analysis of a human I-A homologue using a monoclonal antibody that recognizes an MB3-like specificity. J Exp Med 157:1461–1470
38. Goyert SM, Shively JE, Silver J (1982) Biochemical characterization of a second family of human Ia molecules, HLA-DS, equivalent to murine I-A subregion molecules. J Exp Med 156:550–566
39. Goyert S, Silver J (1984) Monoclonal antibodies cross react with products of multiple class II gene loci: shared epitopes among DR, DS, and SB loci. Dis Markers 2:47–55
40. Grutzmann R, Hammerling GJ (1982) Idiotypic relationship of anti-Ia.2 antibodies. Eur J Immunol 12:307–312
41. Guy K, Van Heyningen V, Cohen BB, Deane DL, Steel MC (1982) Differential expression and serologically distinct subpopulations of human Ia antigens detected with monoclonal antibodies to Ia alpha and beta chains. Eur J Immunol 12:942–948
42. Hall BM, Bishop GA, Duggin GG, Horvath JS, Philips J, Tiller DJ (1984) Increased expression of HLA-DR antigens on renal tubular cells in renal transplants: relevance to the rejection response. Lancet II:247–250
43. Hanafusa T, Pujol-Borrell R, Chiovato L, Russell RCG, Doniach D, Bottazzo GF (1983) Aberrant expression of HLA-DR antigen on thyrocytes in Graves' disease: relevance for autoimmunity. Lancet II:1111–1115
44. Hansen JA, Martin PJ, Kamoun M, Nisperos B, Thomas ED (1981) A supertypic HLA-DR specificity (DR4+5) defined by murine monoclonal antibody. Hum Immunol 2:103–111
45. Herlyn M, Clark WH Jr, Mastrangelo MJ, Guerry D IV, Elder DE, LaRossa D, Hamilton R, Bondi E, Tuthill R, Steplewski Z, Koprowski H (1980) Specific immunoreactivity of hybridoma-secreted monoclonal anti-melanoma antibodies to cultured cells and freshly derived human cells. Cancer Res 40:3602–3609
46. Herlyn M, Lange B, Bennicelli J, Blaszczyk M, Guerry D IV, Koprowski H (1984) Increased levels of circulating HLA-DR antigen in sera of patients with acute lymphoblastoid leukemia. Leuk Res 8:323–334
47. Hoang-Xuan M, Charron D, Zilber M-T, Levy D (1982) Gene antigen register. Biochemical characterization of class II bovine major histocompatibility complex antigens using cross-reactive antibodies. Immunogenetics 15:621–624
48. Holmes NJ, Parham P (1983) Enhancement of monoclonal antibodies against HLA-A2 is due to antibody bivalency. J Biol Chem 258:1580–1586
49. Horibe K, Flomenberg N, Pollack MS, Adams TE, Dupont B, Knowles RW (1984) Biochemical and functional evidence that an MT3 supertypic determinant defined by a monoclonal antibody is carried on the DR molecule on HLA-DR7 cell lines. J Immunol 133:3195–3202
50. Houghton AN, Thomson TM, Gross D, Oettgen HF, Old LJ (1984) Surface antigens of melanoma and melanocytes. Specificity of induction of Ia antigens by human γ-interferon. J Exp Med 160:255–269
51. Hurley CK, Nunez G, Winchester R, Finn OJ, Levy R, Capra JD (1982) The human HLA-DR antigens are encoded by multiple β-chain loci. J Immunol 129:2103–2108
52. Igarashi M, Obata F, Endo T, Yoshii M, Kashiwagi N, Ferrone S (1985) Serological and structural heterogeneity of HLA-DR and DQ antigens in HLA-DR4 homozygous B lymphoid cells. Transplantation (submitted)
53. Indiveri F, Wilson BS, Natali PG, Pellegrino MA, Ferrone S (1980) Immunogenicity of DR antigens isolated from body fluids. Transplant Proc 12:121–124

54. Iwaki Y, Terasaki PI, Kinukawa T, Thai TH, Root T, Billing R (1983) Crossreactivity between human and canine Ia antigens using a mouse monoclonal antibody (CIA). Transplantation 36:189–191
55. Jemmerson R, Morrow PR, Klinman NR, Paterson Y (1985) Analysis of an evolutionarily conserved antigenic site on mammalian cytochrome c using synthetic peptides. Proc Natl Acad Sci USA 82:1508–1512
56. Johnson JP, Meo T, Riethmuller G, Schendel DJ, Wank R (1982) Direct demonstration of an HLA-DR allotypic determinant on the low molecular weight (beta) subunit using a mouse monoclonal antibody specific for DR3. J Exp Med 156:104–111
57. Ju S-T, Benacerraf B, Dorf ME (1980) Genetic control of a shared idiotype among antibodies directed to distinct specificities. J Exp Med 152:170–182
58. Kalil J, Hyafil F, Crevat D, Bono R, Fellous M (1980) Monoclonal antibodies directed to MHC products. In: Preud'homme JL, Hawken VAL (eds) Abstracts of Fourth International Congress of Immunology, Paris, July 1980 (abstract 8.1.17)
59. Kalil JE, Fellous M (1982) Monoclonal antibodies to HLA-DR antigens. In: Ferrone S, David C (eds) Ia antigens. Vol II. Man and other species. CRC Press, Boca Raton, Florida, pp 55–80
60. Karol B, Reichlin M, Nobel RW (1978) Idiotypic cross-reactivity between antibodies of different specificities. J Exp Med 148:1488–1497
61. Kasahara M, Ogasawara K, Ikeda H, Okuyama T, Ishikawa N, Takenouchi T, Wakisaka A, Kikuchi Y, Aizawa M (1983) A monoclonal antibody that detects a polymorphic determinant common to HLA-DR1 and 2. Tissue Antigens 21:105–113
62. Kasahara M, Takenouchi T, Ogasawara K, Ikeda H, Okuyama T, Ishikawa N, Moriuchi J, Wakisaka A, Kikuchi Y, Aizawa M, Kaneko T, Kashiwagi N, Nishimura Y, Sasazuki T (1983) Serologic dissection of HLA-D specificities by the use of monoclonal antibodies. Immunogenetics 17:485–495
63. Koide Y, Awashima F, Yoshida TO, Takenouchi T, Wakisaka A, Moriuchi J, Aizawa M (1982) The role of three distinct Ia-like antigen molecules in human T cell proliferative responses: effect of monoclonal anti-Ia-like antibodies. J Immunol 129:1061–1069
64. Koning F, Schreuder I, Giphart M, Bruning H (1984) A mouse monoclonal antibody detecting a DR-related MT2-like specificity: serology and biochemistry. Hum Immunol 9:221–230
65. Laemmli UK (1970) Cleavage of structural proteins during the assembly of the head bacteriophage T4. Nature 227:680–685
66. Larhammar D, Schenning L, Gustafsson K, Wiman K, Claesson L, Rask L, Peterson P (1982) Complete amino acid sequence of an HLA-DR antigen like β chain as predicted from the nucleotide sequence: similarities with immunoglobulins and HLA-A, -B, and -C antigens. Proc Natl Acad Sci USA 79:3687–3691
67. Linch DC, Nadler LM, Luther EA, Lipton JM (1984) Discordant expression of human Ia-like antigens on hematopoietic progenitor cells. J Immunol 132:2324–2329
68. Liu Y-N, Bona CA, Schulman JL (1981) Idiotypy of clonal responses to influenza virus hemagglutinin. J Exp Med 154:1525–1538
69. Lunney JK, Osborne BA, Sharrow SO, Devaux C, Pierres M, Sachs DH (1983) Sharing of Ia antigens between species. IV. Interspecies crossreactivity of monoclonal antibodies directed against polymorphic mouse Ia determinants. J Immunol 130:2786–2793
70. MacLean GD, Seehafer J, Shaw ARE, Kieran MW, Longenecker BM (1982) Antigenic heterogenicity of human colorectal cancer cell lines analyzed by a panel of monoclonal antibodies. I. Heterogeneous expression of Ia-like and HLA-like antigenic determinants. J Natl Cancer Inst 69:357–363
71. Maeda H (1984) Mouse monoclonal antibody detects a new polymorphic Ia determinant other than HLA-DR antigen: a possible allele of DC-1. Tissue Antigens 23:163–170
72. Maeda H, Hirata R, Okuyama M, Thompson A, Tohyama H (1984) Two-dimensional gel analysis of a second family of class II molecules by polymorphic HLA-DR4,5 and w9 monoclonal antibodies. J Immunol 132:2478–2484

73. Malavasi F, Milanese C, Fabbi M, Richiardi P, Caligaris-Cappio F, Ferrero E, Roggero S, Dellabona P, Ceppellini R (1984) Generation and characterization of murine monoclonal antibodies against HLA class II molecules. Diagn Immunol 2:53–62
74. Marder P, Hinson A, Russo C, Ferrone S, Ades E (1984) Heterogeneity of human peripheral blood mononuclear cells detected by monoclonal antibodies to monomorphic determinants of human Ia antigens. Immunobiology 167:483–494
75. Marti GE, Tosato G, Blaese RM, Nadler L, Kindt TJ (1982) A monoclonal antibody directed against a human B lymphoid cell activation antigen. In: Vitetta ES (ed). B and T cell tumors. Academic, New York, pp 85–89
76. Marti GE, Nadler LM, Chused TM, Tosato G, Blaese RM, Kindt TJ (1985) Cellular distribution of a human I-A-like (DS/DC) antigen on normal and neoplastic lymphoid cells. Hum Immunol 12:23–35
77. McMaster WR, Williams AF (1979) Monoclonal antibodies to Ia antigens from rat thymus: cross-reactions with mouse and human and use in purification of rat Ia glycoproteins. Immunol Rev 47:117–137
78. Moller G (ed) (1976) Biochemistry and biology of Ia antigens. Transplant Rev 30:3–322
79. Moretta A, Accolla RS (1984) Effect of anti-class II monoclonal antibodies on human T cell function. Dis Markers 2:313–320
80. Muchmore AV, Megson M, Decker JM, Knudsen P, Mann DL, Broder S (1983) Inhibitory activity of antibodies to human Ia-like determinants: comparison of intact and pepsin-digested antibodies. J Immunol 131:725–730
81. Nadler LM, Stashenko P, Hardy R, Tomaselli KJ, Yunis EJ, Schlossman SF, Pesando JM (1981) Monoclonal antibody identifies a new Ia-like (p 29, 34) polymorphic system linked to the HLA-D/DR region. Nature 290:591–593
82. Natali PG, Cordiali-Fei P, Cavaliere R, Di Filippo F, Quaranta V, Pellegrino MA, Ferrone S (1981) Ia-like antigens on freshly explanted human melanoma. Clin Immunol Immunopathol 19:250–259
83. Natali PG, De Martino C, Marcellini M, Quaranta V, Ferrone S (1981) Expression of Ia-like antigens on the vasculature of human kidney. Clin Immunol Immunopathol 20:11–20
84. Natali PG, De Martino C, Pellegrino MA, Ferrone S (1981) Analysis of the expression of I-A^k-like antigens in murine fetal and adult tissues with the monoclonal antibody 10-2.16. Scand J Immunol 13:541–546
85. Natali PG, De Martino C, Quaranta V, Bigotti A, Pellegrino MA, Ferrone S (1981) Changes in Ia-like antigen expression of malignant human cells. Immunogenetics 12:409–413
86. Natali PG, De Martino C, Quaranta V, Nicotra MR, Frezza F, Pellegrino MA, Ferrone S (1981) Expression of Ia-like antigens in normal non lymphoid tissues. Transplantation 31:75–78
87. Natali PG, Segatto O, Ferrone S, Tosi R, Corte G (1984) Differential tissue distribution and ontogeny of DC-1 and HLA-DR antigens. Immunogenetics 19:109–116
88. Natali PG, Bigotti A, Calaviere R, Liao S-K, Taniguchi M, Matsui M, Ferrone S (1985) Heterogeneous expression of melanoma associated antigens and HLA antigens by primary and multiple metastatic lesions removed from patients with melanoma. Cancer Res 45:2883–2889
89. Natali PG, Bigotti A, Cavaliere R, Nicotra MR, Tecce R, Manfredi D, Chen Y-X, Nadler LM, Ferrone S (1985) Gene products of the HLA-D region in normal and malignant tissues of non lymphoid origin. Hum Immunol (in press)
90. Natali PG, Bigotti A, Russo C, Sakaguchi K, Igarashi M, Ferrone S (1985) Monoclonal antibodies to human histocompatibility antigens. In: Ferrone S, Dierich MP (eds) Handbook of monoclonal antibodies: application in biology and medicine. Noyes, Park Ridge, NJ, pp 382–403
91. Neppert J, Mueller-Eckhardt C (1984) Monoclonal mouse antibodies to human MHC class I antigens cocap class II antigens. Tissue Antigens 24:187–189
92. Ng AK, Pellegrino MA, Imai K, Ferrone S (1981) HLA-A,B antigens, Ia-like antigens and tumor-associated antigens on prostate carcinoma cell lines: serologic and immunochemical analysis with monoclonal antibodies. J Immunol 127:443–447
93. O'Farrell PZ, Goodman HM, O'Farrell PH (1977) High resolution two-dimensional electrophoresis of basic as well as acidic proteins. Cell 12:1133–1142

94. Oudin J, Cazenave PA (1971) Similar idiotypic specificities in immunoglobulin fractions with different antibody functions or even without detectable antibody function. Proc Natl Acad Sci USA 68:2616–2620
95. Ozato K, Epstein SL, Bluestone JA, Sharrow SO, Hansen T, Sachs DH (1983) The presence of a common idiotype in anti-H-2 immune sera as detected by anti-idiotype to a monoclonal anti-H-2 antibody. Eur J Immunol 13:13–18
96. Parham P, Ploegh HL (1980) Molecular characterization of HLA-A,B homologues in owl, monkeys and other nonhuman primates. Immunogenetics 11:131–143
97. Pellegrino MA, Indiveri F, Fagiolo U, Antonello A, Ferrone S (1982) Immunogenicity of serum HLA antigens in allogeneic combinations. Transplantation 33:530–533
98. Piatier-Tonneau D, Boyer B, Debre P, Charron DJ (1983) Syngeneic anti-idiotypes against monoclonal anti-HLA-DR antibodies: characterization of recurrent idiotypes. J Immunol 131:1339–1343
99. Piatier-Tonneau D, Viguier M, Debre P, Charron DJ (1984) Idiotypic relationship of 43 monoclonal antibodies to MHC class II antigens. Dis Markers 2:93–100
100. Pierres M, Mercier P, Madsen M, Mawas C, Kristensen T (1982) Monoclonal mouse anti-I-A^k and anti-I-E^k antibodies cross-reacting with HLA-DR supertypic and subtypic determinants rather than classical DR allelic specificities. Tissue Antigens 19:289–300
101. Pollack MS, Heagney SD, Livingston PO, Fogh J (1981) HLA-A,B,C and DR alloantigen expression on forty-six cultured human tumor cell lines. J Natl Cancer Inst 66:1003–1012
102. Quaranta V, Pellegrino MA, Ferrone S (1981) Serologic and immunochemical characterization of the specificity of four monoclonal antibodies to distinct antigenic determinants expressed on subpopulations of human Ia-like antigens. J Immunol 126:548–552
103. Quaranta V, Tanigaki N, Ferrone S (1981) Distribution of antigenic determinants recognized by three monoclonal antibodies (Q2/70, Q5/6 and Q5/13) on human Ia-like alloantigens and on their subunits. Immunogenetics 12:175–182
104. Quaranta V, Zanetti M, Reisfeld RA (1982) A recurrent idiotype on monoclonal anti-human Ia antibodies. J Exp Med 156:1551–1556
105. Quaranta V, Madjic O, Stingl G, Kiszka K, Honigsmann H, Knapp W (1984) A human Ia cytoplasmic determinant located on multiple forms of invariant chain (y_1,y_2,y_3). J Immunol 132:1900–1905
106. Radka SF, Mochamer C, Cresswell P, Kostyu DD, Ward FE, Amos DB (1983) SFR3-DR5, a monoclonal antibodies with HLA-DR5 specificity. J Immunol 130:1863–1866
107. Radka SF, Amos DB, Quackenbush LJ, Cresswell P (1984) HLA-DR7-specific monoclonal antibodies and a chimpanzee anti-DR7 serum detect different epitopes on the same molecule. Immunogenetics 19:63–76
108. Rebai N, Malissen B, Pierres M, Accolla RS, Corte G, Mawas C (1983) Distinct HLA-DR epitopes and distinct families of HLA-DR molecules defined by 15 monoclonal antibodies (mAb) either anti-DR or allo-anti-Ia^k cross-reacting with human DR molecule. I. Cross-inhibition studies of mAb cell surface fixation and differential binding of mAb to detergent-solubilized HLA molecules immobilized to a solid phase by a first mAb. Eur J Immunol 13:106–111
109. Russo C, Pellegrino MA, Ferrone S (1983) A double-determinant immunoassay to quantitate human Ia antigens. Transplant Proc 15:57–59
110. Russo C, Pellegrino MA, Ferrone S (1984) Analysis of the repertoire of anti-HLA antibodies with anti-idiotypes to a murine anti-HLA-A2, A28 monoclonal antibody. Hum Immunol 10:57–67
111. Shaw S, DeMars R, Schlossman SF, Smith PL, Lampson LA, Nadler LM (1982) Serologic identification of the human secondary B cell antigens. Correlation between function, genetics, and structure. J Exp Med 156:731–743
112. Shaw S, Ziegler A, DeMars R (1985) Specificity of monoclonal antibodies directed against human and murine class II histocompatibility antigens as analyzed by binding to HLA-deletion mutant cell lines. Hum Immunol 12:191–211
113. Silver J, Ferrone S (1979) Structural polymorphism of human DR antigens. Nature 279:436–437

114. Spits H, Ijssel H, Thompson A, Vries JE (1983) Human T4+ and T8+ cytotoxic T lymphocyte clones directed at products of different class II major histocompatibility complex loci. J Immunol 131:678–683
115. Spits H, Borst J, Giphart M, Coligan J, Terhorst C, De Vries JE (1984) HLA-DC antigens can serve as recognition elements for human cytotoxic T lymphocytes. Eur J Immunol 14:299–304
116. Spooner RL, Ferrone S (1984) Cross-reaction of monoclonal antibodies to human MHC class I and class II products with bovine lymphocyte subpopulations. Tissue Antigens 24:270–277
117. Steel CM (ed) (1984) Human MHC class II antigens: genetics, structure, and function. Proceedings of the first international workshop on monoclonal antibodies to human MHC class II antigens. Dis Markers 2:9–361
118. Thomas JA, Iliescu V, Crawford DH, Ellouz R, Cammoun M, De-The G (1984) Expression of HLA-DR antigens in nasopharyngeal carcinoma: an immunohistological analysis of the tumour cells and infiltrating lymphocytes. Int J Cancer 33:813–819
119. Thompson CH, Vaughan HA, McKenzie IFC (1983) The definition of an MB related specificity by a monoclonal antibody. Hum Immunol 6:133–150
120. Thompson JJ, Herlyn MF, Elder DE, Clark WH, Steplewski Z, Koprowski H (1982) Expression of DR antigens in freshly frozen human tumors. Hybridoma 1:161–168
121. Toguchi T, Burmester G, Nunez-Roldan A, Gregersen P, Seremetis S, Lee S, Szer I, Winchester R (1984) Evidence for the separate molecular expression of four distinct polymorphic Ia epitopes on cells of DR4 homozygous individuals. Hum Immunol 10:69–81
122. Tosi R, Tanigaki N, Sorrentino R, Accolla R, Corte G (1981) Binding of one monoclonal antibody to human Ia molecules can be enhanced by a second monoclonal antibody. Eur J Immunol 11:721–726
123. Trucco MM, Garotta G, Stocker JW, Ceppellini R (1979) Murine monoclonal antibodies against HLA structures. Immunol Rev 47:219–252
124. Virelizier J-L, Perez N, Arenzana-Seisdedos F, Devos R (1984) Pure interferon gamma enhances class II HLA antigens on human monocyte cell lines. Eur J Immunol 14:106–108
125. Volc-Platzer B, Majdic O, Knapp W, Wolff K, Hinterberger W, Lechner K, Stingl G (1984) Evidence of HLA-DR antigen biosynthesis by human keratinocytes in disease. J Exp Med 159:1784–1789
126. Wilson BS, Indiveri F, Pellegrino MA, Ferrone S (1979) DR (Ia-like) antigens on human melanoma cells. Serological detection and immunochemical characterization. J Exp Med 149:658–668
127. Wilson BS, Indiveri F, Pellegrino MA, Ferrone S (1979) Production and characterization of DR xenoantisera. Use for detection of serum DR antigens. J Immunol 122:1967–1971
128. Wilson BS, Herzig MA, Lloyd RV (1984) Immunoperoxidase staining for Ia-like antigens in paraffin-embedded tissues from human melanoma and lung carcinoma. Am J Pathol 115:102–108
129. Winchester RJ, Wang C-Y, Gibofsky A, Kunkel HG, Lloyd KO, Old LJ (1978) Expression of Ia-like antigens on cultured human malignant melanoma cell lines. Proc Natl Acad Sci USA 75:6235–6239
130. Wong DM, Skelly RR, Walsk WD, Ahmed A, Mittal KK (1985) An anti-I-a murine monoclonal antibody which cross-reacts with HLA-DR2. Hum Immunol 12:37–45
131. Zola H, Bradley J, Macardle P, McEvoy R, Thomas M (1980) A hybridoma antibody which reacts with human cells carrying the DRw4 tissue type. Evidence for heterogeneity of DRw4. Transplantation 29:72–73

Cellular Detection

Cellular Detection of HLA Class II-Encoded Determinants: Subtype Polymorphisms of HLA-D *

F. H. Bach, N. Ohta, A. Anichini, and N. L. Reinsmoen

Table of Contents

Introduction

The introduction of mixed leukocyte culture testing (MLC) [5, 13] combined with the establishment of a one-way method of stimulation in MLC [6], allowed the correlation of proliferative response in MLC with results of serological studies and the suggestion that reactivity in MLC is controlled by the major histocompatibility complex (MHC) in man [4] now known as HLA. That the chromosomal region of HLA which controls the strongest stimulatory determinants for MLC (now known as the HLA-D region) was different from the class I encoding genes was already suggested in two early studies [2, 7]; definitive evidence in this regard came from the studies by Yunis and Amos [46].

* This is paper 420 from the Immunobiology Research Center, University of Minnesota, Box 724 Mayo, Minneapolis, MN 55455. This work was supported in part by NIH grants AI 17687, AI 18326, AM 13083, and AI 19007, ONR contract N14-85-K-0004, March of Dimes grant 6-425, National Multiple Sclerosis Society grant RG 1505-A-1, and the Harry Kay Charitable Foundation.

A series of technical and conceptual advances led to our present day understanding of the D region. Homozygous typing cells (HTCs) [15, 21, 25, 42] were used in MLC, allowing the definition of Dw "specificities," based on the demonstration that response in MLC can be meaningfully quantitated with regard to genetic disparity [1]. In the same year, serological recognition of HLA-D region encoded antigens was accomplished by van Leeuwen et al. [43].

In 1975, the primed lymphocyte typing (PLT) test was described from our laboratories [40] in an attempt to help define T lymphocyte-recognized specificities for which no HTC existed, as well as to obtain a finer analysis of such T lymphocyte-recognized determinants (LD). A further refinement of that test involved the cloning of T cells responsive in MLC/PLT in the mouse [16] and in man [10].

Use of HTCs led to recognition that more than a single Dw specificity could be associated with a serologically defined antigen such as DR4. These Dw specificities were subtypic to the serologically defined antigen, i.e. DR4 could be "split" into a number of Dw specificities. With the recognition that the serologically defined antigens of DR and DQ can be divided into Dw subtypes with HTC testing, it became important to evaluate whether such Dw subtype polymorphisms can be related to DR and DQ protein polymorphisms. Although DR β-chain polymorphism was demonstrated within a single serologically defined DR antigen (e.g., Goyert et al. [19]), we were able to demonstrate that a highly significant correlation existed between the Dw subtype of the cell from which the DR β proteins were taken and the positional variation of those proteins in isoelectric focusing (IEF) [18], a finding independently confirmed by Nepom et al. [26]. These findings support the concept that the Dw subtypes were related to protein differences.

It is our purpose in this paper to discuss our current knowledge of the HLA-D region from the T cell perspective, an area that has been recently reviewed [3]. A brief introduction to the HLA-D region as it is known today may be useful in this regard.

The Genetic Organization of HLA

Within the HLA-D region, there are three different families of genes, called DR, DQ, and DP. Within the DR family, there are three β genes (although this varies) and a single α gene, the product of which associates with the products of DR β genes. The DR α gene is essentially invariant but the β genes are polymorphic to an extent which will be discussed below. The DQ family includes two α genes, DQα_1 and DQα_2, and two β genes, DQβ_1 and DQβ_2. The DP family also consists of two α and two β genes, DPα_1, DPα_2, DPβ_1, and DPβ_2. In addition to the DR, DQ, and DP α and β genes, there is an additional α chain gene, referred to as DZα, the map position of which is not known and which does not appear to fit into any of the three families, as well as recent, and as yet unpublished data (E. Long, personal communication), suggesting the existence of an additional β gene.

Limited data that are available are consistent with the model that (in many cases) the DR Ia specificities (DR1 – DRw14) are present on β-chains encoded by allelic genes. With this model one can, therefore, by convention refer to the DRβ_1 (or $\alpha\beta_1$) genes and their products as carrying these serologically defined specificities. Two serologically defined specificites, DRw52 and 53 (formerly known as MT2 and MT3), appear to be associated, in some cases, with a different DR $\alpha\beta$ dimer that could be referred to as DR$\alpha\beta_2$ [20]. Additional work will be needed before these associations with $\alpha\beta_1$ and $\alpha\beta_2$ can be generalized to the extent just discussed; it is quite possible, if not likely, that there will be exceptions to this rule. We shall, however, use this model to discuss the data to be presented recognizing the caveats that must be considered.

The DQw1 (equivalent to MT1 and MB1), DQw2 (MB2), and DQw3 (MB3) specificities are associated with the expression of DQ $\alpha\beta$ dimers; once again, to the extent that genes encoding these specificities are allelic, they could arbitrarily be assigned to a DQ$\alpha_1\beta_1$ dimer. The products of DP genes are detected by the response of T lymphocytes in the PLT assay [40], on the basis of which the DP polymorphism was defined [39]. Our reference in this paper to DRβ_1 or DRβ_2 genes and DRβ_1 or DRβ_2 proteins is not meant to relate a given gene to a given protein product.

Similar levels of ignorance exist for DQ and DP.

Recognition of Class II Products by T Lymphocytes

Specificities recognized by T lymphocytes are most commonly defined with HTC or PLT reagents; specificities defined with HTCs are referred to as Dw (they are still ill-defined, and thus referred to as "workshop" specificities designated with a "w"); the term LD is used for determinants recognized by T lymphocytes. An LD epitope is associated with a single molecular product; a Dw specificity is defined by the composite response of T lymphocytes to LD epitopes present on all products of HLA-D and thus represents a "haplotype designation."

Can the LD determinants (epitopes) be defined serologically? This is a difficult, if not impossible, question to answer given present knowledge and techniques; nor, at least in the opinion of some, is it the most important question. Given currently available reagents, the determinants most frequently recognized by T cells are usually different from the determinants most readily recognized serologically. If it seems surprising that an epitope is not recognized by both T and B cells, one must remember that certain allogeneic differences recognized strongly by T lymphocytes (such as certain H-2K locus mutants [8, 45]) have been extremely difficult to define serologically, despite very extensive efforts.

The HTC Test

Definition of the HLA-Dw1 through Dw19 specificities is based on proliferative responses of T lymphocytes in a primary MLC to stimulating cells that are putatively homozygous, at least for the DR and DQ products. In some cases the HTCs are autozygous, i.e., the donors are offspring of consanguineous marriage, in which case the cells are almost always homozygous for all HLA-region products; in other cases, HTCs are phenotypically homozygous (allozygous) for DR and DQ, but can be heterozygous for DP. Allozygous HTC may also not be identical in the two haplotypes for the DR and DQ products.

HTCs are chosen as typing reagents if (i) the cells do not stimulate a significant response in the appropriate combinations within the family from which they were derived, (ii) they do not stimulate (or are weak in stimulating) cells of other HTCs used to "define" the same Dw specificity, and (iii) they can be used successfully to "type" an unrelated panel, i.e., to distinguish between unrelated individuals whose cells respond positively in MLC to the HTCs and those who show no response or a weak response, i.e., carry the specificity defined by the HTCs.

With some HTCs, responding cells of the panel form a biphasic response; those responding weakly are assigned the Dw specificity of the HTCs, while those responding strongly are not. More often, however, there is no clear biphasic response, and thus an arbitrary "cut-off" is chosen. It must be emphasized that this arbitrary threshold may represent a substantial amount (30% relative response) of the T cell proliferative response, by those same responding cells, to antigenic differences associated with a full HLA-D disparity. Assignment of Dw specificities, therefore, frequently not just fails to guarantee HLA-D region (including DP) identity between responding and stimulating cells, but leaves a large likelihood of possible nonidentity.

HTC testing has been most useful in defining the series of Dw specificities which represent clusters of antigenic determinants associated with the various class II products. (Class I antigens can, when disparate, also stimulate T lymphocytes to proliferate, albeit weakly.) The response to an HTC represents the aggregate reactions of clones that can recognize determinants associated chiefly with DR, DQ, and DP. It depends not only on the number of determinants carried by the HTC which the responding cell does not have, but also on the "strength" of those determinants, i.e., the frequency of clones that respond to those disparate determinants and the extent of proliferation by cells of those clones.

The ability to define Dw specificities with HTCs, despite the ability of all HLA products to stimulate T cell proliferation, rests to a great extent on three factors. First: the DR product(s) may stimulate most of the proliferating cells in an MLC [11] although there is only a little evidence for this. Second: loose criteria, e.g., a 40%–50% relative response, have been used to designate a typing response; more stringent criteria, such as a 10%–20% relative response, would result in fewer "typing responses." Third: sufficient linkage disequilibrium holds together, on given haplotypes, certain alleles encoding DR, DQ, and other specificities; this linkage disequilibrium leads to sufficient gene, and thus antigen, sharing between the HTCs and the cells of individuals being tested to provide typing responses. To the extent that HLA alleles, such as those of DP, are not in linkage disequilibrium with the DR-DQ combination of a given haplotype, stimulation of proliferation by products of those DP genes creates "noise," which makes more difficult the assignment of a Dw specificity. There is ample evidence that products are held together in linkage disequilibrium with different products in different populations. For instance, DR2 is found with DQw1 in the North American Caucasian population but with DQw3 in Southern American Waru Indians. Related but different Dw specificities may therefore be disclosed in different populations by a single HTC.

Polymorphism Within Serologically Defined DR and DQ (Ia) Specificities

There is polymorphism within single serologically defined (Ia) specificities of DR and DQ. Two major lines of evidence have led to this conclusion. First, individuals expressing a given DR Ia specificity, with the associated DQ Ia specificity (such as DR4-DQw3), can be divided into serveral groups based on assignment of Dw specificities. Second, protein studies of the β chains of DR and DQ have demonstrated a polymorphism in IEF that correlates with the Dw types; this finding will not be discussed further in this paper, although it represents an important link in the overall story.

Certain relationships exist between the class II serologically defined (Ia) and T lymphocyte-defined (Dw/LD) specificities. One speaks of one specificity as being "supertypic" to another (the latter being called "subtypic" to the first) based on population studies. For instance, DQw1 is generally supertypic to DR1, DR2, and DRw6; individuals positive for DQw1 can be divided into those that are positive for DR1, DR2, etc. Any individual typing positively for DR1, DR2, or DRw6 is also likely to carry the specificity DQw1. The DQ Ia and DRw52 and w53 specificities are supertypic to the DR1-DRw15 specificities; in addition, certain of the DR1-DRw14 specificities are supertypic to the various Dw specificities. The relationships of these specificities, including Dw, in terms of their being frequently encoded by a haplotype in the Caucasian population are given in Table 1.

The Dw specificities defined with HTCs were first thought by some to be the equivalent of the serologically defined DR antigens, but there is now much evidence that one serologically defined DR specificity can be associated with several Dw subtypes as defined with HTC or PLT reagents. Although the Dw subtypes are usually referred to as being related to a given DR specificity, they also relate to the supertypic DQ Ia specificities. These subtypes, given Dw designations, represent the aggregate effect of LD-stimulating determinants associated with all of the HLA products. Thus, DQ and DR product-associated LD determinants contribute to the definition of the Dw specificity. One can appropriately speak of DR4-DQw3 or DR2-DQw1 Dw subtypes in the Caucasian population, in which DR4 is generally in linkage disequilibrium with DQw3 and DR2 with DQw1.

Table 1. Established HLA-D region specificities defined by the Ninth International Histocompatibility Workshop 1984

HLA-DR	Specificities	HLA-Dw association	HLA-DQ association
DR1	–	Dw1	DQw1
DR2	–	Dw2	DQw1
	–	Dw12	DQw1
DR3	DRw52	Dw3	DQw2
DR4	DRw53	Dw4,10,13,14	DQw3
		Dw15	DQ blank
DR5	DRw52	Dw5	DQw3
DRw11	DRw52	–	DQw3
DRw12	DRw52	–	DQw3
DR6			
DRw13	DRw52	Dw18,19	DQw1
DRw14	DRw52	Dw9	DQw1
DRw14	DRw53	Dw16	DQw3
DR7	DRw53	Dw7,17	DQw2
	DRw53	Dw11	DQw3
DRw8	DRw52	Dw8	DQ blank
DRw9	DRw53	–	DQw3
DRw10	–	–	DQw1

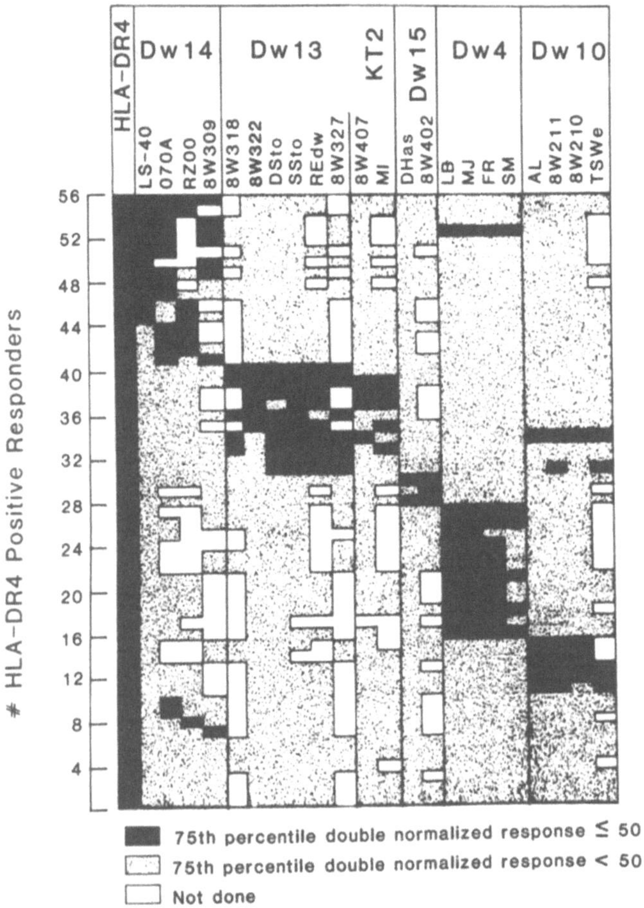

Fig. 1. Five HLA-Dw clusters associated with HLA-DR4: 56 DR4+ cells were typed with 22 DR4+ HTCs defining the Dw clusters Dw14, Dw13 with the associated specificity KT2, Dw15, Dw4, and Dw10

At least four different Dw specificities can be defined within DR4-DQw3: Dw4, Dw10, Dw13 (formerly DB3) and Dw14 (formerly LD40); Dw15 (formerly DYT) is a subtype of DR4, but is not associated with DQw3. In addition, one of these, Dw13, can be further split, using HTCs, into KT2+ and KT2− cells [34]. Some DR4+ or DR2+ individuals carry "blank" (undefined) Dw specificities. This is shown graphically in Fig. 1. Similarly, DR2 can be split into three Dw subtypes; Dw2, Dw12, and a cluster of specificities including MN2 and LD-5a (Fig. 2). We have studied this DR2-associated cluster, LD-5a/MN2, in detail [36]. The subtypes of DR2 and DR4 are listed in Table 2.

Primed Lymphocyte (LD) Typing

The PLT test is an alternative method of defining LD determinants. HTCs are difficult to find and, as discussed above, carry LD determinants associated with class I and class II products that stimulate a proliferative response. In the PLT

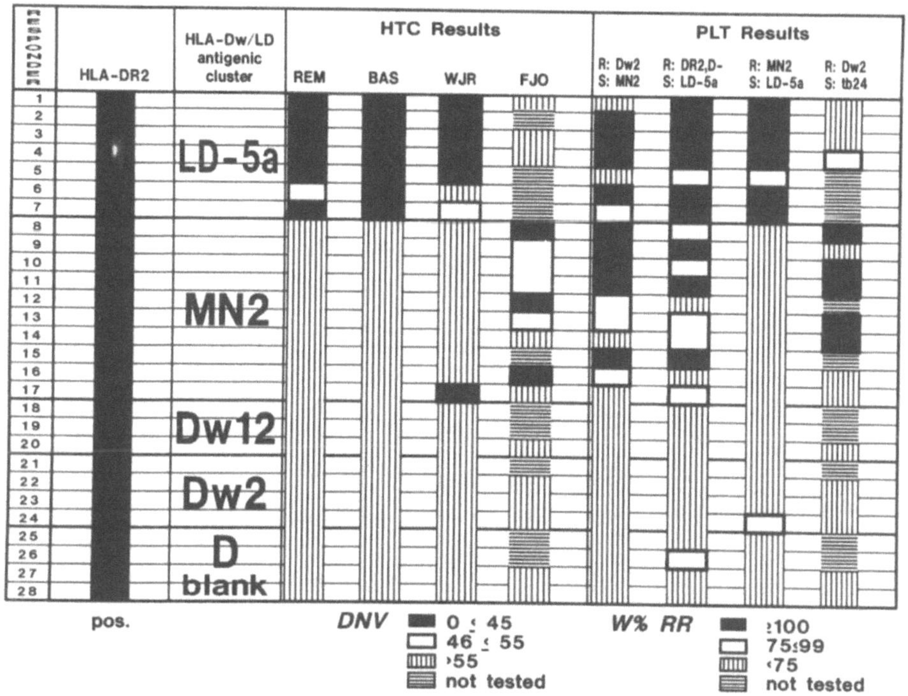

Fig. 2. HLA-DR2-associated Dw clusters: 28 DR2+ cells classified as typing for Dw2, Dw12, MN2, LD-5a, or blank were tested by the LD-5a HTCs REM and BAS as well as a related HTC, WJR, and a fourth DR2+ HTC, FJO. Only LD-5a+ responder cells gave typing responses to the LD-5a HTCs, whereas some, but not all, MN2+ cells gave typing responses to the FJO HTC. When cells were primed against either MN2+ or LD-5a+ haplotypes, both LD-5a+ and MN2+ cells restimulated both these primed reagents, suggesting shared stimulator determinants. By careful selection of the priming cell combinations used to generate additional PLT reagents, stimulatory determinants unique to the LD-5a or MN2 specificities could also be identified

Table 2. HLA-DR2- and DR4-associated Dw specificities (University of Minnesota)

	n	% of DR2 or DR4 haplotypes	Ag frequency	Gene frequency
A. DR2-associated				
Dw2	120	78	0.134	0.069
Dw12	7	5	0.008	0.004
MN2	10	6	0.011	0.006
Dw blank	17	11		
B. DR4-associated				
Dw4	84	43	0.094	0.048
Dw14	41	21	0.046	0.023
Dw10	18	9	0.020	0.010
Dw13	15	8	0.017	0.009
Dw15	4	2	0.004	0.002
Dw blank	32	16		

Total HLA-Dw typed = 896

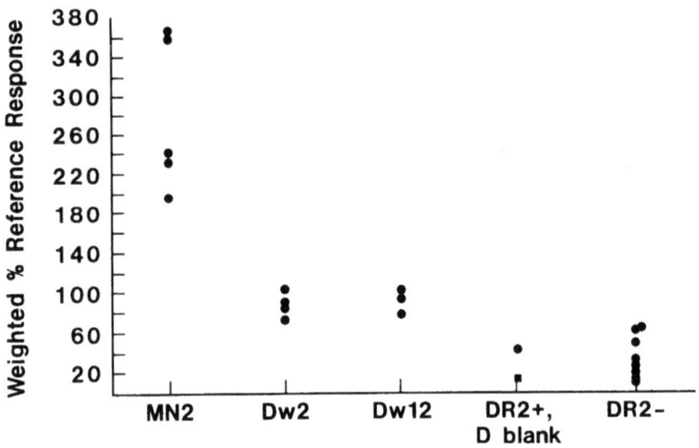

Fig. 3. Definition of the HLA-DR2-associated specificity MN2 ad defined by PLT reagents: PLT reagent generated from responding cell HLA-A3,2; B44,15; DR1; Dw1 primed against stimulator cell HLA-A2, w32; B15, w39; DR1,2; Dw1, MN2 was restimulated by Dw2+, Dw12+, DR2+, DR2+, Dw blank and DR2-negative cells

test there is selective activation of T lymphocytes to determinants associated with single or multiple class I or class II products. In order to develop a PLT reagent, responding and stimulating cells are chosen which differ for various class I and/or class II products. The cells are incubated in a primary MLC for a period of 10 days, providing time for the responding cells to revert to nondividing, but now "primed", cells. These make an accelerated, and very strong, secondary response to the determinants recognized in the priming combination. When third party cells carry the LD specificities recognized in the sensitizing MLC, they will stimulate a proliferative response similar to that evoked by cells of the original sensitizing cell donor; third party cells not carrying those specificities will not evoke such a response.

As illustrated in Fig. 3, PLT reagents can be used to define determinants closely associated with HLA-Dw as defined by HTCs. These reagents are especially useful in defining new HLA-D specificities for which an HTC has not been defined. MN2 is a new HLA-D specificity associated with DR2 which has been defined by PLT, not HTC, reagents.

The "cloning" of PLT-reactive cells has refined the PLT test. Clones presumably define single determinants; cloned reagents, therefore, can define determinants associated with a single product of the class II region. The alleles of DP, for instance, have to date only been defined with PLT reagents. Whereas it is extremely difficult to derive bulk PLT reagents to define the DP antigens, cloning of anti-DP reagents (generated in DR/DQ-"identical" combinations) allows the ready preparation of PLT cells defining the DPw1-DPw3 and DPw5 and DPw6 antigens. Shown in Fig. 4 are results obtained with cloned PLT reagents defining the DPw2 and DPw4 specificities. Most clones primed to DPw2 are restimulated specifically by DPw2. The fact that DPw4, for instance, is usually "split" by using cloned reagents [30, 31, 34] attests further to the power of PLT cell cloning. By choosing appropriate donors for the responding and stimulating cells for the generation of a PLT reagent, it is thus possible to obtain PLT reagents which correspond very closely to the DW specificities defined with HTCs or to define individual LD determinants that make up a part of a Dw specificity.

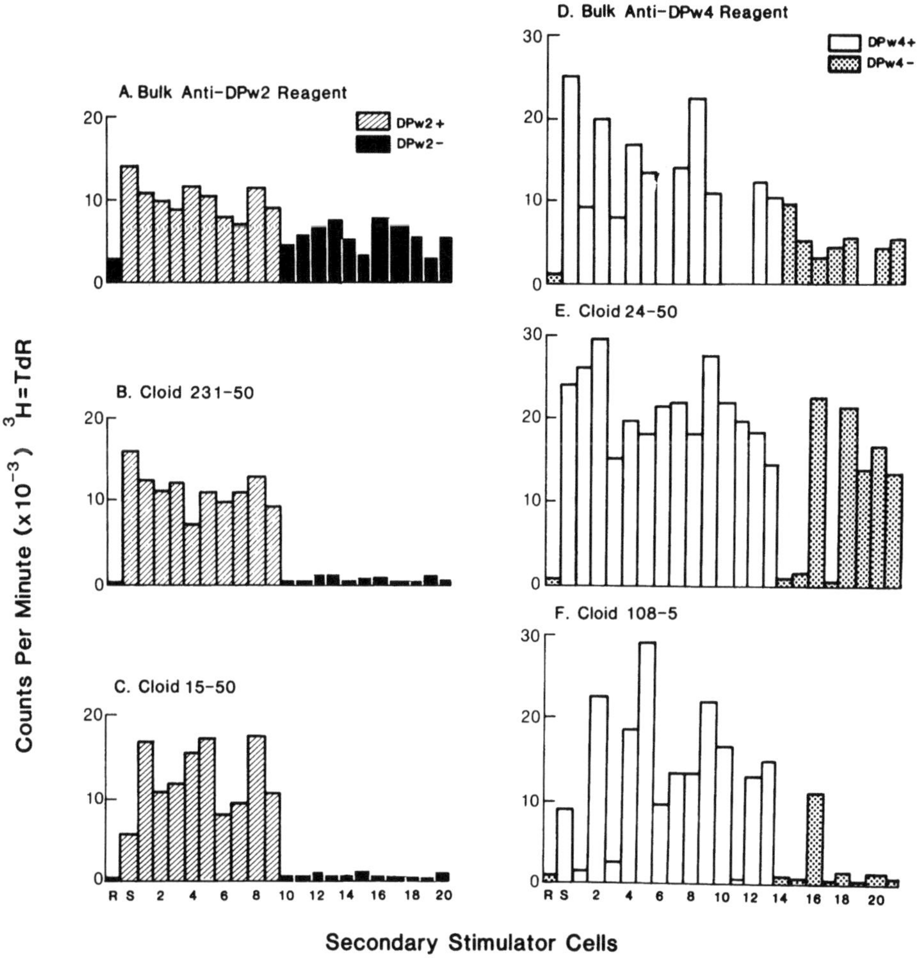

Fig. 4. PLT results of two bulk reagents prepared against DPw2 (*A*) and DPw4 (*D*) and two cloids derived from each bulk reagent (*B, C,* and *E, F* respectively) utilizing the following priming combinations. Anti-DPw2: R = HLA-A2, 11; B7, w35; DR1,7; Dw1,7; DPw3,4; S = HLA-A2, 25; Bw39, w50; DR1,7; Dw1,7; DPw3,2; and anti DPw4: R = HLA-A2; B40; DR4,7; Dw4,7; DPw2; S = HLA-A1, w31; B17, 40; DR4,7i; Dw4,7; DPw2,4. Cloids refer to reagents generated from plating a limited number of cells (i.e. five) per well and are thus probably not true clones

Studies With Cloned T Cells

Although there is some evidence that DR and DQ products can stimulate T lymphocytes, it is not clear whether there are determinants associated with both these products that contribute to the Dw haplotype assignment, i.e., have a population distribution corresponding to the subtypic Dw specificity. We have thus used cloned T cells and panel studies of phenotypically well-characterized cells as well as monoclonal antibody (MoAb) blocking studies, to show that determinants associated with the DR as well as the DQ product appear to contribute to the definition of a Dw specificity [35]. Cloned T cells respond to what are probably two separate DR $\alpha\beta$ dimers, although there is at present no evidence for a further subtype polymorphism of one of these dimers.

Utilizing cells from unrelated donors phenotypically identical for HLA-A and -B, two bulk primed reagents were generated: one against DR4, DRw53, Dw4, DQw3 disparities, the other against DR2, Dw2, DQw1 disparities. The bulk primed reagents were cloned by single cell deposition using the fluorescence activated cell sorter (FACS IV, Becton Dickinson) or by limiting dilution of one cell per three cells. The resulting clonal cell populations were expanded in interleukin-2 (IL-2)-containing medium in the presence of X-irradiated feeder cells [lymphoblastoid cell line (LCL) of the original sensitizing cell]. After 3 weeks expansion, the clones were tested for proliferation in the PLT assay using a panel of well-characterized peripheral blood lymphocyte (PBL) stimulator cells, and for lytic reactivity in a micro-CML assay using a panel of LCL target cells.

Panel Studies and Monoclonal Antibody Inhibition Studies of Cytolytic Clones

Table 3 illustrates the combined results of three CML testings using anti-DR4, -DRw53, -DQw3, and -Dw4 cells. The disparate priming specificities of the original stimulator cell that are shared by the designated LCL targets are underscored, as are cytotoxicity values of 10% or greater. The target cell panel included cells which typed for the five HLA-Dw specificities associated with DR4 (Dw4, Dw10, Dw13, Dw14, and Dw15) as well as DQw3-positive, DR4-negative cells and DQw3-negative, DR4-negative cells. All clones lysed the Dw4-positive targets, including S (the original stimulator cell). Some clones (15, 33) lysed only the Dw4 target cells; other clones (67, 21, 56, 48) also lysed target cells which typed for other DR4-associated Dw specificities. In addition, certain clones (67, 56, 48, 21) lysed targets which did not type for DR4, Dw4, or DQw3 (targets 13, 15, 17, 18, 22).

Of ten clones tested in MoAb inhibition assays, the cytolytic activity of nine was inhibited by the DR-monomorphic MoAb, L243 and Hu4 (representative results illustrated in Table 4). The anti-DQ MoAb Tu22 also appeared to inhibit cytolysis in some cases by some of the clones; this MoAb has been reported to have anti-DR activity [32]. The cytolytic activity of clone 21 is not blocked by the anti-DR or -DQ MoAbs at the concentrations shown but is completely blocked (104% inhibition) at a 1:20 dilution of L243 in addition to being significantly inhibited by an anti-DRw53 MoAb, PL3. This clone lyses eight of eight HLA-DRw53-positive target cells tested, as well as four targets presumed to be DRw53-positive based on DR and DQ phenotyping (14%–51% cytotoxicity), but does not lyse seven DRw53-negative targets or three targets presumed to be DRw53-negative based on DR and DQ phenotyping (Table 3) (−20%–4% cytotoxicity). An intermediate lysis of 9% cytotoxicity was observed with the Dw15 HTC target which does not type as DRw53 with local antisera, but does type as DRw53-positive with Ninth International Histocompatibility Workshop antisera.

Clones were generated against DR2, Dw2, DQw1-disparate specificities using unrelated cells which typed identically for HLA-A and -B and shared the DR3, Dw3, DQw2, and DPw4 specificities. Clones were obtained by single cell deposition (FACS IV) or limiting dilution of one cell per three wells. A total of 123 clones were tested in PLT and CML assays. Table 5 illustrates the combined results of three CML testings. All clones tested lysed the Dw2 targets tested. In addition, some clones (1-12, 3-84) lysed the Dw12 target. Other clones (3-29, 3-27, 1-109) lysed additional DR2-positive targets. Clone 1-17 lysed the Dw2-positive

Table 3. Cytolytic clones: Anti-DR/Dw4 priming[a]

	Targets										
	S1	1	2	3	4	5	6	7	8	9	10
DR	3,4	4,4	4,4	4,4	4,4	4,4	4,4	4,4	4,4	4,4	4,4
DRw	53	(53)	(53)	53	(53)	(53)	53	53	–	53	53
Dw	3,4	4,4	4,4	13,4	13,13	13,13	14,14	14,14	15,15	10,10	10,10
DQ	3	3	3	(3)	(3)	3	3	3	–	3	3
DP	1	4	3,4	NT	NT	5	2,3	3,6	5	NT	4
Clone											
15	18	34	25	15	3	1	–2	–19	2	–2	3
33	43	62	46	34	1	8	8	–10	2	–4	1
67	35	59	44	46	–1	43	–1	–19	3	1	68
21	14	46	24	22	17	14	26	17	9	17	71
56	31	64	35	32	62	24	55	NT	25	–4	3
48	14	46	25	27	34	5	62	64	19	10	3

	Targets											
	11	12	13	14	15	16	17	18	19	20	21	22
DR	5,5	5,5	3,3	2,2	1,9	2,6	2,2	1,1	2,3	3,3	6,6	7,7
DRw	52	NT	52	NT	53	52	–	–	52	NT	52	53
Dw	5,5	5,5	3,3	2,2	1,BSK	6,MN2	2,2	1,1	2,3	3,3	6,6	7,7
DQ	3	NT	2	NT	1	1	1	1	1	NT	1	2
DP	4	4	3,4	4,5	NT	NT	2,5	3,4	4,6	1,3	2,4	4
Clone												
15	–5	–4	6	1	3	–4	–2	–5	–5	–18	–9	–7
33	–6	–7	2	–2	4	–6	–6	3	–4	–2	–3	–4
67	2	6	10	NT	NT	–2	16	2	7	–4	–2	–1
21	–3	–5	–5	4	51	–2	–4	–2	2	–20	–7	29
56	–4	–5	12	8	11	–4	–4	–5	–7	–20	–8	–10
48	–7	–6	4	9	49	–5	–6	55	4	–12	–8	–5

Specificities in parentheses have not been tested but are shown as indicated based on the phenotyping data. See text for definition of underlining
[a] Clones 56, 63, and 46 also demonstrate proliferative reactivity

Table 4. Dissection of determinants associated with different DR dimers: anti-DR4/Dw4/DQw priming combination

	Anti-DR moAb						Anti-DRw53 moAb PL3			Anti-DQ moAb Tu22		
	L243			Hu4								
Clones	80[a]	400	4000	80	400	4000	80	400	4000	80	400	4000
15	113	104	60	121	98	54		NT		14	25	31
37	121	129	121	111	79	57		NT		43	32	67
48	116	106	66	91	81	6	29	− 29	−43	− 3	9	3
67	111	89	38	117	109	57	24	17	24	−13	−11	2
63	97	32	38	145	104	31	− 25	−150	0	38	45	62
21	7	8	14	20	2	10	101	104	76	14	5	29

Results expressed as % inhibition. Values ≧50% are underscored. NT = not tested
[a] Reciprocal moAb dilutions

targets as well as the DR2-negative, DQw1-positive targets tested. Clones 3-27 and 1-109 also lysed some DR2-negative, DQw1-negative targets.

Table 6 demonstrated the patterns of target cell lysis by the three DR-directed and three DQ-directed (based on blocking with MoAbs [35]) clones. Clone 3-19 lysed only Dw2-positive targets, while clone 3-29 lysed all DR2-positive targets and clone 3-27 lysed some additional DR2-negative targets. Two of the DQ-directed clones (3-89 and 3-17) lysed only Dw2-positive targets, while clone 1-17 also lysed two additional DQw1-positive cells (targets 7 and 8).

Our results using cloned T cells are best discussed in the context of the working model that the extensive polymorphism for DR (DR1 – DRw14) is associated with an $\alpha\beta_1$ dimer, and DRw52 and DRw53 with $\alpha\beta_2$. We would suggest that much, or perhaps essentially all, of the polymorphism seen by clones blocked with L243 and Hu4 and within DR4 may also be associated with $\alpha\beta_1$ for DR4. Clones directed as both DR and DQ recognize determinants associated with the subtype polymorphism. This is in concert with findings of DR and DQ β-chain polymorphism correlating with Dw subtypes.

Although we have only one clone putatively reactive with a determinant associated with DRw53 for DR4 haplotypes (blocked by PL3), this clone does not detect a polymorphism subtypic to the DR specificity of the $\alpha\beta_2$ dimer (DRw53). There is increasing, albeit still limited, evidence supporting the concept that the DR β_2 gene/protein is relatively conserved on haplotypes carrying a single serologically defined specificity such as DR4 or DR2. First, Suzuki et al. [41], Nishimura et al. [28], and Knowles et al. [22] have found one DR β spot in IEF that is relatively constant within the subtypes of DR2 and DR4; in the terminology we are using, this would be the DR β_2 protein. Second, the clone (21) described in the present study as reactive with a potential DR $\alpha\beta_2$ dimer reacts with essentially all the DR4-positive cells. Lastly, Cairns et al. [14] in our laboratory have recently sequenced genes from DR4-Dw14 and DR4-Dw13 HTCs; these sequences, taken with a sequence obtained by E. Long from a cell carrying a DR4/Dw4 haplotype (or at least components of Dw4), establish the genetic basis for the DR4-associated, DR β_1 subtype polymorphism. Thus, it may be that the more extensive T lymphocyte-recognized polymorphism is associated primarily with DR$\alpha\beta_1$ and DQ and that DR$\alpha\beta_2$ is relatively conserved.

Table 5. Cytolytic clones: Anti-DR2/Dw2 priming[a]

	Targets																	
	S1	S2	1	2	3	4	5	6	7	8	9	10	11	12	13	14	15	16
DR	2,3	2,3	2,2	2,2	2,2	2,2	2,2	2,2	6,6	1,1	4,4	4,4	4,4	4,4	3,3	3,3	7,7	5,5
Dw	2,3	2,3	2,2	2,2	2,2	12,12	FJO	LD-5a	6,6	1,1	4,4	10,10	14,14	13,13	3,3	3,3	7,7	5,5
DQ	1,2	1,2	1	1	NT	1	1	3	1	1	3	3	3	NT	NT	2	2	3
DP	4,6	4	4,5	2,5	NT	NT	NT	NT	2,4	3,4	6,2	4	6,3	NT	1,3	3,4	4	4
Clone																		
3–89	19.1	38.3	5.2	23.3	41.4	7.8	1.3	−2.8	−7.8	−7.5	2.4	−0.1	−0.7	−0.1	6.4	−16.5	−1.2	0.2
3–17	23.8	25.5	19.4	28.7	29.0	3.5	1.9	−2.8	−3.6	−8.0	3.6	−0.6	−0.9	−0.7	4.2	−19.1	1.7	2.9
1–12	27.7	43.5	35.1	54.0	40.4	19.8	−0.5	−0.6	−5.5	2.0	−0.9	−1.4	−2.1	−2.7	−0.6	−17.3	−3.5	−0.7
3–84	11.1	21.5	13.8	43.5	40.4	30.4	4.1	−2.6	−6.9	−4.9	3.3	−0.2	−0.5	−1.5	1.4	−16.3	−1.2	4.5
3–29	26.8	27.0	21.6	40.9	30.7	29.2	46.6	42.8	−8.3	−7.1	8.1	−0.7	−2.8	−4.2	12.5	−16.3	−2.0	−1.2
1–17	11.2	20.1	22.4	20.0	24.1	0.5	4.7	−3.1	51.0	26.6	0.7	−0.7	−2.0	−2.9	−0.6	−17.1	−1.3	−0.6
3–27	27.2	44.9	17.6	53.1	49.8	35.9	17.7	−1.3	46.9	−4.8	4.4	51.0	−0.2	−1.3	1.8	−15.3	2.0	3.9
1–109	14.6	56.7	33.6	55.0	44.0	8.8	16.1	44.8	12.6	−8.2	14.3	37.4	−3.0	−3.0	5.6	−18.2	22.9	4.3

[a] Clones 3–19, 1–84, 3–91, 3–29, 3–27, and 1–109 also demonstrated strong proliferative reactivity (> 10000 cpm), and clones 3–89, 3–17, and 1–17 demonstrated weaker proliferative reactivity

Table 6. HLA-DR and DQ determinants comprising a "Dw specificity"

		LCL target cells								
		S	1	2	3	4	5	6	7	8
HLA	DR	2,3	2,2	2,2	2,2	2,2	2,2	2,2	6,6	1,1
	Dw	2,3	2,2	2,2	2,2	12,12	FJO	LD-5a	6,6	1,1
	DQw	1,2	NT	1	NT	1	1	3	1	1
	DPw	4,6	4,5	2,5	NT	NT	NT	NT	2,4	3,4
Anti-DR clones	3–19	15	14	40	55	4	1	−2	−2	−5
	3–29	27	22	41	31	29	47	43	−8	−7
	3–27	27	18	53	50	36	18	−1	47	−5
Anti-DQ clones	3–89	19	5	23	41	8	1	−3	−8	−8
	3–17	24	19	29	29	4	2	−3	−4	−8
	1–17	11	22	29	24	1	5	−3	51	26

DP Polymorphism

DP polymorphism has not been discussed in this chapter, as it is reviewed separately elsewhere in this volume (Sanchez-Perez and Shaw). Some comments regarding DP, especially as it may relate to DR and DQ, would seem in order, however. First, reagents to define the DPw1-DPw6 segregant series may be more easily preparable by the "cloning" approach that we have discussed in the past [9]. Second, the protein polymorphism associated with DP could be studied by us following the recognition that the MoAb B7/21 [23] originally described by Royston et al. [37], as an anti-DR MoAb, in fact reacted with the DP dimer. This MoAb was referred to as FA, with the approval of Trowbridge [44], to avoid confusion between LCL 721, with which most of the work was done to define this MoAb as anti-DP, and the MoAb. Third, it has been possible to show formally that FA most probably reacts with the $\alpha\beta$ dimer that expresses the DP determinant, in that anti-FA blocks clones that react with the sensitizing DPw specificity [29]. Fourth, there is some added complexity of determinants recognized by cloned T lymphocytes which may or may not be related to the DP region (as defined with LCL mutants that have lost expression of all class I and of DR and DQ of a given haplotype, but still express DPw2 of that haplotype. Such mutants still express a determinant (called NO1) associated with that same haplotype. NO1 is different from DPw2 in its population distribution. NO1-reactive T cells are blocked with the MoAb Tu39, which is known to react with DP as well as other class II products [29]. Whether determinants recognized by this clone are related to the DP dimer as we currently think of it, or to a new $\alpha\beta$ dimer not previously described, has yet to be determined.

We have suggested that the DP segregant series may be analogous in evolutionary terms to the LD subtype polymorphism related to DR of a single serologically defined specificity, such as DR4 or DR2. This suggestion is based primarily on two findings. First, it is easily shown that restriction fragment length polymorphism (RFLP) patterns detected by Southern blotting are associated with different DR-DQ specificities. It appears more difficult to define RFLP patterns associated with the various Dw/LD subtypes of a given serologically defined DR Ia specificity [27, 38], as is also true for DP [17]. We have suggested that both the subtype polymorphisms of individual DR serologically defined specificities and the DP polymorphism may be of more recent evolutionary origin [3, 27]. Second, there is, to date, no convincing evidence that the several LD specificities of the polymorphism of DP can be reproducibly defined serologically, although some DPw-correlated sera have been found, a situation similar to that which obtained for the DR4 and DR2 Dw subtypes.

Discussion

The use of techniques that allow definition of determinants recognized by T lymphocytes and associated with HLA class II molecules has allowed definition of further polymorphisms not recognized with currently available/characterized serological reagents. Given the intimate relationship thought to exist between T lymphocyte recognition and MHC-encoded molecules, definition of this LD polymorphism may be of the greatest import.

There are several areas of interest in which the respective roles of Dw subtypes and serologically defined DR/DQ specificities have been compared. Two areas, which may well be interrelated, involve (i) studies of HLA class II restriction of nominal antigen for T cell recognition and (ii) HLA antigen association with insulin-dependent diabetes (IDD). We have recently performed/participated in a number of studies in which the class II restricting specificity for several different nominal antigens has been investigated vis-a-vis the serologically defined DR/DQ Ia specificities and the Dw specificities. Subtypes of DR4 and DR2 have been studied for these investigations. In most cases, the restricting specificity was very highly associated with, or identical to, a Dw subtype [33, 36] rather than being associated directly with the serologically defined specificities. (In one case involving a DR2-Dw2-responding cell donor, the bulk reagents recognized the herpes virus in the context of both Dw2 and Dw12, but not in the context of DR2-MN2 or non-DR2 cells [24]. Interestingly, in this immunogenetic situation, we have found several alloreactive clones that were sensitized to a DR2-Dw2 haplotype, but recognized a determinant apparently shared by DR2-Dw2 and DR2-Dw12 target cells. It would thus seem that the T lymphocyte-recognized allo-LD specificities may directly serve, or act as markers for, restricted recognition.

We have also performed a subtype analysis in patients with IDD expressing either DR4 or DR2. In the DR4+ IDD patients, we found a very significantly increased frequency of Dw4 compared to DR4+ normal individuals. In the DR2+ IDD patients, we found a very significantly decreased frequency of Dw2 and increased frequency of MN2 compared to the normal individual [12]. Once again, therefore, it would appear that Dw/LD subtype definition may be of import for what are biologically important phenomena relating to the MHC.

That LD polymorphism, recognized by T lymphocytes, correlates with a protein polymorphism detected in IEF, may well, to a large extent, reflect the functional polymorphism of these MHC loci as it pertains to restricted recognition. It would seem that a correlation between careful definition of class II determinants recognized by T lymphocytes can now be correlated with specific sequences of class II genes encoding those determinants. The tools of molecular biology make the future in this area very exciting indeed.

References

1. Albertini RJ, Bach FH (1968) Quantitative assay of antigenic disparity at HL-A – the major histocompatibility locus in man. J Exp Med 128:639
2. Amos DB, Bach FH (1968) Phenotypic expressions of the major histocompatibility locus in man (HL-A): leukocyte antigens and mixed leukocyte culture reactivity. J Exp Med 128:623
3. Bach FH (1985) The HLA-D region. Immunology Today 6:89
4. Bach FH, Amos DB (1967) Hu-1:major histocompatibility locus in man. Science 156:1506–1508
5. Bach FH, Hirschhorn K (1964) Lymphocyte interaction: a potential histocompatibility test in vitro. Science 143:813
6. Bach FH, Voynow NK (1966) One-way stimulation in mixed leucocyte cultures. Science 153:545
7. Bach FH, Albertini RJ, Amos DB, Ceppellini R, Mattiuz PL, Miggiano VC (1969) Transplant Proc 1:339
8. Bach FH, Widmer SB, Segall M, Bach ML, Klein J (1972) Genetic and immunological complexity of major histocompatibility regions. Science 176:1024
9. Bach FH, Reinsmoen NR (1982) Cloned cellular reagents to define antigens encoded between HLA-DR and glyoxylase. Hum Immunol 5:133
10. Bach FH, Inouye H, Hank JA, Alter BJ (1979) Human T lymphocyte clones reactive in primed lymphocyte typing and cytotoxicity. Nature 281:307
11. Bach FH, Reinsmoen NL, Segall M (1983) Definition of HLA antigens with cellular reactants. Transplant Proc XV:102
12. Bach FH, Rich S, Barbosa J, Segall M (1985) Insulin dependent diabetes – associated HLA-D region encoded determinants. Hum Immunol 12:59
13. Bain B, Vas MR, Lowenstein L (1964) Blood 23:108
14. Cairns S, Curtsinger JM, Dahl CA, Freeman S, Alter BJ, Bach FH (1985) Sequence polymorphism of HLA-DR β_1 alleles relating to T cell-recognized determinants. Nature 317:166
15. Dupont B, Jersild C, Hansen GS, Nielsen S, Thomsen M, Svejgaard A (1973) Typing for MLC determinants by means of LD-homozygous and LD-heterozygous test cells. Transplant Proc 5:1453
16. Fathman CG, Hengartner H (1978) Clones of alloreactive T cells. Nature 272:617
17. Gorski J, Rollin R, Long E, Mach B (1984) Molecular organization of the HLA-SB region of the human major histocompatibility complex evidence for two SB beta chain genes. Proc Natl Acad Sci USA 81:3934
18. Groner JP, Watson AJ, Bach FH (1983) Dw/LD-related molecular polymorphism of DR4 β-chains. J Exp Med 157:1687
19. Goyert SM, Gatti R, Silver J (1982) Peptide map comparisons of similar serologically defined HLA-DR antigens isolated from different lymphoblastoid cell lines. Hum Immunol 5:205
20. Hurley CK, Giles RC, Nunez G, DeMars R, Nadler L, Winchester R, Stastny P, Capra JD (1984) Molecular localization of human class II MT2 and MT3 determinant. J Exp Med 160:472
21. Jorgensen F, Lamm L, Kissmeyer-Nielsen F (1973) An approach to MLC typing. Tissue Antigens 4:323
22. Knowles RW, Flomenberg N, Horibe K, Winchester R, Radka SF, Dupont B (1985) Biochemical characterization of the DR β chains which carry the two distinct HLA-DRw53-related determinants defined by PL3 and 109db and the HLA-DR7-related determinant defined by SFR16-DR7. (submitted)
23. Linner KM, Bach FH (1984) A non-DR, non-DC HLA class II product. In: Albert ED, Baur MP, Mayr WR (eds) Histocompatibility testing 1984. Springer, Berlin Heidelberg New York Tokyo, p 538
24. Linner KM, Monroy L, Bach FH, Gehn RC (1985) Dw subtypes of serologically defined DR-DQ specificities restrict recognition of cytomegalovirus. (submitted)
25. Mempel W, Grosse-Wilde H, Albert E, Thierfelder S (1973) Atypical MLC reactions in HL-A typed related and unrelated pairs. Transplant Proc 5:401

26. Nepom BS, Nepom GT, Mickelson E, Antonelli P, Hansen JA (1983) Electrophoretic analysis of human HLA-DR antigens from HLA-DR4 homozygous cell lines: correlation between β-chain diversity and HLA-D. Proc Natl Acad Sci USA 80:6962
27. Nicklas JA, Noreen HN, Segall M, Bach FH (1985) Southern analysis of DNA polymorphism between Dw subtypes of DR4. Hum Immunol 13:95
28. Nishimura Y, Tsukamoto K, Sone T, Hirayama K, Takenouchi T et al. (1984) Molecular and functional analysis of class II molecules characteristic to HLA-Dw2 and Dw12. In: Albert ED, Baur MP, Mayr WR (eds) Histocompatibility testing 1984. Springer, Berlin Heidelberg New York Tokyo, p 504
29. Ohta N, Bach FH (1985) NO1: An HLA-DQw1 associated determinant present on loss mutants not-expressing DQw1. (submitted)
30. Pawelec G, Shaw S, Wernet P (1982) Analysis of the HLA-linked SB gene system with cloned and uncloned alloreactive T-cell lines. Immunogenetics 15:187
31. Pawelec G, Shaw S, Schneider M, Blaurech M, Frauer M, Brackerts D, Wernet P (1982) Population studies of the HLA-linked SB antigen and their relative importance in primary MLC-typing analysis of HLA-D homozygous typing cells and normal heterozygous populations. Hum Immunol 5:215
32. Pawelec GP, Shaw S, Ziegler A, Muller C, Wernet P (1982) Differential inhibition of HLA-D- or SB-directed secondary lymphoproliferative responses with monoclonal antibodies detecting human Ia-like determinants. J Immunol 129:1070
33. Qvigstad E, Thorsby E, Reinsmoen NL, Bach FH (1984) Close association between the Dw14 (LD40) subtype of HLA-DR4 and a restriction element for antigen specific T cell clones. Immunogenetics 20:583
34. Reinsmoen NL, Bach FH (1983) HLA-D region complexity associated with HLA-DR, Dw, and SB phenotypes. Transplant Proc 15(1):76
35. Reinsmoen NL, Bach FH (1985) Cloned analysis of HLA-DR and -DQ associated determinants: their contribution to Dw specificities. Hum Immunol (in press)
36. Reinsmoen NL, Layrisse Z, Betuel H, Bach FH (1984) A study of HLA-DR2 associated HLA-Dw/LD specificities. Hum Immunol 11:105
37. Royston I, Omary MB, Trowbridge IS (1981) Monoclonal antibodies to human T-cell antigen and Ia-like antigen in the characterization of DR4 β-chains. Transplant Proc XIII:761
38. Segall M, Noreen H, Schluender L, Bach FH (1985) DNA restriction fragment length polymorphism characteristic for Dw subtypes of DR2. Hum Immunol (in press)
39. Shaw S, Johnson AH, Shearer GM (1980) Evidence for a new segregant series of B cell antigen that are encoded in the HLA-D region and that stimulate secondary allogeneic proliferative and cytotoxic responses. J Exp Med 152:565
40. Sheehy MJ, Sondel PM, Bach ML, Wank R, Bach FH (1975) HL-A LD (lymphocyte defined) typing: a rapid assay with primed lymphocytes. Science 188:1308
41. Suzuki M, Yabe T, Satake M, Jeiji T, Hamaguchi H (1984) Two-dimensional gel electrophorite analysis of the MT3 and DR4 molecule from the different D-typed cells. J Exp Med 160:751
42. Van den Tweel JG, Blusse van Oud Alblas A, Keuning JJ, Goulmy E, Termijtelen A, Bach ML, Van Rood JJ (1973) Typing for MLC (LD) I. Lymphocytes from cousin marriage offspring as typing cells. Transplant Proc 5:1535
43. van Leeuwen A, Schuit HRE, Van Rood JJ (1973) Typing for MLC (LD) II. The selection of nonstimulator cells by MLC inhibition tests using DS-identical stimulator cells (MISIS) and fluorescence antibody studies. Transplant Proc 5:1539
44. Watson AJ, DeMars R, Trowbridge IS, Bach FH (1983) Detection of a novel human class II HLA antigen. Nature 304:358
45. Widmer MB, Alter BJ, Bach FH, Bach ML, Bailey DW (1973) Lymphocyte reactivity to serologically undetected components of the major histocompatibility complex. Nature New Biol 242:239
46. Yunis EJ, Amos DB (1971) Three closely linked genetic systems relevant to transplantation. Proc Natl Acad Sci USA 68:3031–3035

Cellular Detection of Human Class II MHC Antigens by Alloreactive T Cell Clones *

R. J. Duquesnoy and A. Zeevi

Table of Contents

Introduction

The Major Histocompatibility Complex (MHC) in humans encodes for cell surface molecules which provide the major stimulus to the alloactivation of human T lymphocytes as demonstrated in the mixed leukocyte reaction (MLR). Especially the HLA-D region controls several types of class II MHC molecules which carry lymphocyte-activating alloantigenic determinants which can be detected in secondary proliferation assays with allogeneically primed lymphocytes. The products of HLA-D have recently been classified into three subsets: HLA-DR, HLA-DQ (formerly MB or DC), and HLA-DP (formerly SB) [4]. Each of these subsets express allelic alloantigenic specificities. In addition, HLA-DR is believed

* Supported by grants AI-21410 and AI-18923 from NIAID, grant AA93 from United Way Health Research Service Foundation, and grant IM373 from the American Cancer Society

to encode for a second system of the HLA-DRw52 and DRw53 specificities which have previously been called MT2 and MT3. Recently developed methodologies to clone alloactivated T cells have provided a powerful immunogenetic tool to analyze the complexity of HLA-encoded lymphocyte-activating determinants.

Alloreactive T cell clones are usually generated from in vitro MLR cultures through soft agar colonies, by limiting dilution, or a combination of these methods. The cloning procedures and the subsequent expansion of alloactivated cloned cells require supplementation of interleukin-2 (IL-2; also referred to as T cell growth factor) and irradiated feeder cells (also called filler cells). Sources of IL-2 are usually supernatants of cultures of phytohemagglutinin (PHA)- or MLR-activated lymphocytes and recently, recombinant DNA IL-2.

The immunogenetic analysis of cellular HLA determinants by alloreactive T cell clones has primarily been performed in two types of assays. The first is the primed lymphocyte typing (PLT) test which is based on the ability of an alloreactive clone to undergo secondary proliferation induced by a stimulator cell carrying a given cellular determinant referred to as a PLT determinant. The other assay is based on the cytolytic activity of certain alloreactive clones which can recognize in cell-mediated lympholysis (CML) assays the so-called CML determinants on target cells. In these CML assays it is important to use target cells which express appropriate HLA antigens. In general, 3-day PHA lymphocytes are proper targets for class I-specific cytolytic cells. On the other hand, 3-day PHA blasts cannot be used in CML assays on class II-specific cytolytic cells because these targets do not express sufficient amounts of class II antigens. To determine class II-specific cytolytic activity, it is necessary to use EBV-transformed lymphoblastoid B cell lines (LCL) which express DR-, DQ-, and DP-encoded class II antigens. It has also been observed that monocytes can serve as targets for class II-specific cytolytic cells [12]. However, it has recently been demonstrated that monocytes express DR but not DQ antigens [25]. This would suggest that monocytes may not be suitable as targets of DQ-specific cytolytic cells. LCL can also be used as stimulators in PLT assays, but it is necessary to inactivate these cells with rather large doses of X-irradiation (generally over 12000 R).

To obtain some understanding about the nature of cellular HLA determinants, several investigators have employed PLT and CML inhibition assays with monoclonal antibodies (MoAb) against various class I and II determinants [14, 36]. These MoAb should be well-characterized in biochemical and serological studies so that sufficient information is available as to which epitopes and which HLA molecules are recognized. Inhibition assays with alloreactive T cell clones may generate distinct "MoAb inhibition profiles" which may yield information about the structural nature of the cellular determinants detected by these clones [11, 33].

The fact that HLA-D contains multiple genes expressing several types of class II molecules must be viewed in context with T lymphocyte MHC recognition. Many laboratories, including ours, have studied alloreactive T cell clones generated from MLR cultures. Such clones may have specificity towards DR, MT, DQ, and DP determinants as measured by PLT [1, 3, 10, 20, 26]. Certain PLT and DP determinants are recognized in association with DR and DQ subtypes [35, 37], while others are novel HLA-D-encoded determinants [8, 9, 23, 27]. These observations demonstrate that HLA encodes many cellular determinants which can activate T cells in MLR.

This paper focuses on data from our laboratory regarding the immunogenetic analysis of cellular determinants encoded by the different HLA-D subregions using PLT and CML assays and MoAb inhibition studies.

PLT Specificity of Alloreactive T Cell Clones Toward HLA-DR-Associated Antigens

T cell clones generated from HLA-D-incompatible MLR combinations frequently show specificity toward DR antigens, suggesting their immunodominance in lymphocyte alloactivation. In some cases, the PLT specificity of a T cell clone is perfectly correlated with the corresponding DR determinant, while other clones recognize allelic PLT determinants merely associated with the DR antigen. Sometimes it is possible to relate these PLT determinants to HLA-D specificities defined by MLR typing with HLA-D-homozygous typing cells. For instance, two DR2-associated clones have been described with PLT specificity for Dw2 and

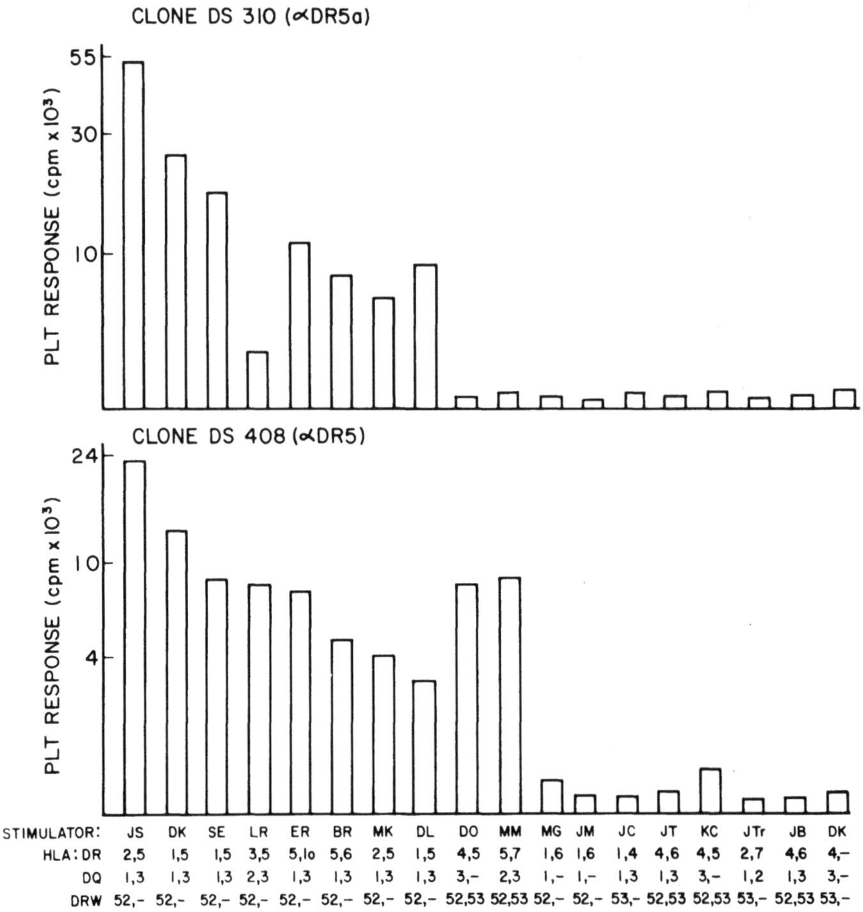

Fig. 1. DR5-associated PLT specificities of alloreactive T cell clones DS310 and DS408. These clones were tested in 3-day PLT assays against an unrelated cell panel. Data are expressed as mean cpm of triplicate cultures

Dw12 respectively [2]. In our laboratory we have identified two clones with identical PLT specificity associated with a subdivision of DR2 [36]. The PLT determinant recognized by these clones was not found on B7-DR2 and B18-DR2 haplotypes and appeared to be unrelated to other previously described DR2-associated cellular or serological specificities. MoAb inhibition studies suggested that the DR2-associated cellular subtype recognized by these PLT clones may reside on a non-DR, perhaps DQ-like molecule [36]. We have studied alloreactive clones which recognize two cellular subtypes of DR5-associated PLT determinants which cannot be distinguished serologically [36]. Figure 1 shows the PLT reactivity patterns of two clones recently generated from a MLR culture with a DR5 stimulator. Clone DS 408 was specific for DR5 and clone DS310 was specific for a DR5-associated PLT determinant previously designated as PC-DR5a [36]. In this cell panel, two DR5 cells, DO and MM, induced strong PLT responses of DS408 but not of DS310. We have previously shown that DO and MM express another DR5-associated PLT determinant, PC-DR5b [36].

PLT inhibition studies were conducted with DR5-associated PLT clones using 15 MoAb against various class II human MHC molecules and a monomorphic class I determinant. These MoAb were previously used by our laboratory as part of a workshop ("Structural and Functional Relationship of Human Class II MHC Molecules," sponsored by the American Society of Histocompatibility and Immunogenetics). The summary report of the participating laboratories, which includes a detailed description of these MoAb has been published by Eckels and Zeevi [11]. Similar MoAb inhibition patterns were observed with both DR5-associated PLT clones DS310 and DS56 (Table 1). Both clones were strongly inhibited by four anti-DR MoAb (243, PA6.231, Q5/6, and Tu35), whereas none of the DQ MoAb (Genox 3.53, Leu 10, and 17.15) or the DRw53 MoAb (1096) showed any significant inhibitory effect. However, quantitative differences in in-

Table 1. Monoclonal antibody[a] inhibition profile of PLT responses of DR5-associated PLT clones DS310 and DS56

MoAb	Specificity	DS310 MoAb dilution			DS56 MoAb dilution		
		1:20	1:100	1:500	1:20	1:100	1:500
243	DR	2	4	5	2	3	2
DA6.231	DR	1	1	2	1	2	14
Q5/6	DR	12	16	56	14	41	79
Tu35	DR	20	26	73	7	13	14
CA2.206	DR	16	44	70	1	2	32
SG465	DR+DQ	37	53	78	1	2	2
SG520	DR+DQ	45	70	100	45	62	94
Q2/70	DR	118	125	122	110	104	129
Q2/80	DR	92	85	72	106	92	86
SG157	DR	72	86	101	70	110	113
Genox 3.53	DQw1	115	118	130	107	116	134
Leu 10	DQw1+3	116	153	142	85	101	94
17.15	DQw3	131	148	139	129	130	127
1096	DRw53	64	80	86	64	62	94
PA2.6	A,B,C	78	115	115	92	105	93

[a] For the sources of MoAb, see [11]

hibition pattern were observed with MoAb CA2.206 and S6465. The PLT activity of clone DS56 was strongly inhibited by these MoAb at all dilutions. On the other hand, the inhibitory effect of these MoAb at various dilutions on the PLT activity of clone 310 varied from moderate to nil. The data on MoAb inhibition profiles of the PLT activity of DR5-associated PLT clones DS310 and DS56 suggested that these clones detect distinct determinants which may reside on the same DR molecule.

Certain MLR combinations may yield several clones with distinctly different PLT reactivity patterns associated with the same DR antigen present on the original stimulator [34, 35]. These findings suggest the presence of multiple PLT determinants associated with the given DR antigen in the same individual. This concept is in concordance with the current understanding of the HLA-DR subregion containing several genes encoding for α and β chains [19].

Detection of DRw52- and DRw53-Associated PLT Determinants by Alloreactive T Cell Clones

The HLA-DR subregion is also believed to encode a subset of DR-like molecules which express the serologically defined DRw52 and DRw53 antigens (formerly MT2 and MT3). Previous studies in our laboratory have demonstrated alloreactive T cell clones specific for DRw53-associated PLT determinants [35]. Table 2 shows the DRw53-associated PLT reactivity patterns of three clones generated from an MLR culture with a DRw53-positive stimulator. It may be seen that the PLT reactivity patterns of these clones were not identical, suggesting the existence of several determinants associated with DRw53. Subsequent studies [37] using MoAb inhibition assays of the PLT activity of two DRw53-associated PLT clones showed that MoAb SG171 and Q5/13 were strongly inhibitory, whereas

Table 2. Reactivity of DRw53-associated PTL clones in secondary proliferation assays with an unrelated cell panel

Stimulator	HLA-D phenotype			PLT (cpm̄)		
	DR	DQ	DRw	HJ1	HJ13	HJ39
JC	4,–	3,–	53,–	18986	13422	26154
SH	4,6	1,3	52,53	3081	18443	23501
DK	4,–	3,–	53,–	7921	19911	48496
JCo	1,4	1,3	53,–	8617	12778	29928
KA	4,7	2,3	53,–	7898	17266	19900
MN	4,7	2,3	53,–	2515	5241	20279
MK	4,7	2,3	52,53	13034	15648	21082
MM	5,7	2,3	52,53	2817	16162	33180
JH	3,7	2,–	52,53	5934	18397	40592
JB	2,7	1,2	52,53	3051	15613	32769
JT	2,7	1,2	53,–	820	12708	27571
RD	5,7	2,3	52,53	875	557	8110
DL	1,5	1,3	52,–	350	5803	175
RL	1,2	1,–	–,–	207	579	9882
Ten DRw53-negative cells				< 300	< 500	< 4000

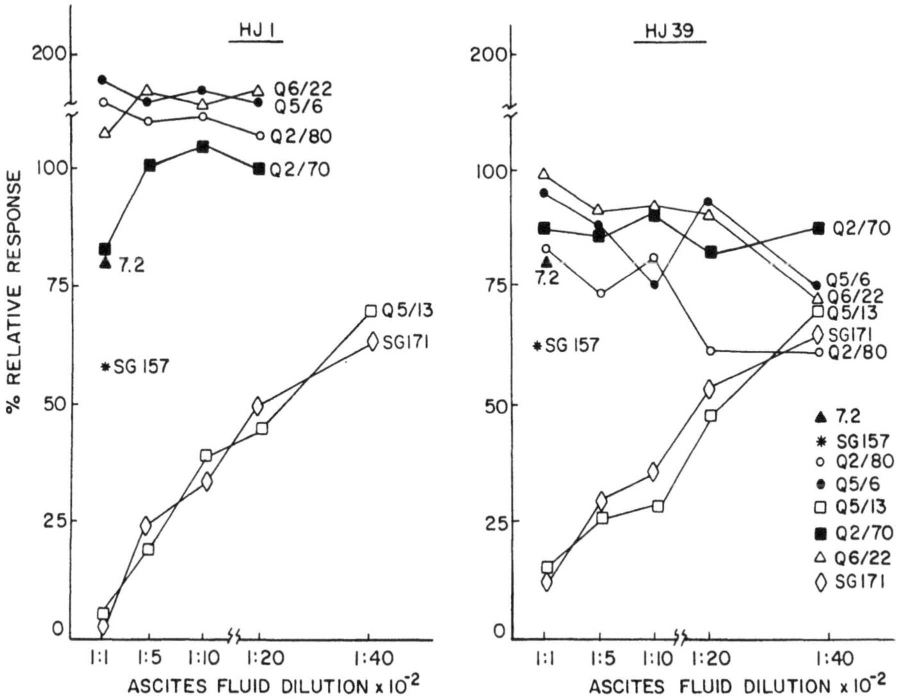

Fig. 2. MoAb inhibition profile of PLT activity of DRw53-associated PLT clones HJ1 and HJ39. All class II MoAb were ascites fluid

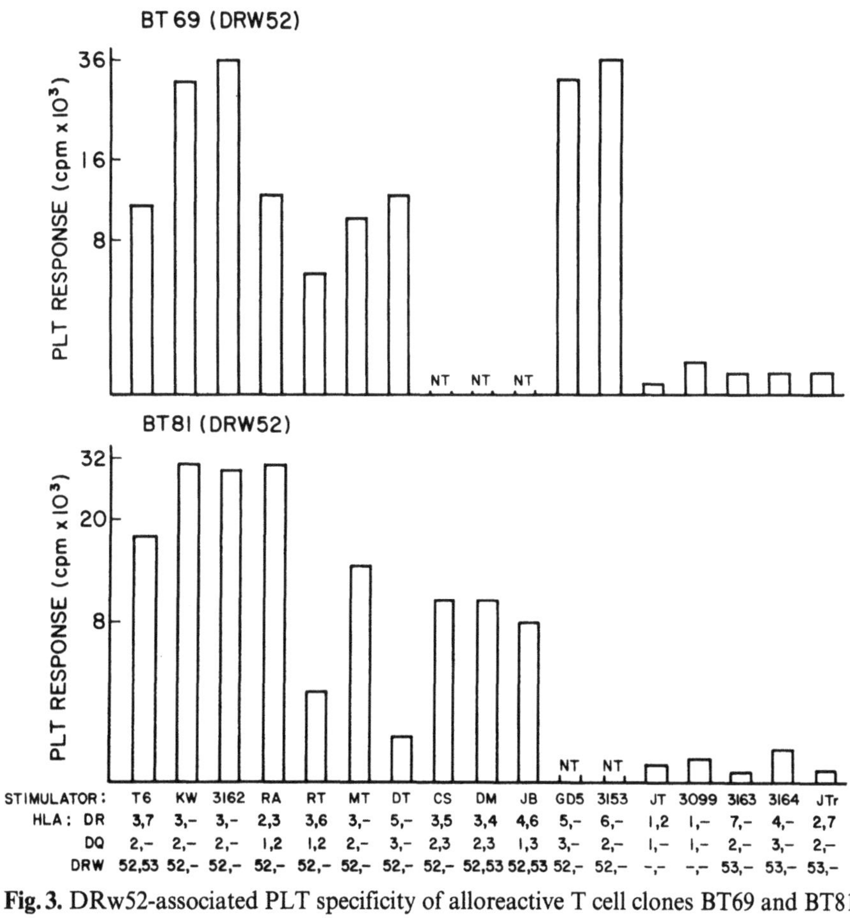

Fig. 3. DRw52-associated PLT specificity of alloreactive T cell clones BT69 and BT81

monomorphic DR MoAb had no effect (Fig. 2). Since SG171 and Q5/13 react with both HLA-DR- and DQ-encoded class II molecules [16, 28], these data suggest that the DRw53-associated PLT determinant detected by clones HJ1 and HJ39 reside on class II molecules which may not express HLA-DR subregion antigens.

We have also recently generated two DRw52-specific clones BT69 and BT81 from an MLR culture with a DR3, DRw52 stimulator (Fig. 3). These data show that DRw52 associates with PLT determinants which can induce proliferation of alloactivated T cells.

Specificity of PLT Clones Toward DQ-Associated Cellular Determinants

The DQ subregion of HLA-D encodes for class II molecules which are equivalent to the murine I-A molecules. These molecules express DQ antigens formerly called MB antigens [6]. Several years ago, we demonstrated the contribution of DQ antigens in primary MLR [5] and in secondary responses of "bulk" PLT cells [7]. The identification of DQ-specific PLT clones firmly established the fact that DQ antigens can induce T cell alloactivation [35]. Table 3 shows the reactivity patterns of two DQw3-associated PLT clones. Clones HJ15 and HJ18 were generated from an MLR culture with a DR4, DQw3 stimulator. Slightly different reactivity patterns were found, suggesting that the DQw3-associated cellular determinants recognized by these clones might be different.

Table 3. Reactivity of DQw3-associated PLT clones in secondary proliferation assays with an unrelated cell panel

Stimulator	HLA-D phenotype			PTL (cpm)	
	DR	DQ	DRw	HJ15	HJ18
JC	4,–	3,–	53,–	21252	29190
SH	4,6	1,3	52,53	13676	9277
JC	1,4	1,3	53,–	24381	20627
KA	4,7	2,3	52,–	21553	26829
MN	4,7	2,3	52,53	25608	20499
MK	4,7	2,3	53,–	18507	21019
TS	4,6	1,3	52,53	10818	13441
RD	5,7	2,3	52,53	11952	10793
MM	5,7	2,3	52,53	6583	2491
JM	5,6	1,3	52,–	25081	11062
NS	2,5	1,3	52,–	11361	10053
LR	3,5	2,3	52,–	3654	15842
DL	1,5	1,3	52,–	3966	12221
AP	1,4	1,3	53,–	230	2308
MKo	2,5	1,3	52,–	19752	1946
JH	3,7	2,–	52,53	15026	1841
KR	2,5	1,–	52,–	8320	2212
AZ	6,7	1,2	52,–	5980	2538
Fourteen and nine DQw3-negative cells				< 500	<2000

Detection of Cellular Antigens Encoded by HLA-DP

The HLA-DP antigens were originally described by Shaw et al. [32] as a group of cellular determinants of the SB system which could be defined by alloactivated T cells in both PLT and CML assays. At present, six DP specificities have been defined by primed T cells generated from bulk MLR cultures of HLA-A, B, C, DR, DQ-identical responder-stimulator combinations from unrelated individuals. Although primed T cells are good "discriminatory" cellular reagents for DP typing, several investigators have cloned these PLT cells by limiting dilution [1, 27]. Several alloreactive T cell clones have been generated which are highly specific for DP determinants [3, 26, 29]. In our experience with more than 500 clones generated from over 20 different MLR cultures of unrelated HLA-A, B, C, DR, DQ-incompatible responder-stimulators, we have not been able to identify a single DP-specific PLT clone. In contrast, DP-specific alloreactive T cells are readily generated from HLA-A,B,C,DR,DQ-identical responder stimulator combinations. Our inability to generate DP-specific PLT clones from HLA-disparate MLR cultures might be due to the fact that DP antigens are weak stimulatory determinants in comparison to DR and DQ. On the other hand, many MLR cultures yield several T cell clones which appear to recognize less well defined (perhaps weak) HLA determinants which are not readily defined either serologically or cellularly by bulk PLT cells. Another explanation for the lack of DP-specific clones from HLA-incompatible MLR cultures is that the alloactivation of DP-specific T cells in primary MLR may require HLA antigen sharing between responder and stimulator, and could, therefore, be HLA-restricted.

Detection of Other HLA-D-Associated PLT Determinants by Alloreactive T Cell Clones

Several investigators, including ourselves, have described alloreactive T cell clones specific for other HLA-D-encoded determinants [9, 23, 27, 37]. Since these determinants were not serologically defined, it seems that alloreactive clones may be useful reagents for defining additional cellular class II polymorphisms. We have recently defined a novel HLA-D-encoded determinant MC1 by a cluster of B cell alloantisera [8]. MC1 can now also be defined by MoAb [31]. The determinant associates with DR1 and DR4 and could also be defined by an alloreactive PLT clone generated from an MLR culture with a DR4, MC1 stimulator (Fig. 4). Clone HJ6 reacted with both DR4, MC1 and DR1, MC1 cells, but not with MC1-negative cells including a DR4-positive cell SH. Two MC1 cells, AP and RL, did not stimulate HJ6. The PLT specificity of this clone was significantly associated with MC1 with correlation value of 0.86. These data suggest that MC1 may also act as a cellular determinant capable of inducing alloactivation of T lymphocyes. Interestingly, MC1 shows a strong association with adult rheumatoid arthritis [8].

STIM	DR	MB	MT	SB	MCI
JC	4,–	3,–	3,–	3,6	+
KA	4,7	2,3	3,–	2,–	+
NK	4,7	2,3	3,–	3,4	+
MN	4,7	2,3	3,–	4,–	+
TS	4,6	1,3	2,3	nd	+
SH	4,6	1,3	2,3	2,–	–
JCa	1,4	1,3	1,3	3,4	+
AP	1,4	1,3	1,3	nd	+
DL	1,5	1,3	1,2	4,–	+
MG	1,6	1,–	1,2	4,–	+
JM	1,6	1,–	1,2	–,–	+
JT	1,2	1,–	1,–	4,–	+
CM	1,6	1,–	1,2	3,–	+
SE	1,5	1,–	1,2	3,–	+
RL	1,2	1,–	1,–	4,–	+
JH	3,7	2,–	2,3	4,–	–
JB	2,7	1,2	1,3	nd	–
NS	2,5	1,3	1,2	4,–	–
JN	5,6	1,3	2,–	–,–	–
KW	7,8	2,3	2,3	–,–	–
JTr	2,7	1,2	1,3	1,4	–
RD	5,7	2,3	2,3	2,4	–
AZ	6,7	1,2	2,–	–,–	–
GB	3,7	2,3	3,–	4,–	–
MKo	2,5	1,3	1,2	3,4	–
KR	2,5	1,–	1,2	2,–	–
MM	5,7	2,3	2,3	2,–	–
LR	3,5	2,3	2,–	2,4	–
BB	2,7	1,2	1,3	4,–	–

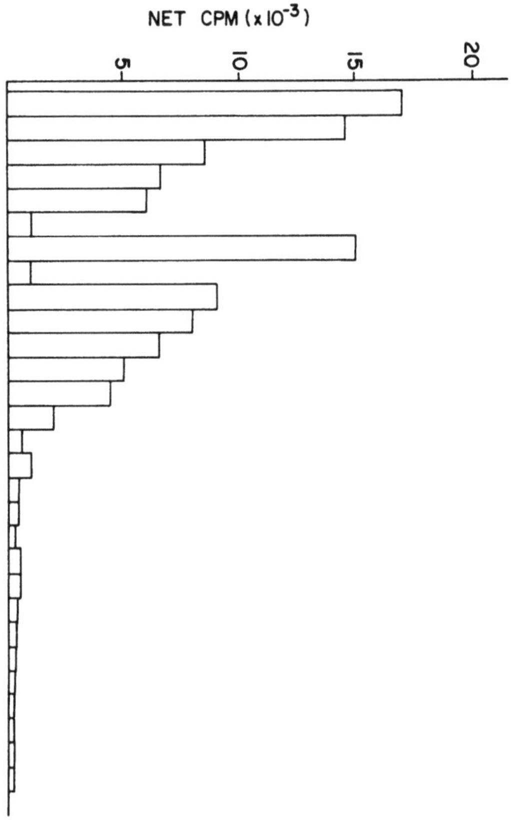

Fig. 4. MC1-associated PLT specificity of alloreactive T cell clone HJ6

PLT Specificity of Alloreactive T Cell Clones Toward Class I HLA Determinants

For many years the class II antigens of HLA-D have been considered to provide the primary stimulus in alloactivation. Until recently, class I HLA antigens were not believed to be directly involved in alloactivation of T cells. Studies on alloreactive T cell clones have shown that class I molecules encoded by HLA-B carry PLT determinants which induce T cell alloactivation [38]. This was demonstrated by clones with PLT specificity strongly associated with B21 and B49 antigens. The PLT reactivity of these clones was inhibited by class I- but not by class II-specific MoAb. These data suggest that class I antigens can directly activate T cells. Similar observations have been made by Reinsmoen et al. [30] and Flomenberg et al. [14]. We have recently described additional clones with specificities for B17, B27, and Bw35 [33]. Certain class I-specific clones show a certain degree of heterogeneity in their PLT response patterns. This was demonstrated with three B27-specific PLT clones generated from the same MLR combination. These clones showed distinctly different PLT reactivity patterns, suggesting the existence of several cellular determinants associated with the same HLA-B27 gene product [33]. Heterogeneity for B27 has also been observed at the serological level with B27-associated MoAb [18].

Specificity of Alloreactive T Cell Clones in CML and PLT Assays

Besides specific immunologic memory, demonstrable in PLT assays, alloactivated T cells have also been shown to exhibit cytolytic activity, as measured in the CML assay. Several investigators have described DR-specific cytolytic T cell clones, some with and others without PLT activity [2, 13, 20, 21, 23, 24]. We have recently described cytolytic T cell clones [33] that are specific for DQ and DR (MT) antigens. Figure 5 shows the CML data on a DQw3-specific clone, DD56, and a DRw53-specific clone, HT72. In view of the concept that DQ represents the human homologue of murine I-A [4, 17, 19], it is evident that human I-A-like molecules carry recognition structures cytolytic T cells. In other words, genes in all three HLA-D subregions DR – (including MT), DQ, and DP – express class II molecules which can be recognized by cytolytic alloreactive T cells.

The availability of cytolytic alloreactive T cell clones has enabled a comparative study of the specificity of these clones in PLT and CML assays. Table 4 shows the results with four clones specific for B17, B21, and B27 antigens. These class I-specific clones were OKT3+, T4−, 8+. Six class II-specific clones were tested which were specific for DR1 and DR5 (I-E-like), DQw3 (I-A-like), DRw52, and DRw53. These class II-specific clones were OKT3+, 4+, and 8−. For each clone, the CML and PLT reactivity showed identical specificity patterns. These data suggested that the specific target alloantigen for cytolytic activity may also induce a proliferative response. Further support of this concept was provided by observations of similar MoAb inhibition profiles of these clones when tested in PLT and CML assays. Figure 6 shows a representative MoAb inhibition profile of the DQw3-specific clone DD56. Class II MoAb SG171, Q2/70, Q5/6, Q5/13, and SG157 induced similar degrees of inhibition of PLT and CML, whereas class II-specific MoAb IIIE3 and IVG1 had no effect. Also, none of the class I-specific MoAb inhibited clone DD56. These similar inhibition profiles for CML and PLT provided additional evidence that the PLT and CML determinants recognized by cloned alloreactive T cells may be closely associated or even identical.

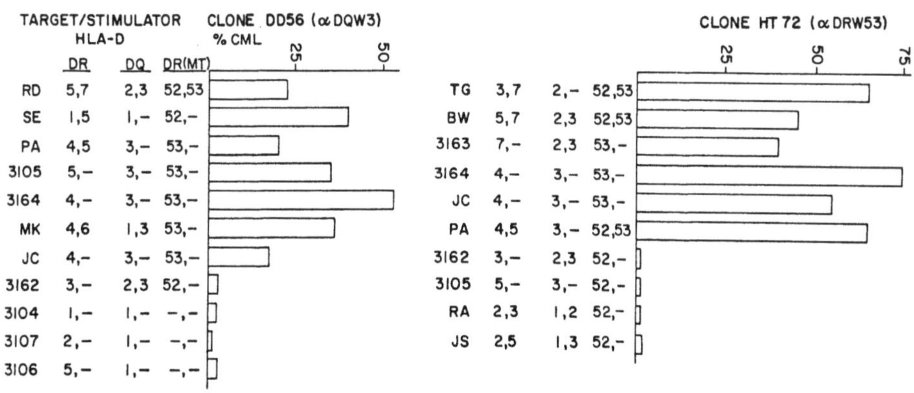

Fig. 5. CML response of clones DD56 (anti-DQw3) and HT72 (anti-DRw53) to an unrelated cell panel

Table 4. Perfect correlation between PLT and CML specificity of allo-reactive T cell clones

Clone	Class	Specificity	PLT vs CML			
			++	+−	−+	−−
DD13	I	B17	7	0	0	13
DD7	I	B17	5	0	0	11
RD3	I	B21	6	0	0	8
DS201	I	B27	6	0	0	10
DL65	II	DR1	3	0	0	9
DS56	II	DR5	6	0	0	8
DD56	II	DQw3	10	0	0	9
BT81	II	DRw52	6	0	0	6
BT69	II	DRw52	6	0	0	4
HT72	II	DRw53	12	0	0	14

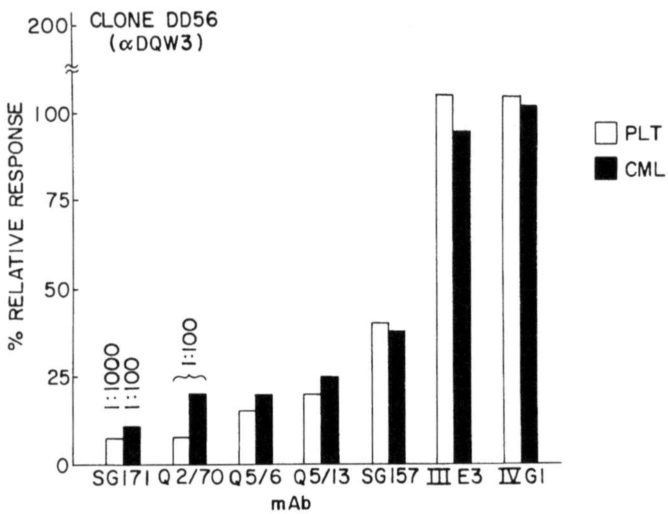

Fig. 6. MoAb inhibition profile of CML and PLT activity of DQw3-associated clone DD56

Allospecificity of IL-2 Release by Alloreactive T Cell Clones

Alloreactive T cell clones, when exposed to alloantigen, have been shown to release various lymphokines, including IL-2 [15]. It is well known that the growth of many cloned T cells is dependent on the presence of IL-2. Also, the ability of cloned alloreactive T cells to proliferate after stimulation with alloantigen alone has been correlated with their ability to release IL-2, athough exceptions have been noted [15]. In context with the present findings regarding identical PLT and CML specificity, we have also compared the specificity of the stimulator inducing IL-2 release and the PLT response of alloreactive clones.

The IL-2 release was analyzed in a three-cell assay whereby irradiated alloreactive T cell clones were incubated with irradiated stimulators in the presence of an

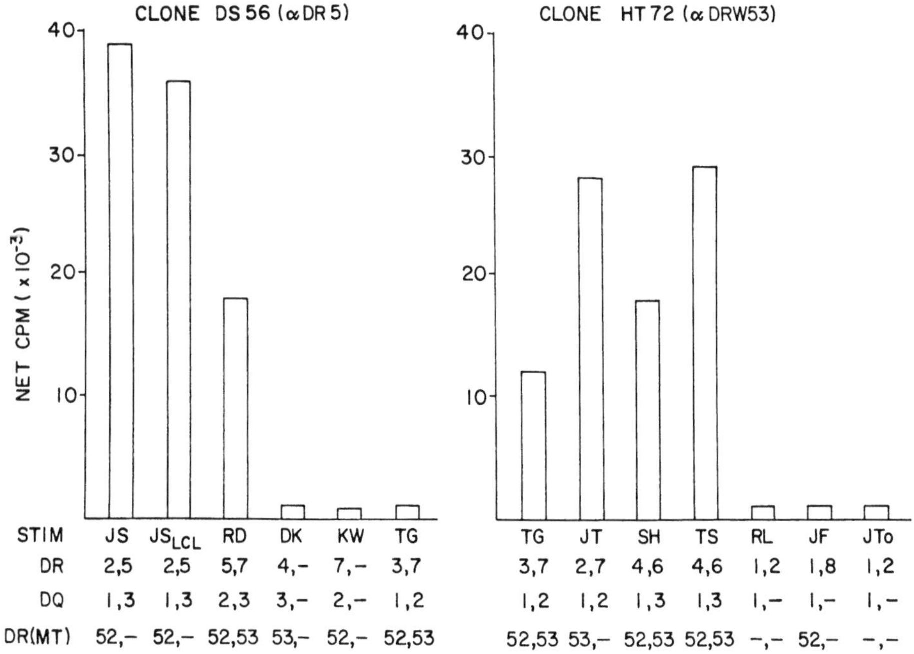

Fig. 7. Induction of IL-2 release from clones DS56 (anti-DR5) and HT72 (anti-DRw53). In these assays, 10^4 irradiated unrelated clones (500 R) were incubated with 10^5 irradiated stimulators (2000 R) and 5×10^3 HT-2 mouse cells

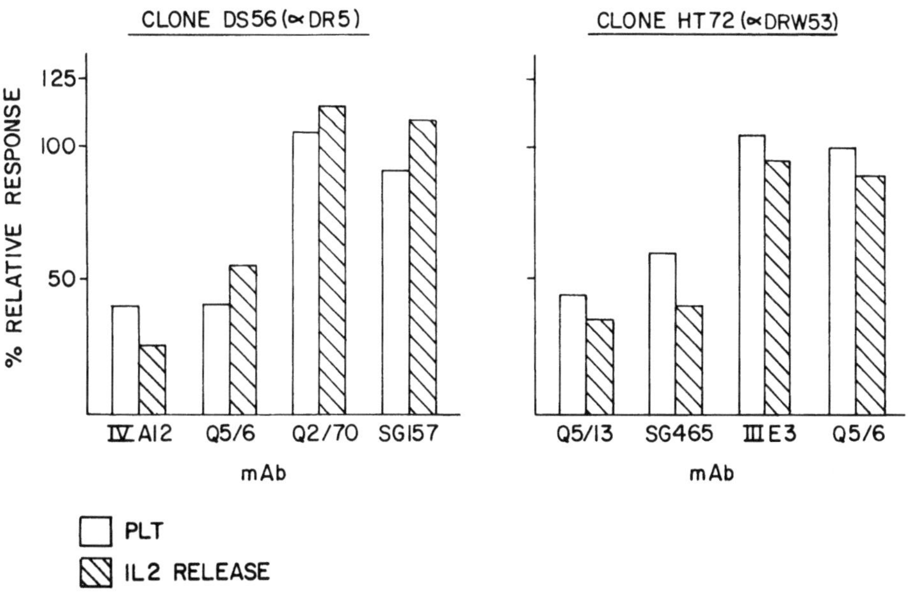

Fig. 8. MoAb inhibition profiles of PLT and IL-2 release from clones DS56 (anti-DR5) and HT72 (anti-DRw53)

IL-2-responsive cell line [33]. Figure 7 shows the results on a DR5-associated clone DS56 and a DRw53-associated clone HT72. Both irradiated peripheral blood lymphocytes (PBL) and LCL from the original stimulator of DS56 can trigger the release of IL-2 of this clone as shown with the proliferation of the IL-2 responsive HT-2 mouse cell line. The stimulatory effect of LCL also seems to rule out PBL as a source for IL-2 release. The DR5-specific IL-2 release by clone DS56 was indicated by the stimulatory effect of the DR5 positive cell RD, but not by any DR5 negative cell. Also, with the DRw53-specific clone HT72, both DR7, DRw53 and DR4, DRw53 stimulators induced IL-2 release, whereas DRw53-negative cells had no effect. These data suggest that the HLA-specificity of IL-2 release was identical to the PLT specificity of these alloreactive T cell clones.

To further analyze the relationship between PLT determinants recognized by alloreactive T cell clones and determinants which induce IL-2 release, we also conducted MoAb inhibition studies. In these assays, the original stimulator was incubated with different MoAb prior to PLT or the three-cell assay for IL-2 release. Figure 8 shows representative results with the DR5-associated DS56 and the DRw53-associated HT72. The two clones showed a similar MoAb inhibition profile in PLT and IL-2 release, suggesting that the same determinant may trigger these T cell functions.

Conclusions

Alloreactive T cell clones have proven to be useful reagents in the immunogenetic analysis of lymphocyte-activating determinants encoded by HLA which otherwise cannot be accomplished by serology or by cellular methods using "bulk" PLT, CML, and homozygous typing cells. It has become apparent that the products of most, if not all, class I and class II HLA loci are directly involved in T lymphocyte alloactivation. Most clones generated from HLA-D-incompatible MLR combinations show specificity for DR or DR-associated determinants (including subtypes) supporting the concept of their dominance in lymphocyte alloactivation. However, many non-DR class II antigens, including the I-A-like DQ antigens, stimulate alloactivated T lymphocytes.

Although a single class I or class II determinant can trigger three properties of an alloactivated T cell, – secondary proliferation, cytotoxicity, and IL-2 release – it is necessary to consider other functions including cellular interactions and production of effector molecules. Studies of the correlation between allospecificity and certain functions of alloreactive clones may provide important information regarding the biological significance of the different products of the human MHC.

References

1. Bach FH, Reinsmoen NL (1982) Cloned cellular reagents to define antigens encoded between HLA-DR and glyoxalate. Hum Immunol 5:133
2. Bach FH, Alter BJ, Widmer MB, Segall M, Dunlap B (1981) Cloned cytotoxic and noncytotoxic lymphocytes in mouse and man: their reactivities and a large cell surface membrane protein (LMP) differentiation marker system. Immunol Rev 54:5

3. Bach FH, Reinsmoen NL, Segall M (1983) The use of cellular reactants in the study of HLA antigens. Transplant Proc 15:102
4. Albert E, Baur MP, Mayr WR (1984) Histocompatibility testing 1984. Springer, Berlin Heidelberg New York Tokyo
5. Duquesnoy RJ (1981) Immunogenetic aspects of the relationship between HLA-DR and the MB and MT system. Transplant Proc 13:1804
6. Duquesnoy RJ, Marrari M, Annen K (1979) Identification of an HLA-DR associated system of B cell alloantigens. Transplant Proc 11:1757
7. Duquesnoy RJ, Zeevi A, Marrari M, Halim K (1982) Immunogenetic analysis of the HLA-D region: serological and cellular detection of the MB system. Clin Immunol Immunopathol 23:234
8. Duquesnoy RJ, Marrari M, Hackbarth S, Zeevi A (1984) Serological and cellular definition of a new HLA-D determinant MC1, and its association with rheumatoid arthritis. Hum Immunol 10:165
9. Eckels DD, Hartzman RJ (1981) Evidence for a new HLA-region determinant by human T-lymphocyte clones. Hum Immunol 3:337
10. Eckels DD, Hartzman RJ (1982) Characterization of human T-lymphocyte clones (TLC's) specific for HLA-region products. Immunogenetics 16:117
11. Eckels D, Zeevi A et al. (1985) Report on monoclonal antibody inhibition of alloreactive T cell clones. Hum Immunol (in press)
12. Feighery C, Stastny P (1979) HLA-D region associated determinants serve as targets for human cell-mediated lysis. J Exp Med 149:485
13. Flomenberg H, Duffy E, Naito K, Dupont B (1983) Two distinct phenotypes of HLA-DR specific cytotoxic T cell lines. Immunogenetics 17:317
14. Flomenberg N, Russo C, Ferrone S, Dupont B (1984) HLA class I-specific T lymphocyte clones with dual alloreactive functions. Immunogenetics 19:39
15. Glasebrook AL, Kelso A, Zubler RH, Ely JM, Prystowsky MB, Fitch FW (1981) Lymphokine production by cytolytic and noncytolytic alloreactive T cell clones. In: Fitch FW, Fathman GC (eds) Isolation, characterization, and vitalization of T lymphocyte clones. Academic, New York, pp 341–354
16. Goyert SM, Shively JE, Silver J (1982) Biochemical characterization of a second family of human Ia molecules, HLA-DS, equivalent to murine I-A subregion molecules. J Exp Med 156:650
17. Goyert SM, Moriuchi J, Winchester R, Silver J (1983) HLA-DS molecules and their relation to supertypic specificities. Hum Immunol 8:53
18. Grumet FC, Fendly BM, Fish FS, Engleman EG (1982) Monoclonal antibody (B27M2) subdividing HLA-B27. Hum Immunol 5:61
19. Hurley CK, Giles RC, Capra JD (1983) The human MHC: evidence for multiple HLA-D region genes. Immunology Today 4:219
20. Kornbluth J, Silver DM, Dupont B (1981) Cloning and characterization of primary alloreactive human T lymphocytes. Immunol Rev 54:111
21. Krensky A, Reiss C, Mier J, Strominger J, Burakoff S (1982) Long-term human cytolytic T cell lines allospecific for HLA-DRw6 antigen are OKT4. Proc Natl Acad Sci USA 19:2356
22. Kristensen T, Malissen B, Johnsen HE (1982) Histocompatibility typing by polyclonal and cloned human cytotoxic T lymphocytes. In: HLA typing methodology and clinical aspects, vol I. CRC, Boca Raton, p 123
23. Malissen B, Charmot D, Mawas C (1981) Expansion of human lymphocyte populations expressing specific immune reactivities. III. Specific colonies, either cytotoxic or proliferative, obtained from a population of responder cells primed in vitro preliminary immunogenetic analysis. Hum Immunol 1:1
24. Meuer SC, Schlossman SF, Reinherz EL (1982) Clonal analysis of human cytotoxic T lymphocyte T4+ and T8+ effector T cells recognize products of different major histocompatibility complex regions. Proc Natl Acad Sci USA 79:4395
25. Nunez G, Giles RC, Ball EJ et al. (1984) Expression of HLA-DR, MB, MT, and SB antigens on human mononuclear cells: identification of two phenotypically distinct monocyte populations. J Immunol 135:1300
26. Pawelec G, Shaw S, Wernet P (1982) Analysis of the linked SB gene system with cloned and uncloned alloreactive T cell lines. Immunogenetics 15:187

27. Pawelec G, Kahle P, Muller C, Rehbein A, Wernet P (1982) Discrete PLT clones detecting HLA-D and new HLA-non-D encoded cell surface determinants. Tissue Antigens 19:269
28. Quaranta V, Pellegrino MA, Ferone S (1981) Serologic and immunochemical characterization of the specificity of four monoclonal antibodies to distinct antigen determinants expressed on subpopulations of human Ia-like antigens. J Immunol 126:548
29. Reinsmoen N, Bach FH (1983) HLA-D region complexity associated with HLA-DR, DW, and SB phenotypes. Transplant Proc 15:76
30. Reinsmoen N, Anichini A, Bach FH (1983) Clonal analysis of T lymphocyte response to an isolated class I disparity. Hum Immunol 8:195
31. Richiardi R, Crepaldi T, Borelly J, Malavasy T, Carbonara AO (1984) A monoclonal antibody detects a new antigenic determinant shared by DR1 and DR4/Dw4 molecules. In: Albert ED, Baur MP, Mayr WR (eds) Histocompatibility testing 1984. Springer, Berlin Heidelberg New York Tokyo, p 431
32. Shaw S, Johnson AH, Shearer GM (1980) Evidence for a new segregant series of B cell antigens that are encoded in the HLA-D region and that stimulate secondary allogeneic proliferative and cytotoxic responses. J Exp Med 152:565
33. Zeevi A, Duquesnoy RJ (1984) Recognition of MHC gene products by human alloreactive T cell clones. In: Von Boehmer H, Haas W (eds) T cell clones. Elsevier, Amsterdam, pp 245–262
34. Zeevi A, Duquesnoy RJ (1985) Recognition of class I and II MHC products by alloactivated human T lymphocytes: the same antigenic determinant stimulates the cytolytic activity, secondary proliferation and interleukin 2 release by alloreactive T cell clones. J Immunogenetics 12:17
35. Zeevi A, Scheffel C, Annen K, Bass G, Marrari M, Duquesnoy RJ (1982) Association of the PLT specificity of alloreactive lymphocyte clones with HLA-DR, MB, and MT determinants. Immunogenetics 16:209
36. Zeevi A, Annen K, Scheffel C, Duquesnoy RJ (1983) Detection of HLA-DR associated PLT determinants by alloreactive lymphocyte clones. Immunogenetics 18:205
37. Zeevi A, Annen K, Scheffel C, Duquesnoy RJ (1983) Detection of non-HLA-DR determinants by alloreactive lymphocyte clones. Hum Immunol 6:97
38. Zeevi A, Scheffel C, Annen K, Duquesnoy RJ (1983) Primed lymphocyte testing specificity of alloreactive lymphocyte clones for HLA-B locus determinants. Proc Natl Acad Sci USA 80:1440

Cellular Detection of Human Class II Antigens: Delineation of a Novel HLA-DP-like Suppressor Restriction System DY *, the Sequential Expression of Class II Antigens, and a Pronounced Functional Flexibility of Class II Alloproliferative T Cell Clones **

P. Wernet, G. Pawelec, and E. M. Schneider

Table of Contents

Cellular Detection of Class II Products

HLA class II gene products, encoded on the short arm of chromosome 6 in the region of 6p21.33 [1], are expressed with limited tissue distribution on the surfaces of immunologically active cells, predominantly B lymphocytes, monocytes, dendritic cells, and macrophages [2, 3]. They are in addition synthesized and expressed by certain other types of cells, notably activated T lymphocytes [4], and various kinds of endothelia and epithelia, especially after induction by agents such as gamma-interferon [5]. Class II antigens are of critical importance for the initiation of immune responses, since at least the majority of T helper cells fails to recognize antigen unless both class II molecules and antigen are available on the surface of the same antigen-presenting cell [6]. Allogeneic class II products stimulate T cell proliferative responses in the apparent absence of additional antigen by virtue of their polymorphism. Although the basis of alloreactivity is not fully understood, the restriction elements for antigen presentation correlate closely with the class II specificities defined by alloreactive T cells, making it fair to assume that the same gene products, and possibly even identical epitopes, are involved in both recognition systems [7, 8]. Alloreactivity provides a method for

* This "DP-like" Restriction System has been named DY
** Supported by SFB 120, A1, B5a, C1

the detection of functionally relevant class II products which would be difficult to establish using MHC-restricted responses to nominal antigen. Hence many of the data on functional activities of class II antigens are based on the measurement of alloreactivity. The proliferative responses of lymphocytes in allogeneic mixed lymphocyte cultures (MLCs), a technique still in use today, for example for transplant donor selection, were first observed more than two decades ago [9]. It rapidly became clear that stimuli for proliferation in MLC are genetically predetermined, usually segregating with the serologically defined HLA-A,B,C class I haplotypes in families, from which they can, however, be separated by genetic recombination events [10]. Methods for typing for these gene products in outbred populations using stimulating cells carrying a majority of the same lymphocyte-activating determinants (LADs) on both haplotypes have been developed. A negative reaction on the part of an untyped donor against such homozygous typing cells (HTCs) is taken to indicate identity between the cells and used as a basis for assignment of that specificity [11]. However, negative reactions are difficult to define, and even with statistical data analysis developed for large international collaborative workshops, a precise definition of specificities has never been forthcoming. Nonetheless, it was possible to define "clusters" of reactivity patterns used to assign specificities, which did behave as an allelic series, and which are termed HLA-Dw types [12]. Similarly, "clusters" of reactivity patterns for alloantisera established a parallel series of specificities, termed HLA-DR, correlating to some extent, but not perfectly, with the cellularly defined HLA-Dw types. In addition, further complexity was introduced by the demonstration of an independent serologically defined allelic system termed HLA-DQ (formerly MB, DC, or DS). HLA-DR, Dw, and DQw specificities are in high linkage disequilibrium and are almost always inherited as a single haplotype, making it difficult or impossible directly to dissect their different functional status as LADs in MLC typing. Nonetheless, some investigators provided data which suggest that both HLA-DR/Dw and HLA-DQ contribute to the overall response stimulated by allogeneic cells in MLC [13].

A technical step forward in clarifying the gene products functioning as LADs was the development of primed lymphocyte typing (PLT) which enabled positive typing responses to be measured [14–16]. Lymphocyte populations sensitized in vitro against alloantigens generate rapid secondary proliferative responses specifically when rechallenged by cells carrying the priming antigens, and can therefore be used as probes to define more precisely the complexity of LADs. Moreover, by establishing priming combinations matched for known LADs, a classical methodology for searching for new LADs was developed. In this way, it was possible to define the products of the HLA-DP (formerly SB) genes, which stimulate such a weak response in primary MLC that they had previously escaped detection above the background "noise" in HTC typing [17]. However, since the HLA-DP products stimulate strong secondary response, their detection by lymphocyte populations primed under appropriate conditions presents a lesser problem.

Although PLT offers many advantages over HTC typing, the responder populations in PLT reagents will represent heterogeneous material capable of responding to multiple stimulatory determinants, thereby reducing the "discriminatory power" for a single LAD. More recently, this problem has been overcome by generating monoclonal PLT populations which presumably respond to a single, or a very limited number of, stimulatory epitopes [18, 19]. Application of cloned PLT reagents by many investigators has clearly demonstrated the existence of LADs closely associated with or identical to the HLA-DR and Dw products, suggesting that these predefined specificities do exist as "immunodominant" stimulatory structures, and not entirely as clustered constellations of different gene products [20–22]. Nonetheless, the situation as a whole is not so simple, since a significant proportion of clones were found to be stimulated by LADs associated with only a particular fraction ("split") of the relevant stimulator cell HLA-DR or Dw type [19, 21–24]. Similar results in both respects have been obtained with HLA-DQw-associated LADs. In addition, stimulatory activity ascribed to both the HLA-DRw52 and DRw53 (formerly MT2 and MT3) supertypic specificities has been reported, as well as proliferative responses against non-class II determinants such as class I HLA-B encoded LADs [21, 24–26]. Clones specific for LADs highly associated with HLA-DPw specificities have also been reported recently by several investigators [22, 27, 28]. To objectify the DP PLT results, a centroid cluster analysis was employed, comparing arithmetical with log-transformed data for the unequivocal assignment of positive and negative responses [17, 27]. With a sharper definition of this allelic group, also more insight concerning the linkage of DP alleles with other class II specificities was obtained [29]. Furthermore, DPw typing of HTCs revealed that of 72 HLA-A,B homozygotes, 23.6% typed for two different DPw specificities, and of 43 HLA-A,B heterozygotes, 27.1% typed for two DPw specificities [30]. This absence of a statistically significant difference for DPw heterozygosity in HTCs further points to a lesser linkage disequilibrium between DP and DR than between DR and HLA-B. It seems that all of the diverse class II gene products may in addition function as target determinants for cytolytic T cells [31–34]. Finally, a number of examples of putative new LAD systems have been proposed on the basis of PLT clone reactivities [35–37]. When such LADs fail to correlate with any currently established HLA specificities, some further indications of their nature may be obtained by employing monoclonal antibodies (MoAb) to inhibit stimulation. Here the assumption is that a MoAb of defined class II specificity is more likely to cross-block stimulation by a similar structure than by a different one. For example, during experiments aimed at generating cloned PLT reagents specific for DP-associated LADs, we noticed that many of the clones derived from HLA-DR/Dw-matched, DPw-mismatched priming combinations showed restimulation patterns which could not be correlated with the presence of the expected DP, or any other, HLA allele [36]. We therefore employed a panel of MoAb made in our laboratory against monomorphic HLA-DR, DQ, and DP determinants [38, 39] to inhibit stimulation of such clones [36]. MoAb reacting only with DQ, DR, or DP all failed to inhibit stimulation of these reagents. The only MoAb which could inhibit were those which had a "broad" reactivity against multiple class II molecules [40]. One of these, designated Tu39, was particularly interesting since it was known preferentially to block stimulation by DP-associated LADs [22, 36, 38]. Moreover, in a study performed in collaboration with Dr. F. Bach's group, it was demonstrated that this MoAb, Tu39, but not an anti-DP MoAb, FA, was able to prevent cytolytic clones with specificity for unknown non-DP gene products centromeric to HLA-DQ from lysing target cells [33]. These data together are thus consistent with the existence of a second, possibly "DP-like" class II product, designated "DY", which, like the other class II products, behaves both as a LAD and as a target determinant for cytotoxic lymphocytes. By a similar approach, utilizing inhibitory activities of MoAb in an antigen (PPD)-presentation system, some evidence for the existence of a functionally relevant, second HLA-DQ-like product has been forthcoming [41].

The application of T cell clones to the study of LADs has also on occassion resulted in the subdivision of certain established class II specificities. This may suggest the existence of multiple epitopes carried on a single class II molecule, or the presence of several different gene products associated with a specificity previously thought to be the product of a single locus. The application of two further techniques, now being initiated in several laboratories, will help in clarifying this matter. In one approach, stimulating cell lines are treated with mutagens and surviving cells selected on the basis of their lack of expression of defined HLA specificities. The availability of panels of such "loss mutants" is valuable for establishing the LAD or target determinant properties of the remaining expressed products, as well as for identifying new ones [1, 33]. The second technique consists of employing stimulator cells normally lacking class II antigens after their transfection with genes encoding single class II molecules. In this way, responses of cloned T cells to a single class II product are assured, and any heterogeneity of responsiveness must then reside at the level of epitopic heterogeneity implicit in a single class II molecule. Thus far, this technique has been applied for DP-restricted presentation of influenza virus antigens to helper T cell clones [42]. There would seem to be no basic reason to expect that such transfectants would not also express class II antigens recognizable by PLT clones, although so far only an example to the contrary has appeared [43]. Supplementary information concerning the question of the number of different epitopes on a particular class II molecule which are recognizable by T cells may again be derived from MoAb stimulation inhibition experiments. Firstly, serological reactivity patterns of anti-class II MoAb already imply an epitopic heterogeneity of class II molecules, at least for the murine anti-human class II B cell repertoire [44, 45]. Regarding T cell recognition, some data do suggest that different clones responding only to a panel of stimulators expressing a particular class II specificity may differ amongst themselves in susceptibility to stimulation inhibition by MoAb [22, 37]. Although other interpretations are possible, for example regarding affinities of the T cell clones' receptors for antigen and/or accessory interaction structures, such results could be interpreted as consistent with a functionally relevant epitopic heterogeneity of the target class II molecule. This is schematically represented in Fig. 1, where clones A and B display identical reactivity patterns in population analyses, correlating with the presence on the stimulating cells of specificity X. From panel studies it would

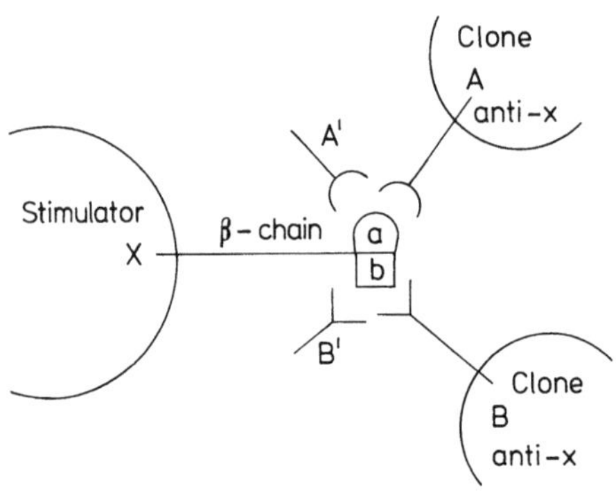

Fig. 1. Epitopic heterogeneity of class II molecules investigated with cloned T cells and monoclonal antibodies. *a,b,* different epitopes of class II molecule: specificity X; *A,B,* T cell clones recognizing stimulator cell specificity X via specific receptors; *A',B'*, monoclonal antibodies recognizing epitopes *a* and *b*, respectively

not be possible to distinguish whether specificity X carried a single, or multiple different, epitopes recognized by the T cell clones. However, by employing appropriate informative MoAb, inhibition of stimulation of clone A but not B, or vice versa, by a particular MoAb would suggest the recognition of different epitopes on the same molecule by the different clones.

The presence of a multitude of functionally active class II determinants is therefore likely to be caused by the generation of heterogeneity at several different levels:

1. The existence of multiple discrete genetic loci
2. The high degree of polymorphism for the products of each locus
3. The existence of multiple epitopes on each molecule
4. Transcomplementation between the products of different class II alpha and beta chain genes [46]

It may be appropriate at this point to ask whether these multiple class II antigens subserve different functions, either directly or in terms of the functions of the T cells which they stimulate. The first part of this question seems quite simple to answer, and the answer is no. That is to say, HLA-DR/Dw-, DQ-, and DP-associated products all seem able to stimulate secondary lymphoproliferative responses, to act as restriction elements for antigen presentation, and to act as target antigens for recognition and lysis by cytotoxic T cells. The second part of the question is more difficult, but may be approached by analyzing the functions of clones stimulated by LADs associated with the different class II products. T helper cell responses stimulated by DR-, DQ-, and DP-associated determinants have all been reported [41, 47–49], although a vigorous characterization of the helper status of the responding cells was not always performed. In one instance, different constellations of lymphokines secreted by influenza virus antigen-specific T helper clones influenced by the DR- or DQ-associated nature of their restriction elements was reported [50], although the correlation between restriction element and secreted lymphokine was not perfect. There are now many instances of the occurrence of class II-specific, interleukin 2 (IL-2)-secreting, proliferative cytotoxic clones, but the target determinants for such clones do not appear to be limited to one or the other type of class II molecule [31–34]. Furthermore, proliferative clones, although they secrete IL-2, may exert suppressive, not helper, effects on cellular reactions [36, 51]. We have found that whilst the majority of PLT clones specific for LADs associated with HLA-DR, Dw, DP, or DQ antigens fail to suppress MLC responses, all clones reacting against the previously mentioned "DP-like" LADs mediate strong suppressive activity [52]. Unlike nonsuppressive PLT clones, such suppressive clones are capable of stimulating rapid primary proliferative responses in unprimed autologous or allogeneic lymphocytes, which are inhibited by MoAb with "broad" anti-class II reactivity, such as Tu39, but not by anti-DR or anti-DQ MoAb [53]. Moreover, this stimulated cell population is itself suppressive when transferred to an MLC, unless the inducing cocultures are performed in the presence of MoAb Tu39, or the responding cells first irradiated to prevent cell division [53, 54]. Thus, at least one mechanism of suppression by PLT clones specific for "DP-like" antigens appears to require induction of suppressive activity in unprimed lymphocytes via the class II determinant defined by Tu39. These results may have significance for the immunoregulatory activity of cell types expressing limited species of class II determinants, as discussed in the following section.

Expression of HLA Class II Antigens on Leukemic Cells and PBMC of Bone Marrow Transplant Patients in the Early Phase of Hematopoetic Reconstitution

Earlier we had demonstrated that Ia antigens not only serve as allodeterminants and restriction elements, but due to their differential expression on leukemic blast cells can also be regarded as differentiation markers [22, 41, 55]. Although it has been shown that a regulatory gene responsible for the induction or repression of the entire HLA-D region is located outside the MHC [56], a differential expression has been noted for HLA-DQ and HLA-DR on certain cells [57]. Recently, using a large panel of granulocytic, lymphatic, and undifferentiated leukemias, we have demonstrated a heterogeneity of HLA-DQ, DP, DR expression and Tu39 binding [58]. The fact that a coordinate sequential expression of class II antigens has been shown on B-ALL [59], which can be manipulated by immune interferon [5], similarly to the induction of HLA-DQ in macrophages [60], or by TPA [61], indicates that individual regulation of expression may occur by a "block" of mRNA transcription. The differential expression of class II molecules on different stages of hematopoetic progenitors has raised the question of their individual relevance in controlling maturation and proliferation via activated T cells and accessory cells in vivo [62].

Results on the differential distribution of HLA class II antigens as defined by Tu22 (HLA-DQ), Tu34 (HLA-DR), Tu39 (broad HLA class II-specific, including HLA-DP-like antigens), and FA (HLA-DP) in human granulocytic and lymphatic leukemia are presented in Table 1. This type of analysis was performed under the general concept that a number of tumor cells of the granulocytic or lymphatic lineage may be considered as arrested stages of normal differentiation. In the case of AML, AUL, as well as certain CML in blast crisis [58], and B-cell leukemias, there are clearly examples where the sum of DQ, DR, and DP expression (i.e. Tu22+Tu34+FA) is less than expression of DR/DP/DP-like (Tu39), suggesting the presence of cells expressing uniquely "DP-like" class II antigens. Leukemic cells with the strongest evidence for this are underlined in the Table. Furthermore, the differential expression and in one case also repression could be shown by in vitro differentiation of leukemic cells. Two of them (one AML* and one T-ALL**) are depicted in Table 1. AML* blasts were almost negative for all class II antigens: 4 days after culture they expressed DQ, DR, FA (to a lesser extent), and DP-like (i.e., Tu39-positive cells). After 11 days culture, differentiation continued towards a mature monocyte phenotype correlating with the occurrence of the LeuM3-defined antigen. At this stage, FA seemed to be repressed, and DQ and DR had returned to the expression levels seen before culture; however, reactivity to Tu39 remained high at 39%. The T-ALL** shown here responded with strong class II antigen expression and quantitatively highest levels of HLA-DR and DP-like (Table 1). Additionally, the phenotype of one B-CLL is included here expressing equal amounts of Tu34- and Tu39-positive cells, but extremely low percentages of Tu22- and FA-positive cells, suggesting that these leukemic blasts express only HLA-DR antigens on their cell surface.

The findings summarized in Table 1 are also of interest in the context of results obtained with quantitative measurements of class II antigen expression on T cell clones derived from normal donors primed to allogeneic stimulators in vitro: 5% –10% of such clones lacked expression of HLA-DQ- and/or HLA-DR-encoded

Table 1. Differential expression of HLA class II antigens on leukemic cells

Leukemia type	Blasts (%)	Tu22 DQ	Tu34 DR	FA DP	Tu39 DR/DP DP-like	LeuM1	LeuM3
AML	60	0	7	15	59	64	nt
AML	50	14	8	9	52	20	45
AML	75	16	20	12	68	48	10
AML	58	15	58	33	33	56	62
AML	90	34	55	54	56	60	18
AML[a]	92	3	5	2	7	96	0
AML[a] (4 days: pp IL-2)	100	28	34	14	39	98	10
AML[a] (12 days: pp IL-2)	100	3	7	0	39	54	24
Pre-B-ALL	95	3	8	10	67	2	0
B-ALL	88	80	90	92	89	0	0
B-CLL	95	90	91	88	85	0	0
B-CLL	95	12	85	19	87	0	0
Burkitt's lymphoma	55	43	50	48	62	32	44
Burkitt's lymphoma	92	2	30	28	86	15	90
T-ALL	92	2	85	56	90	0	0
T-ALL	83	34	80	76	95	0	0
T-ALL[b]	90	0	0	0	2	10	nt
T-ALL[b] (12 days: IL-2)	100	37	93	54	100	0	0
AUL	70	0	17	0	62	4	nt
AUL	90	12	25	13	75	12	4
AUL	98	8	95	92	95	0	0

Results are expressed as percent cells positive in indirect immunofluorescence, counting at least 200 cells per sample

AML[a] and T-ALL[b] were cultured in vitro using partially purified (pp) IL-2 (Lymphokult T-LF, Biotest, FRG) containing the human analogue of IL-3 according to its capacity to drive multilineage differentiation and proliferation of hematopoetic progenitors in vitro. The same type of differentiation did not occur with highly purified IL-2 (Lymphokult T-HP, Biotest, FRG) or recombinant IL-2 (kindly provided by Dr. M. Wrann, Sandoz, Austria). See text for explanation of underlining

molecules but retained reactivity with Tu39, the broad HLA-DR/DP-/DP-like reagent. Furthermore, a selected panel of such T cell clones was able to produce distinct colony-stimulating factor(s) guiding hematopoetic maturation if cultured in the presence of their relevant "target antigens" (unpublished observations).

Results of class II antigen expression detected by Tu22, Tu34, Tu39, and FA on leukemic blasts separated by differential gradient centrifugation [63] showed that quantitative differences were due to distinct blast stages in an individual leukemic cell type, and thus suggest heterogeneity due to cell cycle or maturation (results not shown).

One of the most challenging models to study the development of the immune- and hematopoetic system in vivo is represented by allogeneic bone marrow transplantation (BMT). Early after BMT a solely Tu39-positive monocytoid cell type repopulates peripheral blood together with lymphoid cells of mature and immature phenotype (Table 2). These Tu39-positive cells apparently lacked antigen-presenting capacity for mitogenic and allogeneic responses, although they readily

Table 2. Expression of HLA class II antigens on PBMC after BMT in relation to the content of monocytoid cells

Patient	Days post BMT	Infections		GVHD	Tu22 DQ	Tu34 DR	FA DP	Tu39 DR/DP/ DP-like	Mono- cytoid cells
		Bac- terial	Viral						
HM	11	–	–	–	0	3	2	56	60
HM	17	+	–	–	13	27	10	64	21
BW	12	–	–	–	0	0	0	29	30
BW	18	–	–	+	19	58	63	68	47
GR	61	–	–	–	0	30	4	64	72
GR	88	–	–	–	0	21	0	34	44
RH	19	–	–	–	0	0	0	36	39
HM	10	–	–	–	0	5	0	32	35
HM	17	–	–	+	12	27	25	69	12
KR	12	–	–	+	1	23	9	32	15
KR	19	–	–	+	24	34	32	43	24
MW	12	+	–	–	19	43	47	39	46
BU	19	–	–	–	0	12	6	22	44
BU	229	–	+	–	23	20	30	46	15
DK	45	–	–	+	22	20	18	52	62
DK	824	–	–	–	10	16	16	20	13
OB	52	–	+	–	10	19	14	50	33
OB	229	–	+	–	0	16	31	35	18

Results are expressed as percent cells positive in indirect immunofluorescence, counting at least 200 cells per sample

formed colonies with erythrocytic progenitors (CFU-E), but not BFU-E. Thus it seems likely that they were capable of producing some burst-promoting activity [64]. This monocytoid cell type persisted in patients with delayed or lacking engraftment (unpublished observation).

Maturation of the immune system was indicated by a positive response to phytohemagglutinin (PHA) or allogeneic cells in vitro and correlated with the clinical manifestation of acute graft-vs-host disease (GVHD), severe bacterial or viral infections, or drug allergy in these patients, which were readily overcome thereafter. Interestingly, only then were HLA-DQ-, DR-, and DP-positive cells detected for the first time in peripheral blood mononuclear cells (PBMCs) after BMT (Table 3). If one considers a part of the solely Tu39-positive cells (thus expressing only DP-like antigens) as recipient-derived stromal elements, normally conditioning a successful engraftment of transplanted stem cells, in clinical BMT this could provide the first recognition of class II DP-like incompatibility by the newly developing T cell system. If these stromal cells are not exchanged subsequently by donor type cells, GVDH may fatally impair hematological and immunological reconstitution. Since a recombination between DR and DP and presumably often also DP-like (since DP-like appears to reside centromeric to DR/DQ [33]), is not infrequent even between HLA "identical" siblings, a sizeable proportion of bone marrow transplants is carried out between DP and DP-like incompatible recipient/donor pairs. Manifestation of fatal GVHD could thus be an expression of DP and DP-like incompatibility. Such a case has indeed been documented by Möller and coworkers [65].

Table 3. Surface marker phenotyping of dendritic-like cells in PBMC and bone marrow cultures after allogenic BMT

Source Days in culture	PBMC 14	PBMC 22	BM 16	BM 18
HLA class I	+	+	+	+
Tu22	–	–	–	–
Tu34	–	–	–	
FA	–	–	–	–
Tu39	+	+	+	+

Cultures were performed in 6% partially purified IL-2 (Lymphokult T-LF, Biotest, FRG) with 15% FCS in RPMI 1640. Reactivity to monoclonal antibodies was tested using indirect staining with alkaline phosphatase of adherent dendritic-like cells after removing proliferating T cells and hematopoetic progenitors in the case of bone marrow samples. In addition to the antibodies shown in the table, the following were found consistently negative on dendritic-like cells: CD4–, KiM4–, LeuM1–, LeuM3–, M1/70–, Fc receptor– 3G8, C3b receptor–, Leu7–, Leu8–, anti-TAC–. Antibody OKT10 was found weakly positive on all samples (E. M. Schneider, C. Müller, P. Wernet, unpublished observations). Cytochemicical analysis revealed these cells to be negative for myeloperoxidase, weakly positive for esterase, and strongly positive for acid phosphatase

The distribution of class II-positive cells in BMT patients (Table 2) was attributable not solely to monocytoid cells, but also to in vivo activated T cells positive for the IL-2 receptor and directly responsive to purified IL-2 in vitro. After propagation of such "in vivo-activated" T cells, populations were found positive exclusively for T cell markers (CD3+, CD4+, or CD8+), and expressing HLA class II antigens defined by Tu22, Tu34, FA, and Tu39 mostly in quantitatively equal amounts. However, a few exceptions have been seen, where in vitro propagated T cell lines contained higher percentages of Tu39 positive cells.

Additionally, some patients' PBMC and mononuclear cells from bone marrow samples were distinguished by the presence of dendritic-like cells, which were morphologically and cytochemically identical to those described by Van Voorhis and coworkers [66]. Antigenically, these dendritic-like cells were negative for monocyte-macrophage surface antigens, for CD4, KiM4 [67], complement and Fc receptors, and HLA-DQ, DR, DP antigens but strongly positive for class II antigens detected by Tu39. (Results from three patients' dendritic-like cells are summarized in Table 3.) In the presence of such dendritic-like cells, in vivo activated T cells grew in clusters with this cell type after addition of media containing purified IL-2. Figure 2 shows an electron scanning micrograph of a dendritic-like cell and an activated T cell in suspension. In culture, dendritic-like cells formed an elaborate net of cytoplasmic protrusions.

The differential unique expression of Tu39-positive class II molecules on adherent cell populations, certain T cells, and hematopoetic progenitors opens a new area for the investigation of regulatory events via the novel HLA class II gene products, which we have provisionally referred to as HLA-DP-like ("DY").

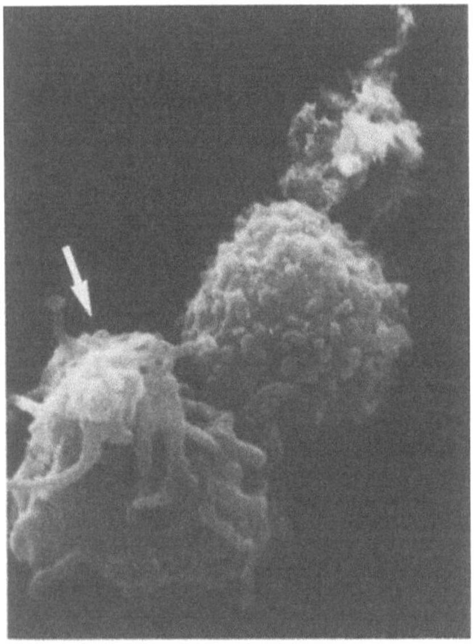

Fig. 2. Scanning electron micrograph of a dendritic-like cell (*arrow*) and an activated T cell in suspension, derived from PBMC of a BMT patient with acute GVHD. ×4700

Mainly on the basis of monoclonal antibody inhibition experiments, we would argue that HLA class II antigens expressed on or recognized by activated T cells serve as restriction elements for their action on defined target cells or – and this could be more important, if class II antigens were differentially expressed on T cell effectors – serve as target populations themselves. Especially the latter would have important implications for the investigation of T cell circuits within the course of the generation of an immune response.

Functional Flexibility in Human T Cell Clones

We would like to point out a pecularity observed with class II-specific T cell clones: When using alloproliferative T cell clones for the study of immunoregulation, it is necessary to retest that the defined clonal function and specificity has remained stable during culture. This statement is based upon our consistent observation of in vitro ongoing differentiation-associated functional alterations of 40 alloreactive PLT clones derived from different donors propagated in a number of ways. All these clones spontaneously lost their alloproliferative capacity after about 30 population doublings in culture. These PLT clones expressed a $CD4^+$, $CD8^-$, $Leu8^-$ phenotype, and secreted IL-2 and other lymphokines which has led to their attribution to the proliferative T "helper" subset. Nonetheless, in 40 of 40 clones examined by us continuously over their total life span, a shift from MHC-specific helper activity to antigen-non-specific suppressor activity was observed without exception. About two-thirds of these clones in addition acquired natural killer(NK)-like activity quite comparable to the NK activity observed in certain clones right from the beginning of their clonal existence in vitro.

The consistent changes in specificity and function of the PLT clones described here occurred at about one-half to two-thirds of their total clonal life span, being clearly dissociated from their eventual demise. These changes were not accompanied by any detectable indications of cellular or karyotypic abnormalities, alteration in cell surface phenotype, or de novo mycoplasma contamination. Therefore our results point to the activation of a mechanism for the preprogrammed cessation of T helper cell activity, representing a further differentiation phase possible in the long-term extrathymic development of antigen-stimulated normal T lymphocytes. This is not surprising if one considers that the totality of specificities expressed by T cells within a given T cell repertoire of an individual is determined not by the genotype of the T cells alone, but also by the environment in which T cell specificities must develop. In this sense, a T cell is quite different in its functional flexibility from a plasma cell which after clonal selection can produce but one specificity of antibody molecules.

There is evidence that the T cell receptor is composed of two chains, alpha and beta, at least one of which is homologous to immunoglobulin. Because the functional T cell receptor appears to be a complex of several other molecules of apparently fixed amino acid sequence, such as CD3, as well as the accessory molecules CD4 and CD8, in addition to the alpha/beta dimer of variable amino acid sequence, different configurations or alterations, for example in glycosylation, of these molecules could lead to a rapid change in specificity.

It has been noted by several investigators [21, 68, 69], and studied more fully by our group [54, 70], that without intermittent recloning procedures, the alloproliferative capacity of "helper" clones appears generally less stable in culture than cytotoxic (CTX) or MHC plus nominal antigen-specific clones. Indeed, clones with both alloproliferative and CTX activity may lose the former with retention of the latter after a period in culture [71, 72]. On the other hand, MHC class II-restricted, virus-specific proliferative clones may acquire specific lytic activity on in vitro culture [73].

In a related context, a high degree of functional heterogeneity in T cell clones may become apparent when periodic restimulation with specific antigen is foregone, and the cells cultured on third-party filler cells or no filler cells at all. Such clones may develop anti-self CTX [74], CTX against limited ranges of third-party target cells [75] (E. M. Schneider, unpublished data), or against target cells primarily susceptible to lysis by NK cells [76–78]. Thus these comparisons of the previous work of other groups indirectly support our conclusion that T cells must continue to diversify in specificity following activation. Possibly this permanently differentiating state can be caused also by somatic variations within the antigen-receptor genes [79]. These would generate cells with new antigenic specificities which are selected for or against according to the culture environment. Even the constant or intermittent presence of specific antigen may not guarantee retention of original clonal specificity and function.

In our hands, change of alloproliferative function of PLT clones was independent of clonal propagation on specific, autologous or third-party filler cells. The use of neither crude, partially purified, or highly purified (Biotest, Lymphocult T-HP) natural IL-2 nor recombinant IL-2 (a gift from Dr. Wrann, Sandoz, Vienna) influenced the loss of alloproliferative specificity. In addition to the stability of phenotypes and karyotypes, growth curves were unaffected. The clones remained completely dependent on filler cells as well as IL-2 for their continuous exponential growth. At the time of loss of class II-specific alloproliferation, those clones which had previously not been suppressive, in addition to their acquisition of a nonspecific suppressive effect for lymphoproliferative responses in MLC and PLT [54, 70], also strongly suppressed Ig secretion in a polyclonal antibody stimulation system [80], and in colony formation assays for granulocytes and macrophages from normal bone marrow (CFU-GM) [81]. The suppressive activity of such ex-PLT clones for CFU-GM was similar in degree and in MHC-nonrestriction to that mediated by suppressor effector clones and primary NK-like clones. Thus the ex-PLT clones that had become refractory to antigen-specific stimulation without exception acquired nonspecific suppressive activity in all these different systems. At least two mechanisms for suppression were demonstrated, one being the class II-DP-like-dependent induction of suppression in unprimed lymphocyte populations [54], and a second being a direct suppressive effect on activated T cell clones. As a hypothesis to be investigated, this latter type of suppression may also be mediated by the same DP-like molecules. Change of function usually occurred in the face of an unchanged morphology which already displayed large granular lymphocyte (LGL) characteristics for the proliferating class II-specific clones before their acquisition of suppressor and NK-like activities. Thus, the ex-PLT clones never displayed the non-LGL morphology nor the highly potent NK capacity shown by certain other NK clones [82].

Stimulation of class II-restricted influenza virus antigen-specific helper clones with high levels of antigen has been found to render them refractory to subsequent stimulation [83]. No studies of possible acquired suppressive activities by these "tolerized" clones have thus far been reported [84]. In the above system, CD3 molecules were found to be modulated by the the tolerogenic process, suggesting the subsequent lack of expression of the T cell receptor for antigen as an explanation for nonreactivity [85]. Our alloreactive clones are maintained in the necessary intermittent presence of antigen, and could perhaps be "tolerized" in the same way. However, this seems unlikely in view of their retention of expression of cell surface CD3 antigens. Indeed, quantitative FACS analysis suggests even an increased density of CD3 on ex-PLT cells as compared to their younger PLT-active counterparts from the same clone. Should CD3 and T cell receptor structure have become decoupled on these clones, lack of receptor would still provide an explanation for nonresponsiveness. However, practically all available evidence to date, particularly T cell antigen receptor gene transfection experiments, seems to suggest that the expression of CD3 structures and of T cell receptor structures is mutually dependent. Certainly CD3 and the T cell receptor appear to be closely associated on the cell surface, and MoAb or antigen-dependent modulation of either structure results in concomitant modulation of the other, and reexpression of both structures is concordant [86]. However, the inability to abrogate CTX function of some $CD3^+$ CTX clones by CD3 modulation has been reported and could be consistent with decoupling of CD3 and the antigen receptor [87].

When alloproliferative, nonsuppressive PLT clones were purposefully rendered non-antigen-reactive by treatment for 18 h with anti-CD3 antibody, followed by 24 h culture in medium with IL-2, they were found to have acquired strong nonspecific suppressive activity for lymphoproliferative responses in MLC (Fig. 3). This treatment and short-term culture protocol resulted in absolutely CD3-negative cells, about 80% of which were able to reexpress CD3 after a further 5 days in culture. For those clones where reexpression of CD3 was associated with regained alloreactivity, such cells no longer suppressed (Fig. 3). A dramatic

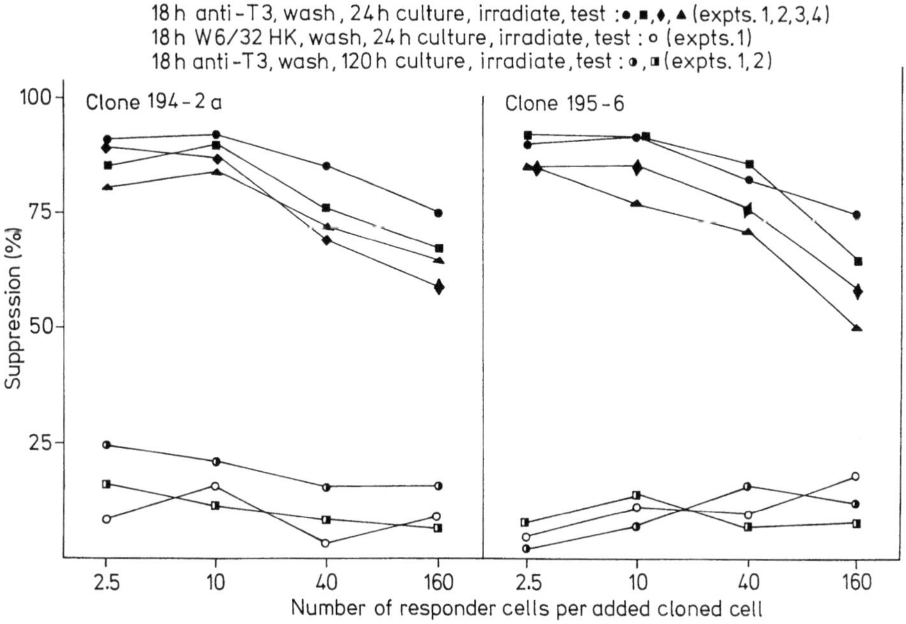

Fig. 3. Reversible induction of MLC suppressive activity in PLT clones by modulation of CD3 antigens: 5×10^6 cells from PLT-active clones 194-2a and 195-6 were cultured for 18 h with 1:100 dilution of ascites from the anti-CD3 monoclonal antibody secreting hybrid SPV-T3b (a gift of J. de Vries, Amsterdam) in medium supplemented with IL-2. The antibody W6/32.HK was employed as a negative control. After washing, the clones were cultured further for 24 h in medium containing IL-2 without antibody. At this point the CD3 antigens were no longer detectable on the cell surface and the clones responded very weakly to alloantigen. They were irradiated and tested for suppression by titration into MLCs, or were cultured for 4-days more in the presence of IL-2 and stimulator-specific filler cells prior to testing for suppression. At this time more than 80% of the cells had reexpressed the CD3 antigens and had regained their specific alloreactivity

modulation of PLT clone reactivity by anti-CD3 antibody had been previously reported by others [88], where NK-like CTX was induced in previously non-CTX cells. It was not investigated whether these clones had also acquired suppressive activity. Murine helper/inducer clones may also rapidly down-regulate antigen receptors after stimulation [89].

More recently, with one particular class II-specific PLT clone we performed systematic recloning experiments at an "age" of 25–28 population doublings (PDs). Surprisingly, the data revealed that about 40% of the recloned PLT clones continued to display solely their alloproliferative specificity after more than 50 PDs. The majority of the recloned cultures, however, had lost alloproliferative capacity as seen in all cases without recloning. Although these results have to be substantiated, they would imply the appearance of a class II-specificity down-regulating influence of certain T cells within a monoclonal population which dominated the total clonal function after about 30 divisions in culture in a preprogrammed fashion. It is not presently clear whether such changes may be reversible, as are the functional consequences of CD3-antibody-induced modulation of the T cell receptor composition on the cell surface. However, if the genes coding for the variable region of the T cell receptor – after analysis with specific cDNA probes in Southern-blot-derived restriction fragment length polymorphisms – should reveal newly detectable rearrangements of alpha and/or beta chain genes, the functional changes correlating to the rearrangement patterns would not be expected to be reversible.

Taking together these data and considerations concerning the changes in specificity of our T cell clones against class II alloantigens, it appears likely that the specific T cell repertoire continues to evolve in activated T cell clones. This conclusion is clearly incompatible with the clonal selection theory in its classical form, but would be compatible with mechanisms generating intraclonal heterogeneity and selecting variants of different functional status from the constantly evolving repertoire.

References

1. Spring B, Fonatsch C, Müller C, Pawelec G, Kömpf J, Wernet P, Ziegler A (1985) Refinement of HLA gene mapping with induced B cell line mutants. Immunogenetics 21:277–291
2. Frelinger JA (1982) Tissue distribution and cellular expression of Ia antigens. In: Ferrone S, David CS (eds) Ia antigens. CRC Press, Boca Raton, pp 37–54
3. Wernet P (1976) Human Ia-type alloantigens: methods of detection, aspects of chemistry and biology, markers for disease states. Transplant Rev 30:271–298
4. Charron DJ, Engleman EG, Benike CJ, McDevitt HO (1980) Ia antigens on alloreactive T cells in man detected by monoclonal antibodies. Evidence for synthesis of HLA-D/DR molecules of the responder type. J Exp Med 152:127s–136s
5. Steeg PS, Moore RN, Johnson HM, Oppenheim JS (1982) Regulation of murine macrophage Ia antigen expression by a lymphokine with immune interferon activity. J Exp Med 156:1780–1793
6. Thorsby E, Berle E, Nousiainen H (1982) HLA-D region molecules restrict proliferative responses to antigen. Immunol Rev 66:39–56
7. Qvigstad E, Thorsby E, Reinsmoen NL, Bach FH (1984) Close association between the Dw14 (LD40) subtype of HLA-DR4 and a restriction element for antigen-specific T cell clones. Immunogenetics 20:583–588
8. Fleischer B, Blaurock M, Wernet P, Pawelec G (1984) Restriction of human influenza A virus-specific T cell clones by HTC-defined subtypes of HLA-Dw6. In: Albert ED, Baur MP, Mayr WR (eds) Histocompatibility Testing 1984. Springer, Berlin Heidelberg New York Tokyo, pp 623–626
9. Bain B, Vas MR, Lowenstein L (1964) The development of large immature mononuclear cells in mixed leukocyte cultures. Blood 23:108–116
10. Yunis EJ, Amos DB (1971) Three closely linked genetic systems relevant to transplantation. Proc Natl Acad Sci USA 68:3031–3035
11. Bradley BA, Edwards JM, Dunn DC, Calne RY (1972) Quantitation of mixed lymphocyte reaction by gene dose phenomenon. Nature 240:54–56
12. Thorsby E, Piazza A (1975) Joint Report. II. Typing for HLA-D (LD-1 or MLC) determinants. In: Kissmeyer-Nielsen F (ed) Histocompatibility Testing 1975. Munksgaard, Copenhagen, pp 414–458
13. Carlsson B, Böhme J, Kalm B, Lundgren G, Möller E, Persson P, Petersen PA, Rask L, Wallin J (1984) HLA-DR and DQ studied with genomic blotting in diabetic families and transplant donor-recipient pairs. In: Albert ED, Baur MP, Mayr WR (eds) Histocompatibility Testing 1984. Springer, Berlin Heidelberg New York Tokyo, p 589
14. Fradelizi D, Dausset J (1975) Mixed lymphocyte reactivity of human lymphocytes primed in vitro. I. Secondary responses to allogeneic lymphocytes. Eur J Immunol 5:295–301
15. Sheehy MJ, Sondel PM, Bach ML, Wank R, Bach FH (1975) HL-A LD (lymphocyte defined) typing: a rapid assay with primed lymphocytes. Science 188:1308–1310
16. Alter BJ, Bach FH, Jaramillo S, Wernet P (1977) Typing an unrelated panel with PLT cells: association with Dw clusters. Scand J Immunol 6:485–489

17. Shaw S, Johnson AH, Shearer GM (1980) Evidence for a new segregant series of B cell antigens that are encoded in the HLA-D region and that stimulate secondary allogeneic proliferative and cytotoxic responses. J Exp Med 152:565–580
18. Bach FH, Inouye H, Hank JA, Alter BJ (1979) Human T lymphocyte clones reactive in primed lymphocyte typing and cytotoxicity. Nature 281:307–309
19. Pawelec G, Wernet P (1980) Restimulation properties of human alloreactive cloned T-cell lines. Dissection of HLA-D-region alleles in population studies and family segregation analyses. Immunogenetics 11:507–519
20. Inouye H, Hank JA, Chardonnens X, Segall M, Alter BJ, Bach FH (1980) Cloned primed lymphocyte test reagents in the dissection of HLA-D. J Exp Med 152:143s–155s
21. Duquesnoy RJ, Zeevi A (1983) Immunogenetic analysis of the HLA complex with T cell clones. Hum Immunol 8:17–23
22. Pawelec G (1983) Allogeneically primed T lymphocyte clones in the analysis of lymphocyte stimulatory determinants. Hum Immunol 8:239–247
23. Eckels DD, Hartzman RJ (1982) Characterisation of human T-lymphocyte clones (TLCs) specific for HLA-region gene products. Immunogenetics 16:117–133
24. Zeevi A, Scheffel C, Annen K, Bass G, Marrari M, Duquesnoy RJ (1982) Association of PLT specificity of alloreactive lymphocyte clones with HLA-DR, MB, and MT determinants. Immunogenetics 16:209–218.23
25. Zeevi A, Duquesnoy RJ (1983) PLT specificity of alloreactive lymphocyte clones for HLA-B locus determinants. Proc Natl Acad Sci USA 80:1440–1444
26. Reinsmoen NL, Anichini A, Bach FH (1983) Clonal analysis of T lymphocytes responding to an isolated class I disparity. Hum Immunol 8:195–206
27. Pawelec G, Shaw S, Wernet P (1982) Analysis of the HLA-linked SB gene system with cloned and uncloned alloreactive T-cell lines. Immunogenetics 15:187–198
28. Bach FH, Reinsmoen NL (1982) Cloned cellular reagents to define antigens encoded between HLA-DR and glyoxylase. Hum Immunol 5:133–138
29. Pawelec G, Shaw S, Schneider M, Blaurock M, Frauer M, Brackertz D, Wernet P (1982) Population studies of HLA-linked SB antigens and their relative importance in MLC typing. Analysis of HLA-D homozygous typing cells and normal heterozygous populations. Hum Immunol 5:215–223
30. Wernet P, Shaw S, Brautbar C, Westphal E, Pawelec G (1983) SB types of HLA-D homozygous typing cells. Immunogenetics 18:547–551
31. Spits H, Borst J, Giphart M, Coligan J, Terhorst C, de Vries JE (1984) HLA-DC can serve as recognition elements for human cytotoxic T lymphocytes. Eur J Immunol 14:299–304
32. Anichini A, Bach FH (1984) HLA-Dw/LD directed cytotoxic T cell clones. Hum Immunol 10:153–164
33. Ohta N, Anichini A, Reinsmoen NL, Strassmann G, Wernet P, Bach FH (1985) Analysis of human class II antigens by cloned cytolytic T cell reagents: a study using loss mutant lymphoblastoid cell lines and monoclonal antibodies detecting the HLA-DP product(s). Hum Immunol 13:21–32
34. Eckels DD, Zeevi A, Beatty PG, Flomenberg N, Goyert S, Knowles RW, Mickelson E, Nepom G, Parham P, Pawelec G, Reinsmoen NL (1985) ASHI workshop summary report: structural and functional relationships of human class II MHC molecules. Hum Immunol (in press)
35. Sheehy MJ, Quintieri FB, Yang SY, Alosco SM, Matsui Y, Yunis EJ, Gabbay KH (1984) HLA antigens of insulin-dependent diabetics. I. PLT colonies detecting Dw10 and a new class II determinant distinct from HLA-D, DR, MB(DC), MT, and SB. Tissue Antigens 23:290–300
36. Pawelec G, Wernet P, Rosenlund R, Blaurock M, Schneider EM (1984) Strong lymphoproliferative suppressive function of clones specific for SB-like antigens. Hum Immunol 9:145–157
37. Zeevi A, Duquesnoy RJ (1985) Recognition of major histocompatibility gene products by human alloreactive T cell clones. In: von Boehmer H, Haas W (eds) T cell clones. Elsevier, Amsterdam, pp 245–262
38. Pawelec G, Shaw S, Ziegler A, Müller C, Wernet P (1982) Differential inhibition of HLA-D- or SB-directed secondary lymphoproliferative responses with monoclonal antibodies detecting human Ia-like determinants. J Immunol 129:1070–1075

39. Wernet P, Ziegler A, Shaw S, Blaurock M, Pawelec G (1983) Monoclonal antibodies against Ia-like antigens inhibiting HLA-D and/or SB-directed secondary proliferative responses. Transplant Proc 15:94–98
40. Crumpton MJ, Bodmer JG, Bodmer WF, Hayes JM, Lindsay J, Rudd CE (1984) Biochemistry of class II antigens: workshop report. In: Albert ED, Baur MP, Mayr WR (eds) Histocompatibility Testing 1984. Springer, Berlin Heidelberg New York Tokyo, pp 29–37
41. Pawelec G, Schneider EM, Wernet P (1985) HLA-DR-, MB- and novel DC-related determinants restrict purified protein derivative of tuberculin (PPD)-stimulated human T cell proliferation. Eur J Immunol 15:12–17
42. Austin P, Trowsdale J, Rudd C, Bodmer W, Feldmann M, Lamb J (1985) Functional expression of HLA-DP genes transfected into mouse fibroblasts. Nature 313:61–64
43. Moen T, de Preval C, Rabourdin-Combe C, Mach B, Gaudernack G, Bondevik E, Thorsby E (1984) Mouse L cells expressing human HLA-DR antigens after transfection with class II genes do not stimulate human T lymphocytes. In: Albert ED, Baur MP, Mayr WR (eds) Histocompatibility Testing 1984. Springer, Berlin Heidelberg New York Tokyo, pp 595–598
44. Rebai N, Malissen B, Pierres M, Accolla RS, Corte G, Mawas C (1983) Distinct HLA-DR epitopes and distinct families of HLA-DR molecules defined by 15 monoclonal antibodies (mAb) either anti-DR or allo-anti-Ia^k cross-reacting with human DR molecule. I. Cross-inhibition studies of mAb cell surface fixation and differential binding of mAb to detergent-solubilised HLA molecules immobilised to a solid phase by a first mAb. Eur J Immunol 13:106–111
45. Beckman IGR, Bradley J, Brooks D, Zola H (1984) Delineation of serologically distinct monomorphic determinants of human MHC class II antigens: evidence of heterogeneity in their topographical distribution. Mol Immunol 21:205–214
46. Charron DJ, Lotteau V, Turmel P (1984) Hybrid HLA-DC antigens provide molecular evidence for gene trans-complementation. Nature 312:157–159
47. Lamb JR, Woody JN, Hartzman RJ, Eckels DD (1982) In vitro influenza virus-specific antibody production in man: antigen-specific and HLA-restricted induction of helper activity mediated by cloned human T lymphocytes. J Immunol 129:1465–1470
48. Qvigstad E, Moen E, Thorsby E (1984) T cell clones with similar antigen specificity may be restricted by DR, MT(DC) or SB class II HLA molecules. Immunogenetics 19:455–460
49. Eckels DD, Lake P, Lamb JR, Johnson AH, Shaw S, Woody JN, Hartzman RJ (1983) SB-restricted presentation of influenza and herpes simplex virus-antigens to human T lymphocyte clones. Nature 301:716–718
50. Rees ADM, Knott G, Lamb JR (1985) Antigen specific human T cell clones: heterogeneity of specificity and function. Behring Inst Mitt 77:75–81
51. Zeevi A, Chiu KM, Duquesnoy RJ (1982) Heterogeneity of cytolytic and suppressor clones of alloactivated cells generated from soft agar colonies. Hum Immunol 5:107–122
52. Pawelec G, Schneider EM, Wernet P (1985) Function of alloproliferative clones correlates better with their class II recognitive specificity than with their cell surface phenotype. Eur J Immunol 15:163–167
53. Pawelec G, Schneider EM, Wernet P (1984) Cloned human T lymphocytes with lymphostimulatory activity preferentially activate suppressor cells. Eur J Immunol 14:335–340
54. Pawelec G, Wernet P (1985) Loss of alloreactivity associated with acquired suppressive and natural killer-like activities of aged T cell clones. In: Feldmann M, Lamb JR, Woody JN (eds) Human T cell clones: a modern approach to immunoregulation. Humana, Clifton, New Jersey p 327–339
55. Wernet P, Betsch C, Barth P, Jaramillo S, Schunter F, Waller HD, Wilms K (1977) Human Ia alloantigens as cell-differentiation markers of normal and pathological leukocyte surfaces. Scand J Immunol 6:563–574
56. Mach B, de Preval C, Gorski J (1984) Molecular genetics of human class II genes and the regulation of their expression. In: Griscelli C, Vossen J (eds) Progress in immunodeficiency research and therapy, vol I. Elsevier, Amsterdam, pp 11–17

57. Newman RA, Delia B, Greaves MF, Navarrete C, Fainboim L, Festenstein H (1983) Differential expression of HLA-DR and DR-linked determinants on human leukemias and lymphoid cells. Eur J Immunol 13:172–177
58. Wernet P, Müller CP, Ostendorf P (1984) Reactivity of lymphocytic and myelocytic leukemia blasts with monoclonal antibodies specific for the different human class II molecules. Dis Markers 2:449–459
59. Long EO, Mach B, Acolla RS (1984) Ia-negative B-cell variants reveal a coordinate regulation in the transcription of the HLA class II gene family. Immunogenetics 19:349–353
60. Goyert SM, Shively JE, Silver J (1982) Biochemical characterization of a second family of human Ia antigens. HLA-DS, equivalent to murine I-A subregion molecules. J Exp Med 156:550–566
61. Wang CY, Al-Katib A, Lane CL, Koznier B, Fu SM (1983) Induction of HLA-DC/DS (Leu 10) antigen expression by human precursor B cell lines. J Exp Med 158:1757–1762
62. Sieff C, Bicknell D, Caine G, Robinson J, Lam G, Greaves MF (1982) Changes in cell surface antigen expression during hematopoietic differentiation. Blood 60:703–713
63. Barth P, Schunter F, Wilms K, Waller HD, Wernet P (1978) Classification of leukemic cells by Ia alloantigens and complement receptors. Bibl Haematologica 45:124–130
64. Gordon LI, Miller WJ, Branda RF, Zanjani ED, Jacob HS (1980) Regulation of erythroid colony formation by bone marrow (BM) macrophages. Blood 55:1047–1050
65. Möller E, Carlsson B, Wallin J (1985) Distinct or overlapping functions of human class II genes? Scand J Immunol 20:483–487
66. Van Voorhis WC, Hair LS, Steinman RM, Kaplan G (1982) Human dendritic cells. Enrichment and characterization from peripheral blood. J Exp Med 155:1172–1187
67. Parwaresch MR, Radzun HJ, Feller AC, Peters K-P, Hansmann M-L (1983) Peroxidase-positive mononuclear leukocytes as possible precursors of human dendritic reticulum cells. J Immunol 131:2719–2725
68. Malissen B, Charmot D, Mawas C (1981) Expansion of human lymphocyte populations expressing specific immune reactivities. III. Specific colonies, either cytotoxic or proliferative, obtained from a population of responder cells primed in vitro. Preliminary immunogenetic analysis. Hum Immunol 2:1–13
69. Effros RB, Walford RL (1984) T cell cultures and the Hayflick limit. Hum Immunol 9:49–65
70. Pawelec G, Wernet P, Rehbein A, Balko I, Schneider EM (1984) Alloproliferative human T cell clones primed and cultured in vitro lose proliferative and gain suppressive activity with age. Hum Immunol 10:135–144
71. von Boehmer H, Kisielow P, Leisseron W, Haas W (1984) $Lyt2^-$ T cell-independent function of Lyt 2^+ cells stimulated with antigen of Concanavalin A. J Immunol 133:59–64
72. Wee S-L, Ochoa AC, Bach FH (1985) Human alloreactive CTL clones: loss and reacquisition of specific cytolytic activity can be regulated by "recombinant" interleukin 2. J Immunol 134:310–313
73. Fleischer B (1984) Acquisition of specific cytotoxic activity by human $T4^+$ lymphocytes in culture. Nature 308:365–367
74. Claesson MH, Miller RG (1985) Functional heterogeneity in allospecific cytotoxic T lymphocyte clones. II. Development of syngeneic cytotoxicity in the absence of specific antigenic stimulation. J Immunol 134:684–690
75. Simon MM, Weltzien H-U, Bühring H-J, Eichmann K (1984) Aged murine killer T cell clones acquire specific cytotoxicity for P815 mastocytoma cells. Nature 308:367–370
76. Acha-Orbea H, Groscurth P, Lang R, Stitz L, Hengartner H (1983) Characterization of cloned cytotoxic lymphocytes with NK-like activity. J Immunol 130:2952–2959
77. Binz H, Fenner M, Frei D, Wigzell H (1983) Two independent receptors allow selective target cell lysis by T cell clones. J Exp Med 157:1252–1260
78. Brooks CG (1983) Reversible induction of natural killer cell activity in cloned murine cytotoxic lymphocytes. Nature 305:155–158
79. Augustin AA, Sim GK (1984) T cell receptors generated via mutations are specific for various histocompatibility antigens. Cell 39:5–12

80. Falcioni F, Pawelec G, Brattig N, Schneider EM, Berg P, Wernet P (1985) Regulation of lymphoproliferation and Ig secretion by lymphocyte clones in man. Immunology 54:685–692
81. Pawelec G, Busch FW, Schneider EM, Rehbein A, Balko I, Wernet P (1985) Acquisition of suppressive and natural killer-like activities associated with loss of alloreactivity in human "helper" T clones. Curr Top Microbiol Immunol (in press)
82. Schneider EM, Pawelec G, Shi LR, Wernet P (1984) A novel type of human T cell clone with highly potent natural killer-like cytotoxicity divorced from large granular lymphocyte morphology. J Immunol 133:173–179
83. Lamb JR, Skidmore BJ, Green N, Chiller JM, Feldmann M (1983) Induction of tolerance in influenza virus-immune T lymphocyte clones with synthetic peptides of influenza hemagglutinin. J Exp Med 157:1434–1447
84. Feldmann M, Zanders ED, Lamb JR (1985) Tolerance in T cell clones. Immunol Today 6:58–62
85. Zanders ED, Lamb JR, Feldmann M, Green N, Beverley PCL (1983) Tolerance of T cell clones is associated with membrane antigen changes. Nature 303:625–627
86. Reinherz EL, Meuer SC, Schlossman SF (1983) The human T cell receptor: analysis with cytotoxic T cell clones. Immunol Rev 74:83–112
87. Moretta A, Pantaleo G, Mingari MC, Moretta L, Cerottini J-C (1984) Clonal heterogeneity in the requirement for T3, T4, and T8 molecules in human cytolytic T lymphocyte function. J Exp Med 159:921–934
88. Spits H, Yssel H, Leeuwenberg J, de Vries JE (1985) Antigen-specific cytotoxic T cell and antigen-specific proliferating T cell clones can be induced to cytolytic activity by monoclonal antibodies against T3. Eur J Immunol 15:88–91
89. Wilde DB, Fitch FW (1984) Antigen-reactive cloned helper T cells. I. Unresponsiveness to antigen restimulation develops after stimulation of cloned helper T cells. J Immunol 132:1632–1638

Regulation and Expression

Modulation of Class II Antigens by Interferons *

F. Ameglio, R. Tosi, N. Tanigaki, A. Dolei

Table of Contents

Introduction

The interferon (IFN) system is composed by a series of antiviral and cell-modulating proteins newly produced by body cells stimulated by foreign substances.

There are three known antigenic types of IFN and a number of subtypes (for a general review see [41]): Alpha-IFN is produced by leukocytes induced by viruses, xenogenic or tumor cells, bacteria, and B-cell mitogens through a mechanism of interactions at cell surface [17], and can prevent spreading of viruses through the bloodstream and enhance the effectiveness of natural barriers (blood-brain, blood-lung, etc.). Beta-IFN is produced by fibroblast and epithelial cells during virus infections, viral RNA being the inducing factor. It diffuses poorly from solid tissues, quickly establishing the antiviral state in the neighboring cells. Gamma-IFN is produced by T cells stimulated by specific antigens or T cell mitogens. All IFNs must be secreted by the producing cell and bind from the outside to specific cell receptor.

The interaction of the secreted IFNs with cell membranes results in the induction of new effector molecules, leading to a multifaceted series of biochemical events resulting in blocking of virus replication and/or spread, regulation of cell growth and differentiation, and modulation of several functions of the immune

* Work supported in part by grants from CNR, Progetto Finalizzato Oncologia, Contratto No 84.00563.44, Progetto Finalizzato Controllo Malattie da Infezione, Contratto No 84.01849.52, and Progetto Finalizzato Ingegneria Genetica e Basi Molecolari delle Malattie Ereditarie, and by USPHS grants AI20251 and CA17276 awarded by the National Institute of Allergy and Infectious Diseases and the National Cancer Institute, Department of Health and Human Services

system. The very potent and widespread immunoregulatory activities of IFNs can be mediated by the effects of inhibition of cell proliferation (long-term effects) and of modulation of specialized functions of cell (short-term effects) independently of cell multiplication. (For a more detailed review of the biological properties of IFNs, see [41]).

Among IFNs, the gamma type presents peculiar features. Its antiviral activity is lower and its modulation of cell functions higher than those of alpha-IFN and beta-IFN. Peculiar to gamma-IFN is the two-step kinetics of cell activation [19]. Moreover, the antitumor activity of this IFN, which is by far the greatest, is due not only to a cytostatic effect, shared by the other two IFNs, but also to a cytocidal action [25]. In addition, IFN-gamma can potentiate, in a synergistic fashion, both the antiviral and the antitumor activities of alpha-IFN and beta-IFN. All these observations imply that gamma-IFN could act as a regulator of cell functions, particularly of those related to the immune system, rather than being a mere antiviral compound.

Since IFNs exert immunoregulatory properties, the possibility arises that these could be performed, at least in part, through the modulation of the expression of the various components of the class I HLA system. Class II antigens of the major histocompatibility complex (MHC) are normally expressed in B cells, activated T cells, macrophages, and other accessory cells. The high complexity of the human class II HLA system is now generally recognized at both DNA and protein levels [1, 37, 67]. At least three families of genes exist: DP, DQ (previously called SB, DC/DS), and DR. At the protein level, three subsets of molecules carrying serologically distinguishable alloantigenic determinants which are quantitatively measurable by immunological methods have been described: DR, DRw52,53 (BR), and DQ. The DR and DRw52,53 (BR) molecules are both controlled by genes of the DR family. They share alpha subunits, but possess different beta subunits [67]. DQ molecules possess distinct alpha and beta chains. (DP molecules are not yet recognizable by specific alloantisera, and therefore cannot be quantitated in our experimental system [15, 35].

In the past 10 years many reports have appeared on the influence of IFNs on MHC products, some of them on the mouse [47, 69], the majority on the human system. The results have been not homogeneous, the variations being attributable to differences in IFN types, cell systems, and detection methods.

The experimental approach which has been most commonly employed is direct cellular binding by polyclonal or, more recently, monoclonal antibodies, utilizing as detection system either fluoresceinated or radiolabeled antibodies. Our experimental approach utilizes a radioimmunoassay (RIA), using either cell lysates or spent culture fluids as competitors of the binding reaction between specific antisera and ^{125}I-labeled class II molecules purified from human lymphoblastoid cell lines [15, 20].

The two methods possess different potentialities and do not always give overlapping results. In fact, by direct binding using cell sorter analysis, the cellular distribution can be defined; by inhibition methods, not only membrane-bound molecules but also cytoplasmic and shed molecules can be quantitated.

In this review we present an outline of our results with RIA and discuss them with reference to the results reported by other groups.

Effects of Interferons on Class II Molecules

Alpha-Interferon

Alpha-interferon has little, if any, effect on class II expression in the cell lines we have tested so far [14, 16, 20–23]. The specificities in the phenotypes of Namalva (lymphoblastoid) and M 14 (melanoma) cell lines were measured in order to test the expression of different loci. Namalva is a DR2, 4; DRw53 (BR4); DQw1, w3 cell. Cell lysates, either before or after IFN treatment, were tested as inhibitors of the specific binding reaction for DR4, DRw53, and DQw1, representing three different loci products. Similarly, M 14 cells [DR4, w6; DRw52 (BR3), DRw53; DQw1, w3] were tested for DR4, DRw53, and DQw1. As shown in Fig. 1, in both cases the effect on all three class II subsets was slight and statistically not significant. In contrast, when either class I molecules (measured by inhibition of binding by a rabbit antiserum directed against the beta chain) or beta$_2$-microglobulin (B-2-M) were tested, an evident increase was seen (Fig. 1 A and B).

The same molecules were also quantitated in the culture fluids, by testing their inhibiting capacity on the different binding reactions. Significant concentrations

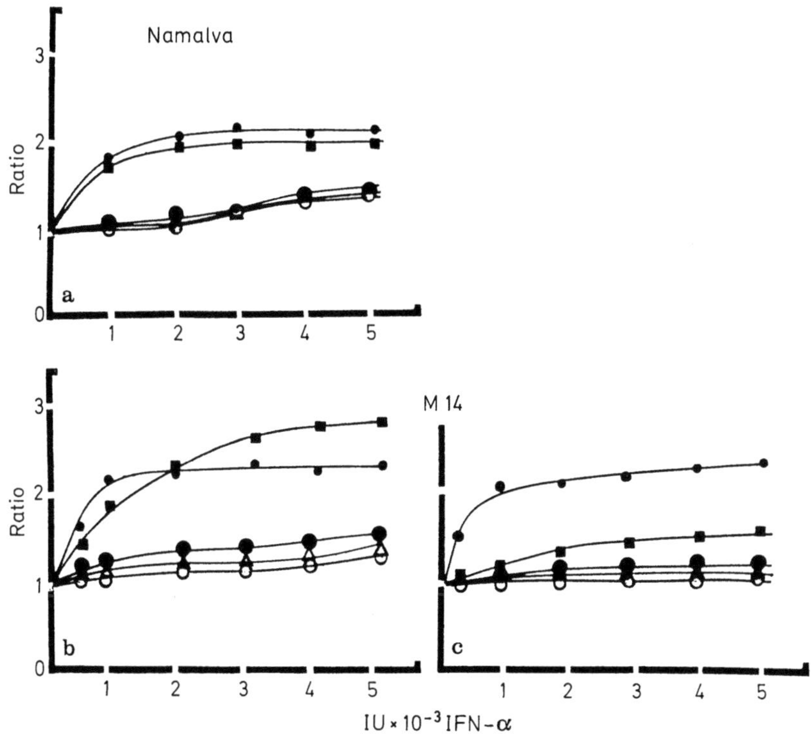

Fig. 1 a–c. Expression of class I (■), B-2-M (●), DR4 (△), DQw3 (●), and DRw53 (○) in Namalva (**a**) and M 14 (**b, c**) cells treated with different amounts of alpha-IFN for 48 h. Results are expressed as ratio of treated/untreated values. Base means (inhibition units $_{50}$/10^6 cells) were: *Namalva:* class I = 12, B-2-M = 11, DR4 = 150, DQw3 = 20, DRw53:126; *M 14:* class I = 13, B-2-M = 98, DR4 = 92, DQw3 = 6, DRw53 = 126. **a, b** cell-associated antigens; **c** shed antigens. Values obtained with 5000 IU/ml alpha-IFN on class I and B-2-M were significantly different from controls ($p < 0.01$). Differences of class II values were not significant of "shed" molecules were found in the media. These varied according to the cell line tested (more "shedding" in M 14 than in Namalva) and the specific locus product, with no defined or predictable pattern. With reference to the cell concentration in the culture, the shed molecules represent a fraction of cell-associated molecules varying from 7% to 100%. Alpha-IFN showed no effect on shed class II molecules (Fig. 1 C). Note the "dissociation" between B-2-M and class I shedding in the same cell line.

There is general agreement in the literature on the increased expression of class I and B-2-M and a lack of effect on class II by alpha-IFN. This was first observed on mouse leukemia L1210 cells, thymocytes, splenocytes, and embryo fibroblasts [44–48], even though in the mouse only mixed alpha- + beta-IFN preparations were used. Subsequent reports on human systems indicated no effect of alpha-IFN on class II or DR antigen expression in melanoma, fibroblastoid, and lymphoblastoid cell lines [3–5, 20, 24, 36, 43, 70, 72, 81]. More recently, however, in melanoma cells, in normal human peripheral blood monocytes, and in myelomonocytoid cell lines, an increase of DR was found follwing treatment with recombinant [6, 29, 66] or native [55] alpha-IFN. These contradictory results may reflect the type and stage of differentiation of the cell exposed to the IFN action.

Interestingly, it has been reported that alpha-IFN and also beta-IFN increased the synthesis of class II HLA mRNAs in several human B lymphoid and melanoma cell lines without increasing membrane expression, indicating that other regulatory mechanisms, operating at the translational and post-translational level, were involved [57].

Beta-Interferon

Beta-interferon was shown to affect class II expression significantly. Dolei et al. [20] reported in 1981 an increased expression and shedding of these molecules in human melanoma and B lymphoblastoid cell lines by pure beta-IFN. A panel of cell lines [14, 20] was tested to see whether the effect of natural beta-IFN on class II molecules was a general phenomenon: M 14 and M 10 (melanoma) and Namalva (B lymphoblastoid) cells were found sensitive to its action. No induction was observed in class II-negative cell lines: E1SM (normal embryo fibroblasts), MG-63 (osteosarcoma), Hep-2 (larynx carcinoma), HeLa (cervical carcinoma), and Molt-4 (T lymphoblastoid) [14, 20, 21].

Figure 2 shows class I, B-2-M, and class II expression in M 14 and Namalva cells treated with graded concentrations of beta-IFN. All three antigens tested were affected by IFN treatment, but class I and B-2-M were more markedly influenced.

Kinetically, expression reached a peak after 48 h treatment and declined thereafter (Fig. 3); the average increase of class II molecules ranged between 1.5-fold and threefold and was lower than that of class I molecules. The shedding of class II molecules in the culture media was also found to be increased. No major differences in the increase of expression of DR, DQ, and DRw52 and 53 products was observed either in Namalva or in M 14 cells.

Enhancement of class II expression by beta-IFN was later confirmed. Giacomini et al. [29] found that recombinant beta-IFN, but not three subtypes of alpha-IFN, enhanced the expression of class II molecules in Colo 38 melanoma cells, the effect being more marked on DQ than on DR antigens. On normal pe-

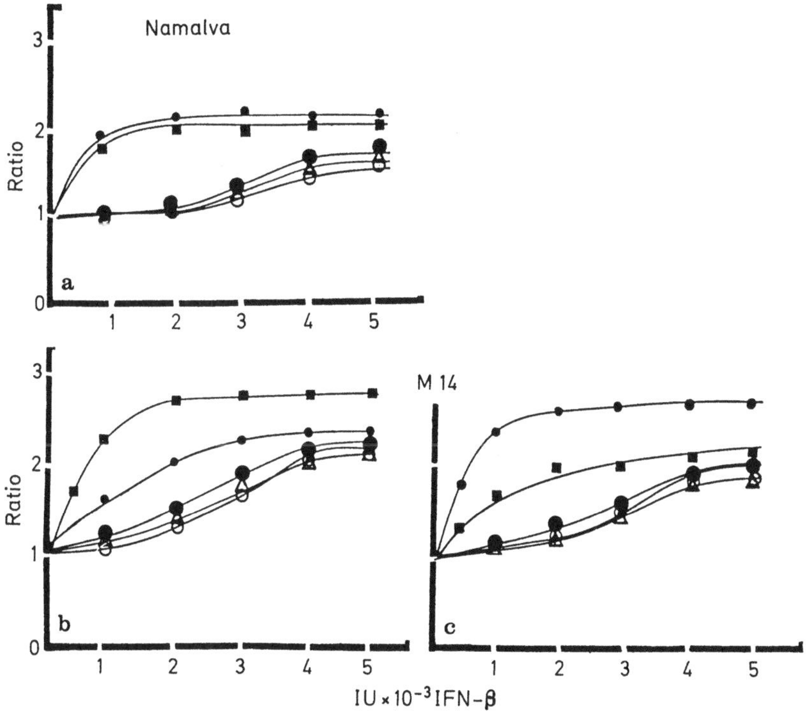

Fig. 2 a–c. Expression of class I (■), B-2-M (●), DR4 (△), DQw3 (●), and DRw53 (○) in Namalva (**a**) and M 14 (**b, c**) cells treated with graded amounts of beta-IFN for 48 h. Results are expressed as ratio of treated/untreated values. Base means are as in Fig. 1. Values obtained with 5000 IU/ml beta-IFN were significantly different from controls ($p < 0.01$ for all products). **A, B** cell-associated antigens; **C** shed antigens

ripheral blood monocytes recombinant Hu-beta-IFN enhanced the expression of DQ and DR [6]. In contrast, no effect of beta-IFN was reported on the Ramos B lympholastoid cell line [72] or on skin Langerhans cells [6]. No change in the percentage of DR-positive cells was found in three myelomonocytoid cell lines (HL60, U937, THP1) treated with native beta-IFN for 3 days by Virelizier et al. [70], nor did beta-IFN induce increased class II expression on bone-marrow-derived macrophages in mouse [59].

Some of these negative results may be due to the particular cell line used, and other cases could possibly be explained by variation in the sensitivity to IFN of different strains from the same cell line. In several reports the antiviral state of the cell was not stated. Another possible explanation of discrepancies could be due to the different methodologies employed.

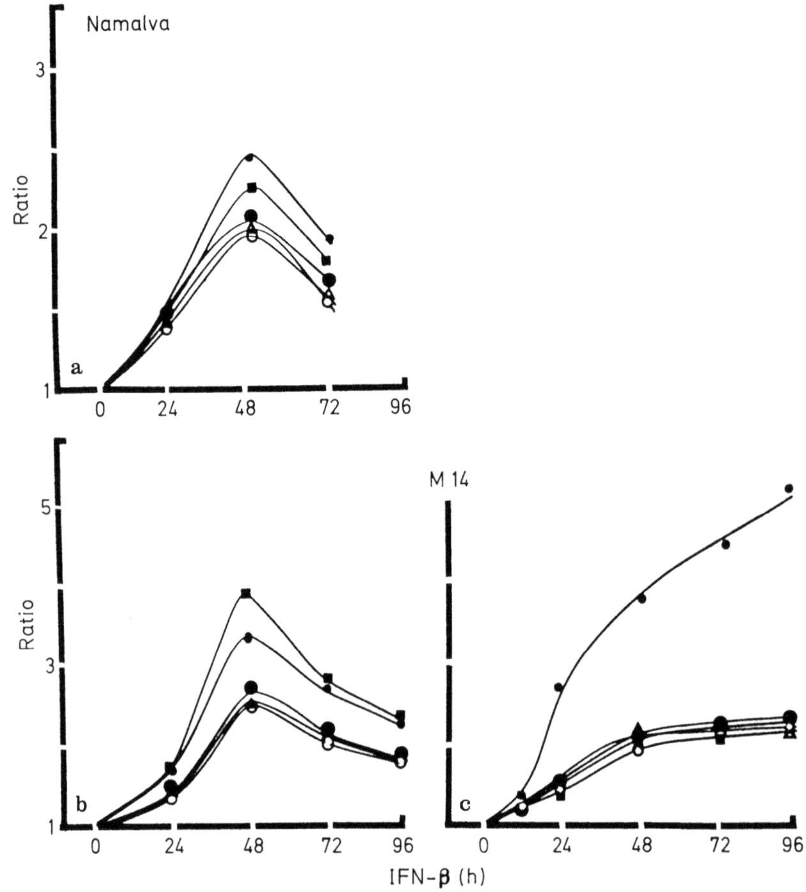

Fig. 3 a–c. Expression of class I (■), B-2-M (●), DR4 (△), DQw3 (●), and DRw53 (○) in Namalva (**a**) and M 14 (**b, c**) cells treated with 5000 IU/ml beta-IFN. Data are expressed as ratio of treated/untreated values. Base levels are as in Fig. 1. **a, b** cell-associated molecules; **c** shed molecules. Statistical significance of increases obtained after 48 h is reported in Fig. 2

Gamma-Interferon

Gamma-interferon has a much greater effect on class II expression than alpha-IFN and beta-IFN [21]. Plateau levels of increase are reached with gamma-IFN concentrations ranging between 50 and 100 IU/ml, as opposed to 2000–5000 IU/ml of beta-IFN. On the basis of the IFN concentration required to obtain 50% of maximum effect, gamma-IFN can be calculated to be 300–600 times more active than beta-IFN as regards class II enhancement [21]. Natural and recombinant gamma-IFN have similar efficiency [1, 15].

Figure 4 shows the effect of recombinant gamma-IFN on M 14 cells. Modulation of the three different class II subsets was separatedly analyzed. DQ is very sensitive to gamma-IFN: up to 14 times more DQ is expressed than in untreated controls. DR and DRw53 (BR4) are also increased, but to a lesser extent (two- to threefold) [1]. A preferential DQ enhancement was observed also in Namalva cells (Fig. 4, lower part) but the differences between DR and DQ, although sta-

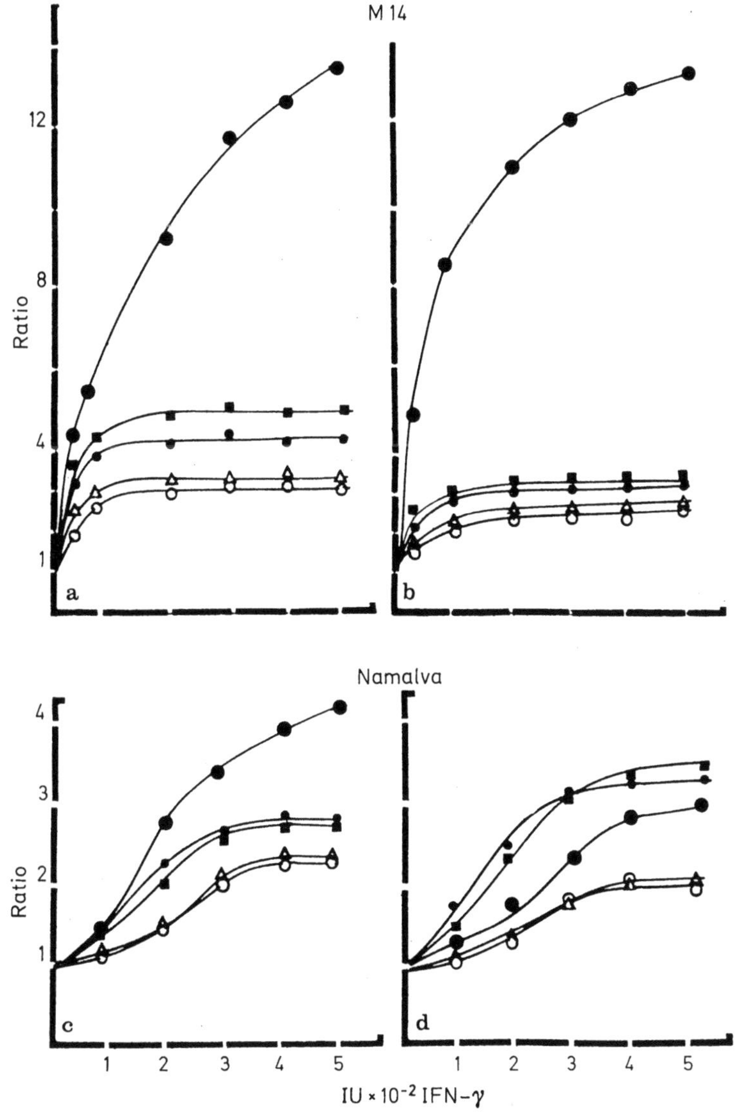

Fig. 4 a, b. Increase of cell-associated (**a**) and shed (**b**) class I (■), B-2-M (●), DR4 (△), DQw3 (●), and DRw53 (○) in M 14 and Namalva cells treated with recombinant gamma-IFN for 48 h. Data are expressed as ratio of treated/untreated values. Base values are as in Fig. 1. Statistical significance for M 14 cells was $p<0.01$ for all antigens except DQ ($p<0.001$), and in Namalva cells, $p<0.01$ for all products

tistically significant, are smaller. Gamma-IFN determines essentially the same effects on normal cells too, as shown by the data of Fig. 5, obtained in normal peripheral blood mononuclear cells (PBMC).

M 14 and Namalva cells are heterozygous at both DR and DQ loci. Thus, it was possible to follow the behavior of both allelic products. As shown in Table 1, the extent of enhancement by gamma-IFN of the two alleles at each locus is modified in a parallel fashion. The same comparison could not be performed on

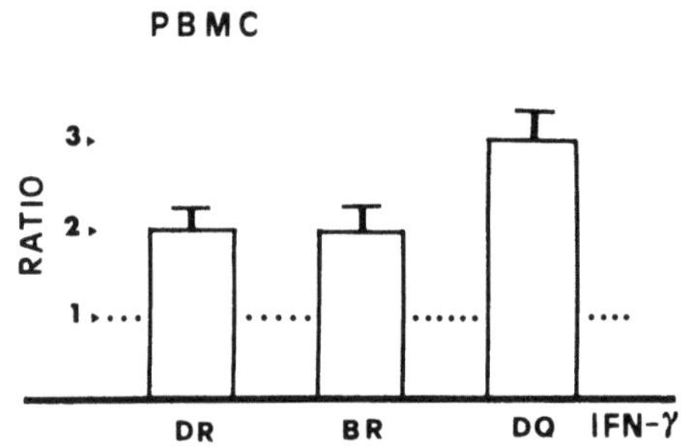

Fig. 5. Expression of DR, DQ, and DRw53 (BR4) in PBMC treated with/without recombinant gamma-IFN (300 IU/ml) for 48 h. Data are expressed as ratio of treated/untreated values and represent the mean increases ± standard deviation for six donors with different haplotypes

Table 1. Expression of allelic products at the DR and DQ loci in M 14 and Namalva cells with and without treatment with 300 IU/ml recombinant Hu-gamma-IFN for 48 h

M 14				Namalva			
	Without gamma-IFN	With gamma-IFN	R	IFN	Without gamma-IFN	With gamma-IFN	R
DR4	92±4	244±10	2.7	DR4	150±7	310±12	2.1
DRw6	75±3	188± 8	2.5	DR2	17±3	33± 5	1.9
DQw3	6±1	64± 5	10.7	DQw3	20±3	63± 7	3.2
DQw1	26±2	262±12	10.0	DQw1	6±1	19± 3	3.1

Data are expressed as inhibition units$_{50}$/10^6 cells (mean ± SD of five experiments). R, ratio of expression by treated/untreated cultures. No statistical significance was found between the increase of the two alleles at each locus

DRw52 and 53 (BR) molecules, because to date only a single DRw BR specificity, DRw53 (BR4), can be quantitated by RIA.

The preferential effect on DQ is also shown by kinetic studies (Fig. 6). A significant enhancement is detectable after as little as 6 h treatment, and plateau levels are not reached even after 3–4 days of culture. As to the DR locus, the action of gamma-IFN is detectable after a 20-h interval, and plateau levels are reached. The same is found for DRw53 (BR4) products [15].

In conclusion, gamma-IFN seems to act on different class II genes by a fine tuning modulation and not by an uniform variation of their expression. Class I antigens and B-2-M are also increased by IFN-gamma to about the same extent as by alpha-IFN and beta-IFN, but lower concentrations are required.

All tested MHC products are shed and accumulate in the culture fluids in a pattern that closely resembles their cellular expression.

In the literature there is almost general agreement concerning the enhancing effects of gamma-IFN on class II products in class II-positive cells. In 1980, using mouse-lymphokine-enriched supernatants, Beller et al. [8, 58] showed an increase of class II-positive macrophages. This effect was subsequently shown to be due to gamma-IFN. IFN-containing lymphokine preparations were also effective in enhancing class II expression in monocytes and macrophages [39, 49, 60, 61, 63–65]. In 1981, Sonnenfeld et al. [62] reported an increase in the number of thymocytes bearing high levels of class II, Ly-1, and Ly-2,3 after treatment with partially purified mouse type II IFN. In the past 2 years several reports have appeared in-

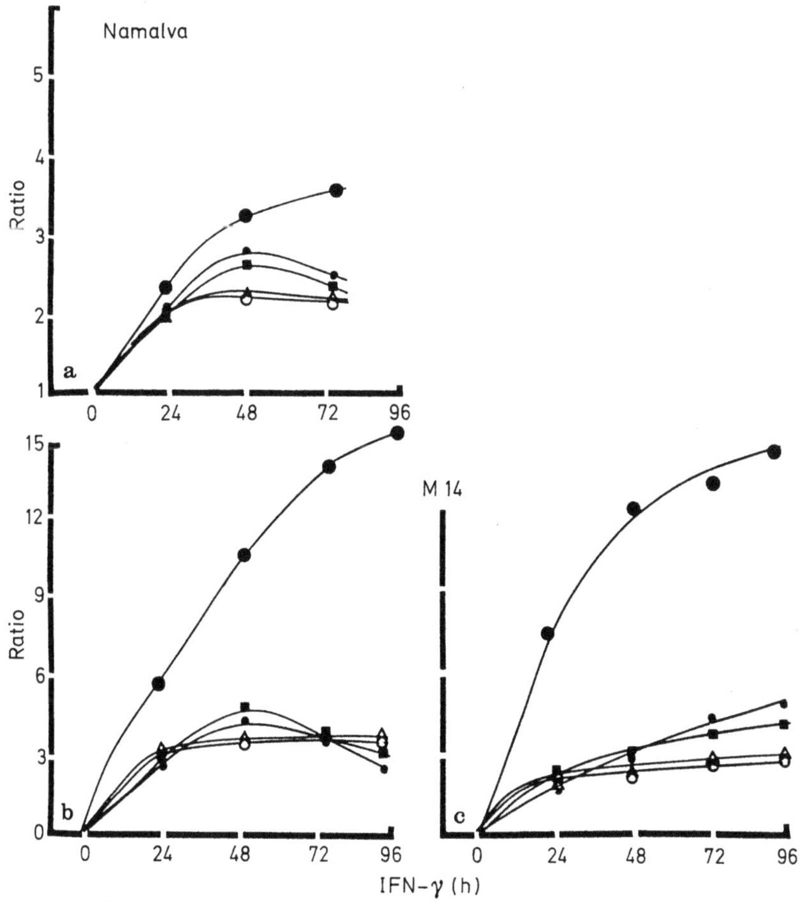

Fig. 6 a–c. Expression of class I (■), B-2-M (●), DR4 (△), DQw3 (●), and DRw53 (○) in Namalva (**a**) and M 14 (**b, c**) cells treated with 300 IU/ml gamma-IFN. Data are expressed as ratio of treated/untreated values. Base levels as in Fig. 1. **A, B** cell-associated molecules; **C** shed molecules

dicating an increase of expression of class II antigens in cells treated with native [1, 7, 21, 34] or recombinant gamma-IFN [6, 7, 15, 18, 31, 32, 34, 66, 70], most of them in human systems, using normal monocytes, PBMC, thymocytes, or cell lines of melanoma, B lymphoid, and monocytoid origin.

IFN doses ranged between 50 and 2000 IU/ml, although results were obtained with as few as 2 IU/ml [34, 70]. One report by Wallach et al. [72], using 200 IU/ml gamma-IFN, indicated no change in surface DR antigens or in 2-5(A)-synthetase activity in Ramos B lymphoblastoid cells, even though another paper by the same group showed increased levels of class II mRNAs in several human B lymphoid and in some melanoma cell lines [57].

The preferential effect of gamma-IFN on DQ [1, 2, 23] was confirmed by Basham and coworkers [6] in human monocytes and by Giacomini et al. [30] in Colo 38 melanoma cells. Robbins et al. [56], analyzing the effect of gamma-IFN on normal human monocytes, reported a parallel increase of DR and DQ, though a close examination of their data may suggest a preferential *relative* DQ enhancement.

As for the mechanism of enhancement of class II antigen expression by gamma-IFN, the increase was not due to decreased shedding, as shedding was also increased [15, 21]. All published data indicated increased synthesis of class II mRNA in gamma-IFN-treated cells [5, 50, 57] and a transcriptional control by gamma-IFN [52]. Moreover, when class II genes are transfected in different host cells, they are regulated by gamma-IFN from the same species as the host cell [26].

Up to now, we have been considering the enhancing of IFNs in cells which already expressed appreciable amounts of class II molecules. A biologically distinct effect is the more recently described phenomenon of gamma-IFN-induced class II induction. This was shown in mast cell progenitors [74], in precursor B cell lines [73], in T-dependent mast cells [42, 76] (in which the effect is opposed by P cell stimulating factor and glucocorticoids), and in hemopoietic, lymphoid, epithelial, fibroblastic, and neuronal cells [75, 77]. Brain cells can be induced by gamma-IFN to express class II antigens both in vitro and in vivo [78]. Vascular endothelial cells [53, 54], macrophages [38, 40] and normal embryo fibroblasts [23, 54, 77] can also be induced by gamma-IFN to produce high levels of class II antigens. The most extensive analysis of gamma-IFN induction on human cell lines has been performed by Houghton et al. [34]. Class II-negative melanoma and other tumor cell lines were induced to express class II antigens by gamma-IFN. An example of class II induction is shown in Table 2. Basal levels of class II molecules on normal diploid fibroblasts were under the detection limits of RIA, and upper limits only are given. Treatment of cells with 200 IU/ml recombinant gamma-IFN induced levels of class II antigens comparable, on a per cell basis, to those in normal B lymphocytes.

Some cell lines cannot be induced by gamma-IFN to express class II antigens, notably class II-negative lines of T lymphoid origin [2, 23] and choriocarcinoma, teratocarcinoma, and neuroblastoma cells [34] even though the last-named could be induced to express class I products.

Collins et al. [18] analyzed gamma-IFN induction of DP, DQ, and DR expression separately and found levels of expression of DQ comparable to those of the other subsets.

Gonwa and Stobo [32] reported that normal monocytes become DR-negative and DQ-negative when kept in culture for at least 4 days; class II expression could be reinduced by subsequent treatment of the cells with recombinant gamma-IFN, up to levels similar to those observed in fresh cells. Another antigen, MAC 120, correlated strictly with DQ antigen expression. Whether or not gamma-IFN cause true induction in this system is hard to define, however, as less than 30000 DQ molecules/cell is not detectable by the flow cytometry assay used.

Table 2. Expression of overall class II molecules in normal diploid E1SM fibroblasts plus IFNs for 96 h

	Control	Alpha-IFN	Beta-IFN	Gamma-IFN
Inhibition $units_{50}/10^6$ cells	<0.3	<0.3	<0.3	28.5

Alpha-IFN and beta-IFN (native): 5000 IU/ml
Gamma-IFN (recombinant): 500 IU/ml

Possible Biological Significance

After summarizing the data concerning the relationship between IFNs and class II antigens, one should consider the biological meaning of such interactions. A starting point is necessarily the role of class II molecules in antigen presentation. This has been determined in functional studies involving interaction with the T cell receptor, the antigen, or both [68], but there is no convincing biochemical evidence for such interactions. Thus the mechanism and regulation of this process can only be matters of speculation.

It is tempting to seek a role of class II molecule enhancement in antiviral defenses, since more efficient antigen presentation in the presence of IFN could be biologically important. This is especially likely in the case of macrophages, the cells normally involved in this phenomenon, for which it has been shown that antigen presentation correlates with class II levels [7, 9, 10, 27, 28, 50, 71]. However, it is possible that also other cell types, upon induction of class II molecules, may become antigen-presenting cells [31, 33]. Good candidates may be endothelial and fibroblast cells [33, 54]. The antigen-presenting ability of mouse fibroblasts [51] transfected with human class II genes has recently been demonstrated.

As to the preferential enhancement of DQ expression by gamma-IFN which was observed in class II-positive cells, it must be remembered that DQ has been attributed a major role in antigen presentation by macrophages, since DQ-positive cells are especially involved in this function [31]. It should be noted, however, that induction in class II-negative cells is preferentially exerted on DP and DR rather than DQ [18].

A further biolgical implication concerns autoimmune diseases. It can be hypothesized that the immune response against self antigens is produced by either presentation at a higher level of efficiency or by cells which normally do not act as presenting cells [12, 13]. If this is the case, the class II-enhancing property of gamma-IFN, which in turn is produced during responses to infections, could facilitate induction of autoimmunity. This is in keeping with the high levels of IFN observed in autoimmune diseases [80].

References

1. Ameglio F, Capobianchi MR, Dolei A, Tosi R (1983) Differential effects of gamma interferon on expression of HLA class II molecules controlled by the DR and DC loci. Infect Immun 42:122–125
2. Ameglio F, Dolei A, Capobianchi MR, Tosi R (1984) Preferential increase of expression and release of DC molecules in human cells treated with interferon. In: Albert ED, Baur MP, Mayr WR (eds) Histocompatibility testing 1984. Springer, Berlin Heidelberg New York Tokyo, p 549
3. Attallah AM, Strong DM (1979) Differential effects of interferon on the MHC expression of human lymphocytes: enhanced expression of HLA without effect on Ia. Int Arch Allergy Appl Immunol 60:101–107
4. Basham TY, Bourgeade MF, Creasey A, Merigan TC (1983) Interferon increases HLA synthesis in melanoma cells: interferon resistant and sensitive cell lines. Proc Natl Acad Sci USA 79:3265–3269
5. Basham TY, Merigan TC (1983) Recombinant interferon gamma increases HLA-DR synthesis and expression. J Immunol 130:1492–1494

6. Basham TY, Smith W, Lanier L, Morhenn V, Merigan T (1984) Regulation of expression of class II major histocompatibility antigens on human peripheral blood monocytes and Langerhans cells by interferon. Hum Immunol 10:83–93
7. Becker S (1984) Interferons as modulators of human monocyte-macrophage differentiation. I. Interferon gamma increases HLA-DR expression and inhibits phagocytosis of zymosan. J Immunol 132:1249–1254
8. Beller DI, Kiely JM, Unanue ER (1980) Regulation of macrophage populations. I. Preferential induction of Ia-rich peritoneal exudates by immunologic stimuli. J Immunol 124:1426–1432
9. Beller DI (1984) Functional significance of the regulation of macrophage Ia expression. Eur J Immunol 2:138–143
10. Birmingham JR, Chesnut RW, Kappler JW, Marrak P, Kubo R, Grey HM (1982) Antigen presentation to T cell hybridomas by a macrophage cell line: an inducible function. J Immunol 128:1491–1492
11. Bodmer JG, Bodmer WF (1984) Monoclonal antibodies to HLA determinants. Br Med Bulletin 40:267–275
12. Bottazzo GF, Pujol-Burrel R, Hanafusa T, Feldmann N (1983) Role of aberrant HLA-DR expression and antigen presentation in induction of endocrine autoimmunity. Lancet II:1115–1119
13. Bondei M, Lamb JR, Bottazzo GF, Feldmann M (1984) Epithelial cells expressing aberrant MHC class II determinants can present antigen to cloned human T cells. Nature 312:639–641
14. Capobianchi MR, Ameglio F, Dolei A, Tosi R (1982) Expression of MHC products in human cell lines treated with interferons. In: Revoltella R, Pontieri GM, Basilico C, Rovera G, Gallo RM, Subak-Sharpe JH (eds) Expression of differentiated functions in cancer cells. Raven, New York, pp 457–487
15. Capobianchi MR, Ameglio F, Tosi R, Dolei A (1985) Differences in the expression and release of DR, BR, and DQ molecules in human cells trated with recombinant interferon gamma. Comparison to the other interferons. Hum Immunol 13:1–11
16. Capobianchi MR, Ameglio F, Tosi R, Dolei A (1984) Modulation of Ia antigens by interferons in human lymphoblastoid cells. In: Aaronson S, Frati L, Verna R (eds) Genetic and phenotypic markers of tumors. Plenum, New York, pp 217–222
17. Capobianchi MR, Facchini J, Di Marco P, Antonelli G, Dianzani F (1985) Induction of alpha interferon by membrane interaction between viral surface and peripheral blood mononuclear cells. Proc Soc Exp Biol Med 178:551–556
18. Collins T, Korman AS, Wake CT, Boss JM, Kappes DJ, Fiers W, Ault KA, Gimbrone MA Jr, Strominger JL, Pober JS (1984) Immune interferon activates multiple class II histocompatibility complex genes and the associated invariant chain gene in human endothelial cells and dermal fibroblasts. Proc Natl Acad Sci USA 81:4917–4921
19. Dianzani F, Zucca M, Scupham A, Georgiades JA (1980) Immune and virus-induced interferons may activate cells by different derepression mechanisms. Nature 283:400–402
20. Dolei A, Ameglio F, Capobianchi MR, Tosi R (1981) Human beta type interferon enhances the expression and shedding of Ia-like antigens. Comparison to HLA-A,B,C and Beta$_2$-microglobulin. Antiviral Res 1:367–381
21. Dolei A, Capobianchi MR, Ameglio F (1983) Human interferon gamma enhances the expression and shedding of class I and class II MHC products in neoplastic cells better than interferon alpha and interferon beta. Infect Immun 40:172–176
22. Dolei A, Ameglio F, Capobianchi MR, Tosi R (1984) Membrane changes induced by interferons in human neoplastic cells. In: Aaronson S, Frati L, Verna R (eds) Genetic and phenotypic markers of tumors. Plenum, New York, pp 211–216
23. Dolei A, Ameglio F, Tosi R (1985) DQ locus products are the preferential Ia target for recombinant interferon gamma. In: Kirchner H, Schellekens H (eds) The biology of the interferon system. Elsevier, Amsterdam, pp 437–440
24. Fellous M, Nir U, Wallach D, Merlin G, Rubinstein M, Revel M (1982) Interferon-dependent induction of mRNA for the major histocompatibility antigens in human fibroblasts and lymphoblastoid cells. Proc Natl Acad Sci USA 79:3082–3086
25. Fleischmann RW (1982) Potentiation of the direct anticellular activity by mouse interferons: mutual synergism and interferon concentration dependence. Cancer Res 42:869–872

26. Folsom V, Gold DP, White J, Marrack P, Kappler J, Tonegawa S (1984) Functional and inducible expression of a transfected murine class II major histocompatibility complex gene. Proc Natl Acad Sci USA 81:2045–2049
27. Gerrard TL, Jurgensen CH, Fauci AS (1983) Differential effect of monoclonal anti-DR antibody on monocytes in antigen- and mitogen-stimulated responses: mechanisms of inhibition and relationship to Interleukin 1 secretion. Cell Immunol 82:394–402
28. Gerrard TL, Cupps TR, Jurgensen CH, Fauci AS (1984) Hydrocortisone-mediated inhibition of monocyte antigen presentation: dissociation of inhibitory effect and expression of DR antigens. Cell Immunol 85:330–339
29. Giacomini P, Aguzzi A, Pestka S, Fisher PB, Ferrone S (1984) Modulation by recombinant DNA leukocyte (alpha) and fibroblast (beta) interferons of the expression and shedding of HLA and tumor-associated antigens by melanoma cells. J Immunol 133:1649–1655
30. Giacomini P, Aguzzi A, Ferrone S (1984) Changes in synthesis of MHC antigens induced by recombinant immune interferon (IFN gamma) in human melanoma cells. ASBC/AAI Meeting, St Louis, June 3–7, 1984
31. Gonwa TA, Picker LJ, Raff HV, Goyert SM, Silver J, Stobo JD (1983) Antigen-presenting capabilities of human monocytes correlates with their expression of HLA-DS, an Ia determinant distinct from HLA-DR. J Immunol 130:706–711
32. Gonwa TA, Stobo JD (1984) Differential expression of Ia molecules by human monocytes. J Clin Invest 74:859–866
33. Hirschberg H, Braathen LR, Thorsby E (1982) Antigen presentation by vascular endothelial cells and epidermal Langerhans cells: the role of HLA-DR. Immunol Rev 66:57–77
34. Houghton AN, Thomson TM, Gross D, Oettgen HF, Old LJ (1984) Surface antigens of melanoma and melanocytes. Specificity of induction of Ia antigens by human gamma interferon. J Exp Med 160:255–269
35. Hurley CK, Show S, Nadler L, Schlossmann S, Capra JD (1982) Alpha and beta chains of SB and DR antigens are structurally distinct. J Exp Med 156:1557–1569
36. Imai K, Ng AK, Glassy C, Ferrone S (1982) Differential effect of interferon on the expression of tumor-associated antigens and histocompatibility antigens on human melanoma cell: relationship to susceptibility to immune lysis mediated by monoclonal antibodies. J Immunol 127:505–508
37. Kauffman JF, Auffray C, Korman AJ, Shackelford DA, Strominger J (1984) The class II molecules of the human and murine major histocompatibility complex. Cell 36:1–26
38. Keley WE, Fiers W, Strom TB (1984) Cloned human interferon gamma, but not interferon-beta or -alpha, induces expression of HLA determinants by fetal monocytes and myeloid leukemic cell lines. J Immunol 132:240–244
39. Kim KJ, Chaouat G, Leiserson WM, King J, Maeyer E (1983) Characterization of T-cell soluble factors modulating the expression of Ia and H-2 antigens on BALB/c B lymphoma cell lines. Cell Immunol 76:253–267
40. King DP, Jones PP (1983) Induction of Ia and H-2 antigens on a macrophage cell line by immune interferon. J Immunol 131:315–318
41. Kirchner H, Schellekens H (eds) (1985) The biology of the interferon system. Elsevier, Amsterdam
42. Koch N, Wong GHW, Schrader JW (1984) Ia antigens and associated invariant chain are induced simultaneously in lines of T-dependent mast cells by recombinant interferon gamma. J Immunol 132:1361–1369
43. Liao SK, Kwong PC, Khosravi M, Dent PB (1982) Enhanced expression of melanoma associated antigens and Beta$_2$-microglobulin on cultured human melanoma cells by interferon. J Natl Cancer Inst 68:19–26
44. Lindhal P, Leary P, Gresser I (1972) Enhancement by interferon of the specific cytotoxicity of sensitized lymphocytes. Proc Natl Acad Sci USA 69:721–725
45. Lindhal P, Leary P, Gresser I (1973) Enhancement by interferon of the expression of surface antigens on murine L_{1210} cells. Proc Natl Acad Sci USA 70:2785–2788
46. Lindhal P, Gresser I, Leary P, Tovey M (1976) Interferon treatment of mice: enhanced expression of histocompatibility antigens on lymphoid cells. Proc Natl Acad Sci USA 73:1284–1287

47. Lonai P, Steinman L (1977) Physiological regulation of antigen binding to T cell: role of a soluble macrophage factor and of interferon. Proc Natl Acad Sci USA 74:5662–5666
48. Lu CY, Unanue ER (1982) Spontaneous T-cell lymphokine production and enhanced macrophage Ia expression and tumoricidal activity in MLR-Lpr mice. Clin Immunol Immunopathol 25:313–222
49. McNicholas JM, King DP, Jones PP (1983) Biosynthesis and expression of Ia and H-2 antigens on a macrophage cell line are stimulated by products of activated spleen cells. J Immunol 130:449–456
50. Nakamura M, Manser T, Pearson GDN, Dalay MJ, Gefter ML (1984) Effect of the interferon-gamma on the immune response in vivo and on gene expression in vitro. Nature 307:381–382
51. Norcross MA, Bentley DM, Margulies DH, Germain RN (1984) Membrane Ia expression and antigen-presenting accessory cell function of L cells transfected with class II major histocompatibility complex genes. J Exp Med 160:1316–1337
52. Peterlin BM, Gonwa TA, Stobo JD (1984) Expression of HLA-DR by a human monocyte cell line is under transcriptional control. J Mol Cell Immunol 1:191–200
53. Pober JS, Gimbrone MA, Cotran RS, Reiss CS, Burakoff SJ, Fiers W, Ault KA (1983) Ia expression by vascular endothelium is induced by activated T cells and by human gamma interferon. J Exp Med 157:1339–1353
54. Pober JS, Collins T, Gimbrone MA, Cotran RS, Gitlin JD, Fiers W, Clayberger C, Krensky AM, Burakoff SJ, Reis CS (1983) Lymphocytes recognizes human vascular endothelial and dermal fibroblasts Ia antigens induced by recombinant immune interferon. Nature 305:726–729
55. Rhodes J, Stokes P (1982) Interferon-induced changes in the monocyte membrane: inhibition by retinol and retinoic acid. Immunology 45:531–538
56. Robbins PA, Brodsky FM, Warner NL, Maino VC (1984) Induction of class II antigens on monocytes cultured with gamma interferon. Dis Markers 2:267–279
57. Rosa F, Hatat D, Abadie A, Wallach D, Revel M, Fellous M (1983) Differential regulation of HLA-DR mRNAs and cell surface antigens by interferon. EMBO J 9:1585–1589
58. Sher MG, Beller DI, Unanue ER (1980) Demonstration of a soluble mediator that induces exudates reach in Ia-positive macrophages. J Exp Med 152:1684–1690
59. Schook LB, Guttman DH, Marlin ME, Niederhuber JE (1984) In vitro-derived bone marrow macrophages. Expression of Ia antigens during macrophage differentiation. Transplantation 37:585–590
60. Smith BR, Ault K (1981) Increase of surface Ia-like expression on human monocytes independent of antigenic stimuli. J Immunol 127:2020–2027
61. Snyder DS, Lu CY, Unanue ER (1982) Control of macrophage Ia expression in neonatal mice: role of a splenic suppressor cell. J Immunol 128:1458–1465
62. Sonnenfeld G, Meruelo D, McDevitt HO, Merigan TC (1981) Effect of type I and type II interferons on murine thymocytes surface antigens expression: induction or selection? Cell Immunol 57:427–439
63. Steeg PS, Moore RN, Oppenheim JJ (1980) Regulation of murine macrophage Ia antigen expression by an immune interferon-like lymphokine: inhibitory effect of endotoxin. J Immunol 129:2402–2406
64. Steeg PS, Moore RN, Johnson HM, Oppenheim JJ (1982) Regulation of murine macrophage Ia antigen expression by a lymphokine with immune interferon activity. J Exp Med 156:1780–1796
65. Steinmann RM, Nogueira M, Witme MD, Tydings JD, Mellman IS (1980) Lymphokine enhances the expression and the synthesis of Ia antigens on cultured mouse peritoneal macrophages. J Exp Med 152:1248–1261
66. Sztein MB, Steeg PS, Johnson HM, Oppenheim JJ (1984) Regulation of human peripheral blood monocyte DR antigen expression in vitro by lymphokines and recombinant interferons. J Clin Invest 73:56⁵65
67. Tanigaki N, Tosi R (1982) The genetic control of human Ia alloantigens: a three-loci model derived from immunochemical analysis of "supertypic" specificities. Immunol Rev 66:5–37
68. Thorsby E (1984) The role of HLA in T cell activation. Hum Immunol 9:1–7

69. Vignaux F, Gresser I (1978) Enhanced expression of histocompatibility antigens on interferon-treated mouse embryonic fibroblasts. Proc Soc Exp Biol Med 157:456–460
70. Virelizier JL, Perez N, Arenzana-Seisdedas F, Devos R (1984) Pure interferon gamma enhances class II HLA antigens on human monocyte lines. Eur J Immunol 14:106–108
71. Walker EB, Lanier LL, Warner NL (1982) Concomitant induction of the cell surface expression of Ia determinants and accessory cell function by a murine macrophage tumor cell line. J Exp Med 155:629–634
72. Wallach D, Fellous M, Revel M (1982) Preferential effect of gamma interferon on the synthesis of HLA antigens and their mRNAs in human cells. Nature 299:833–836
73. Wang CY, Al-Katib A, Lane CL, Kozinei B, Fu SM (1983) Induction of HLA-DC/DS (Leu 10) antigen expression by human precursor B cell lines. J Exp Med 158:1757–1762
74. Wong GHW, Clark-Lewis I, McKimm-Breschkin JL, Schrader JW (1982) Interferon-gamma-like molecules induce Ia antigens on cultured mast cell progenitors. Proc Natl Acad Sci USA 79:6989–6993
75. Wong GHW, Clark-Lewis I, McKimm-Breschkin JL, Harris AW, Schrader JW (1983) Interferon gamma induces enhanced expression of Ia and H-2 antigens on B lymphoid, macrophage, and myeloid cell lines. J Immunol 131:788–793
76. Wong GHW, Clark-Lewis I, Hamilton JA, Schrader JW (1984) P cell stimulating factor and glucocorticoids oppose the action of interferon gamma in inducing Ia antigens on T-dependent mast cells (P cells). J Immunol 133:2043–2050
77. Wong GHW, Clark-Lewis I, Harris AW, Schrader JW (1984) Effect of cloned interferon-gamma on cell lines of hemopoietic, lymphoid, epithelial, fibroblastic, and neuronal origin. Eur J Immunol 14:52–56
78. Wong GHW, Bartlett PF, Clark-Lewis I, Battye F, Schrader JW (1984) Inducible expression of H-2 and Ia antigens on brain cells. Nature 310:688–691
79. Yem AW, Parmely MJ (1981) Modulation of Ia-like antigen expression and antigen-presenting activity of human monocytes by endotoxin and zymosan A. J Immunol 127:2245–2251
80. Ytterberg SR, Schnitzer TJ (1982) Serum interferon levels in patients with lupus erythematosus. Arthritis Rheum 25:401–410
81. Zlotnik A, Shimonkevitz RP, Gefter ML, Kappler J, Marrack P (1983) Characterization of the gamma-interferon-mediated induction of antigen presenting ability in P388D1 cells. J Immunol 131:2814–2820

Changing Antigenic Profiles of HLA Class II Antigens on Activated T Cells and Their Biological Effects

H. Festenstein, L. Fainboim, D. Jaraquemada, and C. Navarrete

Table of Contents

Introduction

When the immune system is activated, complex cell-cell interactions are initiated which ultimately lead to one or more of several well-known kinds of response. The quality and extent of these responses depend largely upon the particular subset of immune cells which are activated and the balance between the various subsets of activated and other cells involved. The cells which participate in the immune response interact through MHC and other cell membrane molecules. An important consequence of activation is the appearance of molecules on the cell surface which are not normally detectable on resting cells. T cells, for example, when activated, undergo profound changes such as increases in RNA, DNA and rate of protein synthesis, accompanied by the appearance of large nucleoli and abundant euchromatin and a vast increase in the amount of endoplasmic reticulum. These processes culminate in phenotypic variations, including changes in the MHC antigenic profile.

The importance of MHC molecules in immune interactions is well documented, and they are known to be involved in the development and function of helper, suppressor, amplifier and killer cells. Thus MHC class II gene products of the same haplotype should be shared by macrophages and T cells for the effective presentation of antigen by macrophages to T cells [7]. T cell cytotoxicity, on the other hand, requires that the target and effector cell share the class I (H-2K/D/L; HLA-A/B/C) molecules. This is true for virally infected cells, chemically modified cells and for effector cells sensitised against a variety of minor histocompatibility antigens, including the H-Y antigen. These requirements for the sharing of MHC antigens are known as MHC restriction [47]. Because of MHC restriction, discussion of the cell interactions in the immune response involving MHC antigens must refer not only to T cells, but also to other cells of the immune system and the target cells with which they interact in the development of the immune response.

This article is a review of the relevant work carried out in this laboratory and discusses possible implications of the changing profiles of MHC antigens on cells involved in the immune response, with particular reference to the appearance of HLA class II antigens on activated T cells.

There are two main ways of considering the functional potential of these class II molecules on the activated T cells – one is that the antigens themselves are involved in the specific functions, the other is that they either provide access to or characterise a particular T cell subpopulation with a specific functional role in the immune response. The original impetus for this study arose from our studies first in the mouse, and then in man, which showed that certain subpopulations of T cells (with no detectable level of class II antigens on the membrane) become MHC class II-positive (and acquire suppressor properties) when activated by a mixed lymphocyte reaction (MLR) or by mitogens.

Although it was previously believed that lymphocyte subpopulations with different phenotypes were relatively stable, it is now clear that their proportions in mixed leucocyte populations can change because of the expansion of particular subpopulations having characteristic antigenic profiles [35]. The balance of the cells with differing antigen phenotypes may also change upon activation as a result of the derepression of genes which are normally silent and not expressed in the resting cells of that lineage [36]. When both these kinds of changes occur simultaneously, the cells acquire functional characteristics which may be attributed to these phenotypic changes (see below). A derepression mechanism was invoked to explain the results of our early experiments, in which we showed for the first time the appearance of characteristic "B cell (Ia) antigens" on mature T cells following activation in mixed lymphocyte culture (MLC). We showed that anti-Thy 1.2, as well as heterologous rabbit anti-mouse bone marrow lymphocyte (MBLA) antisera, reacted with the activated T cells (Figs. 1 and 2).

We also investigated cells that were activated in vivo. It had been reported that lymph node cells taken from oxazolone-painted animals at one stage (day 3) contain actively dividing cells, the great majority of which are T cells [19]. Table 1 shows the results of an experiment performed with such in vivo-activated T cells. It was found again that anti-MBLA was as cytotoxic to these cells as anti-Thy

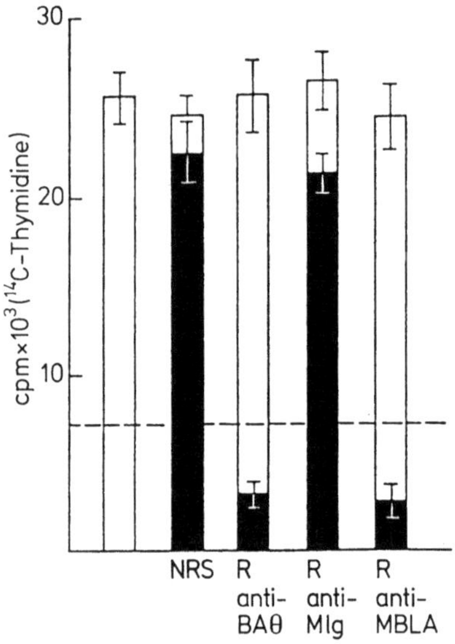

Fig. 1. Specific lysis of activated T lymphocytes by heterologous anti-B cell serum but not by anti-mouse immunoglobulin. CBA/H lymphocytes were activated in a one-way MLC by co-incubating them for 2 days with lymphocytes from (CBA/H × DBA/2)F_1 mice and then labelled with ^{14}-thymidine for a period of 16 h. The activated cells (three tubes per group) were treated with the various sera indicated, in the presence of complement, and then trypsinized to disrupt the membranes from specifically lysed cells in order to release the ^{14}C-labelled DNA. The radioactivity that remained associated with the carefully washed cells was then determined by harvesting the cells onto a filter using a semi-automatic cell harvester. The columns illustrate the mean cpm (±SD indicated by the *vertical bars*) obtained in the various groups. *First column:* untreated control: *Second to fifth columns: white,* cells treated with the various sera plus complement but not trypsinized; *black,* cells treated with the various sera plus complement and then trypsinized. *NRS,* normal rabbit serum (absorbed with mouse spleen cells). The *broken line* shows the counts obtained in non-stimulated control cultures. The sera used in the experiments shown in Fig. 1 and 2 were absorbed and tested for specific anti-B cell activity. After five absorptions with T cells they still reacted with B cells and after absorption with B cells from nude mice they were no longer reactive [36]. See Refs. 36 and 37. Reproduced from Ref. 36

Table 1. Cytotoxic activity of R anti-MBLA against lymph node cells activated in vitro by skin painting with oxazolone

Pretreatment with			cpm (mean±SD)	^{14}C-thymidine release (%)
Antibody	C′	Trypsin		
–	–	–	3552±595	
–	+	+	2767±639	
Anti-H-2[b]	+	+	71± 7	98
Anti-Thy 1.2	+	+	829± 70	70
R anti-MIg	+	+	2773±172	18
R anti-MBLA[a]	+	+	735±358	70

C57BL/6 mice were shaved at the lateral sides of the chest and painted with oxazolone (2% solution in methanol). After 3 days cells were taken from the draining axillary lymph nodes and labelled for a 16-h period in vitro with ^{14}C-thymidine. The isotope uptake in control cultures with cells from non-painted animals was 350±52

[a] Eight times absorbed with mouse thymus cells. Reproduced from Ref. 36

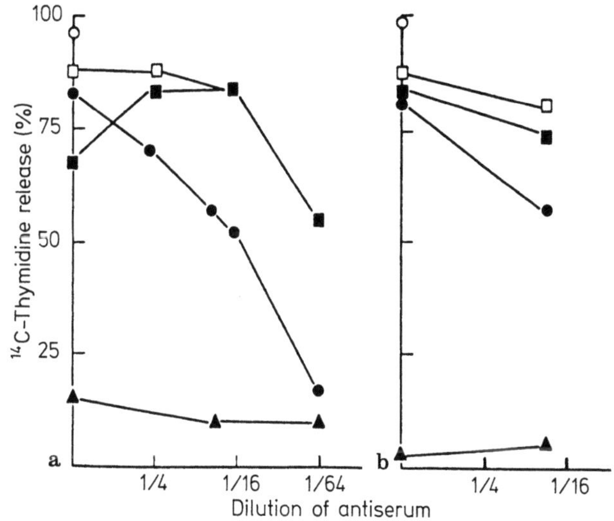

Fig. 2 a, b. Cytotoxicity of various antisera tested against CBA/H lymphocytes activated either in MLC by co-incubation with (CBA/H × DBA/2)F_1 lymphocytes (**a**) or by PHA (**b**). Cytotoxicity was determined as described in Fig. 1 by treating the ^{14}C-thymidine-labelled cells with antibody and complement followed by trypsinization [37]. The results are expressed as % ^{14}C-thymidine release (incorporated into DNA) as a function of antiserum dilution. Note that (i) maximal release observed with anti-Thy 1.2 (anti-Θ) and R anti-MBLA was about the same (approximately 80%), (ii) there was virtually no additive effect when the two sera were used together and (iii) R anti-MIg had very little, if any, cytotoxic activity. The mean cpm of the MLC-activated cells was 9586, as compared to 3174 in the control cultures. The mean cpm of the PHA-activated cells was 47948, as compared to 4378 in cultures without PHA. ○, Anti H-2; □, anti-Θ + R anti-MBLA; ●, R anti-MBLA; ■, anti-Θ; △, R antiMIg. Reproduced from Schirrmacher and Festenstein (1975) Ref. 36

1.2 serum (70% ^{14}C-thymidine release), while R anti-MIg had no significant cytotoxic effect. Even eight absorbtions with mouse thymus cells had not removed the cytotoxic activity R anti-MBLA against the activated T lymphocytes.

Expression of HLA Class II Antigens on Human Activated T Cells

The study of the expression of class II antigens was done on human T cells activated by mitogen and by MLR. The activated cells were typed both by heteroantisera to purified HLA class II glycoprotein from B cells and by HLA class II alloantisera [15].

In these experiments, peripheral blood lymphocytes (PBL) from different people were cultured with various allogeneic lymphocytes and seminal samples. PBL were also stimulated with phytohaemagglutinin (PHA), concanavalin A (ConA), and purified protein derivative of tuberculin (PPD) for 2 days, harvested and washed. After 7 days the allo- or mitogen-activated T cells were treated with various antibodies and incubated with fluoresceinated rabbit anti-human Ig (Fig. 3). Fluorescence reactions were scored by both visual examination and by the fluorescence-activated cell sorter (FACS-I). In all the mitogen-activated T cells, and particularly in the allogeneically activated T cells, there were substantial increases in the proportions of HLA class II-positive, Ig-negative T cells as characterised

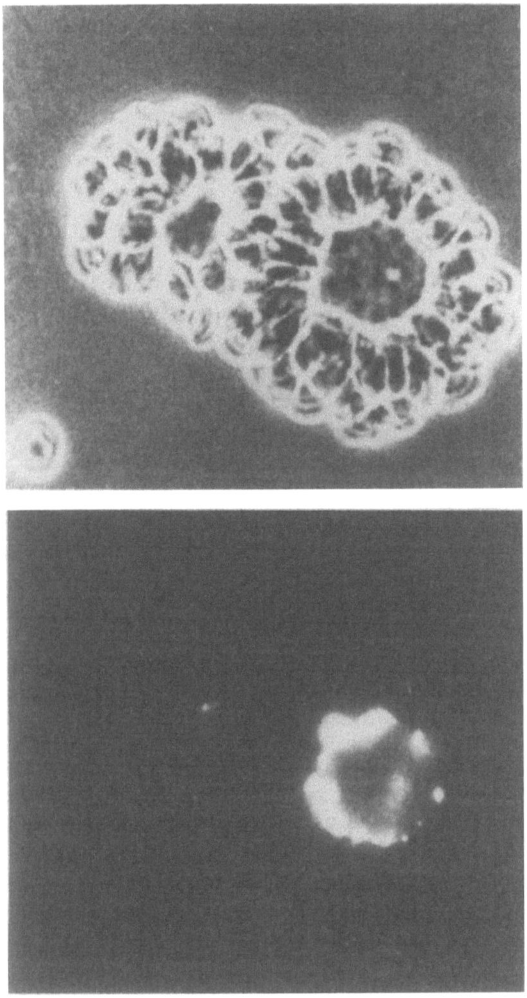

a

b

Fig. 3 a, b. Detection of HLA class II antigens on (activated) human T cells. Cells were first incubated with heterologous anti-human class II antigens (30 min, 4 °C) followed by a combination of sheep anti-human Ig (fluorescein) and sheep anti-rabbit (or anti-chicken) Ig (rhodamine). After a further 30 min at 4 °C, the cells were washed twice and E rosettes formed. Following resuspension, the cells and rosettes were fixed by the addition of 0.5% glutaraldehyde. Class II-positive activated T cells were scored as large lymphoid cells that were E^+, $smIg^-$, Ia^+. **a** Phase contrast observation showing E^+ cells. **b** Same field as in **a** using excitation and barrier filters for rhodamine excitation and observation [= anti-class II (p28, 33) antiserum]. Only one of the two T cells is staining in **b**. Note: these cells were not fluorescent with anti-human Ig when viewed under conditions for fluorescein excitation. Adapted from Greaves et al. (1979) Ref. 15

Table 2. Detection of cell surface class II antigens on activated human T cells

Experiment no.	Stimulus	Class II positive activated T cells (%)
1–4	Allogeneic lymphocytes two-way MLR	17.2–20.0
5	Class II-positive cells responding to T-dcplctcd stimulus (mitomycin C)	31.1
6,7	Unseparated lymphocytes responding to allogeneic seminal cells	19.4, 34.4
8–11	PHA	0, 6.5, 22.7, 7.1
12, 13	Con A	1.0, 3.0
14–17	PPD	56.2, 19.4, 34.5, 39.1
	Control cultures (17)	0.5–1.5

Cultured cells were stained with $F(ab')_2$ sheep anti-human Ig (fluorescein) sheep anti-human (see Fig. 3) plus rabbit $F(ab')_2$ or chicken anti-Ia followed by sheep anti-rabbit or chicken Ig (rhodamine). E rosettes were then formed. All E^+ cells were checked for smIg staining and all Ig^- (approx. 95%) E^+ cells then checked for Ia staining. For these experiments, an arbitrary distinction between large and small rosette-forming cells was made so as to bias recording as far as possible toward activated T cell blasts.
Adapted from Greaves et al. (1979) Ref. 15

by the rabbit (anti-T) or chicken (anti-class II) heteroantisera (Table 2). The activated T lymphocytes did not react with rabbit anti HLA class II heteroantibodies which had been preabsorbed with a B cell line (BRi7) (data not shown). These results were then confirmed and extended by testing the activated T cells with specific anti-HLA-DR alloantisera in complement-dependent cytotoxicity. The results showed that the same allospecificities were detected on activated T cells as on autologous B cells [15, 33] (see Table 2). The possibility of passive acquisition of allogeneic stimulator HLA-DR antigens by the activated T cells was thus ruled out. These results have since been confirmed by several investigators [14, 17, 20, 45]. Furthermore, the appearance of class II-positive T cells in an MLC activation experiment in which the responder T cell population was first depleted of HLA class II-positive cells provided the first clear evidence for the induced endogenous expression of HLA class II antigens in activated human T cells [15]. The endogenous synthesis of class II antigens by both human [2, 3] and mouse [38] activated T cells has also been since demonstrated.

In summary, activation by allogeneic lymphocytes, seminal cells, or PPD substantially increased the proportion of HLA class II-positive T cells. HLA-DR typing indicated that these specificities on the activated T cells were not acquired passively from the stimulator cells, but resulted from derepression of silent genes and/or activation of hidden HLA-DR locus gene products during T cell activation. The functional significance of HLA class II-positive T cell subsets remained to be elucidated. By analogy with results in the mouse [40], we expected them to include suppressor T cells. This possibility was supported by our finding [15] that a higher proportion of the class II-positive T cells belonged to the T_G rather than the T_M subset [25]. These experiments were carried out in collaboration with Dr. Greaves group at ICRF.

Changing MHC Antigenic Profiles of Activated T Cells: Correlating the Phenotypic Changes with Function

Further experiments in our laboratory were then designed to find out what are the precise phenotypic changes on the T cells which are either responsible for or associated with changes in the functional properties of the activated cells. Three different approaches were taken to study and to correlate the phenotypic changes in these T cells with the changes in their functional properties by activating them with:

1. Mitogens
2. Allogeneic HLA class I- and class II-associated suppressor-activating determinants in MLC
3. Allogeneic HLA class II lymphocyte-activating determinants in MLC

The Suppressor Effect of PHA-Activated T Cells

The first of this new series of experiments undertaken with human T cells were performed using PHA as the activator. For this, PBL from healthy donors were stimulated in vitro with PHA and maintained in culture using conditioned medium (TCGF). On successive intervals up to 23 days, 5×10^6 activated cells were taken from the suspension cultures and divided into two aliquots – one for experiments to assay the suppressor activity in culture, the other for serological investigation of surface antigens on the activated cells.

To study their influence on the reactivity of autologous cells, PHA-activated cells were irradiated and mixed with equal numbers of autologous lymphocytes prior to stimulation in culture by PPD.

PBL which were mixed with autologous irradiated 11- and 18-day PHA-activated lymphocytes and then stimulated by PPD responded very poorly compared with cultures without activated cells. While this effect was apparent in most instances only after adding the "11-day" and "18-day" activated cells (Fig. 4), suppression was already evident with "8-day" activated cells in other experiments (data not shown).

Similar results were obtained when the effects of unfractionated irradiated PHA-activated cells were assayed in an allogeneic MLC. In these experiments, irradiated 23-day PHA-activated cells were tested straight out of culture. Representative results are shown in Fig. 5. The suppressor effects were evident when the PHA-activated cells were added to both syngeneic and allogeneic responders in MLC. Serological assays for MHC class II, T4 and T8 antigens were performed on the activated T blasts and on resting T cells (day 0). Activated T cells which were negative for the class II antigens when tested on days 0 and on days 3 and 4 became positive on day 8 and expressed the same HLA-DR specificities present on the syngeneic B cells, confirming our initial results (Table 3) [10]. To find out how these changes related to the development of suppressor function, kinetic experiments were carried out and the number of class II antigen-positive T cells tested with the monoclonal antibodies (MoAbs) DA2 and 62-3-34 were scored at different times after incubation (Fig. 6). Corresponding functional assays were also carried out. The activated T cell populations from "18-day" and "23-day" cultures were assayed for their potential suppressor properties as indicated above. Although T8-positive, HLA class II-positive cells were present in both "14-day"

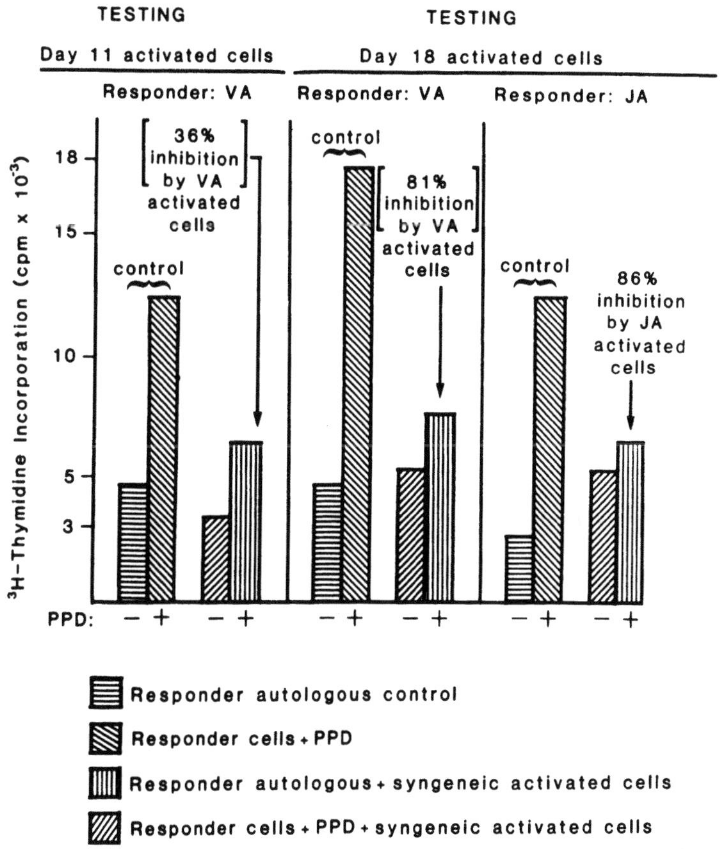

Fig. 4. Suppressor effect of unfractionated PHA-activated T cells on PPD stimulation. PBL from JA and VA were stimulated in culture (10^6 cells/ml) with 1 : 100 final dilution of PHA for 36 h. The supernatant (conditioned medium, CM) was decanted and the cells resuspended in fresh medium (RPMI 1640 plus 10% AB serum) containing 30% CM (v/v final dilution). The cultures were maintained for up to 30 days by changing the medium with CM every 3–4 days. The suppressor effect of the activated T cells (>95% E-rosetting-positive cells) on the response of resting cells to PPD was studied as follow: At 11 and 18 days after PHA activation, 5×10^4 activated cells in 50 µl medium (without CM) were irradiated with 4000 rad and mixed with 5×10^4 syngeneic resting lymphocytes (50 µl) in the presence or absence of 0.6 µlG PPD (50 µl). As a control, 5×10^4 resting cells were mixed with an equal number of syngeneic irradiated resting cells, in the presence of PPD. ^{3}H-thymidine uptake was measured on day 4.5, and percentage inhibition calculated as follows:

$$\% \text{ inhib.} \frac{\text{cpm activated cells } (+\text{PPD}) - \text{cpm activated cells } (-\text{PPD})}{\text{cpm resting cells } (+\text{PPD}) - \text{cpm resting cells } (-\text{PPD})} \times 100$$

Adapted from Fainboim et al. (1980) Ref. 9

and "23-day" activated cells, there were a much larger number in the "23-day" culture than in the "14-day" culture. When the suppressor properties of the "18-day" and "23-day" activated cells were compared, the "23-day" cells were more potent than the "18-day" cells. These results suggest that the class II-positive, T8-positive subpopulation are active suppressors (Fig. 7). This possibility was further confirmed in subsequent experiments, where fractionated T8- and class II-posi-

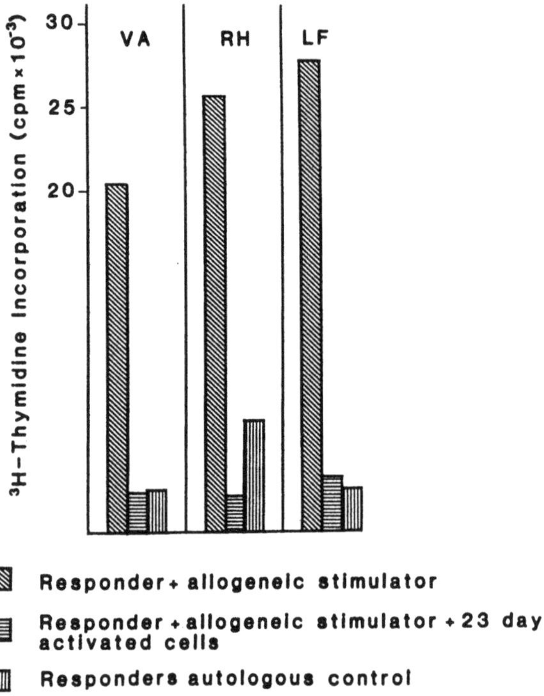

Fig. 5. Suppressor capacity of "23-day" unfractionated PHA-activated T cells in allogeneic MLC. Fifty microliters of responder PBL (5×10^4) were cultured in quadruplicate on microtitre V-well plates in RPMI plus 10% AB serum, then 2×10^4 irradiated autologous normal PBL or "23-day"-activated cells were added in 50 μl of the same medium. Activated autologous VA and RH were added to the VA and RH responders, while RH allogeneic activated irradiated cells were added to LF responders. 5×10^4 allogeneic cells were added to each well of this mixture. For each experiment, the cultures were pulsed for 16 h with 1 μCi ^{3}H-thymidine after 5 days culture, and results expressed in median cpm of quadruplicate cultures.
HLA phenotypes of responder and stimulator cells:

VA, responder VA: A2,A3; B35,B44; DR1,DR2; Dw1,2
stimulator LF: A26,-; B38,-; DR4,DR5; Dw10,5;DQw3.

RH, responder RH: A1,-; B8,-; DR3,DR7; Dw3,7;DQw2
stimulator LF: as above

LF, responder LF: as above
stimulator KH: A3,11; B35,44; DR2,4; Dw2,4

Adapted from Fainboim et al. (1980) Ref. 9

Fig. 7. Suppressor effect of different subsets of "23-day" PHA-activated T cells on MLR. 20×10^7 "23-day" activated cells were treated with 1:25 (final dilution) DA2 for 30 min at room temperature, washed twice and incubated with 1:20 dilution of a rabbit anti-mouse FITC conjugated IgC. The cells were fractionated into weakly reactive (the lower 20% of fluorescence Ia −) and strongly reactive (the upper 60% of fluorescence Ia +) in a FACS-1. Different concentrations of irradiated normal syngeneic cells ( ), class II-positive cells ( ) or total unfractionated activated cells ( ) were added to the MLC

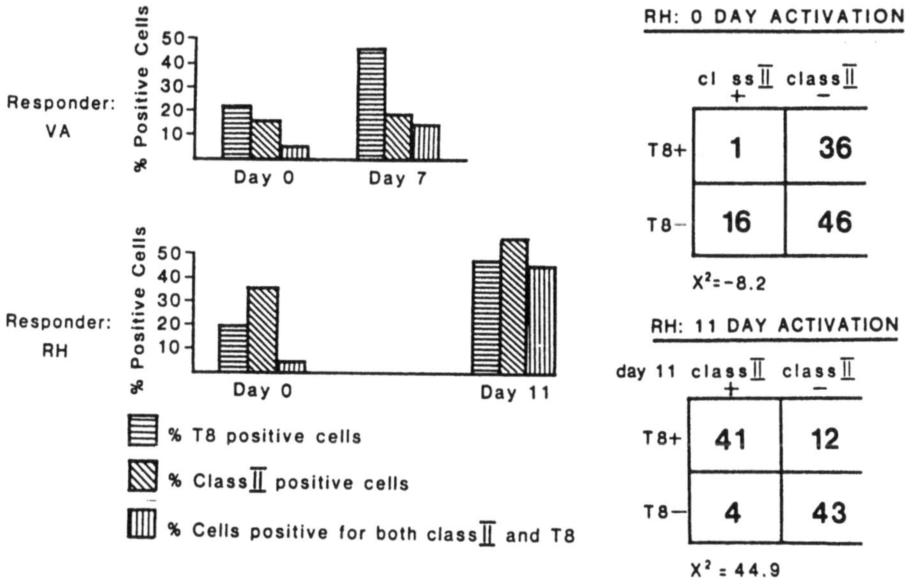

Fig. 6. Expression of T8 and class II on PHA-activated cell surface. Indirect immunofluorescence was used to analyse cell surface markers. Resting or activated cells were treated with 1:50 (final dilution) horse anti-human TH2 ("T8-like") (see [11]) and with two HLA class II MoAbs (DA2 and 63-3-34, both mouse anti-class II monomorphic) at 1:25 final dilution. After 20 min incubation, 1:25 swine anti-horse FITC-labelled or 1:10 goat anti-mouse rhodamine conjugate antibodies were added to the second layer. Observations were made using a standard 14 Zeiss photomicroscope with epi-illumination (iv F1 epi-fluorescence condenser) and 2F1 reflector sleeve, equipped with exciter and barrier filters, for selective excitation and observation of fluorescence and rhodamine

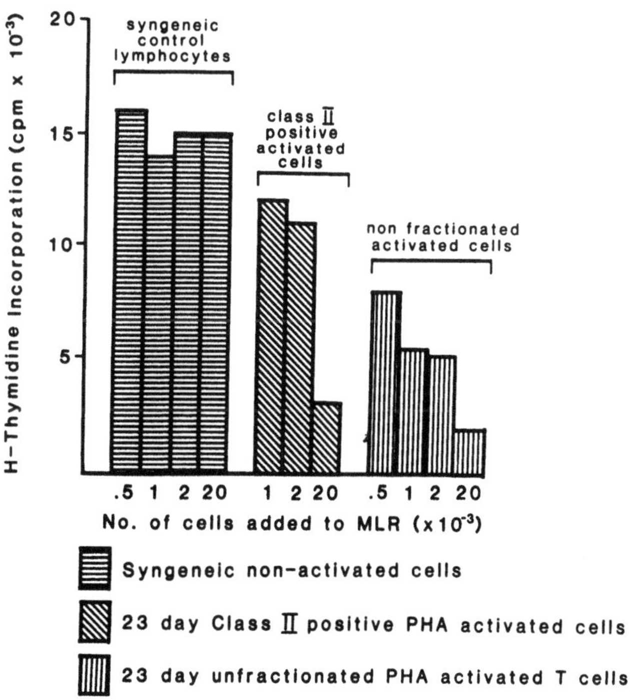

Table 3. HLA-DR typing of PHA-activated human T cells

	Day of culture	AB serum	Heter-ologous and B cell serum	8W432	7W11	277	8W474	7W50+6	7W119+6	8W456	7W34	8W401	8W383	8W1030	8W508	8W1202	8W14+B8=B14	8W509	7W44+5	7W910+5	8W919	8W971	7W98	8W822	8W592	8W1221	8W441
		%		DR1			DR2			DR3			DR4			DR5			DR6			DR7			DR8		
RH	0	10	8	–	–	–	–	–	–	8	8	8	–	–	–	–	–	–	4	–	4	8	8	8	–	–	–
A1,X/B8,X/	3	10	–	–	–	–	–	–	–	–	–	–	–	–	–	–	–	–	–	–	–	–	–	–			
DR3,7	8	13	6	–	–	2	–	–	–	6	–	4	–	–	–	2	–	–	–	–	6	2	4	6	–	–	–
	11	15	6	4	–	4	6	–	6	6	2	6	–	–	–	–	–	–	–	–	4	6	4	4	–	–	–
	18	10	6	–	–	2	–	–	–	6	2	6	–	–	–	–	–	–	–	–	–	4	4	6	–	–	–
	24	10	4	–	–	–	–	–	–	6	2	6	–	–	–	2	–	–	–	–	–	2	4	6	–	–	2
JA	0	10	6	6	6	8	8	8	8	–	–	–	–	–	–	–	–	–	–	–	–	–	–	–	–	–	–
A1,11/B44,27/	8	10	4	–	2	6	4	2	2	–	–	–	–	–	–	–	–	–	–	–	–	–	–	–	–	–	–
Cw2,5/DR1,2	11	10	4	2	2	–	2	2	2	2	2	4	–	–	–	–	–	–	–	2	–	–	–	–	–	–	–
	18	10	4	–	2	6	6	4	4	–	–	–	–	–	–	–	–	–	–	–	–	–	–	–			
VA	0	5	8	8	4	8	4	8	8	–	–	–	–	–	–	–	–	–	–	–	–	–	–	–	–	–	–
A2,3/B35,44/	3	10	–	–	–	–	–	–	–	–	–	–	–	–	–	–	–	–	–	–	–	–	–	–	–	–	–
Cw4,X/DR1,2	8	10	2	2	–	2	–	–	–	–	–	–	–	–	–	–	–	–	–	–	–	–	–	–	–	–	–
	11		2	2	2	2	2	2	2	–	–	–	–	2	–	–	–	–	–	–	–	–	–	–	–	–	–
	18	5	6	6	4	6	8	6	6	–	–	–	2	4	–	–	–	–	–	–	–	–	–	–	–	–	–

Anti-DR sera from the Seventh and Eighth International Histocompatibility Workshop (7W, 8W) were used. Reactions were scored as follows: 2 (20–40% killing); 4 (40–60%); 6 (60–80%); 8 (80–100%). The cells were tested using the complement-dependent cytotoxic test. Acridine orange and ethidium bromide were added at the end of the incubation period to see the live and dead cells respectively tive cells tested independently were actively suppressive in MLC [9]. However, these experiments do not exclude the presence of additional suppressor subpopulations.

MHC Class I-Associated Suppressor-Activating Determinants

The second group of experiments were designed to investigate the functional relevance of the changing antigenic profiles of activated T cells of a specific genotype in response to a particular consanguineous homozygous typing cell (HTC) FPA (DR5, Dw'F5'). FPA's cells were found to be able to induce the expansion of specific suppressor cells in some responders in MLC. This ability to induce suppressor cells was attributed to its suppressor-activating determinant (Sad-W1) which maps to the HLA-B-A telomeric end of chromosome 6. It is separate from the class II genes and is associated with HLA-B35 homozygosity [10]. Only FPA and the HLA-B35-homozygous members of the FPA family, including the three HLA-identical siblings and an HLA-B/DR-recombinant sibling, induced suppressors in the specific responding cells, whereas the HLA-B35-heterozygous family members failed to do so. The response to this Sad is specific, as only cells of a particular MHC genotype (inferred from a family study) produced MHC-restricted T suppressor cells after activation. Thus cells from two HLA-identical siblings, JW and BW, gave discordant typing responses to this HTC as well as to stimulating cells from the HLA-B35-homozygous family members. JW's cells responded well, while BW's cells gave only a weak response [10]. After 6 days culture, most of BW's cells were T8-positive, and of these, 95% were also class II-positive (Fig. 8a) [12]. When BW's lymphocytes were added to JW's cells and then stimulated by FPA, there was no response by JW's cells. This result is attributed to the suppressor effect of BW's cells on JW's cells. [The suppressor effect was not due to the killing of the irradiated stimulating cells (FPA) by potential effectors of BW's lymphocytes, as shown by a negative direct CML test against FPA targets.] Thus the suppression is most likely to be due to the T8-positive, HLA class II-positive suppressor cell subpopulation. This activated T cell subpopulation's antigenic profile is similar to that of the "23-day" PHA-activated T cells described above, but in contrast to those experiments, the suppressor effect of BW's cells was abrogated by irradiation. These results indicate that viable cells were needed for suppression while the PHA suppressor population was radiation-resistant. The suppressor properties of BW's unfractionated responding T cells were eliminated by removing T8-positive cells prior to stimulation with FPA in MLC using antibody and complement. Experiments were then done to further prove that the suppressor effect was due to a T8-positive suppressor lymphocyte subpopulation, which expressed class II antigens after stimulation in MLC. Two T-cell subpopulations were obtained by fractionating BW's cells into T4-positive and T4-negative, using the FACS-1. These two kinds of cell populations were added separately to MLC in which JW's cells were stimulated by FPA. The results showed that only the T4-negative (T8-positive) cells had suppressor properties. When as few as 10^3 of these T4-negative BW lymphocytes were added to 5×10^4 of JW's responder cells, they produced a 72% suppression of her lymphocytes' response to FPA. This suppressor effect was thus highly efficient and specific (Fig. 9). Once the T8-positive resting presuppressor cells which responded to FPA's Sad-W1 were removed (using the FACS-1), the remainder of BW's PBL

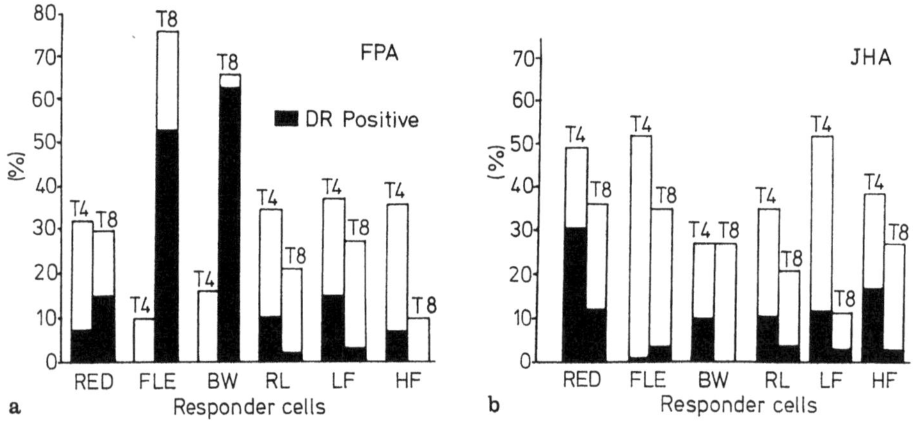

Fig. 8 a, b. Percentage of activated T blast cells expressing either T4 or T8 and DR antigens. Different patterns of expression of T4, T8, and class II antigens on T cells after allostimulation by two different stimulating HLA homozygous cells. The ratio of T4-postitive to T8-positive blasts was similar (>1) for most responders after stimulation. A proportion of both these blasts were class II-positive. However, several "abnormal" phenotypes were observed which corresponded to abnormal responses in MLR. **a** FPA as stimulator. The majority of BW's blasts after stimulation were T8-positive, class II-positive. FLE and RED's cells, which are HLA-identical, had different phenotypes after stimulation. RED's blasts showed the normal T4:T8 ratio, whereas FLE's response was similar to BW's, with a higher proportion of the blasts being of the T8-positive, class II-positive phenotype. **b** JHA as stimulator. FLE and RED are both HLA-D/DR-identical to JHA. After stimulation, FLE's cells showed a normal T4:T8 ratio, but very low expression of class II antigens (see text).

HLA phenotypes of responder cells:

RED: A2; Bw63; Cw-; DR4; DQw3; Dw13, DPw4
FLE: A2; Bw63; Cw-; DR4; DQw3; Dw13; DPw4
BW: A25,32; B18,39; Cw3,-; DR2,7; DQw1,2; Dw2,7
RL: A3,26; B38,-; Cw-; DR4,w6; DQw1,3; Dw10,18
LF: A26,-; B38; Cw-,-; DR4,5; DQw3,-; Dw10,5
HF: A1,28; B37,w65; Cw6,8; DR5,1; DwX,X; DPw2,3

Stimulator HTCs:

FPA: A1; Bw35; Cw4; DR5; DQw1; Dw'F5'; DPw2
JHA: A31; B51; Cw-; DR4; DQw3; Dw13; DPw3

Table 4. Response of BW's purified T cell subpopulation to FPA's lymphocytes in MLC

Responder lymphocytes	Autologous control	Stimulator lymphocytes		
		FPA	LF[a]	PHA
BW total	8993 ± 1470	17542 ± 6248	31602 ± 4977	111458 ± 6995
BW OKT4+	7230 ± 5437	45674 ± 5074	55735 ± 4909	82748 ± 2050
BW OKT4−	979 ± 436	5173 ± 2670	23455 ± 2145	60981 ± 1323

Results expressed as cpm ± sd
BW's total lymphocytes gave a low response to FPA's irradiated cells, but not to LF's or to PHA. However, BW's OKT4-positive lymphocytes responded to FPA as strongly as to the third-party stimulator cells. BW's OKT4-negative lymphocytes were capable of responding to LF and to PHA, but did not respond to FPA. This population was thus responsible for the suppression of BW's response to FPA
[a] LF is heterozygous Dw5/Dw10

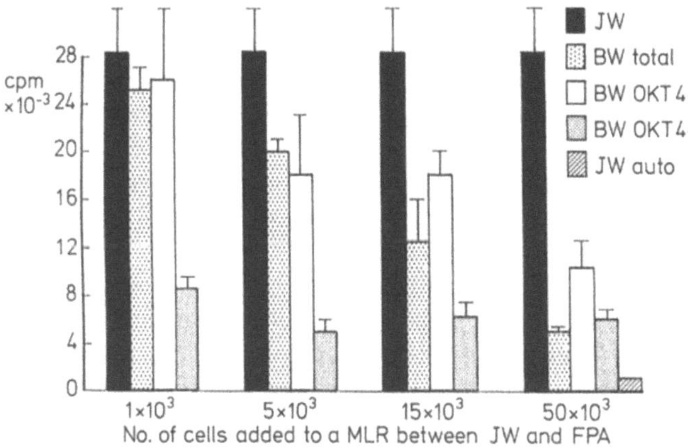

Fig. 9. Suppressor effect of different subpopulations of BW's cells. As few as 10^3 OKT4-negative BW's lymphocytes added to 50000 JW's responder cells produced a suppression of 72% of JW's response to FPA. The OKT4-positive cells were not capable of significant suppression unless 50000 cells were added to the culture (probably due to OKT4-negative contamination). The OKT4-negative subpopulation consisted of more than 95% OKT8-positive cells

proliferated quite normally in response to FPA (HLA-DW'F5') (Table 4). In this experiment only the brightest T4-positive cells were sorted to avoid any contamination with T4-negative cells. The median response of 17,542 cpm of the unseparated BW lymphocytes was increased to 45,674 cpm when the T4-negative (T8-positive) cells were removed. As expected, these T4-negative lymphocytes, which responded normally to PHA and to third-party stimulator cells, failed to respond to the HTC FPA, confirming the T8 specificity of the suppressor effect. BW's T4 cells (Dw2/Dw7) behaved normally in culture in the absence of the suppressor T8 subpopulation and could be HLA-D-typed by a standard panel of Dw2 and Dw7 HTC. The "pseudotyping responses" were thus eliminated.

The finding of a T8-positive, class II-positive suppressor cell subpopulation following stimulation of BW's cells by FPA cells permits differentiation between the two distinct properties of the FPA cells: one to stimulate MLR by the FPA HLA-Dw'F5', the other to stimulate the production of T8-positive, class II-positive suppressor cells by the suppressor-activating determinant Sad-W1, which is associated with B35 homozygosity [12].

Four other HTC were found to induce similar responses by BW's and FW's cells. Three of these were Dw1-B35-homozygous cells, indicating that the Sad-W1 association with B35 is not unique to the FPA HTC. An earlier report by McMichael and Sasazuki [22] described the unexpected outcome of an MLC experiment in a family in which the mother's DW2-homozygous lymphocytes failed to respond to her husband's cells. The husband was Dw1-B35-homozygous. However, in contrast with our data, her offsprings' B35-heterozygous cells also induced only a low response from the mother's cells.

HLA Class II-Associated Suppressor-Activating Determinants

Another pair of HLA-identical siblings, FLE and RED (both Dw13-DR4-homozygous) (see Fig. 8), gave discordant typing responses to FPA: FLE's cells did not respond to FPA, while RED's cells did. The predominant phenotype of the non-responding FLE's cells after FPA activation was T8-positive, class II-positive, the same as BW (Fig. 8a). Furthermore, in a study of a large panel of responders, we observed pseudotyping responses to a small number of HTC in addition to FPA and the Bw35/Dw1 HTC. There was no correlation between their HLA phenotypes, and this was further evidence for non-MHC control of the response to class I-associated Sads.

Abnormally high responses were also observed in cases of D/DR identity betwen responder and stimulators. One such abnormal response was obtained between FLE and JHA. FLE's cells, but not RED's cells, were stimulated by JHA HTC (all Dw13-DR4, HTC). Thus FLE's cells gave an unexpected high response to JHA's cells despite their sharing HLA-D/DR. FLE's cells' response to other DW13 HTCs was low, as expected, and her HLA-identical sibling's cells (RED) also gave a low response to JHA and all other Dw13 HTCs. Data not shown [18].

After activation with JHA, the T4/T8 ratio of FLE's cells was not different from that of other responders (see Fig. 8b), but only a very small proportion of these cells expressed class II antigens (1% T4-positive, class II-positive; 2% T8-postive, class II-positive). The possible lack of active suppressors could be an explanation for the abnormal high response of FLE's cells to JHA's cells. This could be related to the absence of T8-positive, class II-positive T cells after stimulation, thus giving support to the idea that class II expression is needed for T cells to acquire full functional capacity. However, this stimulation could also be explained by an HLA-restricted non-HLA lymphocyte-activating determinant analogous to the mouse [13].

Further Studies of the Expression of HLA-DR and DQ Antigens on Alloactivated T Cells

Several HLA class II molecules have now been identified using a variety of serological, cellular and biochemical techniques (HLA-DR/DQ/DP). The kinetics of the expression of the different class II determinants – HLA-DR and DQ – in addition to T4 and T8, was further studied on alloactivated T cells.

Three different responder cells were stimulated with irradiated allogeneic cells and maintained in culture by IL2 and allogeneic feeder stimulation. The responder cells were tested on days 4, 8, 12, and 16 of culture for the expression of T4, T8, DR, and DQ molecules using the double-immunofluorescence test described. The results are shown in Fig. 10.

The T4/T8 patterns of expression were very similar at all stages after stimulation, but the simultaneous expression of T4, T8, DR, and DQ varied between individuals and between days after activation. The number of T4-positive, DR-positive cells was always higher than the number of T4-positive, DQ-positive cells for all responders. In addition, whereas a proportion of T8-positive cells expressed DR antigens, no T8-positive, DQ-positive cells were detected on any of the responder cells. The kinetics of the expression of these antigens on the different days after activation is shown in Fig. 11.

In both T8-positive and T4-positive subpopulations of cells, the expression of DR occurred earlier than that of DQ. HLA-DR antigens were expressed on the T4-positive cells as early as day 4, and on the T8-positive cells by day 8. The HLA-

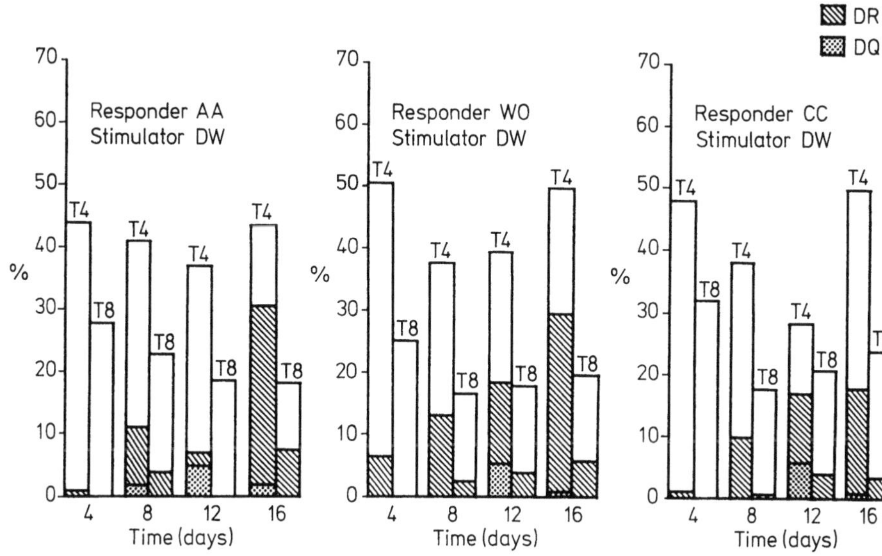

Fig. 10. Different patterns of T4, T8, DR, and DQ antigen expression after alloantigen stimulation. Equal numbers (10×10^6) of responder and irradiated stimulator cells were cultures in 20 ml RPMI medium supplemented with 10% human AB serum at 37 °C in an atmosphere of 5% CO_2 in air. On days 9 and 13,50% of the medium was substituted by a medium containing 20% IL-2 and 10% AB serum. On the same days, 5×10^6 pooled irradiated PBL containing cells of the original stimulators were added to the culture. Samples of the cells were taken on days 4, 8, 12, and 16. The expression of T4, T8, DR, and DQ antigens was measured by the double immunofluorescence technique (see Fig. 11).

Responder and stimulator phenotypes:

AA: A2,26; B51,w65; Cw8,-; DR1,2; DwX,X; DQw1
WO: A1,32; B8,38; Cw7,-; DR3,6; Dw3,18; DQw1,2
CC: A2,11; B35,51; DR1,w14; Dw1,9; DQw1,-
DW: A2,29; B44,60; Cw3,-; DR7,w9; Dw7,DB5

DR expression was very intense and remained up to day 16. However, only a small proportion of T4-positive cells expressed DQ antigens: this expression was weak, occurred between days 8 and 12, and decreased considerably on day 16 despite stimulation being maintained. Again, no T8-positive cell expressed DQ antigens at any stage of the activation process.

The differential expression of HLA-DR and HLA-DQ antigens on activated T cells may have molecular functional relevance, in view of the results obtained indicating heterogeneity of function of the HLA class II DR and DQ molecules described below. In these experiments we have used anti-HLA-DR and DQ MoAbs to study the functional properties of these molecules with respect to lymphocyte activation and the generation of suppressor and cytotoxic effectors.

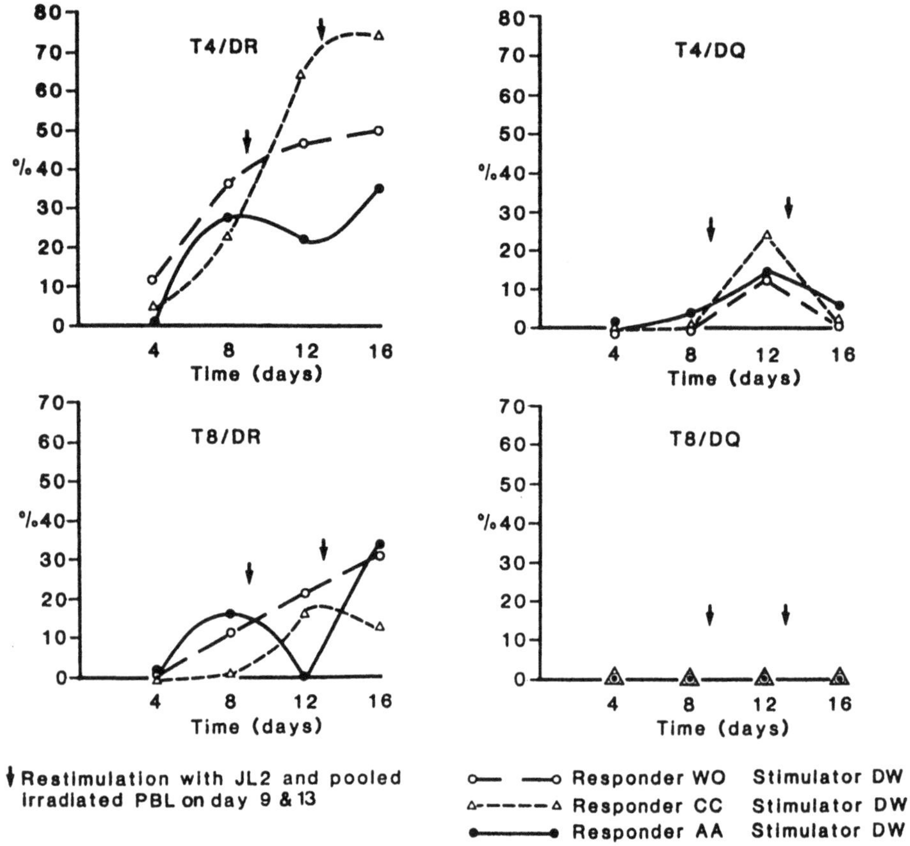

Fig. 11. Kinetic experiments showing the percentage of T4- and T8-positive cells expressing HLA-DR and DQ molecules after alloantigen stimulation. Samples of responder cells cultures as in Fig. 10 were taken on days 4, 8, 12, and 16. The expression of T4, T8, DR, and DQ was measured by double immunofluorescence as follows: Half a million cells were resuspended in 50 µl PBS/BSA (0.2%)/Azide (0.02%) buffer and incubated for 1 h at 4 °C with a mixture of MoAbs at the appropriate dilutions, i.e. anti-HLA-DR (IgG1) and anti-OKT4 (IgG2). After the first incubation the cells were spun and washed three times in PBS/BSA/Azide, resuspended in 50 µl medium and incubated for 20 min at 20 °C with rabbit anti-mouse IgG1 conjugated with rhodamine TRICT and rabbit anti-mouse IgG2 FITC. The cells were then washed three more times in the PBS/BSA/Azide buffer and then examined on a slide using a standard 14 Zeiss microscope (Zeiss, Oberkochen Ltd., West Germany) with an epifluorescent condenser and equipped with a selective filter for FITC (green) and TRICT (red) and a planapochromat 63/1.4 oil pH objective.

Responder and stimulator phenotypes:

AA: A2,26; B51,w65; Cw8,-; DR1,2; DwX,X; DQw1
WO: A1,32; B8,38; Cw7,-; DR3,6; Dw3,18; DQw1,2
CC: A2,11; B35,51; DR1,w14; Dw1,9; DQw1,-
DW: A2,29; B44,60; Cw3,-; DR7,w9; Dw7,DB5

The following MoAbs were used:

OKT4 } IgG2
OKT8 }
DQw1 Genox 35.3 } (IgG1)
DR DA6-231 }

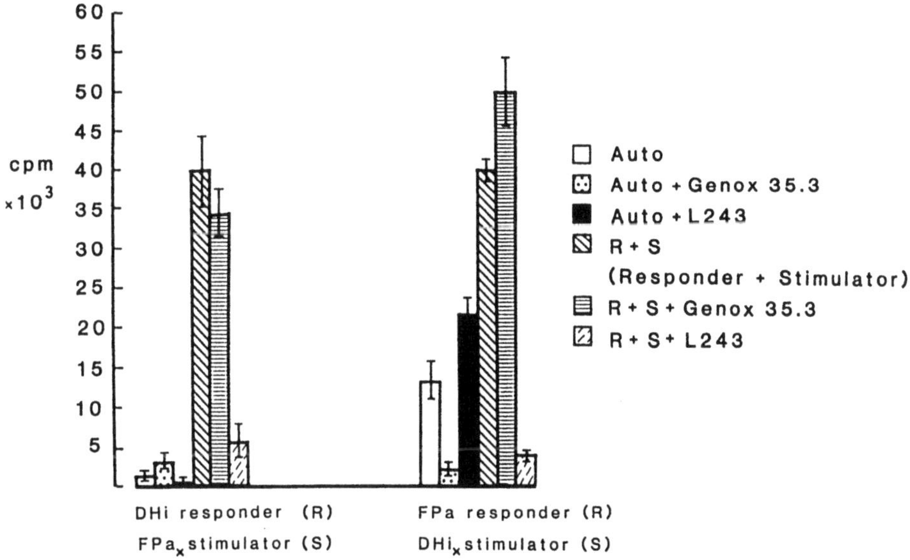

Fig. 12. Effect of adding DR (L243) and DQw1 (Genox 35.3) MoAbs to the FPA/DHI reciprocal MLCs: experiments showing blocking of proliferation with HLA-DR MoAbs. Responder cells (5×10^4) and irradiated (4000 rad) stimulator cells (5×10^4) were cultured in 100 μl RPMI plus 10% normal human serum for 6 days. Autologous controls consisted of 50000 responder cells in 50 μl medium. MoAb supernatant (25% v/v) was added to the relevant cultures

The Effect of HLA-DR and DQ MoAbs in Primary MLR

MoAbs reacting with a monomorphic DR determinant, L243, [21] and the DQw1 determinant Genox 3.53 [1] were used to attempt to block specific functions in primary MLC. For this, two DR-identical, DQ-incompatible consanguineous Caucasoid HTC were used, DHI (DRw11, DQw3) and FPA (DRw11, DQw1). These two cells stimulate each other in MLC. To study whether the DQ incompatibility was responsible for the primary MLR, we used anti-DR and anti-DQw1 MoAbs to try to block the stimulation. Figure 12 shows that the strong reciprocal MLR between FPA and DHI was not blocked by the addition of the DQw1-specific MoAb Genox 3.53. Furthermore, when FPA (DRw11, DQw1) was used as a responder, the addition of Genox 3.53 enhanced the response. In contrast, the addition of the monomorphic DR MoAb L243 to the MLC reduced the response to background level. These results indicated that although FPA's and DHI's DR determinants were identical, their mutual stimulation was due to incompatibility for a DR-related determinant (HLA-Dw) and not to the DQ incompatibility [28].

The Effect of DR and DQ MoAbs on the Induction of Suppressor Cells

The effect of DR and DQ MoAbs on the specific induction of suppressor cells by FPA was also studied. As seen in Fig. 9, BW's cells did not respond to FPA's cells, due to the specific induction of suppressor cells. After the addition of the DQw1 antibody to the MLC, BW's cells reacted normally to FPA, indicating that the induction of suppressor cells had been abolished (Table 4). This effect was maintained if the antibody was added to the culture 8 h after it was set up, but if it was added after 24 h, BW's cells again did not respond. The control MLR between other responder cells (HF) and FPA showed no difference when the DQw1 MoAb was added. In contrast, the DR antibody did not change the low response of BW to FPA, but reduced that of HF's cells to background level. The addition of the antibody 8 h after setting up the culture also blocked the response, whereas if it was added after 24 h, no blocking was observed. Although the induction of BW's suppressor cells by FPA appears to be genetically controlled by class I determinants, DQ molecules could have a role in the initial phase of this induction.

In addition, when the DQw1 MoAb was added to MLC between responder and stimulator, both DQw1-negative, an enhancement of the response was also observed. Preliminary experiments to explain these results suggest some cross-reactivity between the T8 and DQw1 antigens (unpublished data).

The Effect of DR and DQ MoAbs on the Induction of Cytotoxic Cells

The addition of anti-DQw1 MoAb, but not anti-DR MoAb, blocked the induction of cytotoxic effectors in MLR. Figure 13 shows the results of a CML using

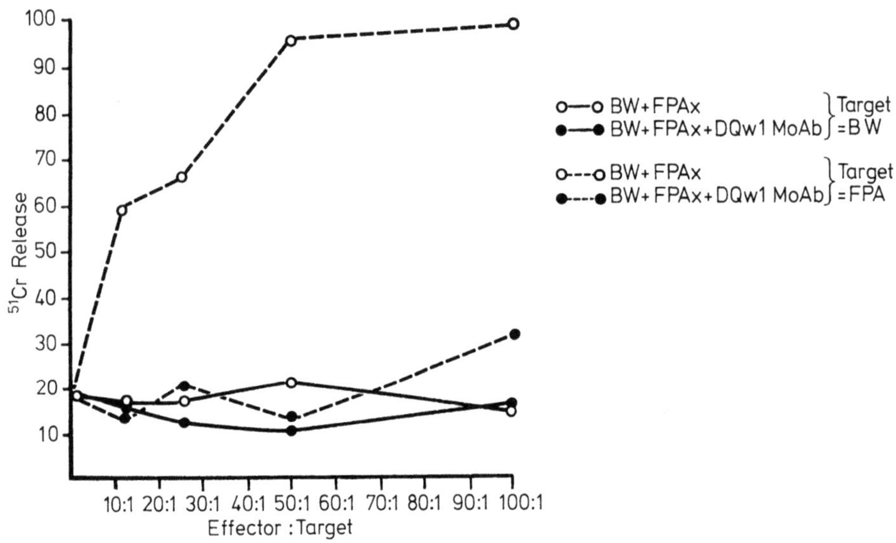

Fig. 13. Effect of adding DQw1-specific MoAb (Genox 35.3) to the cytotoxic T lymphocyte activity of effector cells induced in MLC: specific blocking of cytotoxic T lymphocyte production by DQw1-specific MoAbs. Effector cells were generated in MLC. Ten million responder cells (BW A25,Aw32 / B18,Bw39 / DR2,DR7 / DQw1,Dqw2) were cultured with then million irradiated (4000 rad) stimulator cells (FPA A1 / Bw35 / DRw11 / DRw52 / DQw1) in RPMI plus 10% heat-inactivated normal human serum with or without 10% v/v of DQw1-specific MoAb Genox 35.3 supernatant. The effector cells were harvested on day 6. Normal peripheral blood lymphocytes were incubated with PHA for 3 days at 37 °C in 5% CO_2 and were used as CML targets. CMLs were set up at the effector-to-target ratio of 100:1, 50:1, 25:1, and 12.5:1. Specific chromium release was measured after 4 h and calculated according to the following formula:

$$\% \text{ of cytotoxicity} = \frac{\text{experimental release} - \text{spontaneous release}}{\text{total release} - \text{spontaneous release}} \times 100$$

Table 5. The effect of DQw1 MoAb on the induction of suppressor cells by FPA

Responder cells	Genox 3.53 added (h)	L243 added (h)	Autologous control	Stimulator cells (FPA)
BW	–		2746 ± 1014	3751 ± 1159
Dw2, DB1	0			22943 ± 1688
DR2,7	8			21138 ± 2600
DQw1,2	24			2977 ± 1703
		0		3519 ± 475
		8		8037 ± 1206
		24		3734 ± 2142
HF	–		3676 ± 2131	39104 ± 1842
DwX,X	0			28380 ± 7699
DR1,5	8			NT
DQw1,3	24			36436 ± 4747
		0		3251 ± 1154
		8		7698 ± 1245
		24		23994 ± 1063

Results expressed as mean cpm ± sd from triplicate experiments
FPA's cells are capable of inducing a false typing response by BW's cells due to the production of specific T8-positive suppressor cells. The addition of DQw1 MoAb to the MLC between BW and FPA's cells blocked such a response. If the antibody was added 8 h after the culture was set up, it still blocked the induction of suppressor cells, but this was not the case if it was added after 24 h. No significant differences were observed when the DR MoAb was added to the culture at different times

BW effector cells induced in MLC against FPA, with and without anti-DQw1 MoAb. As previously mentioned, after 6 days stimulation with FPA, the majority of BW's cells are T8-positive, class II-positive (see Table 5), and are capable of specific suppression in MLR. In addition, this population has a strong cytotoxic activity against FPA and other targets sharing FPA's class I antigens after CML following an MLR. However, no specific killing of FPA target cells by BW's effector cells was observed when the DQw1 MoAb was added during the induction phase, i.e. to the MLC. The induction of cytotoxic cells had thus been blocked by the DQw1 MoAb [4, 27].

It is not clear whether the same T8-positive, class II-positive cell subset is responsible for both the suppressor and cytotoxic functions. However, whereas the suppressor effect is specific only for the response of BW's HLA-identical sibling's cells (JW) to FPA in MLC, the cytotoxic effect is specific not only against FPA, but also against third-party targets sharing class I determinants with FPA.

The effect of the DQw1 MoAb thus appears to be relevant for the induction of functional T8-positive, class II-positive cells irrespective of the specificity they can recognise.

From the functional studies mentioned above, it appears that although the DR and DQ antigens are involved in T cell functions, both the DR and DQ molecules have to be present at the same stage of the initiation of the response for it to be complete. Thus the absence of any of the class II molecules (DR/DQ/DP) on antigen-presenting cells may impair the total T cell response.

Expression of HLA Class II Antigens on T Cell Leukaemias

Early studies in our laboratory demonstrated that there is differential expression of the HLA-DR and DQ antigens on the majority of acute leukaemias [26, 29, 30]. Since then, there has been several reports confirming these results [8, 16, 32]. However, all T cell leukaemias of immature (thymic) T cell phenotype have been found to be HLA class II-negative (DR/DQ) [28, 31].

In the experiments reported here, we have confirmed and extended these findings by testing a panel of T cell leukaemic lines of immature, thymic (Molt 4, HSB2, JM, and CEM) and mature, post-thymic (HUT 78) phenotypes for the expression of HLA-DR (L243) [21], DQ (Tu22) [46], and DP (B7/21) [43] antigens, using MoAbs reacting with each of these molecules. A MoAb (L227) [21] reacting with a monomorphic class II determinant was also used (Table 6).

None of the MoAbs used reacted with any of the acute leukaemic cell lines of immature phenotype. In contrast, the T cell line HUT 78, derived from a patient with Sézary syndrome, reacted strongly with the HLA-DR, DQ, and DP MoAbs. It is most likely that the HLA class II expression on the cell line HUT 78 is due to an activation of these cells during the course of the leukaemic process, e.g. viral infection.

Based on the functional and serological data presented above, it is possible to suggest that the absence of DQ antigens on DR-positive acute leukaemias may be responsible for the lack of T cell-mediated autologous anti-tumor cytotoxicity observed in the majority of leukaemias and tumors. In this context, it is interesting to mention that HLA-restricted anti-tumor cytotoxic cells have been described in patients with HTLV leukaemia [23], and it has been shown that HTLV T cell blasts express class II (DR) molecules [39]. Although no data are available with regard to the expression of DQ molecules, it is most likely that these antigens are also expressed on these cells. Their expression would thus contribute to the induction of cytotoxic T cells.

Conclusion

Although the majority of resting T cells appear to be HLA class II-negative, it has now been demonstrated, using MoAbs reacting with class II determinants, that a small proportion of resting T cells do express class II antigens [2, 3, 15].

In contrast, most T cells express class II antigens upon activation with mitogens or alloantigens [15, 20]. Also, class II-positive activated T cells are capable of inducing autologous and allogeneic primary and secondary MLR [6, 34, 44]. In addition, the data reported here show that the induction of HLA class II antigens on activated T cells coincided with the acquisition of suppressor properties, i.e. these suppressor properties become evident only after the expression of the HLA class II antigens. The T cell subpopulation responsible for the suppressor effect was shown to be T8-positive, class II-positive [11] (T8-positive cells that were class II-negative were not suppressors in this system). Thus the progressive expansion of T8-positive subpopulations over 8 days in culture, followed by the emergence of MHC class II antigens on these cells, was the sequence of events observed during the induction of the suppressor properties.

Table 6. Expression of HLA class I and class II antigens on leukaemia- and lymphoma-derived cell lines

Cell line	Cell type	Origin	Class I	Class II			
			Common HLA-A/B/C	Common HLA-DR/DQ/DP	Monomorphic HLA-DR	Monomorphic HLA-DQ	Monomorphic HLA-DP
			W6/32	L227	L243	Tu22	B7/21
MOLT 4	T blast II	ALL	100	–	–	–	–
CCRF-HSB-2	T blast II	ALL	100	–	–	–	–
JM	T blast II	ALL	95	–	–	–	–
CCRF-CEM	T blast II	ALL	98	–	–	–	–
HUT 78	Activated T cell	Sézary cell leukaemia	100	90	85	80	95

ALL, acute lymphoblastic leukaemia
Results are expressed as percentage of cells stained with $F(ab')_2$ FITC goat anti-mouse immunoglobulin (IgG)

Recent studies on the expression of class II antigens on T cell clones have shown that class II-positive T cell clones are capable of presenting soluble antigen to specific T cell clones in a restricted fashion [41], and that these antigens are expressed in every T cell clone irrespective of its function [24]. Furthermore T cell responses to alloantigens and the T cell production of interleukin-2 seem to be a process that indirectly or directly involves the HLA class II molecules [42].

However, the observation that HLA class II MoAbs are not able to block the effector capacity of class II-positive cytotoxic T cells when added to a cell-mediated lympholysis [6] indicate that although the expression of HLA class II molecules on T cells is necessary for these cells to acquire full functional capacity, the specific functional role of the class II molecules on these effector cells is still unresolved. It is possible that the expression of HLA class II molecules on T cells may act as a feedback mechanism for the continuous activation and clonal expansion of these cells once the specific immune response has been selected and initiated.

Interactions between cells resulting in different functions (i.e. helper, suppressor and cytotoxic) depend not only on the class II genetic determinants expressed on the activated cells, but also on the MHC and non-MHC genetic control of these responder cells. These interactions may thus be particularly important in the pathogenesis of HLA-associated diseases.

New nomenclature for T4 and T8 antigens is CD4 and CD8 respectively.

Acknowledgements. We would like to thank all those who contributed monoclonal antibodies and cells lines for this work. We would also like to thank Khalid Razak for technical assistance and Denny Williams for typing the manuscript.

We gratefully acknowledge The Leukaemia Research Fund, Medical Research Council and the Cancer Research Campaign of Great Britain for financial support.

References

1. Brodsky FM, Parham P, Bodmer WF (1980) Monoclonal antibodies to HLA-DRw determinants. Tissue Antigens 16. 30
2. Brown G, Walker L, Ling NR, MacLennan ICM, Richardson P, Johnson GD (1984) Expression of MHC Class II antigens on human blood lymphocytes; studies in relation to B cell neoplasia and cell proliferation. Dis Markers 2:305
3. Brown MF, Cook RG, Van M, Rich RR (1984) Cloned human T cells synthesize Ia molecules and can function as antigen presenting cells. Hum Immunol 11:219
4. Corte G, Moretta A, Cosulich ME, Ramarli D, Bargellesi A (1982) A monoclonal anti-DC1 antibody selectively inhibits the generation of effector T cells mediating specific cytolytic activity. J Exp Med 156:1539
5. Dongworth DW, McMichael AJ (1984) Inhibition of human T lymphocyte function with monoclonal antibodies. Br Med Bull 40:254
6. Engelman EG, Benike CJ, Charron DJ (1980) Ia antigen on peripheral blood mononuclear leukocytes in man. II. Functional studies of HLA-DR positive cells activated in mixed lymphocyte reactions. J Exp Med 152:114
7. Erb P, Feldman M (1975) The role of macrophages in the generation of helper cells. II. The genetic control of the macrophage-T-C interaction for helper induction with soluble antigens. J Exp Med 142:460

8. Faille A, Turmel P, Charron DJ (1984) Differential expression of HLA-DR and HLA-DC/DS molecules in a patient with hairy cell leukaemia: restoration of HLA-DC/DS expression by (12-0-tetradecanoyl-phorbol-13-acetate), 5-azacytidine, and sodium butyrate. Blood 64:33
9. Fainboim L, Navarrete C, Festenstein H (1980) Precursor and effector phenotypes of activated human T lymphocytes. Nature 288:391
10. Fainboim L, Jaraquemada D, Festenstein H, Sachs JA (1981) MHC specified lymphocyte activating and suppressor activating determinants in human mixed lymphocyte reactions. Scand J Immunol 14:655
11. Fainboim L, Navarrete C, Spitz M, Festenstein H (1981) Relationship between "DR" expression and suppressor effect of activating T cells. In: Hraba T, Hasek M (eds) Cellular and molecular mechanisms of immunologic tolerance. Dekker, New York, p 127
12. Fainboim L, Jaraquemada D, Festenstein H (1983) Responder phenotypes after alloactivation with suppressor activating determinants. Transplant Proc 15:771
13. Festenstein H (1976) The Mls system. Transplant Proc 8:339
14. Gerbase-Delima M, Kraemer MH, Novo NF, Paiva ER, Mendes NF (1980) Expression of HLA-DR antigens on T lymphocytes. Tissue Antigens 15:257
15. Greaves MF, Verbi W, Festenstein H, Papasteriadis C, Jaraquemada D, Hayward A (1979) "Ia-like" enigens on human T cells. Eur J Immunol 9:356
16. Guy K, van Heyningen V, Cohen BB, Deane DL, Steel CM (1982) Differential expression and serologically distinct sub-populations of the human IA antigens detected with monoclonal antibodies to Ia alpha and beta chains. Eur J Immunol 12:942
17. Hansen JA, Atkinson K, Martin PJ, Storb R, Longton G, Thomas ED (1983) Human T lymphocyte phenotypes after bone marrow transplantation. Transplantation 36:277
18. Jaraquemada D, Ollier W, Okoye RC, Sachs JA, Festenstein H, Grosse-Wilde H (1983) HLA-DB3: population distribution and family studies of a new HLA-D antigen associated with HLA-DR4 in Caucasoids. Tissue Antigens 22:315
19. Kerbel RS, Doenhoff MJ (1974) Resistance of mitotic B lymphocytes to cytotoxic effects of anti-Ig serum. Nature 250:342–344
20. Ko HS, Fu SM, Winchester RJ, Yu DTY, Kunkel HG (1979) Ia determinants on stimulated human T lymphocytes. Occurrence on mitogen and antigen activated T cells. J Exp Med 150:246
21. Lampson LA, Levy R (1980) Two populations of Ia-like molecules on a human B cell line. J Immunol 125:293
22. McMichael AJ, Sasazuki T (1977) A suppressor T cell in human mixed lymphocyte reaction. J Exp Med 146:368
23. Mitsuya H, Matis LA, Megson M, Bunn PA, Murray C, Mann DL, Gallo RC, Broder S (1983) Generation of an HLA-restricted cytotoxic T cell line reactive against cultured tumour cells from a patient infected with human T cell leukaemia/lymphoma virus. J Exp Med 158:994
24. Moretta A, Accolla RS (1984) Effect of anti-class II monoclonal antibodies on human T cell function. Dis Markers 2:313
25. Moretta L, Ferrarini M, Cooper MD (1978) Characterisation of human T cell subpopulations as defined by specific receptors for immunoglobulins. Contemp Top Immunobiol 8:19
26. Navarrete C, Fainboim L, Festenstein H, Lister A, Amess J, Greaves MF (1981) Selective expression of HLA-DR and HLA-MB antigens on acute leukaemic cells. In: Knapp W (ed) Leukaemia markers. Academic, London, p 65
27. Navarrete C, Jaraquemada D, Fainboim L, Karr R, Hui K, Awad J, Bagnara M, Festenstein H (1985) Genetic and functional relationship of the HLA-DR and HLA-DQ antigens. Immunogenetics 21:97
28. Navarrete C, Jaraquemada D, Hui K, Awad J, Okoye R, Festenstein H (1985) Different functions and associations of HLA-DR and MB(DC) antigens shown by serological, cellular and DNA assays. Tissue Antigens 25:130
29. Navarrete C, Fernandez N, Groves AV, Festenstein H (1985) Differential expression of the HLA-MB(DC) antigens on acute leukaemic blasts. In: Albert ED, Baur MP, Mayr WR (eds) Histocompatibility testing 1984. Springer, Berlin Heidelberg New York Tokyo, p 640

30. Navarrete C, Fernandez N, Alonso C, Festenstein H (1985) Ontogenic and functional implications of the differential expression of HLA-DQ antigens on leukaemic cells. Hum Immunol (in press)
31. Newman RA, Greaves MF (1982) Characterisation of HLA-DR antigens on leukaemic cells. Clin Exp Immunol 50:41
32. Newman RA, Delia D, Greaves MF, Navarrete C, Fainboim L, Festenstein H (1983) Differential expression of HLA-DR and DR-linked determinants on human leukaemias and lymphoid cells. Eur J Immunol 13:172
33. Pachoula-Papasteriadis C, Jaraquemada D, Festenstein H (1979) Modulation of antigen expression on sperm-activated T cells in culture. Transplant Proc 11:1331
34. Pawelec G, Blaurock M, Schneider EM, Shaw S, Wernet P (1982) Alloactivated long-term cultured human T lymphocytes express both HLA-DR and SB antigens but lack lymphocyte stimulation capacity. Eur J Immunol 12:967
35. Pawelec G (1983) Allogeneically primed T lymphocyte clones in the analysis of lymphocyte stimulatory determinants. Hum Immunol 8:239
36. Schirrmacher V, Festenstein H (1975) Activated lymphocytes express surface determinants which react with heterologous anti-B cell serum. J Immunogenet 2:337
37. Schirrmacher V, Festenstein H (1976) ^{14}C-Thymidine release assay: a new test for the study of surface determinants on activated lymphocytes. Tissue Antigens 7:183
38. Singh SK, Abramson EJ, Kreo CJ, David CS (1984) Endogenous synthesis of Ia antigens by a cloned T cell line. J Mol Cell Immunol 1:147
39. Suciu-Foca N, Rubenstein P, Popovic M, Gallo RC, King DW (1984) Reactivity of HTLV-transformed human T-cell lines to MHC class II antigens. Nature 312:275
40. Tada T, Taniguchi M, David CS (1976) Properties of the antigen-specific suppressive T cell factor in the regulation of antibody response of the mouse. IV. Special subregion assignment of the gene(s) that codes for the suppressive T cell factor in the H-2 histocompatibility complex. J Exp Med 144:713
41. Triebel F, Missenard-Leblond V, Autran B, Couty MC, Charron DJ, Debre P (1984) Antigen-specific proliferative human T cell clones with specificity for diphtheria toxoid: genetic and molecular restriction by class II antigens. Eur J Immunol 14:697
42. Triebel F, Missenard-Leblond V, Couty MC, Charron DJ, Debre P (1984) Differential inhibition of human antigen-specific T cell clone proliferative responses by distinct monoclonal anti-HLA-DR antibodies. J Immunol 132:1773
43. Watson AJ, DeMars R, Trowbridge IS, Bach FH (1983) Detection of a novel human class II HLA antigen. Nature 304:358
44. Wollman E, Cohen D, Fradelizi D, Sasportes M, Dausset J (1980) Different stimulating capacity of B and T lymphocytes in primary and secondary allogenic reactions: cellular detection of HLA-D products on T lymphocytes. J Immunol 125:2039
45. Yu DTY, Winchester RJ, Fu SM, Gibofsky A, Ko HS, Kunkel HG (1980) Peripheral blood Ia-positive T cells. J Exp Med 151:91
46. Ziegler A, Uchanska-Ziegler B, Rosenfelder G, Braun DG, Wernet P (1981) Heterogeneity of established human hematopoietic cell lines surface antigens detected by MoAbs and glycosphingolipid patterns. In: Knapp W (ed) Leukemia markers. Academic, London, p 317
47. Zinkernagel RM, Doherty PC (1974) Restriction of in vitro T cell-mediated cytotoxicity in lymphocytic choriomeningitis within a syngeneic or allogeneic system. Nature 248:701

Tissue Distribution of Class II Transplantation Antigens: Presence on Normal Cells *

L. Klareskog and U. Forsum

Table of Contents

Introduction

Expression of class II transplantation antigens has during recent years been described on many cell types, both within the lymphoid system and in nonlymphoid organs. Constitutive expression of class II molecules occurs in some cells of bone marrow origin, but in most cells, class II antigen expression is inducible and transient. For both these categories of cells, important functions in immune reactions have been implicated.

The scope of this review is mainly to describe the expression of class II transplantation antigens on certain normal, nonlymphoid cells without a constitutive expression of class II antigens. The role of class II antigens expressed on hematopoetic cells, including dendritic cells and macrophages, and on endothelial cells

* The studies from our own laboratories referred to in this review wre supported by funds from the Swedish Medical Research Council, the King Gustaf V 80th Birthday Fund the Swedish Association Against Rheumatism and the Swedish work environmental fund

will be discussed in other chapters within this volume (P. Stastny et al., V.C. Broudy and J.H. Fitchen, B. Torok-Storb and F.W. Springton). In addition to reviewing current literature on the distribution of class II antigens in humans, we shall also refer to some studies on class II antigen expression in animals. Such references are in particular made to studies where a new feature of class II antigen distribution has first been described in animals.

A substantial difficulty in defining the distribution of class II antigens is connected with the fact that the reactivities of the used antibodies have only rarely been defined in detail. Thus, despite the fact that the genetic region coding for human class II antigens is now well described, most monoclonal antibodies, as well as heteroantisera used to detect class II antigens, have not been defined as to their reactivity with distinct molecules [see comment in 25]. This shortcoming is further emphasized by the demonstration of more than one alpha and beta chain being coded for by the three different class II loci that are as yet defined (see short review by Bodmer and Bodmer [7]). Furthermore, monoclonal anti-class II antibodies can react with two or more different chains coded for by the class II genes (see Rebai et al. [79]), something that is natural considering the amino acid sequence homologies that have been demonstrated for the different polypeptide chains that constitute the various class II antigens [2, 52, 80]. Many of the antibodies hitherto used can, however, be supposed to be capable of further analysis as to fine specificity, thereby resolving some of the current problems. In the studies from our own laboratories that are referred to, we have in many cases used rabbit antisera that were produced against human class II antigens obtained from spleen cells [40] and for which the gross reactivities are the same as for an earlier described antiserum [39] produced in a similar way. It was later demonstrated by analyses on RNA transcripts that these antisera react at least with a beta chain of the DQ (DC) locus and an alpha chain of the DR locus, and thus with intact class II antigens coded for by at least these two loci (see also [51]). Whether these antisera in addition react with DP (SB) antigens is as yet not known. Like many other anti-class II antisera, these particular sera have been shown to react with class II antigens from a number of different species, including rat, mouse, and guinea pig [49]. The reactivity in these species with class II antigens coded for by different loci is, however, not known.

The first demonstration that class II transplantation antigens may be expressed not only on hematopoetic cells as B lymphocytes, activated T cells, and macrophages/dendritic cells was with rabbit antisera in two different systems. First, immunofluorescence studies were performed on frozen sections of tissue from outbred, free-living guinea pigs. Class II antigens defined by the rabbit anti-class II sera were observed not only on lymphoid cells, but also on a number of epithelial cells, i.e., in the intestine, in bile ducts, in salivary glands, and thymic epithelial cells [22, 102]. Using the same animal system, it was also demonstrated that class II antigens could be expressed on mammary gland epithelium and on mammary gland duct cells in lactating animals, but hardly at all in the epithelium of virgin female guinea pigs [42]. In a second series of experiments, human class II antigens were shown to be expressed on keratinocytes in two different inflammatory conditions, namely mycosis fungoides and lichen planus, both in situ [61, 62] and after dispersion of cells [63]. Concomitantly, it was reported by Hirschberg et al. [30] that human endothelial cells can under certain circumstances express class II transplantation antigens. Shortly thereafter is was convincingly demonstrated that supernates containing gamma-interferon produced by activated T cells can induce class II expression on previously class II-negative cells (first shown for macrophages [92, 93]). These findings had two implications: First, far more cells than hitherto believed have the capacity to express class II transplantation antigens. Second, the expression of class II antigens is not constant, but is influenced at least by inflammatory and hormonal stimuli. Subsequently, a large number of studies on the detailed tissue distribution of class II antigens in different condictions and in different species have been carried out. In particular, an enhanced expression of class II antigens has been demonstrated in various autoimmune conditions and in infectious diseases, and many propositions have been made as to the functional role of the class II antigens in these states. One main conclusion to be derived from these studies is that the variable and inducible amount of class II antigens seen on many nonlymphoid cells, are part of a normal homeostasis in the body; thus, normal individuals subjected to the daily environmental infectious and chemical challenges are subjected to stimuli that may provoke class II induction in some fully normal cells. We will in this review summarize data on class II antigen expression in various organs in health and during various nonmalignant, mainly inflammatory conditions, and finally try to indicate which implications these tissue distribution studies may have for our understanding of the functions of class II transplantation antigens.

Tissue Distribution of Class II Antigens in Various Organs

Skin

The skin, and particularly the epidermis, represents an easily accessible model system for the study of class II antigen expression as it contains both epidermal Langerhans cells that express a constant and high amount of class II antigens [38, 81] and keratinocytes that can be induced to express class II antigens. Epidermal Langerhans cells appear to belong to the family of bone-marrow-derived [95], dendritic, and strongly class II-positive cells that are described in detail by P. Stastny et al. in this volume. As to keratinocytes, the first observations on class II expression of keratinocytes, in mycosis fungoides [61] and in lichen planus [62], were soon followed by observations in graft-vs-host reactions both in the rat [64] and in man [51]. In time, an expanding number of clinical syndromes were described where keratinocytes from affected skin express class II antigens: contact hypersensitivity reactions, discoid lupus erythematosus, tuberculoid psoriasis, pityriasis rosea, Tuberculid and bullous dermatosis [1, 2a, 50, 60, 91]. In normal skin from healthy persons, class II antigen expression on keratinocytes has only been observed in a minor number of flattened ductal keratinocytes and in adjacent cuticular cells that form the asyringial lumen of dermal eccrine ducts [68].

Some information on the mechanisms responsible for the induction of class II antigens on keratinocytes can be gained both from studies on tissue distribution of induced lesions and from in vitro studies on isolated cells. Thus, the tuberculin reaction that has for a long time been used as a prototype for a delayed-type hypersensitivity reaction was used to investigate the cell patterns typical for such a reaction [76, 82, 83] (Scheynius and Tjernlund 1985, submitted for publication). Induction of class II antigens on keratinocytes can in the tuberculin reaction first

Table 1. Distribution of human class II transplantation antigens on nonlymphoid cells

Organ	Condition/disease	Cell type	Ref.
Skin	Mycosis fungoides	Keratinocyte	[61, 63]
	Lichen planus	Keratinocyte	[62]
	Graft-vs-host reaction	Keratinocyte	[51]
	Tuberculin reaction (DTH)	Keratinocyte	[82]
	Contact hypersensitivity	Keratinocyte	[60]
	Various dermatoses	Keratinocyte	[1, 2a, 50, 91]
Intestine	Normal	Epithelium	[18, 69, 84]
	Celiac disease	Epithelium	[86]
	Dermatitis herpetiformis	Epithelium	[58]
	Ulcerative colitis	Epithelium	[88]
	Crohn's disease	Epithelium	[88]
Buccal mucosa	Melkerson-Rosenthal syndrome	Epithelium	Rönnblom et al. (1985), submitted for publication
Tongue	Normal	Epithelium	[18]
Respiratory system	Normal	Epithelium	[18]
Liver and bile ducts	Primary biliary cirrhosis	Bile duct epithelium	[3], Karlsson-Parra et al. (1985) submitted for publication
Thyroid gland	Grave's disease	Thyrocytes	[27]
	Hashimoto's thyroiditis		[35]
	Nodular goiter		
Salivary glands	Sjögren's syndrome	Duct epithelium	[57]
Mammary gland	Normal, lactating	Epithelium	[18, 69, 70, 71]
Placenta	Normal	Epithelioid cells	[9]
Kidney	Normal	Tubular cells (faint staining)	[23, 28]
	Allografted and rejected	Tubular cells (strong staining)	[15, 16, 26, 97]
Lower urinary tract	Normal	Transitional epithelium	[18, 33]
Synovium	Normal	Lining cells (A and B cells)	[34, 43, 89]
	Rheumatoid arthritis and other types of synovitis	Lining cells, fibroblastoid cells, etc.	[11, 34, 43, 44–47, 75, 104]
Muscle	Myositis	Sarcolemma	[72]

For a more complete set of references and for details of distribution and reagents used, see text

be seen at about 4 days after challenge with tuberculin, i.e., 3–4 days after the first appearance of T lymphocytes in the adjacent tissue. The class II antigen expression on keratinocytes reaches a maximum with a confluent intense reactivity in the epidermis around day 8–10 after injection. Class II antigens are still seen patchwise on keratinocytes at day 17, but all have disappeared by day 30 after challenge. It thus appears that infiltration by lymphocytes, mainly T cells, in the dermis and epidermis, as well as by macrophages and other inflammatory cells in the dermis precedes the keratinocyte class II antigen expression and that class

II expression does not vanish until after the lymphocytes have disappeared from the lesion. As in vitro experiments have demonstrated that gamma-interferon released from activated T lymphocytes can induce class II antigen expression on keratinocytes [5], it is reasonable to believe that products released from invading T lymphocytes are responsible for the induced class II antigen expression. Whether other molecules than gamma-interferon can also mediate this effects is unknown.

There appears to be at least a quantitative difference as to expression of different class II antigen molecules in keratinocytes and Langerhans cells [99] (Scheynius and Tjernlund 1985, submitted for publication). Thus, the monoclonals and heteroantisera that recognize the HLA-DR antigens react equally well with Langerhans cells and keratinocytes observed in the tuberculin reaction, and in certain dermatoses with induced class II expression on keratinocytes. Leu 10, an antibody that reacts with HLA-DQ class II products [13], on the other hand reacts only with Langerhans cells and not with keratinocytes on frozen sections of tissue from the actual lesions [99] (Scheynius and Tjernlund 1985, submitted for publication).

No functional in vitro studies have so far been carried out on class II antigen expression on keratinocytes devoid of Langerhans cells. Cell populations containing both class II-expressing keratinocytes and epidermal Langerhans cells obtained from mycosis fungoides lesions have, however, like cells from normal epidermis [8], been efficient stimulators in both the allogeneic and autologous mixed leucocyte culture reactions [63].

Epithelial cells, which, like keratinocytes, line specialized organs such as the eye and orifices, have only been investigated to a limited extent as to class II antigen expression. Thus, the cells within the cornea display many similarities to those of the epidermis, but so far no expression of class II antigens on corneal epithelial cells has been reported. Instead, class II-expressing Langerhans cells, which are present at different densities in all parts of the epidermis [59], are normally present only in the peripheral limbus region of the cornea, as shown both in the guinea pig [41] and in man [18, 101]; in the latter case it has been suggested that corneal grafts taken to avoid the presence of class II-expressing Langerhans cells should relatively easily escape rejection [96).

The flattened epithelial cells of the buccal mucosa appear to have the same capacity for class II expression as, for example, keratinocytes. Thus, class II expression in buccal mucosa epithelial cells has been observed in the rare inflammatory condition Melkerson-Rosenthals syndrome (Rönnblom et al. 1985, submitted for publication), and a limited expression of class II antigens was noted in basal squamous epithelium of normal human tongue [18].

Intestine

The intestine is, like the epidermis, subjected to a number of exogenous stimuli, both from resident bacteria and from alimentary contents. Thus it is difficult to define any "normal", unstimulated state from which states of induction of class II antigens can occur, and it is feasible that class II-inducing stimuli also act in the normal animal and human intestine, where class II antigens have been observed on epithelial cells. In these studies on normal intestinal tissue, a weak to moderate class II expression was noted on intestinal epithelial cells of the small and large bowel of both humans and in animals such as the guinea pig and the rat [18, 22, 65, 69, 70, 73, 84, 86, 102]. The class II antigens in intestinal epithelium are mainly restricted to the top of the villi and to the apical parts of the columnar epithelial cells. The staining patterns indicate that a high proportion of the class II antigens in these cells reside intracellularly. As to the mechanisms responsible for induction of class II antigens on intestinal epithelial cells, studies on the origin and ontogeny of class II-expressing cells have been performed in the rat, and studies on the class II antigen distribution in various pathological conditions have been carried out in the rat and in man. Thus, intestinal epithelial cells from fetal and young rats (up to 4 weeks) do not express class II antigens [65]. In the adult rat, class II antigen expression in intestinal epithelial tissue is primarily seen close to intraepithelial lymphoid infiltrates [4, 12]. In vitro cultured, primarily class II-negative intestinal epithelial cells were, in the study by Cerf-Bensussan et al. [12], shown to express class II antigens within 48 h after incubation with supernates from activated lymphocytes. It was suggested that all epithelial class II antigen expression in the gut may be secondary to the release of gamma-interferon produced by activated T lymphocytes. An argument against such a mechanism as the only one responsible for intestinal epithelial class II antigen expression is, however, provided by the demonstration that intestinal epithelial cells of nude rats also express class II antigens [65]. In their series of experiments, however, evidence was also provided for the involvement of other factors such as luminal contents and perhaps hormones in intestinal epithelial class II expression, as syngeneic grafts of fetal gut transplanted under the kidney capsule failed to express class II antigens at that time when the same tissue subjected to the alimentary content in the gut showed marked class II antigen expression in epithelial cells [65]. These studies also demonstrated that epithelial class II-expressing cells are not of bone marrow origin, that the rat equivalents to both I-A and I-E/C antigens are similarly expressed, and that substantial differences exist between different strains as to epithelial class II antigen expression. The last-named differences were linked to genes outside the MHC. Recent studies on differential class II expression in man have, unlike the results in the rat, indicated that primarily HLA-DR antigens are expressed in intestinal epithelial tissue, with no expression of HLA-DQ antigens being seen [70].

In pathological conditions, a substantial difference in intestinal epithelial class II antigen expression was first noted in the graft-vs-host reaction in the rat [4]. Thus, transfer of both T helper and T suppressor/cytotoxic T cells to F_1 hybrid recipient rats induced class II expression in the epithelial cells of the gut as well as in the keratinocytes of the skin [4]. Similarly, infection with *Trichinella spiralis* in the gut of rats provoked an increase in epithelial class II antigen expression, thereby providing additional evidence for the physiological nature of epithelial class II induction [4].

In humans, increased expression of class II antigens in intestinal epithelial cells has been described in active stages of dermatitis herpetiformis and celiac disease [58, 86], as well as in ulcerative colitis and Crohn's disease [88]. No functional studies on these cells have so far been carried out to support the suggestions that increased local class II antigen expression might enhance immune responsiveness towards local antigens, for example in celiac disease.

Respiratory System

Staining of the ciliated pseudostratified columnar epithelium in the trachea has been noted both in the guinea pig [22, 102] and in man [18]. No reports exist so far on class II antigen expression on respiratory epithelium in inflammatory disease.

Liver and Bile Ducts

In normal liver tissue obtained from humans, as well as from different animals such as guinea pigs, class II antigens are mainly expressed on nonparenchymal cells assumed to be Kupffer cells [22, 55, 69]. Class II antigen expression has been reported on segments of gall bladder epithelium of guinea pigs [22], whereas no class II antigens were seen on normal human gall bladder epithelial cells [69]. In most liver biopsies from patients suffering from primary biliary cirrhosis, there is, however, an intense expression of class II antigens coded for by both HLA-DR and DQ loci [3] (Karlsson-Parra et al. 1985, submitted for publication), whereas no such class II antigen expressing is seen in patients with recurrent secondary cholangitis [3].

Thyroid Gland

The thyroid gland is one of many organs where expression of class II antigens on epithelial cells, here thyrocytes, is seen in certain kinds of disease, but not normally. It also represents one of the few tissues for which the newly induced class II-expressing cells have been investigated functionally. Thus, in Graves' disease, in Hashimoto's disease, and in certain case of nodular goiter, class II antigens can be seen, particularly in those areas of the gland that harbor many infiltrating lymphocytes [27, 35]; often a sharp demarcation zone is seen between class II-positive and class II-negative thyrocytes. As was described for keratinocytes, in vitro cultured human thyrocytes can be induced to express class II antigens. Such induction of class II antigens was demonstrated to occur after incubation of the cultures with the lectins phytohemagglutinin, concanavalin A or pokeweed mitogen [77].

In functional studies, the thyrocytes with an induced class II expression can be shown to present polypeptide antigens from influenza virus, bot not from the intact virus itself, to polypeptide-specific cloned human T-cell hybridomas [59]. This antigen presentation was found to be dependent on the expression of the correct class II antigen on the cell surface of the thyrocytes. These data indicate that epithelial cells, here thyrocytes, can under certain circumstances present antigen to T cells and thereby probably contribute to a local antigen-specific T lymphocyte activation. The results also indicate, however, that there are qualitative differences between class II-expressing thyrocytes and other class II-expressing cells, for example macrophages, as to processing and presentation of antigens to T cells: peripheral blood leukocytes could in these experiments present antigen to polypeptide-specific T cell hybridomas after incubation also with intact influenza virus particles [59].

Salivary Glands

It was initially demonstrated in the guinea pig that both the parotid and the submandibular gland may in certain cases contain class II-expressing epithelial cells [22, 102]. A recent report describes that class II antigen expression can also be seen in the human submandibular gland in both primary and secondary Sjögren's syndrome [57]. As is the case for intestinal epithelial cells and for thyrocytes (see above), a correlation was noted between epithelial class II antigen expression and lymphocytic infiltrates.

Mammary Gland

Expression of class II antigens on glandular cells and duct cells of lactating mammary epithelium has been described both in the guinea pig and in man by means of rabbit anti-class II sera [42, 71] and in man with monoclonal anti-class II antigen antibodies [18, 69, 70]; from these latter studies [70] it was suggested that HLA-DR, but not HLA-DQ, antigens are expressed on lactating mammary epithelium. The staining of epithelium varied between different areas of the mammary gland, the most intense staining being seen in the membranes close to the lumen and intracellularly in the apical parts of the secreting cells. As mentioned at the beginning of this chapter, there is evidence both in animals and in man that class II antigen expression in mammary gland epithelial cells is under hormonal control, as only lactating glands, not glands from nonpregnant females, contain class II-expressing epithelial cells [42, 71]. Furthermore, it was demonstrated in the guinea pig that exogenous administration of lactotropic hormones to virgin female animals induced class II antigen expression in the epithelial cells [42].

Whether epithelial class II expression has anything to do with homing of IgA-producing cells to the mammary gland, as was initially suggested [42], is as yet unknown. It is feasible, however, that class II-expressing mammary gland epithelial cells can, as has been shown for class II-expressing thyroid epithelial cells (see above), present antigens to T cells, and thereby contribute to the local immune defense, for example in mastitis. It is also possible that class II antigens present on milk fat globules [70, 103] may fulfil immunological functions in the suckling offspring.

Placenta

In the human placenta, expression of class II antigens has been reported on cell membranes of suspended polygonal epitheloid cells and trophoblasts [9]. In cryostat sections of placenta, however, only a faint staining for class II antigens was observed after the sections had been subjected to 10 min treatment with trypsin [9].

Kidney and Lower Urinary Tract

In normal kidneys, class II expression has been found primarily on certain dendritic cells and on endothelial cells, whereas conflicting reports have been published as to the expression of class II antigens on tubular epithelium. Thus, some authors have reported a faint homogeneous staining for class II antigens in epithelial cells of proximal tubules [23, 28, 29, 78], whereas other investigators have failed to detect any such reactivity [33, 69, 85]. Later, it has been demonstrated that class II antigen expression in proximal tubular cells occurs in transplantation in rats and mice [6, 15, 16, 100] as well as in man [15, 26, 97]. In the rat, induced class II antigen expression in proximal tubular cells has also been reported in experimental pyelonephritis [32]. The earlier demonstration of a variable expression of class II antigens on proximal tubules also in normal rats, and of variability between different rat strains [65], may indicate that earlier conflicting results on class II antigen expression in normal human kidneys may be due in part to variable genetic backgrounds of investigated individuals (see also [23]). Interestingly, recent observations with monoclonal antibodies defined as to reactivities with DR and DQ locus products indicate that expression of only certain class II products, i.e., DR antigens, is induced during rejection (Claesson et al. 1985, submitted for publication). As is the case for the other epithelial class II-expressing cells, kidney tubular cells have also been suggested to participate in the activation of alloreactive recipient T cells. If this is so, a more detailed knowledge of the differential expression of class II antigens in kidneys might be of clinical significance, but no functional studies on kidney tubular cells in this respect have yet been reported.

In the transitional epithelium in the lower urinary tract, only limited information is available as to class II antigen expression on epithelial cells. Limited expression of class II antigens in certain parts of the epithelium, particularly in the basal layers, has been reported in rat and in guinea pig [22, 33, 102], as well as in man [18]. A somewhat increased number of class II-expressing cells in the epithelium was seen during experimental urinary tract infection with *E. coli* in the rat [32]. It was in this study not definitively ascertained, however, whether these cells were indeed epithelial. In man, some epithelial cells present in the urine of healthy individuals can be shown to express class II antigens [33].

Synovial Tissue

Synovial tissue in normal individuals and in individuals with various inflammatory arthritic conditions have been rather extensively investigated for the presence of class II transplantation antigens. The rationale behind this interest in the potential involvement of different class II-expressing synovial cells in the local activation of immune reactions that may contribute to the development of arthritis. It was initially demonstrated that a relatively high number of cells within the synovial intima of normal individuals subjected to meniscectomy expressed class II transplantation antigens [43], and that a large number of cells in the rheumatoid synovial tissue were class II-positive [34, 43, 112]. Subsequently, it was also demonstrated that the increased class II antigen expression in the synovial tissue of rheumatoid arthritis patients occurs concomitantly or subsequent to infiltration of T cells, particularly T helper cells, into the synovium [19, 20, 34, 44, 45, 56, 75]. When the phenotypes of human class II-expressing cells were further investigated, it appeared that both the previously characterized macrophage-like (type A) cells and fibroblast-like lining (type B) cells could express class II antigens [89]. In suspensions of cells obtained from rheumatoid synovial tissue, it was also possible to identify at least three different class II-expressing cell types, of which one was fibroblastoid and lacked macrophage markers and the other two represented various forms of macrophage-like/dendritic cells [11]. Thus, synovial tissue provides strong support for the idea that fibroblast-like cells can also be induced to express class II antigens; in this case it is feasible that class II expression is induced on macrophage-like cells, fibroblastoid cells, and endothelial cells by products released from the many activated T lymphocytes [10, 21, 43] that can be found in the synovial tissue of patients with active rheumatoid arthritis as well as other arthritic condictions.

Furthermore, detailed immunomorphological studies of synovial tissue and particularly of the pannus found at the interface between cartilage and synovial tissue in individuals with rheumatoid arthritis, have demonstrated that a large number of class II-expressing cells both with and without macrophage markers are present close to the synovial cavity and/or penetrating the cartilage [47]. It also appears that antibodies that recognize DR antigens react with a larger proportion of cells close to the cartilage than is the case for monoclonal specific for DQ gene products [47]. It is thus feasible that differentiated class II antigen expression can preferentially be seen in cells that are induced to express class II antigens, such as certain of the synovial cells, as well as keratinocytes and intestinal and renal tubular cells, as discussed above. Notably, however, expression of DR as well as DQ antigens has been convincingly demonstrated on fibroblasts grown in vitro after incubation with gamma-interferon, indicating that differentiated class II antigen expression may not necessarily represent a general phenomenon [17]. Nevertheless, further detailed studies on the differential expression of different class II gene products in synovial tissue if of considerable interest, not least in view of the possibility that locally distributed antigens of autoantigenic or exogenous nature may have distinct class II molecules as restriction elements during T cell activation.

Cells from inflamed synovial tissue can relatively easily be obtained and studied functionally after therapeutic synovectomies performed in rheumatoid arthritis patients. As the phenotypic patterns display considerable similarities between different inflammatory lesions, particularly those occurring in disease with a suspected autoimmune background, rheumatoid synovial cells may to some extent constitute a model system where functions of different inflammatory cells can be studied. Using this system, it appears that a subpopulation of class II-expressing cells may act as very potent activators of T cells [21, 43, 44, 46] as has been proposed from the above-mentioned immunomorphological in situ studies. This subpopulation encompasses a population of strongly class II-expressing cells with a dendritic morphology, as well as fibroblastoid class II-expressing cells and a small number of cells with macrophage markers. In contrast, other major populations of class II-expressing rheumatoid adherent cells, separated from the stimulatory populations by means of Percoll density gradient centrifugation, may mainly suppress T cell responses [44, 46]. These data support earlier observations, made in more defined systems, that activated macrophages may, even if they express high amounts of class II antigens, suppress T lymphocyte activation [66]. Whether the class II antigens themselves, or products such as prostaglandins released from the activated cells [see 46], are responsible for the suppression of T cell activation is, however, not known. Nevertheless, these two observations emphasize the need for further functional investigations of cells with induced class II antigen expression. Teleologically speaking there should be good arguments both for an enhanced antigen-presenting capacity to T cells and for an induced suppressive function carried out by cells with gamma-interferon-induced class II expression. The need for enhanced responsiveness in, for example, local bacterial infections is obvious, and such a reaction might well provoke subsequent autoimmune reactions [34, 43, 44]. If, on the other hand, local immune reactions are provoked by persistent stimuli of exogenous or autoimmunogenic nature, there should be a need for local suppressive mechanisms, which thus might possibly be mediated by identical cells in different stages of activation and differentiation.

Muscle

The myocyte represents still another type of nonepithelial cell in which class II antigen expression can be induced in inflammatory conditions, such as different kinds of myositis [72], or in transplantation [67]. As is the case for cells from other tissues, sharp demarcation zones can be seen between areas with and without myocyte class II expression; class II expression is closely correlated to distribution of T lymphocyte infiltrates. Notably, some segment of myocytes can express class II antigens on the surface while other segments of the surface of the same cells are class II-negative.

Concluding Remarks

Class II transplantation antigens have, since their definition in the 1970s, attracted great interest, mainly in view of their role as restriction elements when T4/Leu 3-expressing T lymphocytes recognize antigens on class II-expressing cells [48]. Even though the known molecular complexity of class II antigens has increased with the development of new serological and molecular biology techniques, it appears that all class II antigens so far investigated may serve as restriction elements in this context [see 37]. Concerning this aspect of the tissue distribution of class II antigens, there are two points that merit particular attention. First, the differentiated tissue distribution of different class II antigens means that the local conditions for antigen presentation and T cell activation towards a particular immunogen may vary according to the locus that codes for the actual restriction molecule. This issue may increase considerably in complexity if the hitherto defined class II popypeptide chains are shown to be differentially expressed in patterns more complex than has as yet been possible to show with currently available monoclonals. Second, there is evidence to suggest that the ability to process and present different antigens to T lymphocytes may vary considerably between different class II-expressing cells (for a general discussion see [102, 106]). Thus, there is evidence that many different class II-expressing cells, such as clones of B cells, endothelial cells, and epithelial cells from thyroid glands, can in certain cases present antigen to lines and clones of antigen-specific T cells [14, 24, 31, 59], and that many nonlymphoid cells with induced class II expression, including fibroblasts, can stimulate allogeneic T cells to proliferate [74]. On the other hand, there is circumstantial evidence that the efficiency in antigen presentation, as well as the capacity for antigen processing, may vary between most investigated antigen-presenting cells, such as macrophages and dendritic cells and class II-expressing epithelial cells (see for example [59]). In order to better understand the implications of increased class II expression in the great number of conditions, particularly those of autoimmune or infectious nature, where class II induction has been demonstrated to occur, more functional studies are needed on these particular cells.

It should also be pointed out, however, that class II transplantation antigens probably fulfill a number of additional functions besides their role as restriction elements in T cell activation. For example, distinct functions are suggested for the class II antigens that are expressed on the surface of activated T cells as well as constitutively on B lymphocytes [90]. It is possible that class II expression on a large number of nonlymphoid cells might also be involved in a number of other recognition phenomena. Further investigations in this field should be possible when a number of nonlymphoid cells can be induced to express class II antigens in vitro after stimulation with defined molecules such as gamma-interferon, and when distinct class II antigen coding genes can be introduced and expressed in cells previously not expressing these molecules.

References

1. Aiba S, Tagami H (1984) HLA-DR antigen expression on the keratinocyte surface in dermatoses characterized by lymphocytic exocytosis (e.g. pityriasis rosea). Br J Dermatol 111:285–294
2. Auffrey C, Korman A, Roux-Dosseto M, Bono R, Strominger JL (1982) cDNA clone for the heavy chain of the human B cell alloantigen DC1: strong sequence homology to the HLA-DR heavy chain. Proc Natl Acad Sci USA 79:6337–6341

2a. Baker BS, Swain AF, Fry L, Valdimarsson H (1984) Epidermal T lymphocytes and HLA-DR expression in psoriasis. Br J Dermatol 110:555–564

3. Ballardini G, Mirakian R, Bianchi FR, Pisi E, Doniach D, Bottazzo GF (1984) Aberrant expression of HLA-DR antigens in bile duct epithelium in primary biliary cirrhosis: relevance to pathogenesis. Lancet II:1009–1013
4. Barclay N, Mason DW (1982) Induction of Ia antigen in rat epidermal cells and gut epithelium by immunological stimuli. J Exp Med 156:1665–1676
5. Basham TY, Nickoloff BJ, Merigan TC, Morhenn VB (1984) Recombinant gamma interferon induced HLA-DR expression on cultured human keratinocytes. J Invest Dermatol 83:88–90
6. Benson EM, Colvin RB, Russell PS (1985) Induction of Ia antigens in murine renal transplants. J Immunol 134:7–9
7. Bodmer J, Bodmer W (1984) Histocompatibility (1984) Immunology Today 5:251–254
8. Braathen LR, Thorsby E (1980) Studies on human epidermal Langerhans cells. Scand J Immunol 11:401–408
9. Brami C, Sanyal MK, Dwyer JM, Johnson CC, Naftolin F (1983) HLA-DR antigens on human trophoblast. Am J Reprod Immunol 3:165–174
10. Burmester GR, Yu DTY, Irani AM, Kunkel HG, Winchester RJ (1982) Ia+ T cells in synovial fluid and tissue of patients with rheumatoid Carthritis. Arthritis Rheum 24:1370–1376
11. Burmester GR, Dimitriu-Bona A, Waters SJ, Winchester RJ (1983) Identification of three major synovial cell populations by monoclonal antibodies directed to Ia antigens and antigens associated with monocytes/macrophages and fibroblasts. Scand J Immunol 17:69–82
12. Cerf-Bensussan N, Quaroni A, Kurnick JT, Bhan AK (1984) Intraepithelial lymphocytes modulate Ia expression by intestinal epithelial cells. J Immunol 132:2224–2252
13. Chen Y-X, Evans RL, Pollack MS, Lanier LL, Phillips JH, Rousso C, Warner NL, Brodsky FM (1984) Characterization and expression of the HLA-DC antigens defined by anti-Leu 10. Hum Immunol 10:221–235
14. Chesnut RW, Colon SM, Grey HM (1982) Requirements for the processing of antigens by antigen-presenting B cells. J Immunol 129:2382–2388

15. Claesson K, Forsum U, Tufvesson G, Klareskog L, Larsson E, Frödin L (1983) Inflammatory cell phenotypes and Ia antigens in irreversibly rejected kidney grafts. In: Kreis H, Borz B (eds) Renal transplant cytology, 2nd International Workshop, Paris. Wichtig, Milan, pp 137–142
16. Claesson K, Forsum U, Klareskog L, Andreen T, Larsson E, Frödin L, Tufvesson G (1985) Tissue distribution of T-lymphocytes and Ia-expressing cells in rat kidney grafts. Scand J Immunol 22:273–278
17. Colins T, Korman AJ, Wake CT, Boss JM, Kappes DT, Fiers W, Ault KA, Gimbrone MA, Strominger JL, Pober JS (1984) Immune interferon activates multiple class II major histocompatibility genes and the invariant chain gene in human endothelial cells and dermal fibroblasts. Proc Natl Acad Sci USA 81:4917–4921
18. Daar AS, Fuggle SV, Fabre JW, Ting A, Morris PJ (1984) The detailed distribution of MHC class II antigens in normal human organs. Transplantation 38:293–298
19. Duke O, Panai GS, Janossy G. Poulter LW (1982) An immunohistochemical analysis of lymphocyte subpopulations and their microenvironment in the synovial membrane of patients with rheumatoid arthritis using monoclonal antibodies. Clin Exp Immunol 49:22–30
20. Forre O, Thoen J, Lea T, Dobloug JH, Mellbye OJ, Natvig JB, Pahle J, Solheim BG (1982) In situ characterization of mononuclear cells in rheumatoid tissues using monoclonal antibodies. Scand J Immunol 16:315–319
21. Forre O, Egeland T, Dobloug JH, Kvien TK, Natvig JB (1982) Autologous mixed lymphocyte reactions in patients with rheumatoid arthritis and juvenile rheumatoid arthritis: both non-T and in-vivo-activated T cells can act as stimulator cells. Scand J Immunol 16:173–179
22. Forsum U, Klareskog L, Peterson PA (1979) Distribution of Ia-antigen-like molecules on non-lymphoid tissues. Scand J Immunol 9:343–349
23. Fuggle SV, Errasti P, Daar AS, Fabre JW, Ting A, Morris PJ (1983) Localization of major histocompatibility complex (HLA-ABC and DR) antigens in 46 kidneys. Transplantation 35:385–390
24. Grey HM, Colon SM, Chesnut RW (1982) Requirements for the processing of antigen in B cell tumors and macrophages. J Immunol 129:2389–2395
25. Guy K, Steel CM (1985) Interpretation of the specificities of monoclonal antibodies recognizing human MHC class II antigens. Clin Exp Immunol 59:251–254
26. Hall BM, Bishop GA, Duggin GG, Horvath JS, Philips J, Tiller DJ (1984) Increased expression of HLA-DR antigens on renal tubular cells in renal transplants: relevance to the rejection response. Lancet II:247–251
27. Hanafusa T, Pujol-Borrell P, Ciovato L, Russell RCG, Doniach D, Bottazzo GF (1983) Aberrant expression of HLA-DR antigen on thyrocytes in Graves-disease: relevance for autoimmunity. Lancet II:1111–1115
28. Hancock WW, Kraft N, Atkins RC (1982) The immunohistochemical demonstration of major histocompatibility antigens in the human kidney using monoclonal antibodies. Pathology 14:409–414
29. Hart DN, Fabre JW (1981) Endogenously produced Ia antigens within cells of convoluted tubules of rat kidney. J Immunol 126:2109–2113
30. Hirschberg H, Moen T, Thorsby E (1979) Specific destruction of human endothelial cell monolayers by anti-DRw antisera. Transplantation 28:116–120
31. Hirschberg H, Braathen LR, Thorsby E (1982) Antigen presentation by vascular endothelial cells and epidermal Langerhans cells: the role of HLA-DR. Immunol Rev 66:57–77
32. Hjelm EM (1984) Local cellular immune response in ascending urinary tract infection: occurrence of T-cells, immunoglobulin-producing cells and Ia-expressing cells in rat urinary tract tissue. Infect Immun 44:627–632
33. Hjelm E, Forsum U, Klareskog L (1982) Anti-Ia-reactive cells in the urinary tract of man, guinea-pig, rat, and mouse. Scand J Immunol 16:531–538
34. Janossy G, Panai G, Duke O, Bofill M, Poulter LW, Goldstein G (1981) Rheumatoid arthritis: a disease of T-lymphocyte macrophage immunoregulation. Lancet II:839–843
35. Jansson R, Karlsson A, Forsum U (1984) Intrathyroidal HLA-DR expression and T lymphocyte phenotypes in Graves' thyrotoxicosis, Hashimoto's thyroiditis and nodular colloid goitre. Clin Exp Immunol 58:264–272

36. Karlsson-Parra A, Nyberg A, Tötterman TH, Lööf L, Forsum U (1984) Primary biliary cirrhosis – phenotypic characterization of immunocompetent cells in peripheral blood and liver tissue. Ups J Med Sci 89:254–265
37. Kindt TJ (1984) Identical or distinct functional roles for products of the HLA-DR, DC, and SB loci. Scand J Immunol 20:471–473
38. Klareskog L, Malmnäs Tjernlund U, Forsum U, Peterson PA (1977) Epidermal Langerhans' cells express Ia antigens. Nature 268:248–250
39. Klareskog L, Trägårdh, Lindblom JB, Peterson PA (1978) Reactivity of a rabbit antiserum against highly purified HLA-DR antigens. Scand J Immunol 7:199–208
40. Klareskog L, Trägårdh L, Rask L, Peterson PA (1979) Isolation and characterization of detergent solubilized HLA-DR transplantation antigen. Biochemistry 18:1481–1489
41. Klareskog L, Forsum U, Malmnäs Tjernlund U, Rask L, Peterson PA (1979) Expression of Ia-antigen-like molecules on cells in the corneal epithelium. Invest Ophthalmol Vis Sci 18:310–313
42. Klareskog L, Forsum U, Peterson PA (1980) Hormonal regulation of the expression of Ia antigens on mammary gland epithelium. Eur J Immunol 10:958–863
43. Klareskog L, Forsum U, Malmnäs Tjernlund U, Kabelitz D, Wigren A (1981) Appearance of anti-HLA-DR reactive cells in normal and rheumatoid synovium. Scand J Immunol 14:183–192
44. Klareskog L, Forsum U, Scheynius A, Kabelitz D, Wigzell H (1982) Evidence in support of a self-perpetuating HLA-DR-dependent delayed type of cell reactions in rheumatoid arthritis. Proc Natl Acad Sci USA 79:3632–3636
45. Klareskog L, Forsum U, Wigren A, Wigzell H (1982) Relationships between HLA-DR-expressing cells and T lymphocytes of different subsets in rheumatoid synovial tissue. Scand J Immunol 15:501–507
46. Klareskog L, Holmdahl R, Rubin K, Victorin Å, Lindgren J-Å (1985) Different populations of rheumatoid adherenct cells mediate activation vs suppression of T-lymphocyte proliferation. Arthritis Rheum 28:863–873
47. Klareskog L, Johnell O, Hulth A (1985) Expression of HLA-DR and HLA-DQ antigens on cells within the cartilage-pannus junction in rheumatoid arthritis. Rheumatol Int 4 (suppl):11–15
48. Krensky AM, Reiss CS, Mier JW, Strominger JL, Burakoff SJ (1982) Long-term human cytolytic T-cell lines allospecific for HLA-DR6 antigen are $OKT4^+$. Proc Natl Acad Sci USA 79:2365–2369
49. Kvist S, Klareskog L, Peterson PA (1978) Identification of H-2 and Ia-antigen analogues in several species by immunological corssreactions of xenoantisera. Scand J Immunol 7:447–452
50. Lampert IA (1984) Expression of HLA-DR (Ia like) antigen on epidermal keratinocytes in human dermatoses. Clin Exp Immunol 57:93–100
51. Lampert IA, Janossy G, Suitters AJ, Bofill MB, Palmer S, Gordon-Smith E, Prentice HG, Thomas JA (1982) Immunological analysis of the skin in graft versus host disease. Clin Exp Immunol 50:123–131
52. Larhammar D (1983) Class II transplantation antigens: molecular genetic studies. Acta Univ Usp, Abstr Ups Diss Fac Med 477, p 1
53. Larhammar D, Gustafsson K, Claesson L, Bill P, Wiman K, Schenning L, Sundelin J, Widmark E, Peterson PA, Rask L (1982) Alpha chain of HLA-DR transplantation antigens is a member of the same protein superfamily as the immunoglobulins. Cell 30:153–161
54. Larhammar D, Schenning L, Gustafsson K, Wiman K, Claesson L, Rask L, Peterson PA (1982) Complete amino acid sequence of an HLA-DR antigen-like beta-chain as predicted from the nucleotide sequence: similarities with immunoglobulins and HLA-A,B,C antigens. Proc Natl Acad Sci USA 79:3687–3691
55. Lautenschläger I, Häyry P (1981) Expression of the major histocompatibility complex antigens on different liver cellular components in rat and man. Scand J Immunol 14:421–426
56. Lindblad S, Klareskog L, Hedfors E, Forsum U, Sundström C (1983) Phenotypic characterization of synovial tissue cells in situ in different types of synovitis. Arthritis Rheum 26:1321–1332

57. Lindahl G, Hedfors E, Klareskog L, Forsum U (1985) Epithelial HLA-DR expression and T lymphocyte subsets in salivary glands in Sjögren's syndrome. Clin Exp Immunol 61:475–482
58. Ljunghall K, Lööf L, Forsum U (1982) T lymphocyte subsets in the duodenal epithelium in dermatitis herpetiformis. Acta Derm Venerol (Stockh) 62:485–489
59. Londei M, Lamb JR, Bottazzo GF, Feldmann M (1984) Epithelial cells expressing aberrant MHC class II determinants can present antigen to clones of human T cells. Nature 312:639–641
60. MacKie RM, Turbitt ML (1983) Quantitation of dendritic cells in normal and abnormal human epidermis using monoclonal antibodies directed against Ia and HTA antigens. J Invest Dermatol 81:216–220
61. Malmnäs Tjernlund U (1978) Epidermal expression of HLA-DR antigens in mycosis fungoides. Arch Dermatol Res 261:81–86
62. Malmnäs Tjernlund U (1980) Ia-like antigens in lichen planus. Acta Derm Venerol (Stockh) 60:309–314
63. Malmnäs Tjernlund U, Scheynius A, Kabelitz D, Klareskog L (1981) Anti-Ia reactive cells in mycosis fungoides: a study of skin biopsies, single epidermal cells and circulating T lymphocytes. Acta Derm Venerol (Stockh) 61:291–301
64. Mason DW, Dallman M, Barclay AN (1981) Graft-versus-host disease induced expression of Ia antigen in rat epidermal cells and gut epithelium. Nature 293:150–151
65. Mayrhofer G, Pugh CW, Barcley AN (1983) The distribution, ontogeny and origin in the rat of Ia-positive cells with dendritic morphology and of Ia antigen in epithelia with special reference to the intestine. Eur J Immunol 13:112–122
66. Metzger Z, Hoffeld JT, Oppenheim JJ (1980) Macrophage-mediated suppression. I. Evidence for participation of both hydrogen peroxide and prostaglandins in suppression of murine lymphocyte proliferation. J Immunol 124:983–988
67. Milton AD, Fabre JW (1985) Massive induction of donor-type class I and class II major histocompatibility complex antigens in rejecting cardiac allografts in the rat. J Exp Med 161:98–112
68. Murphy GF, Shepard RS, Harrist TJ, Bronstein BR, Bhan AK (1983) Ultrastructural documentation of HLA-DR antigen reactivity in normal acrosyringial epithelium. J Invest Dermatol 81:181–183
69. Natali PG, Martino C, Quaranta V, Nicotra MR, Frezza F, Pellegrino MA, Ferrone S (1981) Expression of Ia-like antigens in normal human nonlymphoid tissue. Transplantation 31:75–78
70. Natali PG, Segatto O, Ferrone S, Tosi R, Corte G (1984) Differential tissue distribution and ontogeny of DC-1 and HLA-DR antigens. Immunogenetics 19:109–116
71. Newman RA, Ormerod MG, Greaves MF (1980) The presence of HLA-DR antigens on lactating human breast epithelium and milk fat globule membranes. Clin Exp Immunol 41:478–486
72. Olsson T, Henriksson KG, Klareskog L, Forsum U (1985) HLA-DR expression, T lymphocyte phenotypes, OKM1 and OKT9 reactive cells in inflammatory myopathy. Muscle Nerve 8:419–425
73. Parr EL, McKenzie FC (1979) Demonstration of Ia antigens on mouse intestinal epithelial cells by immunoferritin labeling. Immunogenetics 8:499–508
74. Pober JS, Collins T, Gimbrone MA, Cotran RS, Gitlin JD, Fiers W, Clayberger C, Krensky AM, Burakoff SJ, Reiss CS (1983) Lymphocytes recognize human vascular endothelial and dermal fibroblast Ia antigens induced by recombinant immune interferon. Nature 305:726–729
75. Poulter LW, Duke O, Hobbs S, Janossy G, Panai G (1982) Histochemical discrimination of HLA-DR positive cell populations in the normal and arthritic synovial lining. Clin Exp Immunol 48:381–388
76. Poulter LW, Seymour GJ, Duke O, Janossy G (1982) Immunohistological analysis of delayed type hypersensitivity in man. Cell Immunol 74:358–369
77. Pujol-Borrell R, Hanafusa T, Chiovato L, Bottazzo GF (1983) Lectin-induced expression of DR antigen on human cultured follicular thyroid cells. Nature 304:71–73
78. Raftery MJ, Poulter LW, Janossy G, Sweny P, Fernando ON, Moorhead JF (1983) Heterogeneity of HLA-DR$^+$ cells in normal human kidney. Immunohistological and cytochemical characterization of discrete cell populations. J Clin Pathol 36:734–741

79. Rebai N, Malissen B, Pierres M, Accolia RS, Corte G, Mawas C (1983) Distinct HLA-DR epitopes and distinct families of HLA-DR molecules defined by 15 monoclonal antibodies (mAb) either anti-DR or allo-anti-Ia$^+$ crossreacting with human DR molecule. Eur J Immunol 13:106–111
80. Roux-Dosseto M, Auffrey C, Lillie JW, Boss JM, Cohen D, DeMars R, Mawas C, Seidman JG, Strominger JL (1983) Genetic mapping of a human class II antigen beta-chain cDNA clone to the SB region of the HLA complex. Proc Natl Acad Sci USA 80:6036–6040
81. Rowden G, Lewis MG, Sullivan AK (1977) Ia antigen expression on human epidermal Langerhans cells. Nature 268:247–249
82. Scheynius A, Tjernlund U (1984) Human keratinocytes express HLA-DR antigens in the tuberculin reaction. Scand J Immunol 19:141–147
83. Scheynius A, Klareskog L, Forsum U (1982) In situ identification of T lymphocyte subsets and HLA-DR expressing cells in the human skin tuberculin reaction. Clin Exp Immunol 49:325–330
84. Scott H, Solheim BG, Brandtzaeg P, Thorsby E (1980) HLA-DR-like antigens in the epithelium of the human small intestine. Scand J Immunol 12:77–82
85. Scott H, Brandtzaeg P, Hirschberg H, Solheim B, Thorsby E (1981) Vascular and renal distribution of HLA-DR antigens. Tissue Antigens 18:195–202
86. Scott H, Brandtzaeg P, Solheim BG, Thorsby E (1981) Relation between HLA-DR-like antigens and secretory component (SC) in jejunal epithelium of patients with coelic disease or dermatitis herpetiformis. Clin Exp Immunol 44:233–238
87. Selby WS, Janossy G, Goldstein G, Jewell DP (1981) T lymphocyte subsets in human intestinal mucosa: the distribution and relationship to MHC-derived antigens. Clin Exp Immunol 44:453–458
88. Selby WS, Janossy G, Mason DY, Jewell DP (1983) Expression of HLA-DR antigens by colonic epithelium in inflammatory bowel disease. Clin Exp Immunol 53:614–618
89. Shiozawa S, Shiozawa K, Fujita T (1983) Presence of HLA-DR antigen on synovial type A and B cells: an immunoelectron microscopic study in rheumatoid arthritis, osteoarthritis and normal traumatic joints. Immunology 50:587–594
90. Singer A, Asano Y, Shigeta M, Hathcock KS, Ahmed A, Fathman CG, Hodes RJ (1982) Distinct B cell subpopulations differ in their genetic requirements for activation by T helper cells. Immunol Rev 64:137–160
91. Smolle J (1985) HLA-DR antigen bearing keratinocytes in various dermatological disorders. Acta Derm Venerol (Stockh) 65:9–13
92. Steeg PS, Moore RN, Oppenheim JJ (1980) Regulation of murine macrophage Ia expression by products of activated spleen cells. J Exp Med 152:1734–1744
93. Steeg PS, Moore RN, Johnson HM, Oppenheim JJ (1982) Regulation of murine macrophage Ia antigen expression by a lymphokine with immune interferon activity. J Exp Med 156:1780–1793
94. Steinman RM, Nussenzweig MC (1980) Dendritic cells: features and functions. Immunol Rev 53:125–148
95. Stingl G, Tamaki K, Katz SI (1980) Origin and function of epidermal Langerhans cells. Immunol Rev 53:149–174
96. Streilein JW, Toews GB, Bergstresser PR (1979) Corneal allografts fail to express Ia antigens. Nature 282:326–327
97. Tuvesson G, Forsum U, Claesson K, Klareskog L, Larsson E, Karlsson-Parra A, Frödin L (1983) T-lymphocyte subsets and HLA-DR-expressing cells in rejected human kidney grafts. Scand J Immunol 18:37–40
98. Unanue ER (1984) Antigen-presenting function of the macrophage. Ann Rev Immunol 2:395–428
99. Volc-Platzer B, Majdic O, Knapp W, Wolff K, Hinterberger W, Lechner K, Stingl G (1984) Evidence of HLA-DR antigen biosynthesis by human keratinocytes in disease. J Exp Med 159:1784–1789
100. Wadgymar A, Urmson J, Baumal R, Halloran PF (1984) Changes in Ia expression in mouse kidney during acute graft-vs-host disease. J Immunol 132:1826–1832
101. Whitsett CF, Stulting RD (1984) The distribution of HLA antigens on human corneal tissue. Invest Ophtalmol Vis Sci 25:520–524

102. Wiman K, Curman B, Forsum U, Klareskog L, Malmnäs Tjernlund U, Rask L, Trägårdh L, Peterson PA (1978) Occurrence of Ia antigens on tissues of non-lymphoid origin. Nature 276:711–713
103. Wiman K, Curman B, Trägårdh L, Peterson PA (1979) Demonstration of HLA-DR-like antigens on milk fat globules membranes. Eur J Immunol 9:190–195
104. Winchester RJ, Burmester G (1981) Demonstration of Ia antigens on certain dendritic cells and on a novel elongated cell found in human synovial tissues. Scand J Immunol 14:441–447

Class II MHC Antigens on Human Monocytes, Endothelial Cells, and Dendritic Cells

P. Stastny, G. Nuñez, and C. Pettaway

Table of Contents

Introduction

One of the distinguishing features of class II MHC antigens is that their expression is regulated differently in different tissues. Thus, while class I antigens can be modulated quantatively in many cells under the influence of factors such as gamma-interferon [7, 25, 59], there are many types of cells in which class II antigens are undetectable under normal unstimulated conditions. In addition, in some cells, as for example in monocytes, expression of HLA-DQ antigens and HLA-DR antigens may be discordant. Thus, as will be seen, there are monocytes in human peripheral blood that express HLA-DR, as well as HLA-DP, but do not have detectable HLA-DQ on their surface [58]. In this chapter we will describe the data pertaining to the expression of surface class II antigens on cells isolated from normal donors and studied under resting conditions. In addition, some information will be given about the changes that take place when such cells are stimulated by lymphocyte factors in vitro.

Historically, the human class II antigens were first recognized by employing cellular techniques such as mixed lymphocyte cultures and typing with homozygous typing cells. Other cellular techniques that have been utilized to detect human class II antigens are the primed lymphocyte test, HLA restricted antigen presentation to specific T cell lines or clones, and assay with cytotoxic T cells recognizing class II antigens. Serologic methods were developed using first alloantisera and later monoclonal antibodies reactive with class II antigens. In addition, structural information has been obtained using techniques of protein chemistry as well as of the DNA and RNA of the corresponding genes, using the technology of molecular genetics. We shall discuss available information regarding class II antigens in monocytes, endothelial cells, and dendritic cells obtained with each of these techniques.

Monocytes

In most studies monocytes have been isolated from human peripheral blood by taking advantage either of their ability to adhere to glass or plastic surfaces or of their size and density characteristics in density gradients. Either of these techniques can yield cell preparations which are sufficiently enriched (>80%) to perform meaningful studies. To check the purity of monocyte preparations, investigators have used staining for nonspecific esterase [41], staining with euchrysine [87], or analysis with one of several monoclonal antibodies that react with differentiation antigens specific for monocytes [17, 56].

Serology of Class II Antigens on Monocytes Using Alloantisera

Several investigators have tested isolated monocytes from human peripheral blood with anti-DR sera and found them to be reactive [49]. In our laboratory we tested monocytes and B cells from 40 donors with the DR typing set of the Seventh International Histocompatibility Workshop [75]. We found that monocytes gave strong cytotoxicity reactions with these typing sera and that there was a good correlation with the results of B cell typing for the antigens DR1, 2, 3, 4, and 7. In further work [16], it was reported that monocytes could be used for DR typing. Similarly, in a more recent study, Merdrignac and coworkers [49] tested monocytes and B cells from 57 donors with a panel of typing sera defining the specificities DR1–7 and found an excellent correlation ($r > 0.81$) between the results obtained with the two kinds of cells. In none of these studies were the monocytes tested with typing reagents for HLA-DQ antigens. However, Nuñez and coworkers [58] have observed that monocytes react very poorly with sera defining DQw1–DQw3. These results are in agreement with reports of studies with monoclonal antibodies, to be discussed below, indicating that more than half of the monocytes from human peripheral blood do not have detectable DQ antigens.

The third kind of human class II antigens, the HLA-DP antigens, have been detected mostly by cellular techniques [71], but recently some preliminary evidence has suggested that these antigens can also be recognized by alloantisera (Johnson et al., unpublished, 1984) and with monoclonal antibodies [52, 70, 86]. In an interesting study from Leiden [83], four pregnancy typing sera were found to react with monocytes defining a specificity closely correlated with HLA-DPw4.

Expression of Class II Antigens on Human Monocytes/Macrophages Detected with Monoclonal Antibodies

Monoclonal antibodies have been extremely useful for studying the expression of class II antigens on human mononuclear cells [55, 73]. Using monomorphic murine monoclonal antibodies against HLA-DR antigens and indirect immunofluorescence, it was shown that virtually all monocytes in human peripheral blood were stained, as detected either by fluorescence microscopy or by flow cytometry [55].

When it became clear that in addition to the DR antigens, the DQ molecules (initially called DC or DS) were detectable and distinct structures [27, 80], it was of interest to investigate their distribution on different cells. It was first reported by Gonwa and coworkers [26] that only about 50% of the peripheral blood monocytes appeared to express DQ in detectable amounts.

In our laboratory [58] we utilized a large panel of monoclonal antibodies to investigate simultaneously the expression of HLA-DR, DP, and DQ. The percentage of cells staining with the various monoclonal antibodies was determined by fluorescence microscopy and also by flow cytometry. In these experiments we used antibody Genox 3.53 specific for DQw1, IVD12 reactive with DQw3, BT3/4, another DQw1 specific monoclonal antibody, and TU22, an antibody reactive with a determinant of DQ molecules of virtually all haplotypes. We observed that the majority of human monocytes expressed DR, including DRw52 (determined with antibody I-LR2) or DRw53 (using antibody 109d6), and DP (characterized with antibody I-LR1), but only a subpopulation had detectable amounts of HLA-DQ. When the determinations were performed in the FACS, monocyte preparations showed about 40% of the cells stained for DQ. By fluorescence microscopy, only about 16% could be seen to be positive with Genox 3.53 and 13% with IVD12. Analysis of staining in the FACS indicated a range of staining intensities, with about 25% of the cells showing only weak staining. Some of the latter were evidently recorded as unstained in the fluorescence microscope.

Using the antibodies Genox 3.53 (anti-DQw1) and IVD12 (anti-DQw3) we found [58] that in heterozygous cells, the antigens recognized by these two antibodies were expressed on the same subset of cells. The experiments were performed with antibodies labelled with either rhodamine (red fluorescence) or fluorescein (green fluorescence) and showed that almost all monocytes with one of the colors also had the other.

Gonwa and Stobo [25] have also analyzed the staining of blood monocytes with anti-DQ monoclonal antibodies in the FACS. They used Genox 3.53 as well as Leu 10, a monoclonal antibody reactive with DQw1 and DQw3, but not with DQw2. About 50% of the adherent mononuclear cells showed staining above control. However, the data could not discriminate between absence of DQ in the remaining cells and low-level expression. Gonwa and Stobo caculated from their results that the DQ-negative subset of monocytes may have expressed DQ, on the average, at a level of 20%–25% of the amount of DR molecules on the same cells [25].

In view of the low level of expression of HLA-DQ molecules on monocytes obtained from peripheral blood, we have attempted to increase their expression by incubation with interferon. In the experiments shown in Table 1, monocytes isolated by adherence to plastic were incubated with gamma-interferon (200 U/ml) for 48 h and then tested in the FACS with several monoclonal antibodies. L203 a monoclonal antibody reacting with DR molecules, stained over 80% of the cells. After they were incubated with interferon there was a two-to threefold increase in staining intensity (not shown). The two antibodies that react with determinants on DQ molecules (TU22 and Leu 10) stained 18.1%–32.8% of the cells. The staining increased on incubation with gamma-interferon but never exceeded 53.5% of the cells. There was no significant change in the staining with 63D3, a monoclonal antibody against a monocyte differentation antigen, or in the control values.

Recent experiments in our laboratory (Nuñez et al., submitted) suggest that there is a correlation between the amount of DQ and DR expressed at the level of single adherent mononuclear cells. These experiments were performed with Leu 10 (anti-DQ) conjugated with phycoerythrin (red fluorescence) and L243

Table 1. Induction of HLA-DQ surface molecules of human monocytes by gamma-interferon (IFN)

Donor of cells	IFN[a] treatment	Monoclonal antibody				
		L203 DR	Tu22 DQ	Leu 10 DQ	63D3 mono	Control antibody
RW	–	87.8	22.2	18.1	94.1	6.9
	+	81.8	53.5	51.8	86.8	3.8
JW	–	81.8	19.1	15.6	92.5	5.5
	+	93.8	40.0	33.1	89.7	5.6
SF	–	92.7	21.7	20.8	96.8	2.8
	+	98.6	36.3	35.7	93.3	4.1
LD	–	95.7	32.8	26.1	91.3	2.6
	+	96.7	50.7	39.9	90.3	2.8

Results expressed as percent positive cells, as determined by flow cytometry
[a] Monocytes incubated for 48 h with 200 U/ml purified IFN (Interferon Sciences Inc., New Brunswick, NJ)

(anti-DR) conjugated with fluorescein (green fluorescence). When the cells were stained separately with either antibody and mixed just prior to flow cytometry, there was excellent separation of the two colors. When the experiment was performed by simultaneously staining the cells with both antibodies, a correlation was observed between the fluorescence intensity of the two colors. The cells staining more intensely for DQ also stained more brightly for DR, and vice versa.

Allogeneic Stimulation by Class II Antigens of Monocytes

Stimulation in the MLR was initially used to detect the human class II antigens on mononuclear cells [18]. But little information was available on the role of individual cell types. In experiments in which the mononuclear cells were fractionated, the adherent cell population appeared to have been more effective in stimulating [2], and monocyte-depleted cells could be reconstituted by addition of small numbers of adherent cells [64].

Recent experiments in our laboratory (Nuñez et al., submitted) have suggested there is a DQ-rich subset of the adherent mononuclear cells which are much more active stimulators of the MLR than the DQ-poor population. These experiments were performed by sorting adherent cells into DQ-rich and DQ-depleted subsets using the monoclonal antibody TU22 in the FACS. Similar results could be obtained by sorting the stimulating cells according to the amount of DR antigens expressed on their surface using the antibody I-LR2 (anti-DRw52) (Table 2). In view of the correlation observed between the intensity of staining for DQ and DR on peripheral blood monocytes, one possible interpretation of these results is that the higher efficiency of DQ-rich cells in the MLR is due simply to the simultaneous higher density of DR expression. Alternatively, it is possible that increased expression of DQ and DR identifies a cellular subset that is functionally more active in the MLR.

Other workers have suggested that dendritic cells may be more important accessory cells than monocytes [85]. Information about dendritic cells will be discussed in detail below. We have used a monoclonal antibody against a monocyte differentiation antigen to further characterize the DQ-rich adherent mononuclear cell subset. In these experiments we used the antibody Leu M3 to separate the

Table 2. Proliferation of T cells induced by allogeneic adherent cells that express different levels of HLA-DR antigens[a]

Experiment	Level of fluorescence	Number of adherent cells ($\times 10^{-3}$)		
		20	10	5
1	High	50952	34121	28080
	Medium	16454	9427	8110
	Low	1881	4297	3240
2	High	88263	49172	44252
	Medium	32092	20227	13470
	Low	26726	18154	11686

[a] Antibody I-LR2 (anti-DRw52) was used to sort for cells with high, medium, or low level of fluorescence in the FACS. Results expressed in 3HTdr uptake (cpm)

DQ-rich population of adherent mononuclear cells into monocyte-marker-positive and -negative subsets. The results indicated that both the DQ-rich monocytes and the DQ-rich cells lacking the monocyte-specific antigen were very effective stimulators in the MLR.

Another way to look at MLR stimulation is to utilize as responders T cells that have been primed to respond to a given HLA-D region antigen. In our experiments we have used cloned T cells, the response of which were characterized by testing against a panel of stimulating cells and by inhibition experiments with monoclonal antibodies. We observed (Nuñez et al., submitted) that in the case of T cell lines responding only to an epitope on HLA-DQ molecules, it was absolutely necessary to have DQ expressed on the stimulating cells. Results with DQ-depleted populations in such tests were completely flat. On the other hand, with T cells recognizing epitopes on DR molecules, two patterns have been observed. In some cases, the DR-specific T cell clones responded much more effectively to stimulation by the DQ-rich subset and less so to the DQ-depleted population. In other experiments, certain T cell clones recognized and proliferated also quite well in responses to the DQ-poor subsets, although the DQ-rich cells were always a little more active as stimulators.

Accessory Cell Function of Monocytes in Antigen-Specific HLA-Restricted Responses

It is well established that human class II antigens restricted the responses of T cells to a variety of antigens such as PPD [8, 30], KLH [65], influenza virus [45], mumps virus [4], and others.

With the use of cloned T cells and panel testing, as well as inhibition of the responses with monoclonal antibodies it has been shown that the restricting determinants can be epitopes on DR molecules [4], DP molecules [19], or on DQ [5].

In our laboratory, we have used mumps virus antigen on adherent blood mononuclear cells to stimulate clones of mumps-specific T cells [4]. These T cell responses were found to correlate with DRw53 and were inhibited by the monoclonal antibody 109d6, known to be specific for DRw53.

In other experiments [5], T cell lines responding to the synthetic polypeptide antigen GAT were found to be restricted by an epitope on HLA-DQ molecules. This was demonstrated by the inhibition of the responses by IVD12 (anti-DQw3) and by TU22 (monomorphic anti-DQ). The specificity recognized by this T cell line was found by panel testing to be distributed to a subset of DR5- and a subset of DR4-positive cells. We have called this antigen DSP5X4. It appears to be similar to the specificity TA10 [48].

Class II Antigens on Human Monocytes/Macrophages from Sources Other Than Blood

Spleen cells were examined with several monoclonal antibodies [58]. The anti-DR monoclonal antibody IIIE3 reacted with 32%, the anti-DQw3 antibody IVD12 with 34%. Only 6% of the spleen mononuclear cells were monocytes as determined with the antibody 63D3. The number of cells that were macrophages could not be determined in these experiments, because 63D3 is known to react with an antigen of monocytes that is lost when they develop into tissue macrophages [56].

More recently, Pettaway et al. (unpublished, 1985) have studied the class II antigens on adherent mononuclear cells from the human spleen.

The expression of DR was determined with L203 by counting 200 cells in the fluorescence microscope. It was observed that 64.5% of the adherent cells from spleen stained for HLA-DR and 15.3% of the adherent cells carried the monocyte differentiation marker 63D3.

The ability of spleen mononuclear cells to stimulate in the MLR was also investigated. Adherent cells were further fractionated into firmly adherent and loosely adherent subsets. Both populations were stimulatory, but the loosely adherent cells, which adhered initially at 2 h but became loose overnight, were considerably more active.

When loosely adherent cells were stained by immunofluorescence, about 70% expressed HLA-DR (L203). A large fraction of these appeared to be B lymphocytes as determined by staining with the monoclonal antibody B1.

Alveolar macrophages were tested with L203, a monoclonal antibody against DR antigens [79]. These cells showed intense surface staining and over 80% were positive. TU22 (anti-DQ) was used to investigate the expression of DQ antigens on alveolar macrophages. Again, virtually all of the cells were found to be positive (Lipscomb et al., unpublished). In spite of the rich expression of surface class II antigens on alveolar macrophages, these cells have been found to be relatively less active than peripheral blood adherent cells in presenting antigens to peripheral blood T cells or to T cell lines [79].

Cell-Mediated Cytotoxicity Against Class II Antigens on Monocytes

Although class II antigens had been known for several years to serve as targets for CTL in the mouse, it was not until 1978 that it became clear that also in man, D-region antigens could be recognized by cytotoxic T cells [CTL) [1, 21]. These studies were performed with monocytes as target cells. Previously most of the work with human cell-mediated lysis was done using PHA T cell blasts as targets. It appears that although class II antigens make their appearance on T cell blasts, such cells are not good targets for class II-mediated killing.

Feighery and Stastny [21] raised CTL by stimulating with cells matched for HLA-A and B and mismatched for HLA-D. The specificity of the CTL was defined by panel study and by inhibition with anti-class II antibodies [6, 22].

Interestingly, the majority of the CTL against class II antigens were of the OKT4 phenotype [3], in contrast to CTL against class I antigens which are known to be of the OKT8 type mainly [63].

Other investigators have also observed CTL against class II antigens on monocytes and on B cell lines [10, 31, 39]. Several CTL cell lines specific for class II antigens have been found to be of the OKT4 phenotype [10, 42, 50]. Cytotoxicity appears to have been directed against DR [6], DQ [43], or DP [10] antigens.

Endothelial Cells

Endothelial cells provide the first barrier between circulating cells of the blood and extravascular tissue sites. In addition, the endothelium is a primary site of contact between circulating immune cells and vascularized allografts. For these reasons, endothelial cells could play an active role in local immune reactions and in determining the immunogenicity of allografts. The expression of class II antigens on vascular endothelium might enable endothelial cells to perform tasks traditionally ascribed to monocytes/macrophages or dendritic cells. Furthermore, Ia-positive endothelial cells in vascularized allografts could render such endothelial cell targets susceptible to antibody and cell-mediated immune responses directed at class II determinants.

Detection of Class II Antigens on Endothelial Cells by Conventional Serology

The expression of class II MHC antigens on vascular endothelium has been controversial. Earlier reports of studies using a limited number of alloantisera mainly derived from planned immunization, and broadly reactive xenoantisera, indicated that endothelial cells isolated from umbilical veins expressed HLA-DR antigens [35, 76]. More recent studies, however, have failed to demonstrate class II antigens by serological methods in endothelial cells from umbilical cords [54, 74]. In recent studies, cord vein endothelial cells and B lymphocytes from autologous cords were compared as targets in cytotoxicity tests with a large panel of well-characterized alloantisera. It was concluded that endothelial cells from cord veins lack surface expression of class II antigens [54]. In parallel experiments, HLA-A,B alloantigens were easily demonstrable in the same preparations of endothelial cells [54]. From these studies it was also concluded that unstimulated cord endothelial cells do not express either HLA-DR or HLA-DQ alloantigens [54].

Detection of Class II Antigens on Endothelial Cells Using Monoclonal Antibodies

Given the conflicting results on the expression of class II antigens obtained using conventional alloantisera, we and others have studied the expression of these antigens with monoclonal antibodies specific for HLA-DR, DQ, and DP molecules. In addition, the availability of such reagents allowed the systematic evaluation of vascular endothelium of a variety of organs. Studies with monoclonal antibodies confirmed the lack of expression of class II antigens on unstimulated endothelial cells from umbilical veins [57, 59, 77]. In addition to the lack of HLA-DR, cord endothelial cells did not express HLA-DP or HLA-DQ molecules as detected by flow cytometry [54].

Of particular interest for those involved in renal transplantation is the expression of class II antigens in kidney endothelium. Most studies have concluded that HLA-DR antigens are expressed in endothelial cells of the glomerular tuft and peritubular capillaries, but not in most large vessels of the kidney [23, 32, 53]. Similar conclusions were derived from studies using a xenoantiserum against human class II antigens [69]. This selective expression of class II molecules in small renal vessels is in contrast with the easy demonstration of HLA-A,B,C antigens in arterial, glomerular, and peritubular capillaries and in venous endothelium [20, 23, 32]. Preliminary studies also indicate that in addition to DR, endothelial cells in the glomeruli and peritubular capillaries express HLA-DQ antigens weakly [24]. Most of the class II staining observed in the glomeruli and peritubular capillaries has been attributable to capillary endothelium. However, other Ia-positive cells have been demonstrated in close relation with vascular endothelium of both glomerular mesangium and peritubular interstitium. These cells have been identified as macrophages and interstitial dendritic cells [23, 32]. Since it has been recently demonstrated that expression of class II antigens can be modulated by soluble factors (see below), it is tempting to speculate that these nonendothelial Ia-positive cells might play a role in the regulation of class II antigen expression in vascular endothelium.

Natali et al. [53] studied the expression of class II antigens in endothelium from a variety of vascularized organs. They showed HLA-DR antigens in capillaries of most organs studied, exceptions being the brain cortex and the placenta. Large vessels of the organs studied did not appear to express detectable DR antigens [53].

Modulation of Class II Antigens in Endothelial Cells

It has been demonstrated that a soluble factor(s) derived from activated T lymphocytes can induce the expression of class II antigens in Ia-negative endothelial cells [59, 77]. Such a soluble factor(s), derived from activation of T lymphocytes with mitogen, also enhances the expression of HLA-DR antigens in other cells, such as monocytes [55]. More recent experiments indicate that gamma-interferon is likely to be the factor responsible for the induction of class II antigens in endothelial cells [60, 61]. In Table 3 are shown results in which culture supernatants from several sources were tested for their capacity to induce expression of HLA-DR antigens on Ia-negative endothelial cells. It can be seen that a large percentage of endothelial cells express surface HLA-DR antigens after 48 h incubation with supernatants derived from T lymphocytes stimulated with mitogen, soluble antigen, or alloantigen. Similarly purified or recombinant gamma-interferons are powerful inducers of HLA-DR on endothelial cells (Table 3).

Table 3. Induction of Ia-like antigens on human endothelial cells

Type of inducer[a]	No. of experiments	Ia-positive endothelial cells (%)[b]	
		Mean	Range
None	29	< 1	0– 2
Mitogen	8	39	6–85
Antigen	6	35	12–57
MLR	7	43	15–66
IL2	3	< 1	0– 2
Gamma-interferon	5	66	35–84

[a] Mitogen, supernatants from PHA (1%) or Con A (2 μg/ml) stimulated T cells; Antigen, supernatants from mumps, GAT or TGAL primed T cells; MLR, primary or secondary MLR supernatants; IL2, supernatants from MLA cell line; Gamma-interferon, 200 μ/ml purified from human lymphocytes (Interferon Sciences Inc., New Brunswick, NJ)

[b] Staining with monoclonal antibody L203 (DR framework) after 48–72 h incubation

The biological implications of the induction of class II antigens on endothelial cells are still unclear. It has been shown that endothelial cells induced to express class II antigens after treatment with gamma-interferon can serve as targets for class-II-specific cytotoxic lymphocytes in vitro [60]. This phenomenon is not unique to endothelial cells, since it has also been shown in fibroblasts by Pober et al. [60], who compared gamma-interferon-treated and control-treated endothelial cells for their ability to induce proliferation of allogeneic lymphocytes. Surprisingly, both interferon- and control-treated endothelial cells stimulated equally well the proliferation of allogeneic lymphocytes in a 7-day MLR [61]. The ability of initially Ia-negative endothelial cells to stimulate allogeneic responses can perhaps be explained by the presence of an Ia-positive contaminating cell population that might be responsible for T cell proliferation observed with both control- and interferon-treated preparations [57]. Alternatively, an Ia-positive contaminating cell population might trigger T cells in the culture, leading to gamma-interferon production and induction of Ia in the initially Ia-negative cell population. Lastly, another possibility is that endothelial cells might enhance the autologous MLR in these cultures, as recently shown by Roska et al. [66] and also observed by us (Nuñez et al., unpublished). Recent experiments by Lipsky and coworkers (Roska et al., in press) suggest that endothelial cells which express Ia antigens after exposure to gamma-interferon can indeed stimulate allogeneic T4 lymphocytes in the MLR, while Ia-negative endothelial cells did not.

Endothelial Cells as Antigen-Presenting Cells

In early work, preparations of umbilical cord endothelial cells were shown to induce proliferation of T lymphocytes in response to soluble antigen [14, 33, 36]. Antigen presentation by endothelial cells was HLA-D-region restricted and inhibited by alloantibodies against HLA-DR [14, 33, 37]. Since in later work it was demonstrated that endothelial cells from the umbilical cord were Ia-negative (see above), it was rather surprising that such cells could present antigen to T lymphocytes in an HLA-D-region restricted fashion. In experiments conducted in our laboratory, we found that the endothelial cell preparations after 2–5 days in culture are routinely contaminated with Ia-positive cells. These Ia-positive cells represent less than 1% of the cells in such preparations [57]. We found that preparations of 2- to 5-day cultured endothelial cells were active in presentation of mumps antigen to HLA-D-region-compatible, antigen-specific T cell lines [57]. Antigen presentation by endothelial cells was completely eliminated by treatment of such cell preparations with monoclonal anti-Ia and complement [57]. These results indicated that the small percentage of Ia-positive cells present in the initial endothelial cell preparations were required for T cell proliferation to antigen. It is possible, however, that endothelial cells that have been modulated to express Ia antigens can serve themselves as antigen-presenting cells.

Endothelial Cells as Stimulators of Allogeneic Responses

Preparations of endothelial cells cultured for 2–5 days have been shown to stimulate proliferation of allogeneic lymphocytes [34]. This early observation was interpreted as the recognition by lymphocytes of allogeneic Ia expressed on endothelial cells [34]. In another set of experiments, lymphocytes primed against endothelial cells or cord monocytes were used to detect HLA-D determinants on endothelial cells or monocytes from the same cord. While the use of cord monocytes allowed a clear-cut detection of HLA-D on restimulation, endothelial cells failed to have such discriminatory capacity [51]. Recent experiments (see above), however, have indicated that endothelial cells do not express class II antigens at the beginning of such cultures. The interpretation of these endothelial-lymphocyte interactions has to take into account (a) the role of a small percentage of Ia-positive cells that frequently contaminate such endothelial cell preparations, (b) the possible enhancement of an autologous MLR response that may mimic an allogeneic response, and (c) Ia expression can be induced on endothelial cells by soluble factor(s) produced by activated T lymphocytes. It has been shown that Ia-negative cells turn Ia-positive during MLR responses in culture [61].

Dendritic Cells

The monocyte/macrophage population was long thought to be the main accessory cell population for antigen or mitogen activation of T lymphocytes. More recently, other cells, such as dendritic cells, have been suggested as alternative or perhaps even the main accessory cells [84].

Dendritic-like cells characterized originally in other species and later in humans share many distinctive features, including (a) cell size and irregularity in shape, (b) cytoplasmic projections, (c) close apposition to T lymphocytes, and (d) most notably, the presence of abundant class II HLA antigens on the cell surface. Studies in vitro have suggested that these cells are potent accessory cells.

Cells currently classified as dendritic are shown in Table 4, together with their tissue localization and certain distinguishing characteristics. They include epidermal Langerhans cells, veiled cells and interdigitating dendritic cells, follicular dendritic cells, and dendritic cells of peripheral blood and spleen.

Class II MHC Antigen Expression in Epidermal Langerhans Cells

Stingl and coworkers [78] observed that a subpopulation of epidermal cells stained by immunofluorescence with alloantisera that also reacted with donor B

Table 4. Dendritic-like cells in man

Cell type and localization	Surface markers			
	T6	Fc	C3R	Common leukocyte antigen
Langerhans cells: epidermis, mucosa	+	+	+	+
Veiled and interdigitating cells: lymphoid tissue, synovium	–	?	–	+
Follicular dendritic cells: lymphoid tissue, follicles	–	?	+	+
Blood and lymphoid dendritic cells: blood, spleen	–	–	–	+

lymphocytes. Using opsonized erythrocytes, these workers showed that the same population that stained with B cell alloantisera also formed Fc rosettes. Langerhans cells were known to be the only cells in the epidermis having Fc receptors. Other investigators using rabbit anti-human Ia heterologous antisera also observed Ia antigens on Langerhans cells [40, 67]. More recently, class II antigen expression by epidermal Langerhans cells has been defined with monoclonal antibodies. Expression of DR molecules was observed on most of these cells by several investigators [11, 28, 29].

The expression of HLA-DQ and HLA-DP molecules was recently demonstrated by us in collaboration with Sontheimer et al. (in preparation). We used TU22, Genox 3.53, and Leu 10 for detection of DQ, and L-LR1 and FA for detection of DP. When suitable donor skin biopsies were used, staining was observed with all of these monoclonal antibodies. The cellular localization was determined by two-color immunofluorescence using the antibody OKT6 as a marker of epidermal Langerhans cells.

Class II Antigens on Dendritic Cells from Peripheral Blood and Spleen

Dendritic cells isolated from human peripheral blood have been found to express antigens recognized by rabbit anti-human Ia sera [44, 84], as well as with various monoclonal antibodies against HLA-DR framework determinants [44, 68, 84].

In recent experiments we have isolated dendritic-like cells from human spleen by differential adherence and density gradient centrifugation (unpublished work). The loosely adherent, low-density cells were found to be the most powerful stimulators in the MLR. Staining of these cells with monoclonal antibodies showed that about 70% expressed framework determinants of HLA-DR. However, this population was also found to contain a large number of B lymphocytes (see above).

Class II Antigens on Veiled Cells and Interdigitating Dendritic Cells

Heterologous anti-human Ia sera have been used to study interdigitating dendritic cells in lymph nodes [46] and dendritic-like cells in the medulla of the thymus [38] and in the rheumatoid synovium [62]. The synovial interdigitating cells have also been found to stain with monoclonal antibodies to DR [15, 81].

Class II Antigens on Follicular Dendritic Cells in Human Lymph Nodes and Spleen

Follicular dendritic cells in human lymph nodes and spleen were intensely DR-positive using immunofluorescence with monoclonal antibodies against DR [29, 82].

Accessory Cell Function of Human Dendritic Cells

Interest in dendritic cells has centered around their apparent important contribution as accessory cells in the immune response. Langerhans cells were found to stimulate allogeneic lymphocytes [12, 47] and capable of presenting soluble antigens to T lymphocytes [13]. Both of these functions could be abolished by treatment with anti-Ia and complement. The accessory cell function was found to be HLA-DR-restricted [9].

Dendritic-cell-rich fractions from human blood have been obtained by a variety of techniques [44, 84]. The cells were loosely adherent, of low density, Fc receptor negative and nonspecific-esterase negative. Such preparations have consisted of 60%–80% of dendritic cells by morphological criteria. These studies have been hampered, however, by the lack of a specific marker for the positive identification of these cells. Negative depletion strategies have recently been used by several investigators as another approach to the purification and characterization of human blood dendritic cells. Thus, van Voorhis and coworkers [85] have used monoclonal antibodies to deplete their preparation of monocytes/macrophages and other cells by killing with complement. Santiago-Schwartz and coworkers [68] have used monoclonal antibodies to remove monocytes, B cells, and T cells in the FACs. The resulting preparations of dendritic cells (75%–80%) appeared to be powerful stimulators of the allogeneic and the autologous MLR.

Summary

Expression of class II antigens is an important feature of all cells that can activate T lymphocytes of the T4 phenotype. It is becoming increasingly clear that this property is not limited to monocytes/macrophages. Many different cells have been found to be able to synthesize class II antigens when stimulated by gamma-interferon, which is a powerful modulator of expression of class I and class II MHC antigens in most cells.

Expression of HLA-DR, DQ, and DP does not always go together. A major portion of peripheral blood monocytes express very low levels or no detectable DQ. HLA-DQ-rich adherent cells are also DR-rich, and have been found to be the more powerful stimulators of allogeneic T cells.

Table 5. Expression of class II MHC antigens in various human cell types

Type of cells	Class II MHC antigens investigated		
	HLA-DR	HLA-DQ	HLA-DP
1. Peripheral blood			
Resting T lymphocytes	−	−	−
Activated T lymphocytes	+	+	+
B lymphocytes	+	+	+
Monocytes	+	+/− [a]	+
Dendritic cells	+	NT	NT
2. Tissue sites			
Macrophages [b]	+	+	+
Dendritic cells [c]	+	+	+
3. Large vessel endothelium			
Unstimulated	−	−	−
Gamma-interferon-treated	+	+	+
4. Capillary endothelium	+	+	NT

[a] A subset of monocytes expressed HLA-DQ
[b] Data based on study of alveolar macrophages
[c] Data from study of Langerhans cells of the skin

Current knowledge of the expression of D-region molecules in different lymphoid and endothelial cells is summarized in Table 5. Unstimulated endothelial cells from large vessels do not support the Ia-dependent accessory functions. However, these cells like many others, can be modulated to become Ia-positive under the influence of lymphocyte factors.

It is becoming increasingly clear that the interactions between T lymphocytes and accessory cells are quite complex. They involve, in addition to the MHC restriction antigens and the ability to process nominal antigen and place it appropriately on the cell surface, a variety of other functions and molecules. Some of these factors are secreted into the medium. Others are membrane-bound and appear to control and stabilize the interaction between T cells and accessory cells. It is possible that they also are involved in eliciting certain T cell reactions. Many cells appear to be active in this regard. Dendritic cells appear to be extremely efficient.

Relatively little is known yet about human dendritic cells. They have been difficult to purify, and their study has lagged because of the unavailability of suitable markers. Our best interpretation of available information is that several different cells can act as accessory cells. Expression of class II MHC antigens is a key attribute of all such cells, but other properties are certainly also required.

References

1. Albrechtsen D, Arnesen E, Thorsby E (1979) Cell-mediated lymphocytotoxicity directed against HLA-D gene products. Transplantation 27:338–341
2. Alter BJ, Bach FH (1970) Lymphocyte reactivity in vitro. I. Cellular reconstitution of purified lymphocyte response. Cell Immunol 1:207–218
3. Ball EJ, Stastny P (1982) Cell-mediated cytotoxicity against HLA-D region products expressed in monocytes and B lymphocytes. IV. Characterization of effector cells using monoclonal antibodies against human T-cell subsets. Immunognetics 16:157–169
4. Ball EJ, Stastny P (1984a) Antigen-specific HLA-restricted human T-cell lines. I. An MT3-like restriction determinant distinct from HLA-DR. Immunogenetics 19:13–26
5. Ball EJ, Stastny P (1984b) Antigen-specific HLA-restricted human T-cell lines. II. A GAT-specific T-cell line restricted by a determinant carried by an HLA-DQ molecule. Immunogenetics 20:547–564
6. Ball EJ, Feighery C, Stastny P (1981) Cell mediated cytotoxicity against HLA-D region products expressed in monocytes and B lymphocytes. III. Inhibition by monoclonal antibodies and study of an HLA-B/DR recombinant. Human Immunol 2:305–313
7. Basham TY, Mergian TC (1983) Recombinant interferon increases HLA-DR synthesis and expression. J Immunol 130:1492–1494
8. Bergholtz B, Thorsby E (1977) Macrophage-dependent response of immune human T lymphocytes to PPD in vitro. Influence of HLA-D compatibility. Scand J Immunol 6:779–786
9. Berle EJ Jr, Braathen LR, Thorsby E (1982) HLA-D/DR restriction of Langerhans cell dependent antigen activation of T lymphocytes. The same D/DR determinants are restriction elements on monocytes and Langerhans cells. Scand J Immunol 16:549–552
10. Biddison WE, Rao PE, Talle MA, Goldstein G, Shaw S (1982) Possible involvement of the OKT4 molecule in T cell recognition of class II HLA antigens: evidence from studies of cytotoxic T lymphocytes specific for SB antigens. J Exp Med 156:1065–1076
11. Bjercke S, Lea T, Braathen LR, Thorsby E (1984) Enrichment of human epidermal Langerhans dendritic cells. Scand J Immunol 19:255–263
12. Braathen LR, Thorsby E (1980) Studies on human epidermal Langerhans cells. Scand J Immunol 11:401–408

13. Braathen LR, Berle E, Modeech-Hanssen V, Thorsby E (1980) Studies on human epidermal Langerhans cells: II. Activation of human T lymphocytes to herpes simplex virus. Acta Derm Venereol (Stockh) 60:381–387
14. Burger DR, Ford D, Vetto RM, Hamblin A, Goldstein A, Hubbard M, Dumonde DC (1981) Endothelial cell presentation of antigen to human T cells. Human Immunol 3:209–230
15. Burmester GR, Dimitriu-Bona A, Waters SJ, Winchester RJ (1983) Identification of three major synovial lining cell populations by monoclonal antibodies directed to Ia antigens and antigens associated with monocytes/macrophages and fibroblasts. Scand J Immunol 17:69–82
16. Colbaugh P, Stastny P (1978) Antigens in human monocytes: use of monocytes in typing for HLA-D related (DR) antigens. Transplant Proc 10:871–874
17. Dimitriu-Bona A, Burmester JR, Waters SJ, Winchester RJ (1983) Human mononuclear phagocyte differentiation antigens. I. Patterns of antigenic expression on the surface of human monocytes and macrophages defined by monoclonal antibodies. J Immunol 130:145–152
18. Dupont B, Hansen JA, Yunis EJ (1976) Human mixed-lymphocyte culture reaction: genetics, specificity, and biological implications. Adv Immunol 23:107–202
19. Eckels D, Lake P, Lamb J, Johnson A, Shaw S, Woody J, Hartzman R (1983) SB-restricted presentation of influenza and herpes simplex virus antigens to human T-lymphocyte clones. Nature 301:716–718
20. Evans PR, Trickett LP, Smith JL, Maciver AG, Tate D, Slapak M (1984) Variable expression of HLA-DR antigens in the human kidney. Dis Markers 2:251–253
21. Feighery C, Stastny P (1979) HLA-D region-associated determinants serve as targets for human cell mediated lysis. J Exp Med 149:485–494
22. Feighery C, Stastny P (1980) Cell-mediated cytotoxicity against HLA-D-region products expressed in monocytes and B lymphocytes. I. Blocking by unlabeled cells and inhibition by antisera. Immunogenetics 10:31–38
23. Fuggle SV, Errasti P, Daar AS, Fabre JW, Ting A, Morris PJ (1983) Localization of major histocompatibility complex (HLA-ABC and DR) antigens in 46 kidneys. Transplantation 35:385–390
24. Fuggle SV, Carter NP, Ting A, Morris PJ (1984) Studies on the tissue distribution of class II antigens. Dis Markers 2:235–250
25. Gonwa TA, Stobo JD (1984) Differential expression of Ia molecules by human monocytes. J Clin Invest 74:859–866
26. Gonwa TA, Picker LJ, Raff HV, Goyert SM, Silver J, Stobo JD (1983) Antigen-presenting capabilities of human monocytes correlate with their expression of HLA-DS, an Ia determinant distinct from HLA-DR. J Immunol 130:706–711
27. Goyert SM, Shively JE, Silver J (1982) Biochemical characterization of a second family of human Ia molecules, HLA-DS equivalent to murine I-A subregion molecules. J Exp Med 156:550–566
28. Haftell M, Favre M, Schmitt D, Thirolet J (1983) Langerhans cells in skin from patients with psoriasis: quantitative and qualitative study of T6 and HLA-DR antigen expressing cells and changes with aromatic retinoid administration. J Invest Dermatol 80:481–484
29. Hancock WN, Atkins RC (1984) Immunohistologic analysis of the cell surface antigens of human dendritic cells using monoclonal antibodies. Transplant Proc 15:963–967
30. Hansen G, Rubin R, Sorensen S, Svejgaard A (1978) Importance of HLA-D antigens for the cooperation between human monocytes and T lymphocytes. Eur J Immunol 8:520–525
31. Hansen PW, Madsen M, Christiansen SE, Johnsen HE, Kissmeyer-Nielsen F (1984) Cell mediated PPD specific cytotoxicity against human monocyte targets: evidence for restriction by class II HLA antigens. Tissue Antigens 23:171–180
32. Hart DNJ, Fuggle SV, Williams KA, Fabre JW, Ting A, Morris PJ (1981) Localization of HLA-A,B,C and DR antigens in human kidneys. Transplantation 31:429–433
33. Hirschberg H (1981) Presentation of viral antigens by human vascular endothelial cells in vitro. Human Immunol 2:235–246
34. Hirschberg H, Evensen SA, Henriksen T, Thorsby E (1975) The human mixed lymphocyte-endothelium culture interaction. Transplantation 19:495–504

35. Hirschberg H, Moen T, Thorsby E (1979) Specific destruction of human endothelial cell monolayers by anti-DRw antisera. Transplantation 28:116–120
36. Hirschberg H, Bergh OJ, Thorsby E (1980) Antigen-presenting properties of human vascular endothelial cells. J Exp Med 152:249–255
37. Hirschberg H, Hirschberg T, Jaffe E, Thorsby E (1981) (1981) Antigen-presenting properties of human vascular endothelial cells: inhibition by anti-HLA-DR antisera. Scand J Immunol 14:545–553
38. Janossy G (1979) Differentiation of lymphoid precursor cells. J Clin Pathol [Suppl] 13:48–58
39. Johnsen HE (1980) Human B-blast specific target determinants in CML: a methodological study. Tissue Antigens 15:189–198
40. Klareskog LT, Jernlund UM, Forsum U, Peterson PA (1977) Epidermal Langerhans express Ia antigens. Nature 268:248
41. Koski IR, Poplack DG, Blaese RM (1976) A nonspecific esterase stain for the identification of monocytes and macrophages. In: Bloom BR, David JR (eds) In vitro methods in cell-mediated and tumor immunosity. Academic, New York, pp 359–362
42. Krensky AM, Clayberger C, Reiss CS, Strominger JL, Burakoff SJ (1982) Specificity of OKT4+ cytotoxic T lymphocyte clones. J Immunol 129:2001–2003
43. Krensky AM, Clayberger C, Greenstein C, Greenstein JL, Crimmins G, Burakoff SJ (1983) A DC-specific cytolytic T lymphocyte line is OKT8+. J Immunol 131:2777–2780
44. Kuntz Crow M, Kunkel HG (1982) Human dendritic cells: major stimulators of the autologous and allogeneic mixed leukocyte reactions. Clin Exp Immunol 49:338–346
45. Lamb J, Eckels D, Lake P, Johnson A, Hartzman R, Woody J (1982) Antigen-specific human T-lymphocyte clones: induction, antigen specificity, and MHC restriction of virus-immune clones. J Immunol 128:233–238
46. Lampert IA, Pizzolo G, Thomas A, Janossy G (1979) Immunohistochemical characterization of cell involved in dermatopathic lymphadenopathy. J Pathol 131:145–156
47. Levis WR, Miller AE (1972) Leukocyte/skin cultures as a measure of histocompatibility in man. Lancet II:357–360
48. Maeda H (1984) Mouse monoclonal antibody detects a new polymorphic Ia determinant other than HLA-DR antigen: a possible allele of DC-1. Tissue Antigens 23:163–170
49. Merdrignac G, Fauchet R, Bouhallier O, Genetet B (1981) HLA-A,-B, and -DR specificities on human monocytes. Tissue Antigens 18:299–305
50. Meuer SC, Hussey RE, Hodgdon JC, Hercend T, Schlossman SF (1982) Surface structures involved in target recognition by human cytotoxic T lymphocytes. Science 218:471–473
51. Moen T, Moen M, Thorsby E (1980) HLA-D region products are expressed in endothelial cells. Tissue Antigens 15:112–122
52. Nadler LM, Stashenko P, Hardy R, Pesando JM, Yunis EJ, Schlossman SF (1981) Monoclonal antibodies defining serologically distinct HLA-D/DR related Ia-like antigens in man. Hum Immunol 2:77–90
53. Natali PG, De Martino C, Quaranta V, Nicotra MR, Frezza F, Pellegrino MA, Ferrone S (1981) Expression of Ia-like antigens in normal human non-lymphoid tissues. Transplantation 31:75–78
54. Neppert J, Nuñez G, Stastny P (1984) HLA-A,B,C; -DR; -MT, -MB, and SB antigens on unstimulated human endothelial cells. Tissue Antigens 24:40–47
55. Nuñez G, Stastny P (1983) Cytofluorometric analysis of major histocompatibility antigens on human monocytes using monoclonal antibodies. Hum Immunol 6:1–11
56. Nuñez G, Ugolini V, Capra JD, Stastny P (1982) Monoclonal antibodies against human monocytes. II. Recognition of two distinct cell surface molecules. Scand J Immunol 16:515–523
57. Nuñez G, Ball EJ, Stastny P (1983) Accessory cell functions of human endothelial cells. I. A subpopulation of Ia-positive cells distinct from monocytes is required for antigen presentation. J Immunol 131:666–673
58. Nuñez G, Giles RC, Ball EJ, Hurley CK, Capra JD, Stastny P (1984) Expression of HLA-DR, MB, MT, and SB antigens on human mononuclear cells: identification of two phenotypically distinct monocyte populations. J Immunol 133:1300–1306

59. Pober JS, Gimbrone MA Jr (1982) Expression of Ia-like antigens by human vascular endothelial cells is inducible in vitro: demonstration by monoclonal antibody binding with immunoprecipitation. Proc Natl Acad Sci USA 79:6641–6645
60. Pober JS, Collins T, Gimbrone MA, Cotran RS, Gitlin JD, Fiers W, Clayberger C, Krensky AM, Burakoff SJ, Reiss CS (1983 a) Lymphocytes recognize human vascular endothelial and dermal fibroblast Ia antigens induced by recombinant immune interferon. Nature 305:726–729
61. Pober JS, Gimbrone MA, Cotran RS, Reiss CS, Burakoff SJ, Fiers W, Ault KA (1983 b) Ia expression by vascular endothelium is inducible by activated T cells and by human interferon. J Exp Med 157:1339–1353
62. Poulter LW, Duke O, Hobbs S, Janossy G, Panayi G, Seymour G (1983) The involvement of interdigitating cells in the pathogenesis of rheumatoid arthritis. Clin Exp Immunol 51:247–254
63. Reinherz E, Kung P, Goldstein G, Schlossman S (1980) A monoclonal antibody reactive with the human cytotoxic suppressor subset previously defined by a heteroantiserum termed TH2. J Immunol 124:1301–1307
64. Rode HN, Gordon J (1974) Macrophages in the mixed leukocyte culture reaction (MLC). Cell Immunol 13:87–94
65. Rodey G, Luehrman L, Thomas D (1979) In vitro primary immunization of human peripheral blood lymphocytes to KLH: evidenced for HLA-D region restriction. J Immunol 123:2240–2254
66. Roska AK, Johnson AR, Lipsky PE (1984) Immunologic function of endothelial cells: Guinea pig aortic endothelial cells support mitogen-induced T lymphocyte activation, but do not function as antigen-presenting cells. J Immunol 132:136–145
67. Rowden G, Lewis MG, Sullivan AK (1977) Ia antigen expression on human epidermal Langerhans cells. Nature 268:247–248
68. Santiago-Schwarz F, Bakke AC, Woodward JG, O'Brien RL, Horwite DA (1985) Further characterization of low density mononuclear cells: FACS-assisted analysis of human MLR stimulators. J Immunol 134:779–785
69. Scott H, Brandtzaeg P, Hirschberg H, Solheim BG, Thorsby E (1981) Vascular and renal distribution of HLA-DR-like antigens. Tissue Antigens 18:195–202
70. Shaw S, DeMars R (1984) Binding specificity of anti-human Ia monoclonal antibodies analyzed with HLA-deletion mutant cell lines: patterns of binding to products of two different HLA haplotypes and of three subregions of a single haplotype. Dis Markers 2:183–195
71. Shaw S, Johnson AH, Shearer GM (1980) Evidence for a new segregant series of B cell antigens that are encoded in the HLA-D region and that stimulate secondary allogeneic proliferative cytotoxic responses. J Exp Med 152:565–580
72. Silberberg-Sinakin I, Gigli I, Bae RL, Thorbecks GJ (1980) Langerhans cells: role in contact hypersensitivity and relationship to lymphoid dendritic cells and to macrophages. Immunol Rev 53:203–232
73. Smith BR, Ault K (1981) Increase in surface Ia-like expression on human monocytes independent of antigenic stimuli. J Immunol 127:2020–2027
74. Soulillou JP, Peyrat MA, Guenel J (1981) Studies of pre- and post graft antibodies against endothelial cells (umbilical cord) in kidney allografts. Transplant Proc 13:1551–1555
75. Stastny P (1977) Antigen in human monocytes: Ia antigens detected in monocytes using seventh workshop sera. In: Bodmer WF, Batchelor JR, Bodmer JG (eds) Histocompatibility testing 1978. Munksgaard, Copenhagen, pp 566–568
76. Stastny P (1978) Endothelial monocyte antigens in man. Transplant Proc 10:875–877
77. Stastny P, Nuñez G (1981) The role of endothelial and monocyte antigens in kidney transplantation. In: Torraine JL, Traeger J, Brodner H, Dubervard HM, Revillard JP, Trian R (eds) Transplantation and clinical immunology, vol XIII. Excerpta Medica, Amsterdam, pp 32–139
78. Stingl G, Wolfe-Schreiner E, Pichler, Gschnait F, Knapp W, Wolff K (1977) Epidermal Langerhans cells bear Fc and C3 receptors. Nature 268:245–246
79. Toews GB, Vial WC, Dunn MM, Guzzetta P, Nuñez G, Stastny P, Lipscomb MF (1984) The accessory cell function of human alveolar macrophages in specific T cell proliferation. J Immunol 132:181–186

80. Tosi R, Tanigaki N, Centis D, Ferrara GB, Pressman D (1978) Immunological dissection of human Ia molecules. J Exp Med 148:1592–1611
81. Tyndall AD, Knight SC, Edwards AJ, Clarke JB (1983) Veiled (dendritic) cells in synovial fluid. Lancet I:472
82. van der Valk P, van der Loo EM, Jansen J, Daha MR, Meiser C-JLM (1984) Analysis of lymphoid and dendritic cells in human lymph node, tonsil, and spleen. Virchows Arch [Cell Pathol] 45:169–185
83. van Leeuwen A, Termijtelen A, Shaw S, van Rood JJ (1982) Recognition of a polymorphic monocyte antigen in HLA. Nature 298:565–567
84. van Voorhis WC, Hair LS, Steinman RM, Kaplan G (1982) Human dendritic cells: enrichment and characterization from peripheral blood. J Exp Med 155:1172–1187
85. van Voorhis WC, Valinsky J, Hoffman E, Luban J, Hair LS, Steinman RM (1983) Relative efficacy of human monocytes and dendritic cells as accessory cells for T cell replication. J Exp Med 158:174–191
86. Watson AJ, DeMars R, Trowbridge IS, Bach FH (1983) Detection of a novel human class II HLA antigens. Nature 304:358–360
87. Young MR, Smith AV (1964) The use of euchrysine in staining cells and tissues for fluorescence microscopy. J R Microsc Soc 82:233–244

Class II Antigens: T Cells

V. Corredor, Y. Matsui, and E. J. Yunis

Table of Contents

Introduction

Class II antigens in humans appear as the products of HLA-DR, DQ, and DP genes located in the HLA-D-region [37] and were first defined by allogeneic cellular immune responses as the gene products controlling the proliferative response during mixed lymphocyte reactions (MLRs) [41].

Class II antigens have been recognized to be present on B cells, macrophages, and activated T cells, and required for cellular recognition between antigen-presenting cells (APCs), B cells, and T cells in order to produce an immune response. Activation of T lymphocytes by APCs produces several changes, leading to the acquisition of the T cells' regulatory and cytotoxic functions; expression of class II molecules on T cells has been demonstrated to result from T lymphocyte activation.

Class II molecules are at present relatively well understood with respect to gene structure and biochemistry. Their function, the origin of their polymorphism and the reason for their expression and synthesis on different cell lines, however, are not yet so well understood.

The recently developed murine monoclonal antibodies recognizing different class II gene products, T cell cloning, and DNA probes are important tools which have helped to elucidate the complex structure and function of class II molecules.

However, little work has been done toward explaining the function of class II antigens on activated T cells.

Expression and Synthesis of Class II Antigens on T Cells

Expression of class II antigens on T cells has been shown to occur following alloactivation during MLR [8, 12, 33], exposure to mitogens [15], or soluble antigen activation [28]. In these experiments, HLA-DR-specific heteroantiserum [8] or specific monoclonal antibodies against class II gene products [28] were used to detect these antigens.

Class II Antigens on Alloactivated T Cells

During MLR, T cells are activated by membrane molecules of the stimulator cells, producing a proliferative response [2]. After this allosensitization, these cells express class II molecules on their surfaces. When T cells are examined before allosensitization or at rest, they do not react with class II-specific antibodies and no HLA-DR antigens can be detected. However, when responder cells once come into contact with the stimulator cell population, the expression of class II molecules is initiated [12]. Nonactivated and MLR-activated T cells have been exposed to a specific heterologous antiserum for HLA-D/DR antigens, showing that the specific antiserum did not react against non-activated T lymphocytes and thymocytes, but did react with activated lymphocytes, as determined by indirect immunofluorescence. These experiments and subsequent SDS gel electrophoresis showed, after immunoprecipitation of activated T lymphocytes with heteroantiserum, that the expressed molecule was a 29K and 30K complex [12].

The maximal peak of class II molecule expression after alloactivation has been shown to occur after approximately 6–8 days in culture [8, 15]; after this time antigen expression begins to decrease, disappearing by 16–18 days [8]. However, on restimulation class II molecules reappear, reaching the maximal peak of expression after 2–3 days [8].

Not all T cell populations have been shown to produce class II antigens after activation. Utilization of antigen detection with hetero- and specific responder alloantiserum showed that 40%–60% of alloactivated cells were class II-positive [35], a result similar to the data presented by other groups [26, 28], who used specific monoclonal antibodies against class II antigens to detect class II-positive T cells. Other experiments showed that helper/inducer (CD 4) and cytotoxic/suppressor (CD 8) cells were able to express class II antigens after activation on MLR, but once primed T cells were depleted of class II-positive cells the percentage of cytotoxic/suppressor (CD 8) cells decreased to zero. Thus, all CD 8 cells express class II antigens, but the same is not true of the CD 4 cells [35].

It is not yet known why a percentage of T cells do not express class II antigens after activation.

Mitogen-activated T Cells

Various studies have shown that T cells express class II molecules when activated by different mitogens, such as phytohemagglutinin (PHA), which binds to *N*-acetyl-galactosamine-containing oligosaccharides, concanavalin A (Con A), which binds saccharides with a terminal D – mannose, or pokeweed mitogen (PWM) [15, 38]. The expression has been shown to be initiated approximately 3 days after mitogen activation and to reach maximum levels between 7 and 9 days after PHA, Con A, or PWM activation [15]. However, other laboratories have shown peak expression after 72 h of PHA activation [14].

Analysis of the percentage of activated T cell populations expressing class II molecules have shown that, after PHA activation, 18% of mature T cells (CD 3+), 22% of the helper/inducer T cell subset (CD 4+) and 16% of T cells not expressing the CD 4 phenotype (CD 4−) expressed class II antigens. For Con A activation the corresponding figures are 20% of CD 3+, 16% of CD 4+, and 15% of CD4− cells [28]. In addition, T lymphocyte subpopulations bearing either IgM receptors or IgG receptors appear to be equivalent in their ability to produce class II molecules as detected by indirect rosette microassay with specific monoclonal antibodies [14]. The appearance of class II molecules on T lymphocyte surface coincides with the loss of IgM Fc receptors [14].

A monoclonal antibody against class II molecules has been shown to block interleukin-2 (IL-2) dependent T cell proliferation in cultured T cells, suggesting a relationship between class II antigen expression on T lymphocytes and the production of IL-2 or the synthesis of IL-2 receptor [18].

These results have been interpreted in two different ways: first, that the action of the antibody was to inhibit the IL-2 binding by something like steric hindrance, or alternatively, that class II molecules were participating in the cellular events required by the cell to proliferate and mediated by IL-2 signal. Using monoclonal antibodies against HLA-DR antigens and HLA-DR heteroantisera, Effros et al. [9] showed that DR antigen expression on PHA-activated T cells correlated with the ability of T cells to be maintained in IL-2-dependent long-term culture. According to these authors, this fact supports the concept that class II molecules are involved in the transmission of signals by IL-2.

Soluble Antigen Activation

T lymphocytes activated with Tetanus Toxoid (TT) reach peak class II antigen expression after 7 days in culture in the presence of peripheral blood mononuclear cells (PBMCs); approximately 40%–50% of T cells cultured with TT or purified protein derivative (PPD) have been shown to express class II antigens. Interestingly, TT used in place of other stimulators in T cell activation did not induce the expression of class II antigens in T cells of the CD 4− phenotype, while 20% and 38% of mature T cells (CD 3) and helper/inducer T cells (CD 4) respectively expressed class II antigens after activation [28].

The expression of class II molecules on activated T cells has raised many questions: (1) Do T cells synthesize class II molecules? (2) Are these molecules absorbed from the culture media on MLCs? (3) Or is the increase of the class II-positive T cell population after activation the result of the clonal expansion of a small class II-positive T cell subpopulation?

Passive uptake and expression of the class II antigens of the stimulator cell by the responder cells has been demonstrated by different laboratories in mouse MLC systems [21]. Despite some evidence to the contrary [40], human T cells endogenously synthesize class II molecules after activation [6, 12, 14, 28, 40]. Studies using different heteroantisera and lymphocytotoxicity, showed that class II molecules expressed on responder T lymphocytes after activation were of the responder HLA phenotype and not of the stimulator phenotype [8, 34]. Later, other investigators [6] showed using two-dimensional gel electrophoretic analysis of metabolically labeled proteins that the responder cells were able to synthesize class II antigens different from those of the stimulator cells. These findings supported previous evidence obtained with one-dimensional gel electrophoresis [12].

The possibility that a clonal expansion of class II-positive T cells occurs after activation has been investigated by several groups, based on the evidence that a small percentage (0%–5%) of resting T cells expressed the antigens [6, 14, 28, 32]; however, when resting T cells are treated with specific antisera or monoclonal antibodies plus complement, to avoid the presence of any class II-positive T cell at the moment of activation, and are then alloactivated, class II molecules are expressed. The inability to precipitate class II molecules before alloactivation with monoclonal antibodies also suggests that class II molecules are synthesized by T cells rather than produced by clonal expansion, and are not acquired by passive uptake of HLA molecules produced by the stimulator cells during MLR in the human system.

The Nature of Class II Molecules Expressed on Activated T Cells

Activated T cells are known to express antigens coded by different loci of the HLA-D region [20, 24, 25, 27]; however, little is known concerning the expression, kinetics, and functional significance of the gene products of individual class II loci on activated T cells.

Some laboratories have demonstrated that alloactivated T lymphocytes, when restimulated and expanded for 9–75 days in medium containing IL-2, express DR antigens, and are also able to express DP (SB) antigens [26]; likewise, the expression of DQw1 (DC 1) antigen determinants has been demonstrated after PHA activation using monoclonal antibodies recognizing this antigen. Also, *Chlamydia* – specific human T lymphocytes have been shown to express DR, DP, and DQ antigens, using monoclonal antibodies to detect these antigens by indirect radioimmunoassay. In these studies it was shown that *Chlamydia* – specific T cell clones which develop unresponsiveness to antigen restimulation expressed fewer determinants for DQ and anti-Tac monoclonal antibodies than clones with antigen-specific proliferative capacity [27].

Recently, however, it has been shown that a monoclonal antibody recognizing a class II antigen related to the murine I-A antigen (DQ) reacted with B cells but not with mitogen-activated T cells, suggesting the probability that some class II molecules are not expressed on activated T cells or that the expression varies [16]. Activated T cells apparently express the same HLA-DR molecules as B cells, as shown by peptide maps and partial amino acid sequences after immune precipitation with rabbit antiserum against purified DR antigens [1].

Class II Molecules Expressed on T Cell Clones

Class II molecules have been shown to be expressed in T cell clones derived from mixed leukocyte cultures (MLCs) [25]. However, it was recently demonstrated that expression and synthesis of class II molecules occured on antigen-specific T cell clones sequentially stimulated with Trinitrophenyl (TNP)-modified PBMCs, cloned by limiting dilution, and subcloned and expanded with IL-2 with weekly restimulations. The clones expressing CD 3, CD 4, and CD 2 surface molecules, as detected by flow cytometry, were positive for the activated T cell marker Tac and DR membrane proteins, and were negative for CD 8 and other markers defining B cells and monocytes. The same authors metabolically labeled two different clones with ^{3}H-leucine and ^{3}H-tyrosine, immunoprecipitated the cell lysates with a framework-specific antibody to DR antigens or against murine I-A^b antigen, and demonstrated by two-dimensional gel electrophoresis the presence of the alpha and beta chains (34K and 29K respectively) of the DR molecule [5].

Functional Significance of Class II Molecule Expression on T Cells

Stimulatory Capacity

Activated T cells have been shown to be capable of stimulatory allogeneic MLR. The proliferation of responder cells has been found to be blocked by monoclonal antibodies against class II antigens but not against class I antigens, suggesting that T cells expressing class II molecules could have a role of stimulating allogeneic responses during MLR [39]. It has been shown that anti-DR sera inhibited the stimulating capacity of primed lymphocytes during MLCs, but not the responder capacity [34].

When DR-positive T cells are removed from the T cell population, the secondary proliferative response during MLR is abolished, apparently showing that the memory response capacity resides on class II-positive T lymphocytes [34]; similar results have been obtained by purifying resting T lymphocytes for stimulation of PLT cells or secondary proliferative responses, where no stimulation occurred at all [39]. When purified T lymphocytes are used to stimulate responder-purified T cells, no proliferation is observed unless nonpurified lymphocytes are used as responders. Once T lymphocytes are alloactivated and used as stimulators on PLT cells, a significant proliferative response is developed, showing the role of class II antigens in stimulating secondary proliferative responses [39].

Using a class II-positive T cell subpopulation characterized by the inability to bind sheep red blood cells in the presence of theophylline, stimulation by activated T cells has been shown to be 10-fold more potent than stimulation by the same number of B cells [32]. On the other hand, alloactivated T lymphocytes have also been able to stimulate autologous MLR, but of a lower level than allogeneic T cells [35], while DR-negative T lymphocytes failed to stimulate autologous T cell proliferation. Other investigators have found that T cells displaying HLA-D/DR antigens, when primed with lymphocytes from unrelated donors but sharing the same HLA-D/DR specificities, were able to stimulate proliferation to a degree comparable to that displayed by unrelated donors with different HLA-D/DR specificities. These results suggest that T cell priming can be induced by other HLA class II gene products or even by non-HLA antigens [25, 35]. Homozygous typing cells (HTCs) primed in MLRs (against an HTC, Dw3/DR3) and expressing HLA-D/DR antigens (Dw2) have been shown to fail to be able to restimulate secondary MLR of heterozygous T cells (Dw2, DR2/Dw3, DR5). Suppression appears to be responder-specific, a phenomenon which has been explained by the researchers in terms of a hypothetical expansion during primary stimulation of a HLA-D-restricted suppressor T cell population. In this regard, T cells bearing helper (CD 4) or suppressor (CD 8) phenotypes have been able to express HLA-D/DR antigens and to stimulate MLR, while CD8+ T cells appear to react in a higher proportion with class II antibodies [35]. Nevertheless, it has been shown that 6-day-old cells from MLR and 10-day-old cells from PLT expressing class II antigens on their surfaces are able to stimulate proliferative responses of allogeneic lymphocytes in primary MLC and to restimulate secondary proliferative responses of T cell clones which are HLA-D and DP(SB)-specific. But on one occasion, T cells from 15- to 81-day-old IL-2 cultures, also expressing DR and DP antigens failed to stimulate either primary proliferative responses or HLA-D or DP-specific responses from specific responders. An explanation of the fact that 6-day-old MLC and 10-day-old PLT (non-IL-2-cultured) T cells stimulate proliferative responses, while 15- to 81-day-old IL-2-propagated T cells do not, remains to be found [26].

Antigen Presentation Function

As antigen presentation has been shown in various cells expressing class II molecules in their membranes, the probability that activated T cells develop the same functions has been investigated. When alloactivated T lymphocytes expressing DR antigens were tested for the ability to proliferate in the presence of autologous T cells and TT or diphteria toxoid, a positive response was observed. This observation has permitted researchers to hypothesize that there is an accessory function of T cells, although this function is not as efficient as that tested with non-T cell PBMCs [10].

Further evidence has been provided [5] that trinitrophenyl (TNP)-specific T cell clones synthesize HLA-DR antigens after activation, and once irradiated, these clones serve as stimulators of TNP-specific T cell proliferation by responder clones sharing the same HLA-DR specificity. These findings confirm the antigen-presenting function of activated T cells.

Activated T Lymphocytes and Helper Activity

Interaction between T lymphocytes and B lymphocytes has been shown to be necessary for antibody production. Activated T cells expressing class II molecules have been shown to be required for B cell activity. Primary experiments showed that the generation of plaque-forming cells against sheep erythrocytes in the presence of allogenic tonsillar B cells was lost after elimination of T cells expressing class II antigens [13]. Also, evidence that only helper/inducer (CD 4) cells synthesized class II molecules after soluble antigen activation has stimulated work on CD 4+ and CD 4− subpopulations [28]. Elimination of class II-positive T lymphocytes by complement lysis after TT activation resulted in the elimination of the proliferative response to the specific TT antigen, as well as to the unrelated mumps antigens. When class II-positive T cells were not eliminated, proliferation was not inhibited. Similar results were obtained with class II-negative T cells reconstituted with 10% autologous macrophages and restimulated in a secondary proliferation with specific TT antigen or unspecific mumps antigen. When CD 4+, class II-positive T lymphocytes were cultured with B cells, immunoglobulin production was detected, whereas poor immunoglobulin detection was observed in CD 4+, class II-negative, T cell and B cell cocultures. Surprisingly, a great amount of immunoglobulin production has been shown when CD 4+, class II-positive cells and CD 4+, class II-negative cells were cultured together, suggesting a cooperation between the two types of cells in helper activity [29]. In recent studies, autoreactive T cell clones were obtained from PBMCs primed with an autologous ragweed-specific T helper/inducer (CD 4) cell; the clones expressed CD 4, CD 2, CD 3, class II antigens but not CD 8 antigen, and proliferated with autologous class II antigens from B cells, macrophages, and lymphoblastoid B cell lines. The T cell clones induced autologous B cells to produce high levels of immunoglobulins in the absence of ragweed antigen, while the ragweed-specific T cell clone used for priming needed the presence of exogenous antigen to induce IgG production. Thus it appeared that expression of class II molecules in autologous cells served to amplify the induction of immunoglobulin production [3].

Helper and Suppressor Factors

Antigen-specific and nonspecific factors with helper and suppressor activity, some of which are apparently class II antigen dependents, have been described in the mouse [36].

Suppressor cells are known to release suppressive factors after stimulation by HLA-DR specific stimulator cells. Suppression of proliferation, however, occurs against any stimulating cell, regardless of its HLA-DR specificity [31].

In alloactivated T cells added to a MLR, suppression has been demonstrated for the DR type of stimulator cells, as shown by the observation that cells sharing DR antigen specificities with the priming cell were inhibited in their capacity to stimulate. Supernatants from DR-positive but not DR-negative T cell populations were shown to inhibit fresh cultures, suggesting that the release of soluble suppressor factors is DR-antigen dependent. This inhibition has been shown to be non-antigen-specific [11].

Helper factors produced by human T cells upon activation and facilitating a B cell response to unrelated antigens have also been described [19]. Antigen-specific T helper factor (ASF) from supernatants of TT antigen-stimulated human T cells has been shown to induce anti-TT antibody synthesis in autologous B cells. Also, insolubilized anti-DRw antisera of an ASF donor partially removed the ASF activity, suggesting that soluble factors contain class II-like determinants. Anti-DRw antisera, when added to B lymphocyte cultures, were also able to inhibit B cell responses to ASF [19].

Cell Cycle and Class II Antigen Expression on T Cells

It has been shown, using flow cytometric analysis, that class II molecules appear late in relation to DNA synthesis [7]. Studies performed in our laboratory have shown variations in the cell surface densities of major histocompatibility antigens during the cell cycle on normal and leukemic T cell lines as well as on different lymphoblastoid B cell lines. These studies attempted to determine the amount of surface antigen quantitatively and to correlate that amount with DNA content and cell size by means of dual-beam flow cytometry. Using monoclonal antibodies against class I and class II gene products, antigen quantity on the cell surface was determined by immunofluorescence on resting and PHA-activated T cells, normal T cell clones with cytotoxic, natural killer-like functions and leukemic T cells. As shown previously [17], leukemic T cell lines do not express class

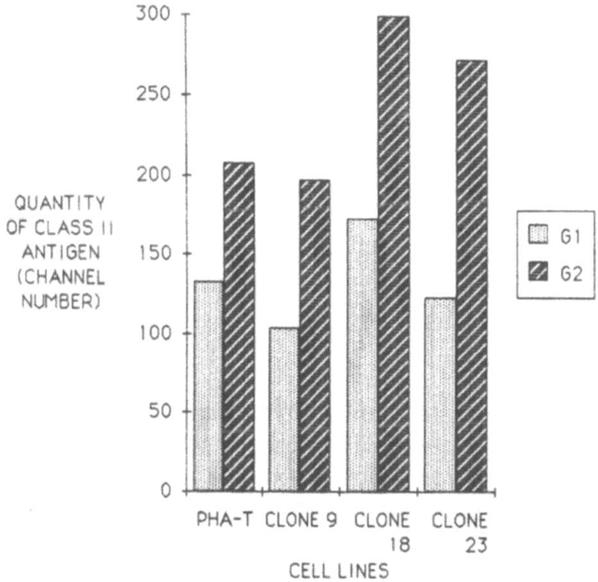

Fig. 1. Comparisons of the relative quantity of MHC class II antigens on the surface of the cell lines. The relative quantities of the surface antigen, or the means of the immunofluorescence intensity, in the G1 phase (*dotted bars*) and the G2 phase (*striped bars*) were obtained from the histograms of the class II antigen expression using a flow cytometer and the window defining the cell cycle. *PHA-T*, activated T cells cultured with PHA for 3 days and maintained with PHA-induced conditioned medium. *Clones 9, 18, 23*, T cell clones with cytotoxic, natural killer-like, and noncytotoxic functions respectively

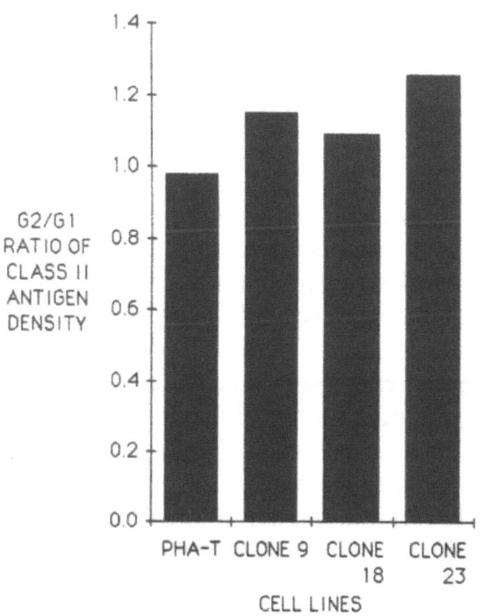

Fig. 2. The G2/G1 ratio of MHC class II antigen density on the surface of the cell lines. The G2/G1 ratio of the surface antigen density was obtained by dividing the G2/G1 ratio of the surface antigen quantity by the G2/G1 ratio of the cell surface area

II molecules. The study demonstrated that T lymphocytes increase the quantity of class I and class II antigens on the cell surface during the cell cycle, more during the G2 phase than during the G1 phase (Fig. 1). The lowest amount of class II antigens was found on the specific cytotoxic T cell clone (clone 9). Noncytotoxic (clone 23) and natural killer (clone 18) clones showed higher amounts of class II antigens during both G1 and G2 than the specific alloreactive cytotoxic T cell clone (clone 9). Similar findings were obtained for class I antigens. Although not shown, the density of class I antigens was found to be less during G2 than during G1. On the other hand, there was a higher density of class II antigens during G2 than during G1 in T cell clones (Fig. 2) (Matsui et al., unpublished results).

Class II Antigens on Thymus

Class II antigens have been detected on the human thymus and on thymocytes activated with a combination of phorbol ester 12-*o*-tetra-decanoyl phorbol-13-acetate (TPA) and the calcium ionophore ionomycin, but not on resting thymocytes [24]. Monoclonal antibodies against class II molecules have been shown to stain small numbers of cells in cortex and medulla. The cells probably represent epithelial cells, suggesting a close relationship between thymocytes and epithelial cells [4]. Similarly, using monoclonal antibodies and rabbit anti-p 23-30 antiserum for immunoelectron-microscopic staining it has been shown that epithelial thymus cells are the predominant class II-bearing cells on thymus, as was previously shown in the mouse. Intense staining of the dendritic array was found throughout the cortex [30].

DQ (DC 1) antigens have been shown to be expressed on thymic reticuloepithelial cells; 8- and 26-week-old embryos expressed DQ and HLA-DR antigens on cortical and medullary thymic dendritic cells as detected by monoclonal antibodies. The authors of this report suggest that DQ antigens can play a role in T lymphocyte–stroma interactions and in the development of the immunologically competent T lymphocyte system. The maturation process during which class II antigens reach maximum expression on the thymus has been reported to require 32 weeks. Thymic cells bearing class II antigens can stimulate MLR, a process which can be blocked by monoclonal antibodies [22, 23].

Summary

Class II antigens are expressed on human T cells after activation by mitogens, soluble antigens, or alloactivation during mixed lymphocyte culture.

Human T cells synthesize class II molecules rather than obtaining them by means of passive uptake from donor cells during mixed culture or by clonal expansion of small class II-positive T cell subpopulation. Although preliminary reports suggested that all class II molecules are expressed on activated T lymphocytes, it is still possible at least that there is a quantitative differential expression of the three different kinds of class II antigens on activated T cells, or even that certain class II molecules are expressed only on B lymphocytes.

It appears that expression of HLA-DR varies in relation to the type of T cell activation; for example, activation by lectins result in the expression of HLA-DR in all CD 8 cells and a proportion of CD 4 cells. In contrast, activation of lymphocytes by soluble antigens results in preferential expression of HLA-DR by CD 4 cells.

We have mentioned in this review that HLA-DR is expressed on the surface of epithelial cells of the thymus, but not on thymocytes. Nevertheless, other class II antigens, i.e., DQ, may be necessary for the maturation of T lymphocytes.

One aspect of the subject of expression of class II antigens on T lymphocytes that requires more study is the relationship of different requirements for class II antigens by specific and nonspecific helper and suppressor factors. Furthermore, the role played by class II antigens in the immune network needs to be elucidated. It is not known, for example, how the class II antigen of a specific activated T cell interacts with the same type of molecule on the surface of B lymphocytes to trigger the production of immunoglobulins and/or specific antibody.

Acknowledgments. The authors would like to thank Dr. H. Slayter, Dr. J. D. Dasgupta, and Mr. Glen B. Glater for their assistance.

References

1. Altevogt P, Fohlman J, Kurnick JT, Peterson P, Wigzell H (1980) Biochemical comparison of HLA-DR molecules derived from autologous human T and B lymphoblasts. Eur J Immunol 10:908–914
2. Bach FH, Voynow NK (1966) One-way stimulation in mixed leukocyte cultures. Science 15:545
3. Bensussan A, Meuer SC, Schlossman SF, Reinherz EL (1984) Delineation of an immunoregulatory amplifier population recognizing autologous Ia molecules. Analysis with human T cell clones. J Exp Med 159:559–576
4. Bhan AK, Reinherz EL, Poppema S, McCluskey RT, Schlossman SF (1980) Location of T cell and major histocompatibility complex antigens in the human thymus. J Exp Med 152:771
5. Brown MG, Cook RG, Van Rich M (1984) Cloned human T cells synthesize Ia molecules and can function as antigen presenting cells. Hum Immunol 11:219–228
6. Charron JD, Engleman EG, Benike CJ, McDevitt HO (1980) Ia antigens on alloreactive T cells in man detected by monoclonal antibodies. Evidence for synthesis of HLA-D/DR molecules of the responder type. J Exp Med 152:127s
7. Cotner T, Williams JE, Christenson L, Shapiro HW, Strom TB, Strominger J (1983) Simultaneous flow cytometric analysis of human T cell activation antigen expression and DNA content. J Exp Med 157:461–472
8. DeWolf CM, Schlossman SFS, Yunis EJ (1979) DRw antisera react with activated T cells. J Immunol 122:1780–1784
9. Effros RB, Dillard L, Zeller E, Naeim F, Walford RL (1983) Strong HLA-DR expression in T cell cultures after activation is necessary for IL-2-dependent proliferation. Hum Immunol 8:249–254
10. Engleman EG, Benike CJ, Charron DJ (1980) Ia antigen on peripheral blood mononuclear leukocytes in man. II. Functional studies of HLA-DR positive T cells activated in mixed lymphocyte reactions. J Exp Med 152:114s
11. Engleman EG, Benike CJ, Grumet C, Evans RL (1981) Activation of human T lymphocytes subsets: helper and suppressor/cytotoxic cells recognize and respond to distinct histocompatibility antigens. J Immunol 127:2124
12. Evans RL, Faldetta TL, Hymphreys RE, Pratt DM, Yunis EJ, Schlossman SF (1978) Peripheral human T cells sensitized in mixed lymphocyte culture synthesize and express Ia-like antigens. J Exp Med 148:1440
13. Fu SM, Chiorazzi N, Wang GY, Moutazeri G, Kunkel HG, Ko HS, Gottlieb AB (1978) Ia-bearing T lymphocytes in man. Their identification and role in the generation of allogenic helper activity. J Exp Med 148:1423

14. Indiveri F, Wilson BS, Russo C, Quaranta V, Pellegrino MA, Ferrone S (1980) Ia-like antigens on human T lymphocytes: relationship to other surface markers, role in mixed lymphocyte reactions and structural profile. J Immuno. 125:2673–2678
15. Ko HS, Fu SM, Winchester RJ, Yu DTY, Kunkel HG (1979) Ia determinants on stimulated human T lymphocytes. Occurrence on mitogen and antigen-activated T cells. J Exp Med 150:246
16. Marti GE, Nadler LM, Chused TM, Tosato G, Blease RM, Knidt TJ (1985) Cellular distribution of a human I-A like (DS/DC) antigen on normal and neoplastic lymphoid cells. Hum Immunol 12:35
17. Martin PJ, Giblett ER, Hansen JA (1982) Phenotyping human leukemic T-cell lines: enzyme markers, surface antigens, and cytogenetics. Immunogenetics 15:385
18. Moretta A, Acolla RS, Cerottini JC (1982) IL-2 mediated cell proliferation in humans is blocked by monoclonal antibody directed against monomorphic determinants of HLA-DR antigens. J Exp Med 155:599
19. Mudawwar FB, Yunis EJ, Geha RS (1978) Antigen-specific helper factor in man. J Exp Med 148:1032–1043
20. Nadler LM, Stashenko P, Hardy R, Tomaselli KJ, Yunis EJ, Schlossman SF, Pesando JM (1981) Monoclonal antibody identifies a new Ia-like (p29,34) polymorphic system linked to the HLA-D/DR region. Nature 290:591–593
21. Nagy ZA, Elliott BE, Nabholz M, Krammer FH, Pernis B (1976) Specific binding of alloantigens to T cells activated in the mixed lymphocyte reaction. J Exp Med 143:648
22. Natali PG, Russo C, Ng AK, Nicotra MR, Apollonj C, Pellegrino MA, Ferrone S (1982) Ontogeny of human Ia antigens. Cell Immunol 73:385–396
23. Natali PG, Segatto O, Ferrone S, Tosi R, Corte G (1984) Differential tissue distribution and ontogeny of DC1 and HLA-DR antigens. Immunogenetics 19:109–116
24. Newman RA, Domenico D, Greaves MF, Navarrete C, Fainboim L, Festenstein H (1983) Differential expression of HLA-DR and DR-linked determinants on human leukemias and lymphoid cells. Eur J Immunol 13:172–176
25. Pawelec G, Kahle P, Wernet P (1982) Specificity spectrum and cell surface markers of mono- and multifunctional mixed leukocyte culture-derived T cell clones in man. Eur J Immunol 12:607
26. Pawelec G, Blaurock M, Schneider EM, Shaw S, Wernet P (1982) Alloactivated long-term cultured human T lymphocytes express both HLA-DR and SB antigens but lack lymphocyte stimulation capacity. Eur J Immunol 12:967
27. Qvidstad E, Bosnes V, Thorsby E, Gaudernack G (1985) HLA class II cell surface antigens on T lymphocyte clones (abstract). Hum Immunol 12:109
28. Reinherz EL, Kung PC, Pesando JR, Ritz J, Goldstein C, Schlossman SF (1979) Ia determinants on human T-cell subsets defined by monoclonal antibody. Activation stimuli required for expression. J Exp Med 150:1472–1482
29. Reinherz EL, Morimoto C, Penta AC, Schlossman SF (1981) Subpopulations of the T4+ inducer T cell subset in man: evidence for an amplifier population preferentially expressing Ia antigen upon activation. J Immunol 126:67–70
30. Rouse RV, Parham P, Grumet FC, Weissman IL (1982) Expression of HLA antigens by human thymic epithelial cells. Hum Immunol 5:21–34
31. Sasportes M, Wollman EE, Cohen D, Carosella E, Bensussan A, Fradelizi D, Dausset J (1980) Suppression of the human allogeneic response in vitro with primed lymphocytes and suppressive supernates. J Exp Med 152:270s
32. Schuurman RKB, Gelfand EW, Matheson D, Zimmerman B, Dosch HM (1980) Identification of Ia on a subpopulation of human T lymphocytes that stimulate in a mixed lymphocyte reaction. J Immunol 124:1924–1928
33. Suciu-Foca N, Susinno E, McKiernan P, Rohowsky C, Wiener J, Rubinstein (1978) DRW determinants on human T cells primed against allogeneic lymphocytes. Transplant Proc 10:845
34. Suciu-Foca N, Khan R, Hardy M, Godfrey M, Susinno E, Reed E, Woodward K, Reemtsma K (1981 a) Expression of HLA-D and DR gene products on in vitro and in vivo primed human T cells. Transplant Proc 13:1020
35. Suciu-Foca N, Rohowsky C, Coburn C, Reed E, Khan R, Lewison A (1981 b) Alloreactive T cells. Expression of HLA-D antigens, stimulation of autologous MLR, and possible immunoregulatory function. Hum Immunol 3:301–312

36. Tada T (1984) Help, suppression, and specific factors. In: Paul W (ed) Fundamental immunology. Raven, New York, pp 481–517
37. WHO-HLA Nomenclature Committee (1985) Nomenclature for factors of the HLA system 1984. Vox Sang 49:42–49
38. Winchester RJ, Kunkel (1979) The human Ia system. Adv Immunol 28:221–292
39. Wollman EE, Cohen D, Fradelizi D, Sasportes M, Dausset J (1980) Different stimulating capacity of B and T lymphocytes in primary and secondary allogeneic reactions: cellular detection of HLA-D products on T lymphocytes. J Immunol 125:2039–2043
40. Yu DTY, McCune JM, Fu SM, Winchester RJ, Kunkel HG (1980) Two types of Ia-positive cells. Synthesis and exchange of Ia antigens. J Exp Med [Suppl] 52:895
41. Yunis EJ, Amos DB (1971) Three closely linked genetic systems relevant to transplantation. Proc Natl Acad Sci USA 68:3031

Class II MHC Antigens and Hematopoiesis *

V. C. Broudy, J. H. Fitchen

Table of Contents

* Supported by Veterans Administration research funds

Burst-Forming Unit–Erythroid (BFU-E): An immature erythroid progenitor which is relatively insensitive to erythropoientin and gives rise to multiple subcolonies or "bursts" of erythroid cells in vitro
Burst-Promoting Activity (BPA): A family of regulatory glycoproteins which stimulate the growth of BFU-E
Colony: A cell population derived from the proliferation of a single ancestral cell in vitro
Colony-Forming Unit–Granulocyte, Macrophage (CFU-GM): The committed progenitor cell which forms colonies of granulocytes and macrophages
Colony-Forming Unit–Erythroid (CFU-E): A relatively mature erythroid progenitor whose proliferation is absolutely dependent on erythropoietin
Colony-Forming Unit–Granulocyte, Erythrocyte, Macrophage, Megakaryocyte (CFU-GEMM): The progenitor which gives rise to mixed colonies containing granulocytes, erythrocytes, macrophages, and megakaryocytes
Colony-Stimulating Activity (CSA): A family of regulatory glycoproteins which stimulate the growth of CFU-GM
Committed Progenitor Cell: An immature hematopoietic cell with limited self-replicative capacity which is committed to a single line of differentiation
Stem Cell: A primitive hematopoietic cell capable of both self-renewal and differential into committed progenitor cells

The Hematopoietic Hierarchy

Pluripotent hematopoietic stem cells have an extensive capacity for both self-renewal and for differentiation into progenitor cells committed to a single line of differentiation (Fig. 1) [1]. These committed progenitor cells have a limited capac-

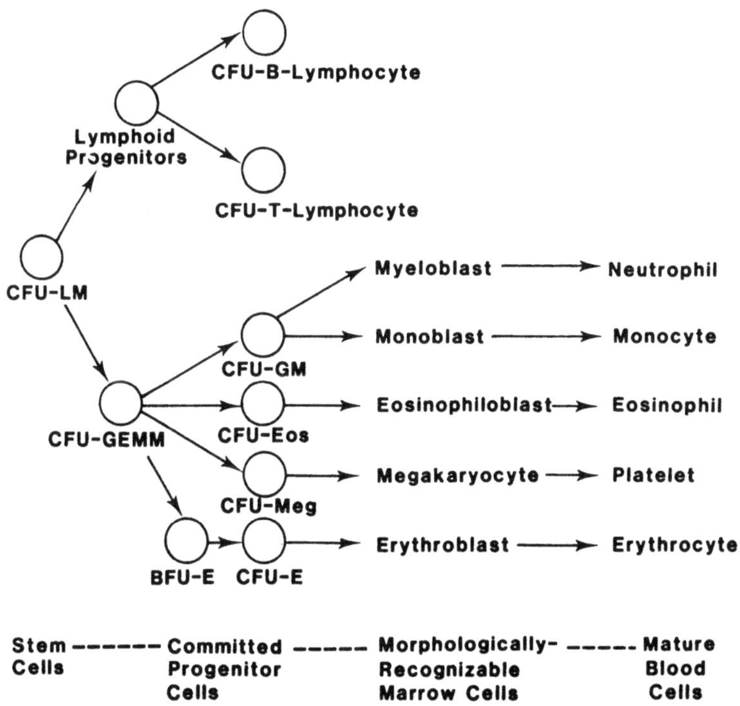

Fig. 1. A model of hematopoiesis

ity for self-renewal, and give rise to the mature cellular constituents of the peripheral blood (leukocytes, erythrocytes, and platelets). Progenitor cells comprise only a small portion (less than 0.1%) of the marrow cells [2]. They are not morphologically recognizable, but can be detected by their ability to form colonies of mature cells in semisolid media in vitro.

There is no direct assay for the pluripotent hematopoietic stem cell in man; its existence is inferred from studies of patients with chronic myelogenous leukemia, polycythemia vera, and sideroblastic anemia. The Philadelphia (Ph-1) chromosome, a balanced translocation between chromosomes 9 and 22, is found in cells of the granulocytic, monocytic, megakaryocytic, and erythroid lineage in patients with chronic myelogeneous leukemia [3, 4]. Polycythemia vera patients with glucose-6-phosphate dehydrogenase (G6PD) mosaicism express only one G6PD isoenzyme in granulocytes, platelets, and erythrocytes; skin fibroblasts and lymphocytes contain both isoenzymes [5]. These observations argue for the existence of a hematopoietic progenitor cell common to the granulocytic, erythroid, monocytic, and megakaryocytic lines which is illustrated in Fig. 1 as the CFU-GEMM. An in vitro assay for the CFU-GEMM has been described [6]. A study of the distribution of G6PD isoenzymes in a heterozygous patient with sideroblastic anemia demonstrates the existence of a primitive pluripotent stem cell common to myeloid and B and T lymphoid lines which is illustrated in Fig. 1 as the CFU-LM [7].

Control of Hematopoiesis

In the human bone marrow, granulopoiesis and erythropoiesis are tightly regulated to maintain peripheral blood counts within a narrow range despite the production of large numbers of mature cells (approximately 10^{11} granulocytes and 2×10^{11} erythrocytes per day). The marrow can also respond briskly and specifically to demands for increased production: bacterial infections lead to a prompt increase in granulopoiesis, and hemolysis produces erythroid hyperplasia.

Hematopoiesis is probably controlled at several levels in the hematopoietic hierarchy. The most primitive stem cells can undergo either self-renewal or commitment to differentiation along various lineages [8]. More mature committed progenitor cells respond to lineage-specific humoral regulators such as colony-stimulating activity or erythropoietin. Other levels of control include regulation of the size of the mitotic pool and the rate of release of mature cells from the marrow.

Models of Stem Cell Committment to Differentiation

Several models of stem cell renewal and committment have been proposed. In the stochastic model [9, 10] self-renewal or commitment occur at random governed by the laws of probability. Potential for each lineage is lost progressively and stochastically during differentiation. Support for this hypothesis comes from studies of single-cell blast colonies which contain variable combinations of cells committed to different lineages [11]. Other theories of stem cell differentiation include the hematopoietic inductive microenvironment model, in which the immediate surroundings of individual stem cells influence commitment [12], and the stem cell competition model in which humoral factors such as CSA and erythropoietin competitively direct stem cell committment [13].

Soluble Regulators of Granulopoiesis and Erythropoiesis

Granulopoiesis in vitro is regulated by a family of glycoproteins known as colony-stimulating activity (CSA) [14]. Sources of CSA include monocytes [15], activated T lymphocytes [16, 17], fibroblasts [18], endothelial cells [19, 20], and marrow stromal cells [21, 22]. There may be different classes of CSA which preferentially stimulate the growth of macrophage colonies [23, 24], granulocytic colonies [24], and eosinophilic colonies [25]. The gene for GM-CSA, a granulopoietic growth factor which stimulates the proliferation of mixed granulocyte-macrophage colonies, has been cloned and sequenced [26].

The growth of primitive erythroid precursors (burst-forming units–erythroid; BFU-E) in vitro is relatively independent of erythropoietin and requires a regulatory glycoprotein called burst-promoting activity (BPA) [27, 28]. BFU-E form large multi-unit clusters in methylcellulose [29] or plasma clot [30] cultures. A number of different cell types can produce BPA, including monocytes [31, 32], T lymphocytes [33], marrow stromal cells [34], and endothelial cells [35]. Recent evidence suggests that interleukin-3 (IL-3) contains burst-promoting activity. The gene for IL-3 has been cloned and sequenced [36].

The more mature erythropoietic cells, colony forming unit-erythroid (CFU-E) have an absolute requirement for erythropoietin for growth [37]. CFU-E form colonies containing 8-32 hemoglobinized cells in methylcellulose or plasma clot cultures [38].

Cell-Cell Interactions in the Regulation of Granulopoiesis and Erythropoiesis

Soluble factors produced by monocytes have been implicated in the regulation of granulopoiesis. Monocyte-derived recruiting activity (MRA) stimulates T lymphocytes, fibroblasts, endothelial cells, and marrow stromal cells to release CSA [17, 18, 20, 29]. Lactoferrin, a product of mature granulocytes and a putative feedback regulator of granulopoiesis [40, 41] inhibits production of MRA [17]. Bacterial endotoxin stimulates direct production of CSA by monocytes, and has an even greater effect on MRA production [35]. Thus, monocytes release an activity which stimulates auxiliary cells to produce CSA, and monokine production is inhibited by lactoferrin and stimulated by endotoxin.

A number of inhibitors of granulopoiesis in vitro have been identified. Prostaglandins of the E series inhibit the growth of CFU-GM [42–44]. Bone marrow cells of patients with acute leukemia produce leukemia-associated inhibitory activity (LIA) which inhibits growth of normal CFU-GM [45]. LIA and acidic isoferritins share several characteristics (both are inhibitory to CFU-GM at low concentrations, are proteins of similar molecular weight, and LIA is blocked by antibody to acidic isoferritin) and may be identical [46]. Normal monocytes constitutively produce acidic isoferritins which may function as physiologic regulators of granulopoiesis [47], although this has been questioned by some investigators [48]. T lymphocytes modulate monocyte release of acidic isoferritins: OKT8-positive lymphocytes inhibit while OKT4-positive lymphocytes stimulate acidic isoferritin production [49].

The relative importance of T lymphocytes and monocytes in the control of erythropoiesis is controversial [50]. Some investigators argue that T lymphocytes play a critical role in erythropoiesis [33, 51], while others suggest that they are not involved [52]. Still other studies suggest that monocyte concentration may be critical [53], and that small numbers of monocytes (as few as 10^4 cells per plasma clot) may stimulate BFU-E growth [32]. Coculture experiments suggest that interactions between monocytes and T lymphocytes result in increased BFU-E growth [54, 55]. A problem with all of these studies is the heterogeneity of target cell populations in which BFU-E represent only a small fraction of the cells. Cultures of single, isolated BFU-E have shown that both a monocytoid cell line and a T cell line can directly produce BPA and stimulate BFU-E growth [56].

Endothelial cells, when stimulated by monokines, produce BPA [57]. Normal human bone marrow microenvironmental cells also produce BPA when stimulated by monokines [39]. Thus, a variety of auxiliary cells have been implicated in the regulation of erythropoiesis in vitro, but the relative importance of each and the manner in which they interact remain to be determined.

Prostaglandin E, a product of monocytes, has been shown to stimulate growth and differentiation of BFU-E [58–60] while acidic isoferritins, also a normal monocyte product, exert a suppressive effect on erythropoiesis in vitro [49].

Expression of Class II MHC Antigens on Hematopoietic Progenitor Cells

The surface antigenic structure of hematopoietic cells changes during the course of differentiation [61]. Some antigens are present on early progenitors and lost with maturation, while others are expressed with differentiation [62]. Study of the representation of cell surface antigens on progenitor cells may result in a better understanding of the process of cell differentiation and the function of specific surface antigens. This knowledge can aid the identification of cells and cell lineages, the classification of hematologic neoplasia, and, potentially, the diagnosis and treatment of hematologic diseases.

Two major methods have been used to investigate the cellular distribution of class II MHC antigens: complement-mediated cytotoxicity and cell sorting [63]. For the cytotoxicity assay, cells are incubated with monoclonal antibody or heteroantiserum, treated with complement, and cultured to detect surviving progenitor cells by their ability to form colonies. Cytotoxicity testing has several limitations: (1) failure of complement-mediated killing of progenitor cells may reflect inefficient complement fixing by antibody, resistance of progenitors to complement lysis, or low antigen density [64]; (2) alterations in colony growth seen with complement-mediated cytotoxicity may reflect elimination of important auxiliary cells (e.g., monocytes, T lymphocytes) rather than hematopoietic progenitors; (3) not all monoclonal antibodies activate complement (although this problem can be circumvented by use of an antiglobulin assay [65]); and (4) antigen density cannot be quantitated by this method.

In the cell sorting method, cells are treated with monoclonal antibody then with a fluorescein-conjugated second antibody. Fluorescence-positive and -negative fractions are then separated on a fluorescence-activated cell sorter (FACS) and cultured to detect progenitor cells. Problems with this approach include (1) the somewhat arbitrary distinction between positive and negative subsets, (2) the limited number of cells which can be sorted per unit of time, and (3) the question of whether increased colony growth in one fraction is due to sorting of critical auxiliary cells into that fraction.

Expression on Pluripotent Stem Cells

Little is known about the antigenic status of the human pluripotent stem cell because of the lack of an in vitro assay for this cell. Moore et al. used a two-layer continuous bone marrow culture method to show that a multipotent stem cell does not express Ia antigens [66]. Methodologic problems, including the use of a nonirradiated stromal layer which could have harbored progenitor cells, prevent strong conclusions from being drawn from this study. Indeed, Andrews et al. [67] have recently reported that when the adherent layer is irradiated (to insure that stem cell proliferation takes place only in the antibody-treated nonadherent layer), regeneration of CFU-GM does not occur if the nonadherent cells are treated with anti-DR monoclonal antibody and complement. However, in another study, long-term human bone marrow cultures, modified for optimal growth without the need for a pre-established adherent layer [68], showed comparable cumulative CFU-GM and BFU-E growth after 5 weeks whether or not marrow cells were treated with anti-Ia monoclonal antibodies and complement [69]. Since all of these studies have necessarily relied upon indirect observations, the expression of class II antigens by human pluripotent hematopoietic stem cells has yet to be conclusively demonstrated.

Expression on CFU-GEMM

The human multipotent progenitor cell (CFU-GEMM) has been shown to express DR antigens using both complement-dependent cytotoxicity and cell sorting techniques [70–72]. Studies using human alloantisera directed against DQ (formerly MB, DS/DC) did not reveal the DQ antigen on CFU-GEMM [72].

In one study it was concluded that Ia antigens were detectable on CFU-GEMM during the S-phase of the cell cycle, but not on noncycling CFU-GEMM [73]. This conclusion was based on tritiated thymidine suicide and cytotoxicity studies. Depletion of S-phase CFU-GEMM by high specific-activity tritiated thymidine removed all CFU-GEMM sensitive to complement-mediated cytotoxicity with an anti-Ia monoclonal antibody (NEI-011). Initial treatment with NEI-011 and complement resulted in no further inhibition when the cells were subsequently exposed to tritiated thymidine.

Expression on CFU-GM

There is strong experimental evidence that human CFU-GM express DR antigens [64, 72, 74–76]. Monoclonal antibodies recognizing DR framework determinants caused greater than 90% inhibition of CFU-GM growth from normal human bone marrow in conjunction with complement [74]. In this study, peripheral blood mononuclear cells were added to the anti-DR-treated marrow prior to culture to exclude the possibility that the decrement in CFU-GM growth was due to elimination of critical auxiliary cells. The presence of DR antigens on a high portion of CFU-GM has been confirmed by cell sorting studies [64, 72]. In earlier studies employing indirect immunofluorescence, it has been shown that myeloblasts and promyelocytes, but not their more mature progeny, are stained by anti-Ia heteroantisera [77].

Conflicting data suggesting that only about 50% of CFU-GM are DR positive have been presented by one group [78, 79], while others using the same monoclonal antibody (New England Nuclear NEI-011, derived from clone 7.2 from Drs. Hansen and Torok-Storb) have found virtually 100% inhibition of CFU-GM growth using complement-mediated cytotoxicity [80]. The discordant findings are probably related to the use of complement-dependent cytotoxicity, different dilutions of monoclonal antibody and the fact that CFU-GM are apparently heterogeneous in DR antigen density. We have recently reported studies showing that the dilutions of complement and antibody are important factors in CFU-GM cytotoxicity assays [65]. Moreover, we have found considerable heterogeneity in DR antigen density on CFU-GM [81]. When marrow cells were incubated with the anti-DR monoclonal antibody OKIa1 and sorted into fractions of negative, low, medium, and high fluorescence intensity, these fractions contained 4%, 17%, 23%, and 56% of the CFU-GM respectively.

Pelus [78] and Broxmeyer [82] have reported that CFU-GM lose DR antigens after as little as 3–6 h in suspension culture. They used cytotoxicity testing and found that CFU-GM were no longer killed by anti-DR monoclonal antibody NEI-011 after maintenance in suspension culture. We have found that complement sensitivity of CFU-GM increases after suspension culture and therefore used cell sorting to analyze the expression of DR antigens on CFU-GM that had been maintained in suspension culture for 24 h. With each of three monoclonal antibodies against framework determinants of DR antigens (OKIa-1, Q5/13, and Q2/80) we found no change in DR antigen density on normal CFU-GM [81]. Our results are in agreement with the findings of Cannistra et al. [83] who detected no loss of DR antigens on partially purified CFU-GM after 6 or 18 h incubation.

Both cell sorting and cytotoxicity studies have shown that human CFU-GM lack DQ (DS/DC, MB) antigens [61, 64, 72]. Linch et al. showed that approximately 40% of CFU-GM are DP (SB)-positive [64].

Expression on BFU-E and CFU-E

The majority of immature erythroid progenitor cells (BFU-E) are DR-positive [62, 64, 71, 72]. Approximately 50% of BFU-E express DP (SB) antigens, but DQ (DC) antigens have not been detected on these cells [61, 64].

Winchester et al. [77] reported that colony formation by both CFU-E and BFU-E is inhibited by heteroantisera to Ia antigens in conjunction with complement. We also observed complement-dependent inhibition of BFU-E and CFU-E-derived colony formation by anti-Ia heteroantiserum, but found no effect on these progenitors with monoclonal antibody against DR antigens, even though the monoclonal antibody potently inhibited CFU-GM [84]. On the other hand, Robinson et al. [62], using non-cytotoxic monoclonal antibodies against Ia antigens and FACS found that a proportion of BFU-E segregated to the fluorescence-positive fraction, while CFU-E did not. Recently, Linch et al. [64] reported that DR antigens are detectable on BFU-E and CFU-E, but that CFU-E are less susceptible to complement-mediated lysis at suboptimal complement concentrations. The contrasting results of experiments involving heteroantisera instead of monoclonal antibodies and using cytotoxicity rather than cell sorting are probably due to technical differences among the various studies. The most convincing data suggest that very primitive erythroid progenitors express DR antigens and that these antigens are lost or decrease substantially in association with differentiation from BFU-E to CFU-E.

Expression on Hematopoietic Cells in Chronic Granulocytic Leukemia

There is dispute regarding the class II antigenic profile of CFU-GM in chronic granulocytic leukemia (CGL). One group has reported that CFU-GM from many patients with CGL are not killed by anti-DR monoclonal antibody and complement, suggesting that they lack DR antigens [78, 82]. Other investigators have found that CFU-GM from normals and patients with CGL are equally sensitive to lysis by anti-DR monoclonal antibody and complement [85, 86]. The divergent results may be explained by our recent findings using gated cell sorting, which suggest that DR antigens are present but decreased on CFU-GM from patients with CGL [87]. Bone marrow cells from five patients with CGL were treated with anti-DR monoclonal antibody Q5/13 and fluorescent second antibody and then sorted into fractions of negative, low, medium, and high fluorescence intensity. In contrast to normals, the majority of marrow CFU-GM from four of the five CGL patients segregated to the negative and low fluorescence fractions (Table 1). The fifth patient showed a bimodal distribution. Particularly interesting were the results with marrow cells from a patient with Ph1-chromosome-negative CGL who underwent a bone marrow transplant from his HLA-identical, MLC-nonreactive brother. Before the transplant, DR antigens could not be detected by cell sorting on 95% of the patient's marrow CFU-GM. When he was re-studied 4 months post-transplant, DR antigens were found on 99% of his marrow CFU-GM, which distributed evenly in the low, medium, and high fluorescence fractions.

Our results contrast with the findings of Cannistra et al. [83], who studied HLA-DR antigen expression on partially-purified CFU-GM from the peripheral blood of patients with CGL. They found that 55%–84% of the CFU-GM expressed monomorphic determinants of DR antigens. Quantitative analysis indi-

Table 1. DR antigen density on bone marrow CFU-GM from patients with CGL

Patient	Ph1 chromosome	% DR+ CFU-GM by cytotoxicity	% CFU-GM recovered in fluorescence fraction			
			Neg	Low	Med	High
H. B.	+	97	10	53	29	8
M. S.	+	48	8	83	8	0
J. V.	+	97	32	57	4	7
M. C.	+	100	1	39	4	56
J. S. (pre-BMT)	–	87	95	5	0	0
J. S. (post-BMT)	–	94	1	30	28	33
Normals ($n=3$)		93 ± 3	2 ± 1	9 ± 2	21 ± 6	68 ± 9

All tests were performed with monoclonal antibody Q5/13 at a dilution of 1:20. BMT, bone marrow transplant cated that DR antigen density on peripheral blood CGL CFU-GM was equivalent to normal monocytes. There are several possible explanations for the apparent discrepancy between the results. First, different anti-DR monoclonal antibodies were employed in the two studies. Second, we compared DR antigen density on CGL CFU-GM and normal CFU-GM, whereas Cannistra et al. compared DR antigen density on CGL CFU-GM and normal monocytes. Finally, we analyzed bone marrow CFU-GM, whereas Cannistra et al. studied peripheral blood CFU-GM. Indeed, Ferrero et al. [88] have presented evidence suggesting that peripheral blood and bone marrow CFU-GM differ antigenically and may have a parent-progeny relationship. Clarification of the DR antigen status of CFU-GM in CGL must await direct comparison of antigen density on peripheral blood and bone marrow progenitors from individual patients.

Expression on Hematopoietic Cells in Polycythemia Vera

Expression of Ia antigens on erythroid progenitors from 11 patients with polycythemia vera has been analyzed [89]. Endogenous growth (i.e., growth without added erythropoietin, a chracteristic of the neoplastic clone) of peripheral blood BFU-E and CFU-E was entirely abrogated by treatment with anti-DR monoclonal antibody 7.2 and complement. Growth of marrow-derived CFU-E was also reduced by more than 90% in the cytotoxicity assay. These data suggest that DR antigens persist to the CFU-E stage in polycythemia vera, whereas they are apparently lost coincident with differentiation from BFU-E to CFU-E in normals [90].

Class II Antigens and Hematopoietic Regulation

Class II Antigens and Prostaglandin E

Prostaglandin E (PGE) has been implicated in the regulation of granulopoiesis and erythropoiesis. Addition of PGE at concentrations of 10^{-6}–10^{-9} M to cultured marrow cells inhibits proliferation of CFU-GM and enhances growth of BFU-E in a dose-dependent fashion [43, 44, 60, 91]. An inhibitory effect on CFU-GM has also been noted with in vivo administration of PGE [92].

One group has reported that PGE preferentially inhibits colony formation by DR-positive CFU-GM. However, a differential effect of PGE on DR-positive and DR-negative CFU-GM depends on the existence of the two populations of progenitors, one with and the other without DR antigens. Since it has been widely reported that nearly all CFU-GM are DR-positive, a differential effect of PGE on DR-positive and DR-negative CFU-GM seems implausible. It is possible, however, that PGE-mediated inhibition of CFU-GM is a function of DR antigen density rather than absolute presence or absence of antigens. We have used two approaches to explore this possibility. First, we used cytotoxicity and suboptimal concentrations of anti-DR monoclonal antibody to kill approximately 50% of the CFU-GM, then exposed the surviving progenitor cells to PGE. Second, we used gated cell sorting to obtain CFU-GM of varying DR antigen density and cultured these cells in the presence or absence of PGE. With neither method were

Table 2. PGE-mediated inhibition of bone marrow CFU-GM from normals and patients with CGL

Bone marrow source	*n*	% CFU-GM inhibition (±SE) at PGE log molar concentration						
		−5	−6	−7	−8	−9	−10	−11
Normals	3	56±6	38±3	30±3	22±3	20±4	9±2	5±1
CGL patients	3	90±6	42±2	19±5	9±2	4±1	2±2	0

we able to demonstrate a relationship between PGE-mediated inhibition and the expression or density of DR antigens on CFU-GM [81]. Possible explanations for the divergent results include the use of different anti-DR monoclonal antibodies and the use of different sources of CSA which could conceivably contain small amounts of PGE (not excluded in either study) or stimulate different subsets of CFU-GM.

Pelus et al. analyzed the antigenic profile of CFU-GM from patients with CGL and found both markedly decreased DR antigen expression and decreased responsiveness to inhibition by PGE [79, 93]. When preincubated in suspension culture with PGE, CFU-GM reexpressed DR antigens and regained sensitivity to the inhibitory effects of PGE. We have detected decreased DR antigen density on CFU-GM from patients with CGL using gated cell sorting (see Table 1), but no correlation between DR antigen density and inhibition by PGE [87, 94]. We also tested the effect of a range of concentrations of PGE on unsorted CFU-GM from normals and patients with CGL. We found that CGL CFU-GM were more sensitive than normal CFU-GM at high PGE concentrations, but less sensitive than normal CFU-GM at low PGE concentrations (Table 2). That is, the dose-inhibition relationship is steeper for CGL CFU-GM than for normal progenitors.

Class II Antigens and Acidic Isoferritins

Acidic isoferritins, a normal monocyte product, suppress the growth of CFU-GM, BFU-E, and CFU-GEMM. This inhibitory effect is reportedly limited to DR-positive progenitors in the S-phase of the cell cycle [47, 73, 82]. Depletion of DR-positive progenitors by cytotoxicity (monoclonal antibody NEI-011) or tritiated thymidine suicide renders the surviving progenitors insensitive to the inhibitory effects of acidic isoferritins. In addition, culture conditions which resulted in loss of DR antigens were associated with loss of sensitivity to acidic isoferritins.

The release of acidic isoferritins from monocytes is modulated by T lymphocytes, and this interaction is reportedly HLA-DR-restricted [49]. Depletion of DR-positive monocytes or T lymphocytes by complement-dependent cytotoxicity prevents both constitutive release of acidic isoferritins by monocytes and T lymphocyte modulation of this release. These effects are seen only with autologous cells or cells from HLA-DR-matched donors. Thus, the production of acidic isoferritins, factors with potential relevance to the regulation of both normal and leukemic myelopoiesis, may be controlled by an HLA-DR-restricted interaction of T lymphocytes and monocytes.

Effect of DR-Positive and DR-Negative T Lymphocytes on Erythropoiesis

Normal peripheral blood T lymphocytes contain at least two functionally distinct populations with opposing effects on erythropoiesis: a DR-positive population which inhibits erythropoiesis, and a DR-negative population which stimulates erythropoiesis [90, 95]. Depletion of DR-positive T lymphocytes by cytotoxicity (monoclonal antibody 7.2) resulted in increased growth of peripheral blood BFU-E. The stimulatory effect of the DR-negative T lymphocyes was seen only when monocytes were present and the cells shared at least one DR haplotype [90]. Further support for the finding that modulation of BFU-E growth by DR-positive T lymphocytes is DR restricted is provided by the study of a patient with a T cell lymphoproliferative syndrome and pure red cell aplasia [96]. Peripheral blood T8-positive, DR-positive T lymphocytes from this patient were found to suppress growth of autologous BFU-E and CFU-E. Erythroid colony growth of cells from two HLA-identical siblings and two unrelated but DR-identical donors was also suppressed: colony growth of cells from two HLA-mismatched individuals was unaffected. These observations suggest that DR-positive and DR-negative T cell populations may modulate erythropoiesis, and that these interactions are limited to cells of a similar DR haplotype.

Summary

That class II MHC antigens are expressed on hematopoietic progenitor cells has been clearly established, but *why* they are expressed on these cells and *how* they are involved in hematopoiesis has not been clearly defined. Does the expression or density of class II antigens on the surface of hematopoietic progenitor cells affect their responsiveness to hematopoietic regulatory factors? Are class II antigens involved in hematopoietic cellular interactions analogous to those which occur in the immune system? Are class II antigens altered in myeloproliferative disorders in such a way that hematopoietic regulation breaks down? Can the expression of class II antigens be modified in the myeloproliferative disorders so that normal regulation is restored?

The answers to these questions are currently unknown, but several lines of circumstantial evidence suggest that class II MHC antigens will prove to be of importance in hematopoietic regulation. First, class II antigens are known to play a regulatory role in the generation of the immune response, and the lymphoid/immune system is closely related to the hematopoietic system (they share a common stem cell, the interacting cell types are similar in the two systems, and they both participate in the defense against infection). Second, class II antigens are restricted in tissue distribution and have been demonstrated principally on cells involved in the generation of the immune response and on hematopoietic progenitor cells. Third, as we have discussed, recent observations suggest that certain hematopoietic cellular interactions may be class II-restricted.

References

1. Quesenberry P, Levitt L (1979) Hematopoietic stem cells. N Engl J Med 301:755, 819, 868
2. Lord BI (1983) Hematopoietic stem cells. In: Potten CS (ed) Stem cells. Their identification and characterization. Churchill Livingstone, New York, p 118
3. Whang J, Frei E, Tjio JH, Carbone PJ, Brecher G (1983) The distribution of the Philadelphia chromosome in patients with chronic myelogenous leukemia. Blood 22:664
4. Golde DW, Burgaleta C, Sparkes RS, Cline MJ (1977) The Philadelphia chromosome in human macrophages. Blood 49:367
5. Adamson JW, Fialkow PJ, Murphy S, Prchal JF, Steinmann L (1976) Polycythemia vera: stem and probable clonal origin of the disease. N Engl J Med 295:913
6. Fauser AA, Messner HA (1979) Identification of megakaryocytes, macrophages, and eosinophils in colonies of human bone marrow containing neutrophilic granulocytes and erythroblasts. Blood 53:1023
7. Prchal JT, Throckmorton DW, Carroll AJ, Fuson EW, Gams RA, Prchal JF (1978) A common progenitor for human myeloid and lymphoid cells. Nature 274:590
8. Ogawa M, Porter PN, Nakahata T (1983) Renewal and commitment to differentiation of hematopoietic stem cells. Blood 61:823
9. Till JE, McCulloch EA, Siminovitch L (1964) A stochastic model of stem cell proliferation, based on the growth of spleen-colony forming cells. Proc Natl Acad Sci USA 51:29
10. McCulloch EA (1983) Stem cells in normal and leukemic hematopoiesis. Blood 62:1
11. Suda T, Suda J, Ogawa M (1983) Single-cell origin of mouse hematopoietic colonies expressing multiple lineages in variable combinations. Proc Natl Acad Sci USA 80:6689
12. Curry JL, Trentin JJ (1967) Hematopoietic spleen colony studies: I. Growth and differentiation. Dev Biol 15:395
13. VanZant G, Goldwasser E (1979) Competition between erythropoietin and colony-stimulating factor for target cells in mouse marrow. Blood 53:946
14. Burgess AW, Metcalf D (1980) The nature and action of granulocyte-macrophage colony stimulating factors. Blood 56:947
15. Golde DW, Cline MJ (1972) Identification of the colony-stimulating cell in human peripheral blood. J Clin Invest 51:2981
16. Ruscetti FW, Chervenick PA (1975) Release of colony-stimulating activity from thymus-derived lymphocytes. J Clin Invest 55:520
17. Bagby GC, Rigas VD, Bennett RM, Vandenbark AA, Garewal HS (1981) Interaction of lactoferrin, monocytes, and T lymphocyte subsets in the regulation of steady-state granulopoiesis in vitro. J Clin Invest 68:56
18. Bagby GC, McCall E, Layman DL (1983) Regulation of colony-stimulating activity production. Interactions of fibroblasts, mononuclear phagocytes, and lactoferrin. J Clin Invest 71:340
19. Quesenberry PT, Gimbrone MA (1980) Vascular endothelium as a regulator of granulopoiesis: production of colony-stimulating activity by cultured human endothelial cells. Blood 56:1060
20. Bagby GC, McCall E, Bergstrom KA, Burger D (1983) A monokine regulates colony-stimulating activity production by vascular endothelial cells. Blood 62:663
21. Harigaya K, Cronkite EP, Miller ME, Shadduck RK (1981) Murine bone marrow cell line producing colony-stimulating factor. Proc Natl Acad Sci USA 78:6963
22. Garnett HM, Cronkite EP, Harigaya K (1982) Regulation of the colony-stimulating activity produced by a murine marrow-derived cell line (H-1). Proc Natl Acad Sci USA 79:1545
23. Stanley ER, Heard PM (1977) Factors regulating macrophage production and growth. J Biol Chem 252:4305
24. Nicola NA, Metcalf D, Matsuomoto J, Johnson GR (1983) Purification of a factor inducing differentiation in murine myelomonocytic leukemia cells. J Biol Chem 258:9017
25. Griffin JD, Meuer SC, Schlossman SF, Reinherz EL (1984) T cell regulation of myelopoiesis: analysis at a clonal level. J Immunol 133:1863

26. Gough NM, Gough J, Metcalf D, Kelson A, Grail D, Nicola NA, Burgess AW, Dunn AR (1984) Molecular cloning of cDNA encoding a murine hematopoietic growth regulator, granulocyte-macrophage colony stimulating factor. Nature 309:763
27. Johnson GR, Metcalf D (1977) Pure and mixed erythroid colony formation in vitro stimulated by spleen conditioned medium with no detectable erythropoietin. Proc Natl Acad Sci USA 74:3879
28. Aye MT (1976) Erythroid colony formation in cultures of human marrow: effects of leukocyte conditioned medium. J Cell Physiol 91:69
29. Ogawa M, Parmley RT, Bank HL, Spicer SS (1976) Human marrow erythropoiesis in culture. I. Characterization of methylcellulose colony assay. Blood 48:407
30. Tepperman AD, Curtis JE, McCulloch EA (1974) Erythropoietic colonies in cultures of human marrow. Blood 44:659
31. Zuckerman KS (1980) Stimulation of human BFU-E by products of human monocytes and lymphocytes. Exp Hematol 8:924
32. Zuckerman KS (1981) Human erythroid burst-forming units. Growth in vitro is dependent on monocytes, but not T lymphocytes. J Clin Invest 67:702
33. Nathan DG, Chess L, Hillman DG, Clarke B, Breard J, Merler E, Housman DE (1978) Human erythroid burst-forming unit: T-cell requirement for proliferation in vitro. J Exp Med 147:324
34. Werts ED, DeGowin RL, Knapp SK, Gibson DP (1980) Characterization of marrow stromal (fibroblastoid) cells and their association with erythropoiesis. Exp Hematol 8:423
35. McCall E, Bagby GC (1985) Monocyte derived recruiting activity: kinetics of production and effects of endotoxin. Blood 65:689
36. Fung MC, Hapel AJ, Ymer S, Cohen DR, Johnson RM, Campbell HD, Young IG (1984) Molecular cloning of cDNA for murine interleukin-3. Nature 307:233
37. Gregory CJ (1976) Erythropoietin sensitivity as a differentiation marker in the hematopoietic system: studies of three erythropoietic colony responses in culture. J Cell Physiol 89:289
38. McLeod DL, Shreeve MM, Axelrad AA (1974) Improved plasma culture system for production of erythrocytic colonies in vitro: quantitative assay method for CFU-E. Blood 44:517
39. Broudy V, Zuckerman K, Jetmalani S, Fitchen J, Bagby GC (1984) The production of burst promoting activity (BPA) and colony stimulating activity (CSA) by adherent fibroblastoid marrow cells (F) is regulated by autologous monocytes. Clin Res 32:305A
40. Broxmeyer HE, Smithyman A, Eger RR, Myers RA, DeSousa M (1978) Identification of lactoferrin as the granulocyte-derived inhibitor of colony-stimulating activity production. J Exp Med 148:1052
41. Broxmeyer HE, DeSousa M, Smithyman A, Ralph P, Hamilton J, Kurland J, Bognacki J (1980) Specificity and modulation of the action of lactoferrin, a negative feedback regulator of myelopoiesis. Blood 55:324
42. Pelus LM, Broxmeyer HE, Kurland JI, Moore MAS (1979) Regulation of macrophage and granulocyte proliferation. Specificities of prostaglandin E and lactoferrin. J Exp Med 150:277
43. Taetle R, Koessler A (1980) Effects of cyclic nucleotides and prostaglandins in normal and abnormal human myeloid progenitor cell proliferation. Cancer Res 40:1223
44. Pelus LM, Broxmeyer HE, Moore MAS (1981) Regulation of human myelopoiesis by prostaglandin E and lactoferrin. Cell Tissue Kinet 14:515
45. Broxmeyer HE, Jacobsen N, Kurland J, Mendelsohn N, Moore MAS (1978) In vitro suppression of normal granulocytic stem cells by inhibitory activity derived from human leukemia cells. J Natl Cancer Inst 60:497
46. Broxmeyer HE, Bognacki J, Dorner MH, DeSousa M (1981) Identification of leukemia associated inhibitory activity as acidic isoferritins. J Exp Med 153:1426
47. Broxmeyer HE, Bognacki J, Ralph P, Dorner MH, Lu L, Castro-Malaspina H (1982) Monocyte-macrophage-derived acidic isoferritins: normal feed-back regulators of granulocyte-macrophage progenitor cells in vitro. Blood 60:595
48. Jacobs A (1983) Do acidic isoferritins regulate hematopoiesis? Br J Haematol 55:199

49. Broxmeyer HE, Juliano L, Lu L, Platzer E, Dupont B (1984) HLA-DR human histocompatibility leukocyte antigens-restricted lymphocyte-monocyte interactions in the release from monocytes of acidic isoferritins that suppress hematopoietic progenitor cells. J Clin Invest 73:939
50. Goodman JW, Goodman DR (1983) Involvement of cells of the immune system in regulation of erythropoiesis. In: Dunn CDR (ed) Current concepts in erythropoiesis. Wiley, Chichester, p 59
51. Mangan KF, Desforges JF (1980) The role of T lymphocytes and monocytes in the regulation of human erythropoietic peripheral blood burst forming units. Exp Haematol 8:717
52. Nomdedeu B, Gormus BT, Banisadre M, Rinehart JJ, Kaplan ME, Zanjani ED (1980) Human peripheral blood erythroid burst forming unit (BFU_E): evidence against T-lymphocyte requirement for proliferation in vitro. Exp Haematol 8:845
53. Gordon LI, Miller WJ, Branda RF, Zanjani ED, Jacob HS (1980) Regulation of erythroid colony formation by bone marrow macrophages. Blood 55:1047
54. Reid CDL, Baptista LC, Chanarin I (1981) Erythroid colony growth in vitro from human peripheral blood null cells: evidence for regulation by T-lymphocytes and monocytes. Br J Haematol 48:155
55. Clarke BJ, Harvey AR, Kaiser J, Leeds C (1984) Quantitative analysis of the role of accessory cells in the development of human blood BFU-E-derived erythroid colonies. Exp Haematol 12:259
56. Linch DC, Nathan DG (1984) T cell and monocyte-derived burst-promoting activity directly act on erythroid progenitor cells. Nature 312:775
57. Zuckerman KS, Bagby GC, McCall E, Sparks B, Wells J, Patel V, Goodrum D (1985) A monokine stimulates production of human erythroid burst-promoting activity by endothelial cells in vitro. J Clin Invest 75:722
58. Rossi GB, Mighiaccio AR, Mighiaccio G, Lettieri F, DiRosa M, Mastroherardino G, Peschle C (1980) In vitro interaction of PGE and CAMP with murine and human erythroid precursors. Blood 56:74
59. DeGowin RL, Gibson DP (1981) Prostaglandin-mediated enhancement of erythroid colonies by marrow stromal cells (MSC). Exp Haematol 9:274
60. Lu L, Pelus LM, Broxmeyer HE (1984) Modulation of the expression of HLA-DR (Ia) antigens and the proliferation of human erythroid (BFU-E) and multipotential (CFU-GEMM) progenitor cells by prostaglandin E. Exp Haematol 12:741
61. Sieff C, Bicknell D, Caine G, Robinson J, Lam G, Greaves MF (1982) Changes in cell surface antigen expression during hematopoietic differentiation. Blood 60:703
62. Robinson J, Sieff C, Delia D, Edwards PAW, Greaves M (1981) Expression of cell-surface HLA-DR, HLA-ABC and glycophorin during erythroid differentiation. Nature 289:68
63. Fitchen JH, Foon KA, Cline MJ (1981) The antigenic characteristics of hematopoietic stem cells. N Engl J Med 305:17
64. Linch DC, Nadler LM, Luther EA, Lipton JM (1984) Discordant expression of human Ia-like antigens on hematopoietic progenitor cells. J Immunol 132:2324
65. Fitchen JH, Russo C, Ferrone S (1984) Complement-dependent killing of human hematopoietic progenitor cells with noncomplement-fixing monoclonal antibodies in an antiglobulin assay. Blood 63:873
66. Moore MAS, Broxmeyer HE, Sheridan APC, Meyers PA, Jacobsen N, Winchester RJ (1980) Continuous human bone marrow culture: Ia antigen characterization of probable pluripotential stem cells. Blood 55:682
67. Andrews RG, Takahashi M, Segal G, Powell J, Bernstein ID, Singer JW (1984) Progenitors of CFU-GM in long term marrow culture (LTBMC) express the 4.1 (HLA-DR) but not the L4F3 antigen. Blood 64 (Suppl 1):110a
68. Gartner S, Kaplan HS (1980) Long-term culture of human bone marrow cells. Proc Natl Acad Sci USA 77:4756
69. Keating A, Powell J, Takahashi M, Singer JW (1984) The generation of human long-term marrow culture from marrow depleted of Ia (HLA-DR) positive cells. Blood 64:1159
70. Fitchen JH, LeFevre C, Ferrone S, Cline MJ (1982) Expression of Ia-like and HLA-A,B antigens on human multipotential hematopoietic progenitor cells. Blood 59:188

71. Bodger MP, Izaguirre CA, Blacklock HA, Hoffbrand AV (1983) Surface antigenic determinants on human pluripotent and unipotent hematopoietic progenitor cells. Blood 61:1006
72. Falkenburg JHF, Jansen J, van der Vaart-Duinkerken N, Veenhoff WFJ, Blotkamb J, Goselink HM, Parlevliet J, vanRood JJ (1984) Polymorphic and monomorphic HLA-DR determinants on human hematopoietic progenitor cells. Blood 63:1125
73. Lu L, Broxmeyer HE, Meyers PA, Moore MAS, Thaler HT (1983) Association of cell cycle expression of Ia-like antigenic determinants on normal human multipotential (CFU-GEMM) and erythroid (BFU-E) progenitor cells with regulation in vitro by acidic isoferritins. Blood 61:250
74. Fitchen JH, Ferrone S, Quaranta V, Molinaro GA, Cline MJ (1980) Monoclonal antibodies to HLA-A,B, and Ia-like antigens inhibit colony formation by human myeloid progenitor cells. J Immunol 125:2004
75. Levine MN, Fay JW, Jones NH, Metzgar RS, Haynes BF (1981) Phenotypic characterization of human bone marrow granulocyte-macrophage forming progenitor cells. Blood 58:1047
76. Greenberg P, Grossman M, Charron D, Levy R (1981) Characterization of antigenic determinants on human myeloid colony forming cells with monoclonal antibodies. Exp Haematol 9:781
77. Winchester RJ, Ross GD, Jarowski CI, Wang CY, Halper J, Broxmeyer HE (1977) Expression of Ia-like antigen molecules on human granulocytes during early phases of differentiation. Proc Natl Acad Sci USA 74:4012
78. Pelus LM (1982) Association between colony forming units-granulocyte macrophage expression of Ia-like (HLA-DR) antigens and control of granulocyte and macrophage production. A new role for prostaglandin E. J Clin Invest 70:568
79. Pelus LM, Saletan S, Silver R, Moore MAS (1982) Expression of Ia-antigens on normal and chronic myeloid leukemia human granulocyte-macrophage colony-forming cells (CFU-GM) is associated with regulation of cell proliferation by prostaglandin E. Blood 59:284
80. Torok-Storb B, Nepom GT, Nepom BS, Hansen JA (1983) HLA-DR antigens on lymphoid cells differ from those on myeloid cells. Nature 305:541
81. Fitchen JH, Burger DR (1983) Heterogeneity of Ia antigen density on human granulocyte-macrophage progenitor cells (CFU-G,M). Blood 62 (Suppl 1):134a
82. Broxmeyer HE (1982) Relationship of cell-cycle expression of Ia-like antigenic determinants on normal and leukemia human granulocyte-macrophage progenitor cells to regulation in vitro by acidic isoferritins. J Clin Invest 69:632
83. Cannistra SA, Daley JF, Larcom P, Griffin JD (1985) Expression of Ia antigens on myeloid progenitor cells in chronic myeloid leukemia: direct analysis using partially purified colony-forming cells. Blood 65:414
84. Belzer MB, Fitchen JH, Ferrone S, Foon KA, Billing RJ, Golde DW (1981) Expression of Ia-like antigens on human erythroid progenitor cells as determined by monoclonal antibodies and heteroantisera to Ia-like antigens. Clin Immunol Immunopathol 20:111
85. Goldman JM, Hibbin J, Kearney K, Orchard K, Th'ng KH (1982) HLA-DR monoclonal antibodies inhibit proliferation of normal and chronic granulocytic leukemia myeloid progenitor cells. Br J Haematol 52:411
86. Griffin JD, Beveridge RP, Schlossman SF (1982) Isolation of myeloid progenitor cells from peripheral blood of chronic myelogenous leukemia patients. Blood 60:30
87. Schwamborn JS, Ferrone S, Burger DR, Fitchen JH (1984) Altered expression of Ia antigens on monocytes and granulocyte-macrophage progenitors (CFU-GM) from patients with chronic granulocytic leukemia (CGL). Blood 64 [Suppl 1]:198a
88. Ferrero R, Broxmeyer HE, Pagliardi GL, Venuta S, Lange B, Pessano S, Rovera G (1983) Antigenically distinct subpopulations of myeloid progenitor cells (CFU-GM) in human peripheral blood and marrow. Proc Natl Acad Sci USA 80:4114
89. Torok-Storb B, Papyannopoulou T (1981) Polycythemia vera: abnormal patterns of cell surface antigen expression on endogenous CFU-E. Blood 58 (Suppl 1):92a
90. Torok-Storb B, Hansen JA (1982) Modulation of in vitro BFU-E growth by normal Ia-positive T cells is restricted by HLA-DR. Nature 298:473

91. Kurland JI, Bockman RS, Broxmeyer HE, Moore MAS (1978) Limitation of excessive myelopoiesis by the intrinsic modulation of macrophage derived prostaglandin E. Science 199:552
92. Gentile P, Byer D, Pelus LM (1983) In vivo modulation of murine myelopoiesis following intravenous administration of prostaglandin E. Blood 62:1100
93. Pelus LM, Gold E, Saletan S, Coleman M (1983) Restoration of responsiveness of chronic myeloid leukemia granulocyte-macrophage colony-forming cells to growth regulation in vitro following preincubation with prostaglandin E. Blood 62:158
94. Schwamborn JS, Ferrone S, Fitchen JH (1984) Prostaglandin E (PGE)-mediated inhibition of granulocyte-macrophage progenitors (CFU-GM) from patients with chronic granulocytic leukemia. Blood 64 [Suppl 1]:198 a
95. Torok-Storb B, Martin PJ, Hansen JA (1981) Regulation of in vitro erythropoiesis by normal T cells: evidence for two T-cell subsets with opposing function. Blood 58:171
96. Lipton JM, Nadler LM, Canellos GP, Kudisch M, Reiss CS, Nathan DG (1983) Evidence for genetic restriction in the suppression of erythropoiesis by a unique subset of T lymphocytes in man. J Clin Invest 72:694

Class II MHC Antigens and Erythropoiesis *

B. Torok-Storb and F. W. Symington

Table of Contents

Introduction

Stem cells are defined by their potential for virtually unlimited self-replication. Their capacity for self-renewal is critical for maintaining tissue systems that are composed of cells with short functional life spans. In the complex process of hematopoiesis, stem cells not only self-replicate but also give rise to a variety of more differentiated progeny, each of which can become committed to one lineage of differentiation. These committed precursor cells are no longer true stem cells, since they are now programed to divide a limited number of times and to mature into functional end-stage blood elements (i.e., red blood cells, granulocytes, monocytes, platelets). A simplified diagram of the hematopoietic system is shown in Fig. 1.

Inherent in any stem cell system are control mechanisms that regulate the rate of cell division to allow self-replication to increase and decrease as the system requires. Besides requiring regulation of stem cell replication, hematopoiesis requires coordinated regulation of stem cell differentiation as well as precise control of the proliferation and maturation of the various independent lineages of committed precursors. The expression of class II molecules by various cellular components of the hematopoietic system has prompted research into the possible role these molecules may play in regulating this system.

* This work was supported by grants CA18221, CA30924, and AM34431 from the NCI and NIADDKD, and by NCI Postdoctoral Fellowship award IF32 CA07461-02 to F.W.S.

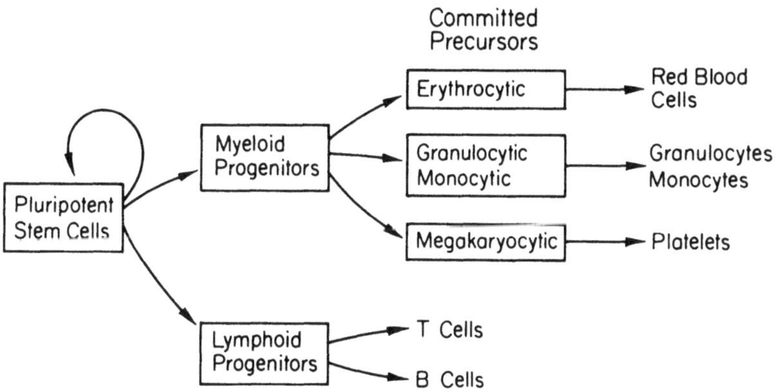

Fig. 1. A simplified diagram of the hematopoietic system showing the precursor-progeny relationships of various classes of progenitor cells. Only the pluripotent stem cells are assigned self-replicative ability

Erythropoiesis Assayed In Vitro

Red blood cells (RBC), being functional end-stage elements with a finite life span and no proliferative potential, are maintained at relatively constant numbers by proliferation and maturation of committed precursors. The immediate precursors of the RBC are erythroblasts, which are the morphologically distinct cells that make up the marrow erythron. Erythroblasts divide a limited number of times and cannot self-replicate. Erythroblast numbers, therefore, are maintained by proliferation and maturation of more immature precursors. These immature precursors cannot be identified morphologically, but they can be assayed in vitro by their ability to form colonies of 8–100 erythroblasts after 5–7 days in culture. On the average, 10^5 normal mononucleated bone marrow cells will contain 200–500 erythroid-colony-forming units (CFU-E) [1, 2].

The CFU-E also lack self-replicative potential; their numbers are maintained by even more immature precursors that can be assayed in vitro by their ability to form a cluster of large colonies, each of which contains hundreds of erythroblasts. Colonies derived from this class of precursor are unusual in that the initial cell divisions yield motile progeny that disperse, so that the final colony is composed of subcolonies, or a "burst" of CFU-E-like colonies [2–4], hence the name BFU-E, for erythroid-burst-forming units. It is important to that marrow-derived precursors are heterogeneous with respect to their maturational state. Therefore, various classes of BFU-E and CFU-E can be identified by proliferative potential that is reflected in colony size. This phenomenon is graphically represented in Fig. 2.

BFU-E obviously have considerable proliferative potential, but the extent to which they are self-maintaining is debated. In replating experiments BFU-E appear to have some self-renewal potential, but this may reflect the known heterogeneity of this compartment. It is generally agreed that BFU-E are not stem cells. BFU-E are believed to proliferate in vivo and in vitro in response to erythropoietin and to give rise to CFU-E [2]. BFU-E are the most immature erythroid precursor identified thus far, and are thought to be produced by multipotent stem cells.

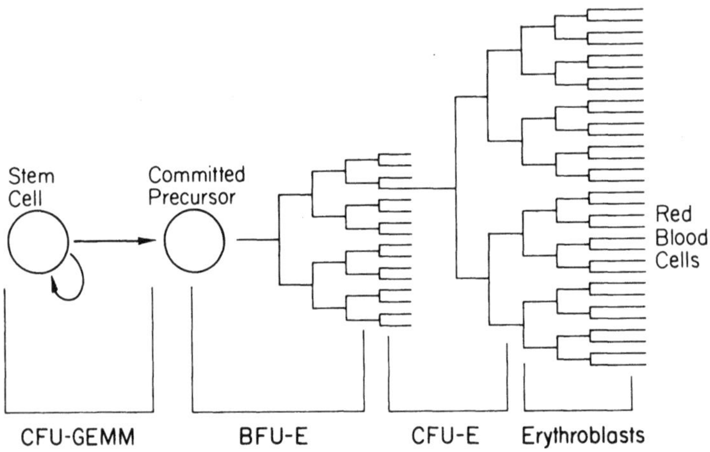

Fig. 2. A simplified diagram of precursor/progeny relationships within the erythroid lineage. The self-replicating stem cell is pluripotent and can also give rise to other lineages. These stem cells are approximated in vitro by growth of CFU-GEMM (see text). Precursors assayed as BFU-E in vitro constitute a heterogeneous population with regard to proliferative potential; to a lesser extent the same is true of CFU-E and erythroblasts

Multipotent stem cells are approximated in vitro by the growth of colonies containing granulocytes, erythroblasts, macrophages, megakaryocytes, and sometimes lymphocytes. A cell giving rise to such a colony is termed a CFU-GEMM [5–7]. Because CFU-GEMM give rise to a variety of differentiated progeny, it has been suggested that these precursors are hematopoietic stem cells. A limited self-renewal capacity of CFU-GEMM has been suggested by replating experiments, but this may merely reflect a tendency of in vitro culture systems to favor differentiation over self-renewal. The relationship between the CFU-GEMM and the true stem cell (i.e., the cell needed for hematopoietic engraftment) is unclear.

Regulation of Erythropoiesis

The complexity of regulation within the erythroid lineage is illustrated well by rendering mice acutely anemic and then measuring the number and cell cycle kinetics of BFU-E and CFU-E. Such studies have shown that only the number of CFU-E is increased in response to increases in serum erythropoietin levels. The production of BFU-E is not increased. In fact the number of BFU-E decreases initially in response to anemia, indicating increased proliferation and production of CFU-E with no commensurate increase in the production of BFU-E. Investigators have concluded from these studies that the regulation of BFU-E production is independent of erythropoietin [2, 8].

The in vivo mechanisms which regulate the production of BFU-E by the multipotent stem cell are unknown. A considerable body of evidence, however, suggests that early events in hematopoiesis, like BFU-E production, may be influenced by auxiliary cells. The demonstration of auxiliary cell function comes from both in vivo and in vitro studies. It has been shown that T lymphocytes, which do not contain any stem cells, can promote erythropoiesis in vivo in mice and enhance marrow engraftment in transplanted dogs [9–12]. In vitro, the addition of T lymphocytes as well as monocytes has been shown to modulate growth of murine, canine and human erythroid colonies [13–17]. Until recently the mechanisms underlying these phenomena have seemed obscure. With the advent of hybridoma technology it should be possible to develop probes which can distinguish various cellular components of the hematopoietic system, making definitive studies of their regulation possible.

Expression of Class II Molecules by Erythroid Precursors

Murine monoclonal antibodies reactive with human HLA-D region gene products have been used by many investigators to determine whether hematopoietic precursors express these molecules [18–21]. Our studies employed two distinct methodologies. The first method used two-stage complement (C′)-mediated cytotoxicity to deplete bone marrow or peripheral blood mononuclear cells of antigen-positive cells prior to culturing for colonies. With this technique, reduction of colony growth from treated cells could be interpreted to indicate either that precursors express class II molecules, or that auxiliary cells critical for colony growth express class II molecules. To distinguish between these two possibilities, we and others used the second methodology, fluorescence-activated cell sorting (FACS) of antibody-labeled cells, to demonstrate that immature precursors could be enriched in the positive population [20, 22–24].

Taken together, both sets of experiments indicated that class II molecules are expressed on immature precursors CFU-GEMM and BFU-E. Our studies also suggested that expression is lost with erythroid maturation, since CFU-E expressed undetectable levels of these molecules. Although there is controversy regarding antigen expression on CFU-E [23, 24], it is certain that erythroblasts as well as RBC are negative for class II molecules, and that expression is ultimately lost with maturation.

Our initial cytotoxicity studies (Table 1) used monoclonal antibodies 7.2 and P4.1, which are specific for monomorphic framework determinants on HLA-DR p29,34 heterodimers [22, 26], and SG465, which has reported specificity for a monomorphic determinant on HLA-DQ molecules [25]. Cytotoxic treatment with each of these antibodies strongly inhibited BFU-E growth. The results with SG465 were unexpected, because other monoclonal antibodies to DQ or DQ-like antigens failed to react with precursor cells (Table 2) [23, 24, 26, 27]. For example, antibody 17.15 reacts with a DQ-related supertypic determinant encoded by DR4, DR5, DRw9, and some DR7 haplotypes. When 17.15 was used in two-stage C′-mediated cytotoxicity with bone marrow and peripheral blood mononuclear cells from individuals who were DR4,4, DR4,5, DR2,4, or DR1,5, B cells from all individuals studied were lysed, whereas growth of CFU-GEMM and BFU-E was not affected (Table 1). Sieff et al. [27] used FACS separation of hematopoietic cells to show that precursor cells do not express the supertypic DQ determinant recognized by antibody Genox 3.53.

These observations suggest that expression of certain class II antigens may be lineage- and/or stage-restricted among marrow-derived cells. Examples of restricted class II antigen expression by mature cells include the lymphoid-specific binding of monoclonal antibodies 17.15 and 33.1 [26, 28] and the binding of anti-

Table 1. Effect of antibody plus complement treatment on the growth of hematopoietic CFU

Antibody	Specificity	Precursor	Inhibition (%)
P4.1	DR framework	CFU-E	11 ± 2.1
		BFU-E	84 ± 7.2
		CFU-GEMM	98 ± 11.2
7.2	DR framework	CFU-E	16 ± 2.3
		BFU-E	80 ± 9.7
		CFU-GEMM	100 ± 0
SG465	DQ framework[a]	CFU-E	ND
		BFU-E	62 ± 14.2
		CFU-GEMM	ND
17.15	Supertypic (DR4,5,7)	CFU-E	ND
		BFU-E	2 ± 1.6
		CFU-GEMM	1 ± 1.1

Ficoll-Hypaque-separated bone marrow mononuclear cells were treated with two-stage (in the case of SG465, three-stage) C'-mediated cytotoxicity, washed, and then cultured for growth of CFU-E, BFU-E and CFU-GEMM. Data expressed as inhibition of antibody-plus-C'-treated cells compared to cells treated with C' only (median ± SE of three to ten separate experiments)
[a] See text

Table 2. Differential expression of class II antigen subsets by BFU-E

Antibody (reactivity)	Relative growth (%)	No. of experiments
None; C' alone	100	6
P4.1 (DR)	6 ± 3	6
I-70 (DP)	3 ± 4	3
TU22 (DQ)	112 ± 17	3
17.15 (DQ-like)	96 ± 4	3

Ficoll-Hypaque-separated peripheral blood mononuclear cells from normal individuals were treated as described for Table 1 with antibody plus C' complement or with C' alone, and BFU-E were counted following 14 days culture. Data are expressed as mean ± S.E. growth (%) relative to control growth obtained in three to six separate experiments. Control BFU-E growth from cells treated with C' alone ranged from 34 to 115 BFU-E/plate. All experiments were plated in triplicate

DQ reagents to subpopulations of DR-positive macrophages [29, 30]. Examples of differential expression by hematopoietic precursors are given in Table 2, which shows that cytotoxic treatment with either DP- or DR-, but not with DQ-reactive antibodies, could deplete precursor activity from cultured peripheral blood lymphocytes (PBL). We have begun to investigate the basis for lineage-restricted class II antigen expression. Unfortunately, hematopoietic precursor cells occur in very low frequencies, such that concentration techniques do not yield sufficient numbers of these cells for biochemical analysis. To circumvent this problem, we have established autologous cell lines to compare expression of class II molecules on erythroid and lymphoid cells.

Expression of Class II Molecules on Erythroid Leukemia Cells and Autologous B Cells

HLA-DR-positive and -negative clones have been derived rom the human erythroid leukemia (HEL) cell line originally described by Martin and Papayanopoulou [31]. We also established an autologous B lymphoblastoid line (B-line) from this patient using Epstein-Barr virus. Fortuitously, this paticnt had an HLA-DR7 phenotype that was recognized by antibody 17.15.

Indirect immunofluorescence labeling and FACS analyses of these cells indicated that, like normal erythroid precursors, the HEL-DR+ cells did not bind antibody 17.15, whereas they were virtually 100% positive after labeling with antibody 7.2 or P4.1. The B-line, like normal B cells, was 100% positive for all three antibodies. FACS histograms summarizing these data are shown in Fig. 3. Other FACS data (not shown) established a DP+/DQ−/DR+ phenotype for HEL-DR+ similar to that of normal erythroid precursor cells. Interestingly, HEL-DR+ cells failed to stimulate primary in vitro alloproliferation, and they were unable to trigger secondary alloproliferation of T cells primed with B-line, normal DR7 PBL, or HEL-DR+ [32]. Coculture and supplementation experi-

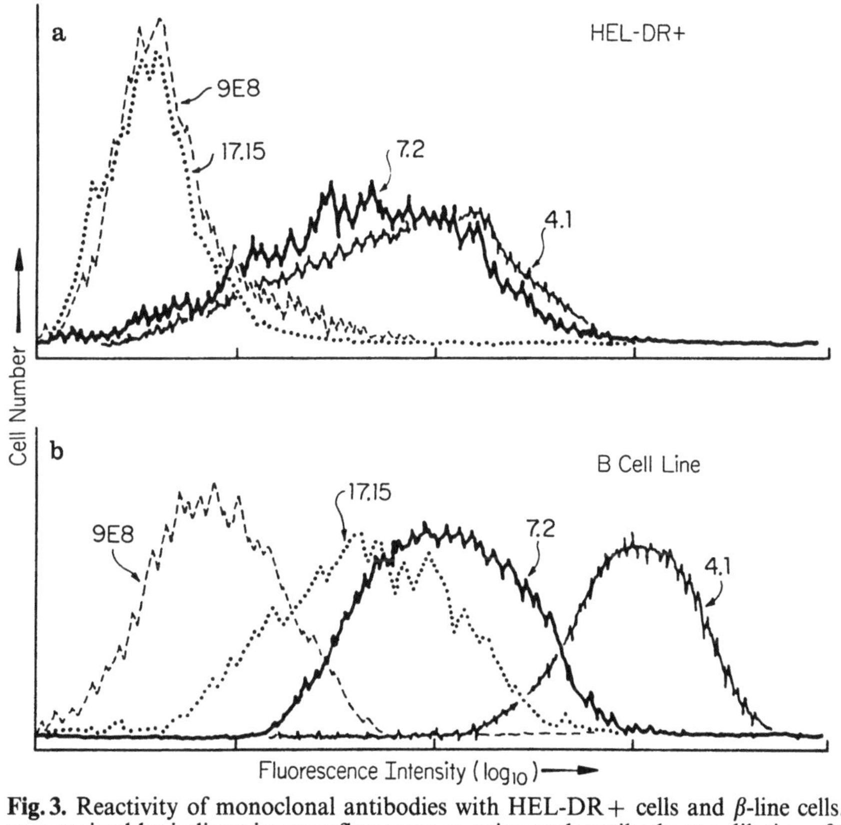

Fig. 3. Reactivity of monoclonal antibodies with HEL-DR+ cells and β-line cells. Cells were stained by indirect immunofluorescence, using each antibody at a dilution of $1:10^2$. Control samples were stained with 9E8, a murine anti-mouse antibody. Samples were analyzed with a FACS IV (Becton-Dickinson) equipped with a four-decade logarithmic amplifier. Each curve depicts an analysis of 10^4 cells

ments did not implicate suppression or lack of lymphokines in the failure of HEL-DR+ to stimulate primary alloproliferation. Evidently the class II molecules expressed by HEL-DR+ cells are qualitatively or quantitatively insufficient for stimulating alloproliferation.

The biochemical nature of the class II antigens expressed by HEL-DR+ and B-line was examined in two-dimensional electrophoresis studies which indicated that the P4.1-reactive antigens of HEL-DR+ closely resemble molecules precipitated from the B-line [32]. These studies also explained the unexpected binding of SG465 to HEL-DR+ and normal erythroid precursor cells on the basis of cross-reactivity of this reagent with DR molecules. Most importantly, molecular genetic data demonstrated that the HEL-DR+ class II phenotype is transcriptionally regulated. Such observations further support the hypothesis that lineage-associated variations in class II molecules occur within the hematopoietic system. The possible functional relevance of these variations is unknown. We can hypothesize, however, that selective expression of variant molecules among different cell types within an organism may influence cell-cell interactions in a tissue-specific manner.

Class II Molecules and the Modulation of Erythropoiesis

The number of BFU-E grown from a given population of mononuclear cells can be increased by coculturing with normal T lymphocytes [33–35]. The magnitude of stimulation varies considerably, with maximum stimulation occurring under stringent culture conditions after other putative auxiliary cells have been depleted. In addition, maximum stimulation is achieved when T cells are cocultured with a population of relatively homogeneous and immature BFU-E derived from the non-T fraction of peripheral blood. Growth of more mature BFU-E and CFU-E, which can only be obtained from bone marrow, is less sensitive to the influences of T cells [36]. The growth-enhancing effect of normal T cells is probably mediated by factors produced by stimulated cells, since mitogen-stimulated lymphocyte-conditioned media could mimic the T cell effect [33].

The growth-enhancing effect of normal T cells was shown to be the net effect of at least two functionally distinct populations of T lymphocytes: one that enhances BFU-E growth, and one that limits this enhancement. The T cells which inhibit enhancing activity were found to express HLA-DR antigens (DR+) [14]. Subsequent studies showed that this T cell effect was dependent on the presence of monocytes, and that the modulation of monocyte-dependent T cell-derived stimulating activity by DR+ T cells is genetically restricted. This was based on a series of experiments which showed that the modulation of T cell effects could only be demonstrated when the BFU-E source and the cocultured T cells shared at least one DR haplotype [37].

There are two possible models by which DR+ T cells could limit the enhancing T cell effect. In the first, DR+ T cells could prevent the in situ elaboration of stimulating activity by interfering with monocyte–T cell collaboration. Genetic restriction in this system could operate at the level of monocyte–T cell collaboration. Schreier and Iscove have shown that collaboration between H-2 (I-A region)-compatible cells is required for elaboration of factors that stimulate the growth of mouse hematopoietic cells [38]. Our hypothesis that a subpopulation of DR+ T cells can suppress monocyte–T cell collaboration falls within the scope of other known T cell suppressor functions.

The second model would suggest that DR+ T cells interact with precursors of BFU-E to limit their responsiveness to monocyte-dependent T cell stimulating activity. This model initially seemed attractive because the genetic restriction of this phenomenon offered a role for the class II molecules preferentially expressed on immature precursor cells. However, subsequent studies of the modulation of auxiliary cell function suggest that the first model is more likely to be correct [39]. Therefore, the function of class II molecules on precursors remains unknown. It is possible that the in vitro assays of hematopoiesis currently in use are inadequate for studying critical interactions between stem cells and other cells which influence their growth.

Clinical Relevance

Immature hematopoietic precursors CFU-GEMM and BFU-E express class II molecules recognized by antibodies specific for framework determinants on HLA-DR- and HLA-DP-encoded antigens. Whether or not the hematopoietic stem cell required for marrow engraftment also expresses these molecules is unknown. This unknown becomes important when considering autologous marrow transplant protocols for treating lymphocytic leukemias which involve treatment of donor marrow with anti-class II monoclonal antibodies and complement. Under the best circumstances, i.e., stem cells are class II negative, engraftment could be expected to be delayed because of the loss of immature committed precursors. If the stem cell does express class II molecules, no engraftment will occur. Either of these outcomes poses considerable risk to the patients. However, the fact that hematopoietic precursor cells differentially express subsets of class II molecules suggests that such risks could be avoided by treating the marrow inoculum with antibodies specific for gene products expressed only by lymphocytes. Such treatments could deplete malignant B lymphoblastoid cells without damaging hematopoietic stem cells and precursor cells. This is an obvious application of the data presented.

The clinical relevance of the in vitro "DR-restricted monocyte-dependent T cell" modulation of erythropoiesis is not yet clear. That these observations may reflect physiological mechanisms is suggested by the ability of T cells to enhance murine erythropoiesis in vivo and to promote marrow engraftment in dogs. In the latter case, donor T lymphocytes were required for successful engraftment of DLA-D-incompatible marrow. The mechanisms by which T cells facilitate engraftment are unknown. The clinical significance of this finding may prove central for predicting the outcome of allogeneic, T cell-depleted marrow transplants, particularly when the donor and recipient are partially mismatched for HLA determinants. It is likely that optimal transplantation methodologies will not be developed until the role of hematopoietic cell subpopulations and the function of their surface molecules in repopulation are more thoroughly understood.

Acknowledgements. The authors are indebted to Susan Brown and Gretchen Johnson for their technical assistance, to Drs. J. Hansen and P. Martin for their generous contributions of antibodies, and to Dr. J. Pesando for supplying antibody I-70 and reviewing the manuscript.

References

1. Stephensen JR, Axelrod AA, McLeod DL, Shreeve MM (1971) Induction of colonies of hemoglobin-synthesizing cells by erythropoietin in vitro. Proc Natl Acad Sci USA 68:1542
2. Gregory CJ (1976) Erythropoietin sensitivity as a differentiation marker in the hemopoietic system: studies of three erythropoietic colony responses in culture. J Cell Physiol 89:289
3. Axelrod AA, McLeod DL, Shreeve MM, Heath DS (1974) Properties of cells that produce erythrocytic colonies in vitro. In: Robinson WA (ed) Hemopoiesis in culture. US Government Printing Office, Washington, DC, p 226
4. Ogawa M, MacEachern MD, Avila L (1977) Human marrow erythropoiesis in culture. II. Heterogeneity in the morphology, time course of colony formation, and sedimentation velocities of the colony forming cells. Am J Hematol 3:29
5. Johnson GR, Metcalf D (1977) Pure and mixed erythroid colony formation in vitro stimulated by spleen conditioned medium with no detectable erythropoietin. Proc Natl Acad Sci USA 74:3879
6. Hara H, Ogawa M (1978) Murine hemopoietic colonies in culture containing normoblasts, macrophages, megakaryocytes. Am J Hematol 4:23
7. Fauser AA, Messner HA (1979) Identification of megakaryocytes, macrophages, and eosinophils in colonies of human bone marrow containing granulocytes and erythroblasts. Blood 53:1023
8. Adamson JW, Torok-Storb B, Lin N (1978) Analysis of erythropoiesis by erythroid colony formation in culture. Blood Cells 4:89
9. Lord BI, Schofield R (1973) The influence of thymus cells in hemopoiesis: stimulation of hemopoietic stem cells in a syngeneic, in vitro, situation. Blood 42:395
10. Resnitzky P, Zipori D, Trainin N (1971) The effect of neonatal thymectomy on hemopoietic tissue in mice. Blood 37:634
11. Deeg HJ, Storb R, Weiden PL, Shulman HM, Graham TC, Torok-Storb BJ, Thomas ED (1979) Abrogation of resistance to DLA nonidentical unrelated marrow grafts in lethally irradiated dogs by thoracic duct lymphocytes. Blood 53:522
12. Storb R, Epstein RB, Bryant J, Ragde H, Thomas ED (1968) Marrow grafts by combined marrow and leukocyte infusions in unrelated dogs selected by histocompatibility typing. Transplantation 6:587
13. Sharkis SJ, Spivok JL, Ahmed A, Misti J, Stuart RK, Wiktor-Jedrzejczok W, Sell KW, Sensenbrenner LL (1980) Regulation of hematopoiesis: helper and suppressor influences in the thymus. Blood 55:524
14. Torok-Storb BJ, Storb R, Graham TC, Prentice RL, Weiden PL, Adamson JW (1978) Erythropoiesis in vitro: effect of normal versus transfusion-sensitized mononuclear cells. Blood 52:706
15. Reid CDL, Baptista LC, Chanarin I (1981) Erythroid colony growth in vitro from human peripheral blood null cells: evidence for regulation by T-lymphocytes and monocytes. Br J Haematol 48:155
16. Wiktor-Jedrzejczok W, Sharkis S, Ahmed A, Sell KW (1977) Theta-sensitive cells and erythropoiesis: identification of a defect in w/w^v anemic mice. Science 196:313
17. Torok-Storb B, Martin PJ, Hansen JA (1981) Cellular interactions in the regulation of in vitro erythropoiesis. In: Stamatoyannopoulos G, Nienhuis AW (eds) Hemoglobins in development and differentiation. Liss, New York, p 137
18. Janossy G, Francis GE, Copellaro D, Goldstone AH, Greaves MF (1978) Cell sorter analysis of leukemia-associated antigens on human myeloid precursors. Nature 276:176
19. Belzer MB, Fitchen JH, Ferrone S, Foon KA, Billing RJ, Golde DW (1981) Expression of Ia-like antigens on human erythroid progenitor cells as determined by monoclonal antibodies and heteroantiserum to Ia-like antigens. Clin Immunol Immunopathol 20:111
20. Robinson J, Sieff C, Delia D, Edwards PAW, Greaves M (1981) Expression of cellsurface HLA-DR, HLA-ABC and glycophorin during erythroid differentiation. Nature 289:68

21. Fitchen JH, Cline MH (1979) Human myeloid progenitor cells express HLA antigens. Blood 53:794
22. Torok-Storb B, Martin PJ, Hansen JA (1981) Cellular interactions in the regulation of in vitro erythropoiesis. In: Stamatoyannopoulos G, Nienhuis AW (eds) Hemoglobins in development and differentiation. Liss, New York, p 137
23. Linch DC, Nadler LM, Luther EA, Lipton JM (1984) Discordant expression of human Ia-like antigens on hematopoietic progenitor cells. J Immunol 132:2324
24. Falkenburg JHF, Jansen J, van der Vaart-Duinkerken N, Veenhof WFJT, Blotkamp J, Goselink HM, Parlevilet J, van Rood JJ (1984) Polymorphic and monomorphic HLA-DR determinants on human hematopoietic progenitor cells. Blood 63:1125
25. Goyert SM, Silver J (1982) Further characterization of HLA-DS molecules: implications for studies assessing the role of human Ia molecules in cell interactions and disease susceptibility. Proc Natl Acad Sci USA 80:5719
26. Torok-Storb B, Nepom GT, Nepom BS, Hansen JA (1983) HLA-DR antigens on lymphoid cells differ from those on myeloid cells. Nature 305:541
27. Sieff C, Bicknell D, Caine G, Robinson J, Lam G, Greaves MF (1982) Changes in cell surface antigen expression during hematopoietic differentiation. Blood 60:703
28. Marti GE, Kuo MC, Shaw S, Chang CC, DeMars R, Sogn JA, Coligan JE, Kindt TJ (1983) A novel HLA-D/DR-like antigen specific for human B lymphoid cells. J Exp Med 158:1924
29. Nunez G, Giles RC, Ball EJ, Hurley CK, Capra JD, Stastny P (1984) Expression of HLA-DR, MB, MT, and SB antigens on human mononuclear cells: identification of two phenotypically distinct monocyte populations. J Immunol 133:1300–1306
30. Gonwa TA, Picker LJ, Raff HV, Goyert SM, Silver JS, Stobo JD (1983) Antigen-presenting capabilities of human monocytes correlates with their expression of HLA-DS, an Ia determinant distinct from HLA-DR. J Immunol 130:706
31. Martin PJ, Papayanopoulou T (1982) A new human erythroleukemia cell line with spontaneous and induced globin expression. Science 216:1233
32. Symington FW, Levine F, Braun M, Brown SL, Erlich HA, Torok-Storb B (1985) Differential Ia antigen expression by autologous human erythroid and B lymphoblastoid cell lines. J Immunol 135:1026–1032
33. Nathan DG, Chess L, Hillman DG, Clarke B, Beard J, Merler E, Housman DE (1978) Human erythroid burst-forming unit: T-cell requirement for proliferation in vitro. J Exp Med 147:324
34. Torok-Storb B, Martin PJ, Hansen JA (1981) Regulation of in vitro erythropoiesis by normal T-cells: evidence for two T-cell subsets with opposing function. Blood 58:171
35. Mangan KF, Chikkappa G, Bieler LF, Scharfman WB, Parkinson DR (1982) Regulation of human blood erythroid burst-forming unit (BFU-E) proliferation by T-lymphocyte subpopulations defined by Fc receptors and monoclonal antibodies. Blood 59:990
36. Lipton JM, Reinherz EL, Kudisch M, Jackson PM, Schlossman SF, Nathan DG (1980) Mature bone marrow erythroid burst-forming units do not require T-cells for induction of erythropoietin-dependent differentiation. J Exp Med 152:350
37. Torok-Storb BJ, Hansen JA (1982) Modulation of in vitro BFU-E growth by normal Ia-positive T-cells is restricted by HLA-DR. Nature 298:473
38. Schreir MH, Iscove NN (1980) Hematopoietic growth factors are released in cultures of H-2 restricted helper T-cells, accessory cells and specific antigen. Nature 287:228
39. Torok-Storb B (1984) T-cell effects on in vitro erythropoiesis: Immune regulation and immune reactivity. In: Young NS, Levine AS, Humphries RK (eds) Aplastic anemia: stem cell biology and advances in treatment. Liss, New York, p 163

Expression of Class II Antigens on Nonhematopoietic Tumor Cells

S. Carrel, J.-P. Mach, P. Ferremi, L. Giuffré, and R.S. Accolla

Table of Contents

Introduction

Class II antigens constitute a heterogeneous and polymorphic family of molecules encoded in the major histocompatibility complex (MHC) and primarily expressed on B cells, macrophages, and activated T cells [1]. However, not only lymphoid cells and macrophages express class II antigens. Hammerling et al. [2] first reported that murine epidermal cells and epididymal sperm cells expressed Ia determinants.

In the human, the first nonhematopoietic cells found to express class II antigens were the skin Langerhans cells [3–5]. These cells present in normal skin are considered to be related to monocytes [6]. All other normal epidermal cells, including melanocytes, Merkel cells, and keratinocytes were found not to express class II antigens. Malignant melanocytes, however, can express class II antigens. Several authors looked for the presence of class II antigens on a number of established melanoma cell lines and found that more than 50% of them reacted either with hetero- or alloantisera specific for class II antigens [7–12]. Immunoprecipitation of detergent-solubilized ^{125}I-labeled membrane proteins from melanoma cell lines confirmed the presence of the known class II bimolecular complex of 33000 and 28000 daltons.

The purpose of this chapter is to review the main literature concerning the expression and function of class II antigens in nonlymphoid solid tumor cells and to present some recent results from our laboratory concerning the structural characterization of the nonlymphoid class II molecules and the modulation of expression of their distinct subsets (HLA-DR and -DC) by interferons. Our findings will be discussed in view of recent data from the literature concerning the biological role of these class II antigens.

Class II Antigen Expression on Nonhematopoietic Tumor Cell Lines

After the demonstration of class II antigen expression by melanoma cell lines [7, 8], we showed that an endometrial carcinoma line (END-1) established in our laboratory expressed large amounts of class II antigens [13]. The biochemical analysis of the class II molecules produced by this cell line is discussed below. We also identified class II antigens on three of eight malignant glioma (astrocytoma) cell lines, both by binding radioimmunoassay and by sodium dodecyl sulphate–polyacrylamide gel electrophoresis (SDS-PAGE) using the monoclonal antibody (MoAb) D1-12, which has been shown to recognize a monomorphic determinant located on the β-chain of the HLA-DR molecule [14]. More recently, a bladder carcinoma cell line, T24 [15], and a liver carcinoma cell line, SK-HEP-1 [15], as well as a subclone of the colon carcinoma cell line LoVo [16], were shown to express HLA-DR antigens (Table 1).

Table 1. Expression of class II antigens in solid tumors and tumor cell lines

Site	Tumor type	Cell line
Skin	Basal cell carcinoma (2/4)	
	Primary melanomas (11/15]	Numerous [26]
	Metastatic melanomas (5/12)	Numerous [27–31]
Brain	Cyctic astrocytoma (4/5)	
	Glioma (7/18)	Numerous [30, 31]
	Ganglioneuroblastoma (1/1)	
	Meningioma (6/6)	
	Neuroblastoma (0/10)	
	Ganglioneuroblastoma (1/1)	
Gastrointestinal tract	Adenocarcinoma	
	stomach (3/3)	
	colon (7/9)	
	sigmoid (4/5)	Clone of LoVo [16, 32]
	rectum (4/8)	
	liver (1/1)	SK-HEP-1 [15]
Female genital tract	Breast (8/14)	T47 [15]
	Ovary (1/2)	
	cystadenocarcinoma of ovary (3/4)	
	adenocarcinoma of endometrium (2/2)	END-1 [13]
Lung	Pulmonary adenocarcinoma (3/4)	
Urogenital tract	Urinary bladder carcinoma (4/5)	T24 [15]

Immunohistological localization of HLA-DR antigens was performed by means of indirect immunoperoxidase or indirect immunofluorescence techniques using fresh frozen tissue fragments. Anti-HLA-DR MoAbs were used for all determinations

With these results obtained essentially on tumor cell lines, it was not clear whether the class II expression on nonhematopoietic cells was related to the in vitro culture conditions, or a phenomenon associated with the malignant phenotype of the cell lines studied, similar to the ectopic production of hormones. A partial answer to this question was reached by testing the expression of HLA-DR antigen on frozen sections from tumor biopsies.

Class II Antigen Expression on Fresh Tissue Biopsies

The expression of HLA-DR on frozen tissue sections was analyzed using a three-layer biotin-avidin-peroxidase system [17]. A representative example obtained with a primary melanoma is shown in Fig. 1. Some of the tumor masses were brightly stained by the anti-HLA-DR MoAb D1-12, while others remained totally unstained. In addition, an intense staining of lymphocytes and macrophages infiltrating the tumor can be seen [18].

The fact that the anti-HLA-DR MoAb stains only some group of cells within a morphologically homogeneous melanoma nodule, suggests the presence of distinct subpopulations of tumor cells. This raises the question of whether this heterogeneity is due to a multicellular origin of the tumor, or to different degrees of differentiation of tumor cells derived from a single malignant clone. Recent results from the group of Fidler, obtained in the B16 mouse melanoma model, seem to favor the second hypothesis [19].

In cancer of epithelial origin, such as colorectal carcinoma, Daar et al. [20] reported that about half of 15 biopsies from different patients contained malignant

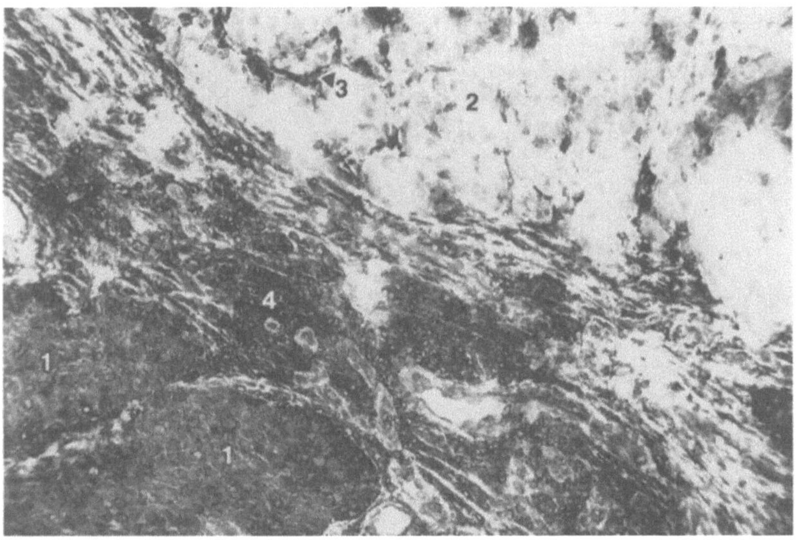

Fig. 1. Immunohistological localization of HLA-DR antigen on a frozen section from a primary melanoma. The anti-HLA-DR MoAb D1-12 was used in indirect immunoperoxidase staining using the biotin-avidin system with aminoethylcarbazole as chromogen. *1*, HLA-DR-positive tumor nodules; *2*, HLA-DR-negative tumor nodules; *3*, HLA-DR-positive inflammatory cells (probably granulocytes and macrophages surrounding the tumor masses); *4*, HLA-DR-positive proliferating T lymphocytes

cells expressing HLA-DR antigens. The positive cells stained by an anti-HLA-DR MoAb were, as in the case of melanoma, not homogeneously distributed within the tumor masses but limited to certain tumor areas. Interestingly, the normal colon epithelial cells adjacent to the tumor were negative. Similarly, Natali et al. [21] detected malignant cells expressing HLA-DR in biopsies of some histological types of breast carcinoma, namely medullary and tubular. The normal breast epithelial cells also expressed HLA-DR antigens, whereas ductal infiltrating breast carcinoma cells were HLA-DR-negative. Thus, it appars that for breast epithelial cells the malignant transformation of these results in a loss of HLA-DR expression.

In 20% of biopsies from malignant astrocytes, we also found that a small percentage of cancer cells did express HLA-DR antigens [22]. This observation lead us to study HLA-DR antigen expression by normal brain tissues obtained at autopsy. We found several clearly positive cells in the white matter (Fig. 2), and by morphological criteria identified them as astrocytes [23]. Furthermore, reactive astrocytes surrounding a brain metastasis (identified by anti-glial-fibrillary acidic protein antibodies) were strongly positive with anti-HLA-DR MoAbs.

From the results discussed and summarized in Table 1, it is clear that malignant and normal cells of nonlymphoid origin can express class II antigens. However, the mechanism of induction and the functional significance of class II molecules in these cells is unknown. Human epidermal Langerhans cells have been shown to stimulated in vitro allogeneic lymphocytes whose proliferation could be blocked by anti-class II MoAbs or anti-DR allosera [24, 25]. To date, however, such stimulation using class II-positive tumor cells has provided no satisfactory results, as will be discussed below (Conclusions).

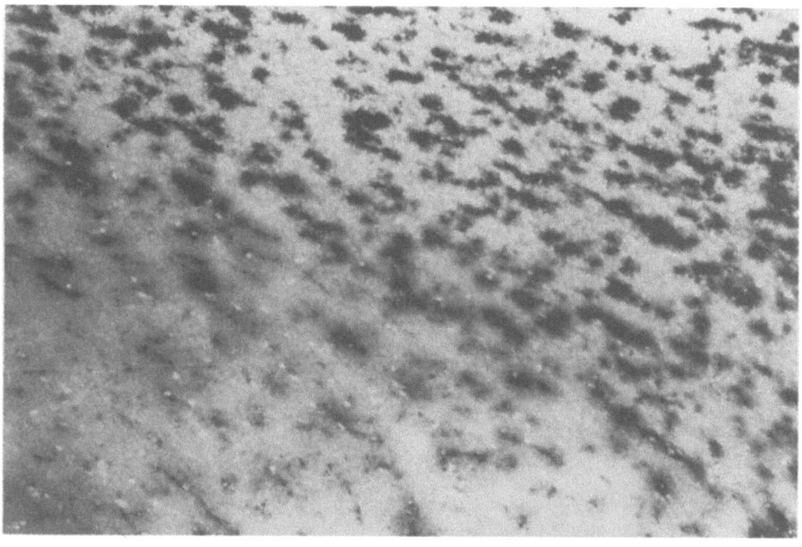

Fig. 2. Immunohistological localization of HLA-DR antigens on a frozen section of normal human brain. The anti-HLA-DR MoAb D1-12 was used in indirect immunoperoxydase staining using the biotin-avidin system with aminoethylcarbazole as chromogen

Biochemical Characterization of Class II Antigens Isolated from Nonlymphoid Tumor Cells

Class II molecules are heterodimeric structures made of two distinct noncovalently linked subunits, the α chain of 34000–36000 daltons and the β chain of 24000–28000 daltons. Both chains are glycosylated; the β chain carries a single complex glycan, whereas the α chain carries both a complex and a high mannose glycan [33].

One of the basic characteristics of the class II molecules is their high degree of polymorphism [34]. In our laboratory we have used a very sensitive two-dimensional peptide mapping technique [35] to assess the degree of structural heterogeneity of class II antigens. Using this approach, we have demonstrated the simultaneous expression on the same B cell lines of various subsets of class II molecules that we operationally called NG1 and NG2 [36] and of at least two DQ-like mol-

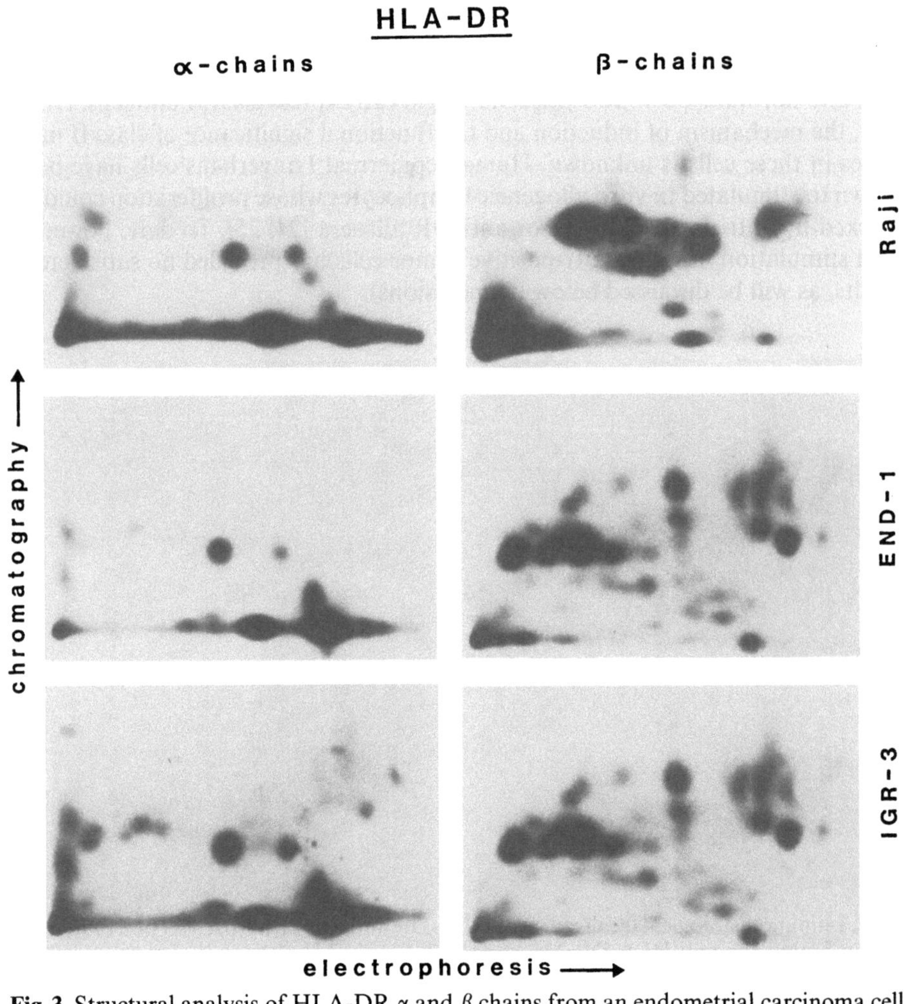

Fig. 3. Structural analysis of HLA-DR α and β chains from an endometrial carcinoma cell line, END-1, and from a melanoma cell line, IGR-3, compared with those from a reference B cell line, Raji. (For details on the two-dimensional peptide mapping technique see [35])

ecules [37]. The NG1 subset appears to be the equivalent of the known HLA-DR antigens, but NG2 does not correspond to a serologically defined subset. NG2 molecules are relatively less polymorphic than DR molecules. They may be included in the previously defined SB antigens or, more likely, constitute a novel type of HLA class II molecules.

The various class II subsets differ from each other at the level of both the α and the β subunits.

In this review, we will restrict ourself to results obtained with an anti-HLA-DR (NG1) MoAb, D1-12. Until recently, little information was available on the biochemical characteristics of Ia antigens in nonlymphoid cells. We present here some data on the structure of the HLA-DR subset isolated from endometrial carcinoma cell line END-1 and from melanoma cell line, IGR-3. The two-dimensional peptide maps of separated α and β chains from the DR subset in the two tumor cell lines were compared with the homologous peptide maps of a B-cell line, Raji, taken as a reference. As shown in Fig. 3, significative differences were observed when the β chain fingerprints of the three cell lines were compared. Since it is known that the chains of HLA-DR molecules carry the polymorphic character, these results are compatible with the different HLA-DR typing of the three cell lines analyzed, Raji (DR 3,6) END-1 (DR2, X) IGR3 (DR 1,7).

However, when the peptide maps of α chains of DR molecules derived from Raji IGR3 and END-1 were analyzed, a striking similarity was observed between them. This structural homology of α chains from cell lines of different DR confirms previous findings of our group and others on the absence of genetic polymorphisms for the large subunit of HLA-DR molecules [38].

Taken together, these results indicate that nonlymphoid tumor cells express class II molecules sharing the basic structural features with homologous molecules in lymphoid cells. The melanoma cells showed polymorphism in the HLA-DR β chain and nonpolymorphism in the HLA-DR and NG2 α chains; structural identity among α chains of different DR and NG2 phenotype. Alexander et al. [39] came to the same conclusions when they compared HLA-DR molecules of autologous melanoma and B lymphoblastoid cell lines. They found only some differences, asparagine-linked oligosaccharide processing with more of the larger complex glycan on the α chain of the HLA-DR from melanoma cells.

Heterogenous Expression of HLA-DR Antigens on Clones and Subclones of A Melanoma Cell Line, Me43

Cells from the class II-negative melanoma line Me43 were cloned and subcloned in methylcellulose and the cell surface antigenic profile analyzed using a panel of MoAbs [40]. The most striking observation concerns the expression of HLA-DR antigens by the various clones. In six of 22 clones more than 15% of the cells expressed HLA-DR antigens, in three of these more than 75%. Representative FACS histograms illustrating the surface phenotype of Me43 cells prior to cloning and of two clones are shown in Fig. 4. The anti-HLA-DR MoAb D1-12 stained about 90% of the cells of clone 16, while cells of the original cell line and of clone 18 were unstained. Cells from clone 16 were also stained by a MoAb raised against a melanoma cell line, Me3-TB7, while the uncloned cells and the cells of clone 18 were unstained.

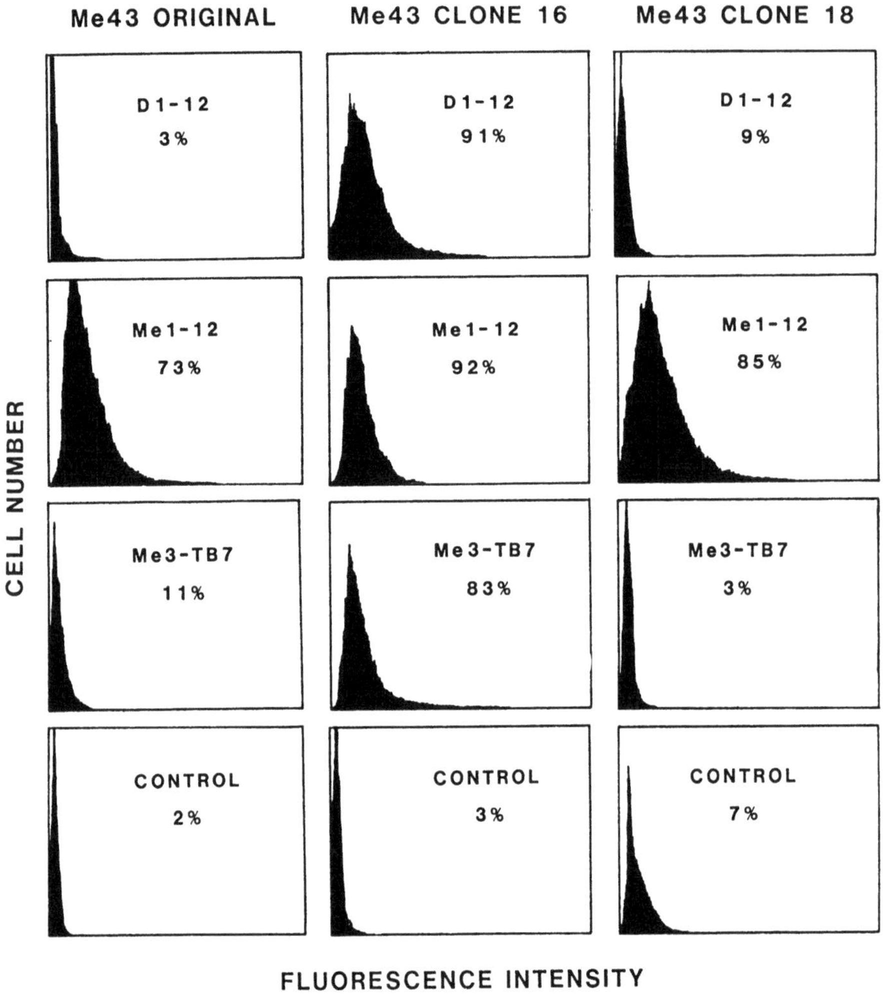

Fig. 4. FACS histograms illustrating the cell surface phenotypes of Me43 melanoma cells prior to cloning (*left*), Me43 clone 16 (*center*), and Me43 clone 18 (*right*). *D1-12,* anti-HLA-DR MoAb; *Mel-12, Me3-TB7,* anti-melanoma MoAb; CONTROL, anti-CEA MoAb

When cells from HLA-DR-positive Me43 clones were subcloned, all the 20 subclones tested were found to be HLA-DR-negative. Furthermore, when cells from HLA-DR-positive clones were kept in culture for more than 12 weeks, a gradual loss of HLA-DR expression was observed.

The great diversity and the lack of stability of the cell surface phenotype, especially the expression of HLA-DR, in the different clones and subclones in vitro sugest that the tumor heterogeneity observed in vivo is not due to stable mutations, but rather to epigenetic factors such as selective differentiation induced by locally produced modulation.

Tumor cell heterogeneity is a subject of increasing interest since the demonstration in the mouse B16 melanoma model [41] that selected subpopulations of tumor cells have markedly different metastatic properties. It has also been shown that antigens expressed by cells from a primary tumor are lost in cells from the corresponding metastases [42], and some recent data indicated that an antibody against a receptor could modify the metastatic potential of a selected subclone [43, 44]. However, no direct relationship between metastatic potential and antigen expression has yet been reported. In this context, it would be of interest to study the antigenic phenotype of cells from a primary melanoma and to follow the phenotype of these cells during the whole dissemination process, giving special attention to the appearance and/or disappearance of class II molecules.

Modulation of Class II Antigen Expression by Interferons

Several authors have shown that interferons can enhance the expression of class I (HLA-ABC) antigens on a wide variety of both murine and human cells [45–48]. The effect of interferons on the expression of class II antigens (HLA-DR) was less clear. Imai et al. [49] reported that incubation of cultured melanoma cells with partially purified interferon-α significantly increased the expression of HLA-ABC and B2-microglobulin, but did not alter the expression of HLA-DR or the expression of two melanoma-associated antigens. Similar results were observed by Liao et al. [50] using another melanoma line. More recently, Basham and Merigan [51] showed that interferon-γ, but not interferon-α, increased the expression of HLA-DR on HLA-DR-positive melanoma cells.

In our laboratory, we have shown that recombinant interferon-γ (IFN-γ) not only enhanced the expression of HLA-DR on DR-positive solid tumor cells, but could also induce the expression of class II antigens (DR and DQ) on tumor cell lines which normally did not express these antigens. As shown in Table 2, IFN-γ induced the expression of HLA-DR and HLA-DQ on the two class II-negative melanoma lines Me43 and GLL-19 and enhanced HLA-DR expression on the HLA-DR-positive line Me1477. IFN-γ also induced the expression of high levels of HLA-DQ (detected by the monoclonal antibody produced by Ziegler et al.

Table 2. Effect of IFN-γ treatment on the expression of class I and class II antigens on melanoma, glioma, neuroblastoma, colon carcinoma, and cervical carcinoma cells

Cell line		Monoclonal antibody			
		Anti-HLA-DR	Anti-HLA-DC	Anti-HLA-ABC	Control
Melanoma	Me1477	4100 (900)	1750 (140)	3300 (1100)	150 (100)
	GLL-19	1340 (145)	600 (160)	3900 (2400)	130 (140)
	Me43	980 (70)	530 (350)	7200 (1950)	120 (65)
Glioma	LN-18	1330 (130)	200 (190)	6200 (4000)	110 (110)
	LN-235	500 (80)	125 (100)	3360 (3400)	80 (50)
Neuroblastoma	LAN-1	180 (130)	90 (110)	1100 (125)	115 (90)
Colon ca	HT-29	2270 (100)	280 (230)	5400 (630)	110 (120)
	LoVo	1800 (140)	750 (500)	500 (200)	100 (200)
Cervix ca	Me180	500 (80)	360 (110)	3580 (1200)	60 (130)

Results are expressed as cpm bound of ^{125}I-labeled rabbit anti-mouse F(ab')2 antibodies to 10^5 target cells incubated with an excess of MoAbs; the numbers in parentheses are the cpm bound to untreated control cells tested in parallel. Cells were treated for 4 days with 500 U/ml IFN-γ

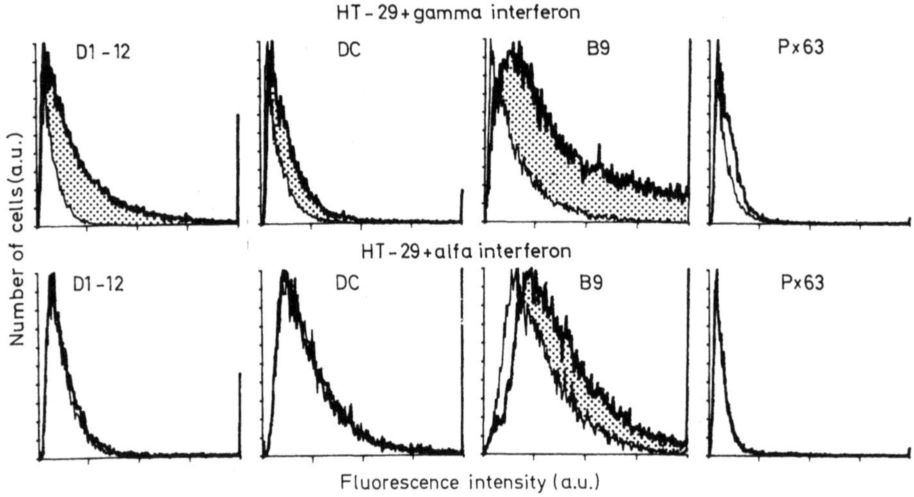

Fig. 5. IFN-γ and IFN-α treatment of HT-29 colon carcinoma cells; effect on the expression of class I and class II HLA antigens. Cells were incubated with 500 U/ml IFN-γ or with 2000 U/ml IFN-α for 4 days and the expression of the antigens tested by 1 h incubation at 4 °C with the relevant MoAb followed by goat anti-mouse/fluorescein isothiocyanate. The results are depicted as FACS histograms plotting fluorescence intensity number of cells. Ten thousand cells were analyzed for each tracing. *D1-12,* anti-HLA-DR MoAb; *DC,* anti-HLA-DC MoAb; *B9,* anti-HLA-ABC MoAb; *P63,* control culture fluid

[52]) on cells from the Me1477 line, while this antigen was undetectable in untreated cells. Finally, as expected, IFN-γ also enhanced the expression of class I antigens on these three melanoma cell lines.

In addition to melanoma cell lines, we found that IFN-γ was also able to induce the expression of HLA-DR antigens on the glioma lines LN-18 and LN-235, on the colon carcinoma cell lines HT-29 and LoVo, and on the cervical carcinoma line Me180 [53]. The analysis by flow microfluorometry of IFN-γ-treated HT-29 colon carcinoma cells showed a homogeneous increase of staining intensity with the anti-class I and -class II antibodies (Fig. 5). The histogram of HT-29 cells stained with the anti-HLA-DR MoAb D1-12 clearly showed that almost all cells became positive for HLA-DR after IFN-γ treatment, while the low level of HLA-DQ detected on untreated cells remained unchanged.

Figure 6 shows that MoAb D1-12 precipitated a classical HLA-DR heterodimer from lysates of HT-29 cells which had been treated for 4 days with 100 U/ml IFN-γ and biosynthetically labeled with ^{35}S-methionine. Untreated control HT-29 cells labeled in parallel showed no detectable HLA-DR bands.

Interesting results were obtained with cells from the neuroblastoma line LAN-1, which without IFN did not express either class I or class II antigens. As shown in Table 2, IFN-γ treatment was not able to induce expression of class II antigens on these neuroblastoma cells, but it did induce the expression of class I antigens. These findings indicate that LAN-1 cells have receptors for IFN-γ, and that the induction of class I and class II antigens expression is regulated by distinct mechanisms.

When HLA-DR-negative tumor cell lines were treated with either IFN-α or IFN-β, enhanced expression of class I antigens only was observed. Neither IFN-α

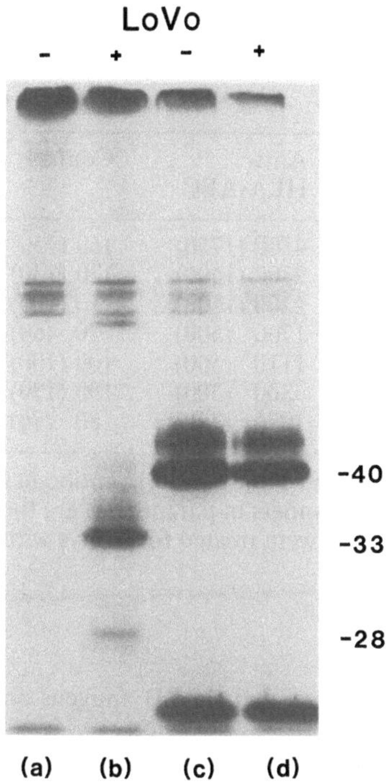

Fig. 6. Autoradiography from an SDS-PAGE of ^{35}S-methionine-labeled proteins from the HLA-DR-negative colon carcinoma line HT-29. The cells were treated for 4 days with 100 U/ml IFN-β and precipitated with the anti-HLA-DR MoAb D1-12 (lane *b*) and with MoAb D1 directed against a colon-carcinoma-associated antigen (lane *d*). Untreated control cells were processed in parallel (lanes *a*, *c*)

nor IFN-β induced the expression of class II antigens (HLA-DR and -DQ) on the cell lines analyzed in this study (Tables 3 and 4). Since class I antigens are enhanced on these cells, the absence of effect of IFN-α and IFN-β on class II antigens is not due to a lack of receptor for IFN-α and β. A study similar to the one described here was recently reported by Houghton et al. [54].

From previous cloning experiments we knew that HLA-DR-positive clones obtained without the addition of IFN from HLA-DR-negative cell lines expressed these class II antigens only for a limited period of time, never exceeding 12 weeks [40]. It was therefore of interest to study the maintenance of the induced HLA-DR phenotype on melanoma cells treated with IFN-γ. Me43 cells were treated for 4 days with 500 U/ml IFN-γ and then further cultured for 8 days in the absence of IFN-γ. The cells were tested for antigen expression at days 0, 4, and 8 after the end of IFN-γ treatment. As shown in Table 5, after 4 days of culture in the absence of IFN-γ the level of HLA-DR antigen expressed had decreased by more than 50% and that of HLA-DQ by more than 40%. After 8 days, the level of expression of both class II antigens had decreased by more than 80%, while the enhanced expression of class I antigens and B2-microglobulin had decreased by more than 40%. A similar decrease of class II antigen expression after withdrawal of IFN-γ was observed for the melanoma line GLL-19. Taken together, these results clearly show that the induction of expression of class II antigens by IFN-γ on class II-negative cells is not a permanent event.

The observation that a large variety of human nonlymphoid tumor cell lines can be induced to express class II antigens by IFN-γ treatment raises the question of whether this induction is a general phenomenon. Preliminary results indicate that IFN-γ is unable to induce the expression of HLA-DR not only on LAN-1

Table 3. Effect of IFN-α treatment on the expression of class I and class II antigens on melanoma, glioma, colon carcinoma, and cervical carcinoma cells

Cell line		Monoclonal antibody			
		Anti-HLA-DR	Anti-HLA-DC	Anti-HLA-ABC	Control
Melanoma	Me1477	3400 (3200)	570 (550)	4300 (1750)	160 (150)
	GLL-19	130 (130)	250 (230)	2300 (1400)	120 (130)
	Me43	150 (190)	330 (280)	2200 (1100)	110 (100)
Glioma	LN-18	95 (110)	160 (120)	1700 (500)	70 (80)
Colon ca	HT-29	140 (150)	130 (125)	1110 (500)	100 (100)
	LoVo	150 (130)	300 (340)	300 (300)	190 (130)
Cervix ca	Me180	95 (80)	120 (120)	1970 (720)	80 (70)

Results are expressed as cpm bound of ^{125}I-labeled rabbit anti-mouse F(ab')2 antibodies to 10^5 target cells incubated with an excess of MoAbs; the numbers in parentheses are the cpm bound to untreated control cells tested in parallel. Cells were treated for 4 days with 10000 U/ml IFN-α

Table 4. Effect of IFN-β treatment on the expression of class I and class II antigens on melanoma and cervical carcinoma cells

Cell line		Monoclonal antibody			
		Anti-HLA-DR	Anti-HLA-DC	Anti-HLA-ABC	Control
Melanoma	Me1477	4920 (2860)	1040 (320)	6780 (1550)	260 (125)
	GLL-19	140 (110)	130 (150)	3100 (1700)	125 (100)
	Me43	160 (170)	260 (130)	4200 (2900)	80 (60)
	IGR-3	2200 (1800)	200 (260)	5200 (1910)	230 (160)
Cervix ca	Me180	250 (210)	320 (220)	5100 (750)	240 (210)

Results are expressed as cpm bound of ^{125}I-labeled rabbit anti-mouse F(ab')2 antibodies to 10^5 target cells incubated with an excess of MoAbs; the numbers in parentheses are the cpm bound to untreated control cells tested in parallel. Cells were treated for 4 days with 10000 U/ml IFN-β

Table 5. Reversibility of IFN-γ-induced enhancement of class I and class II antigens expressed on melanoma Me43 cells

Monoclonal antibody	Untreated control cells	Cells treated for 4 days with 500 U/ml IFN-γ	Four days after treatment	Eight days after treatment
Anti-HLA-DR	120	1380	650	320
Anti-HLA-DC	140	1200	730	270
Anti-HLA-ABC	2700	5800	4600	3100
Anti-B2m	1900	5700	4400	3200
Control	120	110	130	120

Results are expressed as cpm bound of ^{125}I-labeled rabbit anti-mouse F(ab')2 antibodies to 10^5 target cells incubated with an excess of MoAbs cells, but also on several other neuroblastoma lines. This observation indicates that the induction of HLA-DR by IFN-γ is not a general phenomenon.

The molecular mechanisms by which interferons induce and/or increase the expression of surface antigens are poorly understood. It has been shown that the addition of IFN-γ to cultures of a mouse macrophage cell line leads to a tenfold increase in the level of mRNA coding for class II surface molecules [55]. It has also been reported that IFN-α enhances HLA-DR mRNA in each cell line which expresses HLA-DR antigens without increasing the expression of these antigens [56]. Thus, the question remains to what extent the absence of detectable HLA-DR and DQ antigens on the surface of certain solid tumor cells is due to a lack of class II mRNA or to an inhibition of translation. Alternatively, the enhancement of mRNA upon IFN-γ treatment might be restricted to the HLA-DRα, β, or invariant chain which would be produced in insufficient amounts for complete expression of the class II antigen complex. Finally, the expression of class II antigens could be modulated post-transcriptionally [57].

Functional Significance of Class II-Positive Tumor Cells

Very little is known about the functional properties of the class II antigens expressed on melanoma or other class II-positive nonlymphoid tumor cell lines.

Pollack [58] reported on a weak but significant stimulation of allogeneic lymphocytes by HLA-DR-positive melanoma cells. This response was at least partially dependent on the DR type of the responder cells used.

Table 6 shows some of our preliminary data obtained by unidirectional mixed lymphocyte tumor cell cultures (MLTC). Cells from three HLA-DR-positive melanoma cell lines were used as stimulators and peripheral blood lymphocytes (PBL) from seven different healthy donors as responders. Prior to stimulation, the stimulator tumor cells were pretreated with a standard dose of gamma irradiation (4000 R). Proliferation of the responder T cells was measured by ^{3}H-thymidine uptake after 5 days culture. Cells from the melanoma line Juso induced a significant proliferation of the lymphocytes from donors 4, 5, and 7, while Me312 melanoma cells stimulated the proliferation of lymphocytes of donors 1, 4, 5, and 7 and Me8 melanoma cells stimulated the proliferation of the lymphocytes from donors 5, 6, and 7.

Several authors have demonstrated that melanoma cells are capable of stimulating autologous T lymphocytes. Du Pont Guerry IV et al. [59] and Zehngebot et al. [60] showed that melanoma cells from early disease expressed HLA-DR antigens and stimulated autologous T cells, while those from advanced disease did not stimulate autologous T cells, irrespective of HLA-DR expression. In the early disease cases, the stimulatory capacity was proportional to the quantitative expression of HLA-DR antigens. Treatment of the stimulating cells with specific anti-DR serum showed marked inhibition in their capacity to induce blastogenesis. From these experiments it was concluded that expression of HLA-DR is necessary, but not sufficient, for melanoma cells to induce lymphocyte proliferation.

More recently, Fossati et al. [61] reported on positive autologous lymphocyte stimulation observed in all of six HLA-DR-positive primary melanomas, whereas two HLA-DR-negative primary melanomas were unable to stimulate autologous

Table 6. Stimulation of allogeneic lymphocytes by HLA-DR-positive melanoma cells

Responders (donor no.)	S:R ratio	Stimulator cells			
		Mel Juso	Me8	Me312	None
1	1:5	308 (−0.2)	363 (0.08)	*7237* (24)	270
	1:10	560 (1.0)	398 (0.63)	*5118* (175)	
2	1:5	595 (0.2)	1274 (1.1)	2459 (2.1)	847
	1:10	918 (0.7)	1233 (1.2)	1851 (1.7)	
3	1:5	3930 (1.0)	7493 (2.1)	1431 (0.2)	3329
	1:10	4321 (1.2)	5220 (1.5)	4219 (1.1)	
4	1:5	*19769* (40)	535 (0.4)	*4074* (7.1)	485
	1:10	*18227* (37)	1050 (1.7)	*2185* (3.7)	
5	1:5	*14709* (12)	*5001* (3.9)	*4574* (3.3)	1195
	1:10	*27767* (23)	1540 (1.1)	*4453* (3.4)	
6	1:5	*11121* (16)	*4102* (5.6)	1638 (1.5)	672
	1:10	*2970* (4)	1570 (2)	1264 (1.3)	
7	1:5	*16315* (14)	*3578* (3)	*8261* (6.7)	1139
	1:10	*9052* (7.7)	1593 (1.2)	*6085* (5)	
Medium	1:5	369	341	630	
Control	1:10	282	226	390	

Stimulator cells were irradiated with 4000 R. 10^5 PBL per well were cultured in 10% autologous serum. Results are expressed as Mean ^{3}H-thymidine incorporation (cpm), with the stimulation index $\left(\frac{\text{mean cpm in test} - \text{mean cpm of stimulators}}{\text{mean cpm of PBL alone}}\right)$ in parentheses.

lymphocytes. Anti-HLA-DR, but not anti-HLA-DC, MoAbs were able to block the proliferation of lymphocytes induced by autologous primary melanoma. No stimulation was obtained with either HLA-DR-positive or HLA-DR-negative metastatic melanoma. HLA-DR-positive metastatic melanoma cells were, however, able to stimulate allogeneic lymphocytes. These authors further showed that in vitro treatment of HLA-DR-positive primary melanoma cells with IFN-γ induced increased expression of HLA-DR antigens, which caused an increase in the proliferation of allogeneic but not of autologous lymphocytes.

The cytotoxic reactivity of lymphocytes for autologous melanoma cells has been studied by several investigators. In a group of 13 patients with recurrent or metastatic melanoma, Knuth et al. [62] observed no cytotoxicity with lymphocytes freshly isolated from peripheral blood or with lymphocytes cocultured for 7 days with autologous melanoma cells. Most interestingly, however, when these lymphocytes, previously sensitized with autologous melanoma cells in vitro, were cultured in medium containing interleukin-2 (IL-2), cytotoxic reactivity for autologous melanoma cells was observed in seven of the 13 patients. De Vries and Spits [63] reported that activation of PBL from a melanoma patient by cocultivation with autologous melanoma cells resulted in the generation of cytotoxic activity against the autologous melanoma cells. In terms of proliferation, only a slight increase in ^{3}H-thymidine incorporation was observed, with a stimulation index of 2.1.

In neither of the papers mentioned above is there any information about the expression of class II antigens by the stimulating tumor cells. In light of the results of Fossati et al. [61] and Knuth et al. [62], we think that it is mandatory in experiments along these lines to assess the class II cell surface phenotype of the stimulating cells.

Conclusions

From the present knowledge of human class II antigens expressed by nonlymphoid tumors, summarized in this chapter, it is evident that class II genes can be switched on and off depending upon the differentiation stage of a given cell type and its topographic tissue distribution in physiological as well as pathological conditions. The expression of class II genes seems to be under the control of factors encoded by regulatory gene(s) located outside the MHC [64]. The induction of expression of class II antigens by tumor cells might be of benefit for the control of tumor growth, if these antigens could help to "present" tumor-associated antigens to the T lymphocytes.

Primary melanomas often express relatively high levels of HLA-DR antigens and are commonly infiltrated with host T cells, while metastatic melanomas express only minimal or on HLA-DR antigens and are rarely infiltrated by T cells. Investigations of the in vitro interaction between melanoma cells and autologous lymphocytes showed that only HLA-DR-positive tumor cells from primary, and not from metastatic, tumors could stimulate autologous T lymphocytes. Expression of HLA-DR antigens by tumor cells appears therefore necessary, but not sufficient, for melanoma cells to induce T lymphocyte proliferation.

In vitro treatment of melanoma cells by IFN-γ was shown to induce the expression of HLA-DR antigens on DR-negative melanoma cells and to increase its expression on DR-positive cells. It has also been reported that such an increase of HLA-DR antigen expression can enhance lymphocyte proliferation [61]. These findings raise the question of whether treatment of melanoma patients with IFN-γ may help their immune system to recognize antigens on autologous tumor cells. It has also been shown in vitro that IFN-γ can enhance the expression of tumor-associated or differentiation antigens on melanoma cells [49, 53, 54]. If these in vitro observations can be reproduced in vivo, they would give a rationale for IFN-γ treatment of cancer patients.

References

1. Accolla RS, Moretta A, Mach JP (1984) The human Ia system: an overview. Semin Hematol 21:287–301
2. Hämmerling GJ, Mauve G, Goldberg E, McDevitt HO (1975) Tissue distribution of Ia antigens: Ia on spermatozoa, macrophages, and epidermal cells. Immunogenetics 1:428–437
3. Rowden G, Lewis MG, Sullivan AK (1977) Ia antigen expression on human epidermal Langerhans cells. Nature 268:247–248
4. Klarkeskog L, Tjernlund UM, Forsum U, Peterson PA (1977) Epidermal Langerhans cells express Ia antigens. Nature 268:248–250
5. Stingl G, Katz SI, Abelson LA, Mann DL (1978) Immunofluorescent detection of human B cell alloantigens on s-Ig-positive lymphocytes and epidermal Langerhans cells. J Immunol 120:661–664
6. Haines KA, Flotte TJ, Springer TA, Gigli I, Thonbecke GJ (1983) Staining of Langerhans cells with monoclonal antibodies to macrophages and lymphoid cells. Proc Natl Acad Sci USA 80:3448–3451

7. Winchester RJ, Wang C, Gibofsky A, Kunkel HG, Lloyd KO, Old LJ (1978) Expression of Ia-like antigens on cultured human malignant melanoma cell lines. Proc Natl Acad Sci USA 75:6235–6239
8. Wilson BS, Indiven F, Pellegrino MA, Ferrone S (1979) DR (Ia-like) antigens on human melanoma cells. Serological detection and immunochemical characterization. J Exp Med 149:658–668
9. Natali PG, de Martino C, Quaranta V, Bigotti A, Pellegrino MA, Ferrone S (1981) Changes in Ia-like antigen expression on malignant human cells. Immunogenetics 12:409–413
10. Lloyd KO, Ng J, Dippold WH (1981) Analysis of the biosynthesis of HLA-DR glycoproteins in human malignant melanoma cell lines. J Immunol 126:2408–2413
11. Mitchell KF, Ward FE, Koprowski H (1982) DR antigens on melanoma cells: analysis with monoclonal antibodies. Human Immunol 4:15–26
12. Thompson JJ, Herlyn MF, Elder DE, Clark WH, Steplewski Z, Koprowski H (1982) Expression of DR antigens in freshly frozen human tumors. Hybridoma 1:161–168
13. Carrel S, Gross N, Heumann D, Mach JP (1979) Expression of "Ia-like" antigens on cells from a human endometrial carcinoma cell line END-1. Transplantation 27:431–433
14. Carrel S, Tosi R, Gross N, Tanigaki N, Carmagnola AL, Accolla RS (1981) Subsets of human Ia-like molecules defined by monoclonal antibodies. Mol Immunol 18:403–411
15. Pollack MS, Heagney SD, Livingston PO, Fogh J (1981) HLA-A,B,C and DR alloantigen expression of forty-six cultured human tumor cell lines. J Natl Cancer Inst 66:1003–1012
16. MacLean GD, Seehafer J, Shaw ARE, Kieran MW, Longenecker BM (1982) Antigenic heterogeneity of human colorectal cancer cell lines analyzed by a panel of monoclonal antibodies I. Heterogeneous expression of Ia-like and HLA-like antigenic determinants. J Natl Cancer Inst 69:357–364
17. Guesdon JL, Ternynck T, Avrameas S (1979) The use of avidin-biotin interaction in immunoenzymatic techniques. J Histochem Cytochem 27:1131–1139
18. Carrel S, Schreyer M, Schmidt-Kessen A, Mach JP (1982) Reactivity spectrum of 30 monoclonal antimelanoma antibodies to a panel of 28 melanoma and control cell lines. Hybridoma 1:387–397
19. Poste G, Doll J, Fidler J (1981) Interactions among clonal subpopulations affect stability of the metastatic phenotype in polyclonal populations of B16 melanoma cells. Proc Natl Acad Sci USA 78:6226–6230
20. Daar AS, Fuggle SV, Ting A, Fabre JW (1982) Anomolous expression of HLA-DR antigens on human colorectal cancer cells. J Immunol 129:447–449
21. Natali PG, Giacomini P, Bigotti A, Imai K, Nicotra MR, Ng AK, Ferrone S (1983) Heterogeneity in the expression of HLA and tumor-associated antigens by surgically removed and cultured breast carcinoma cells. Cancer Res 43:660–668
22. de Tribolet N, Carrel S, Mach JP (1984) Brain-tumor-associated antigens. Prog Exp Tumor Res 27:118–131
23. de Tribolet N, Hamou MF, Mach JP, Carrel S, Schreyer M (1984) Demonstration of HLA-DR antigens in normal human brain. J Neurol Neurosurg Psychiatry 47:417–418
24. Berle EJ, Braathen LR, Throsby E (1982) HLA-D/DR restriction of Langerhans cell-dependent antigen activation of T lymphocytes. Scand J Immunol 16:549–552
25. Pollack MS, Goldenhersh M, Chin-Louie J, Safai B (1982) The functional study of DR-positive human epidermal Langerhans cells in mixed cell cultures with allogeneic lymphocytes. Clin Immunol Immunopathol 24:12–25
26. Howe AJ, Seeger RC, Molinaro GA, Ferrone S (1981) Analysis of human tumor cells for Ia-like antigens with monoclonal antibodies. J Natl Cancer Inst 60:827–829
27. Lloyd KO, Ng J, Dippold WG (1981) Analysis of the biosynthesis of HLA-DR glycoproteins in human malignant melanoma cell lines. J Immunol 126:2408–2413
28. Natali PG, Bigotti A, Nicotra MR, Viora M, Manfredi D, Ferrone S (1984) Distribution of human class I (HLA-A,B,C) histocompatibility antigens in normal and malignant tissues of nonlymphoid origin. Cancer Res 44:4679–4687

29. Ruiter DJ, Bergman K, Welvaart K, Scheffer E, von Vloten WA, Russo C, Ferrone S (1984) Immunohistochemical analysis of malignant melanomas and nevocellular nevi with monoclonal antibodies to distinct monomorphic determinants of HLA antigens. Cancer Res 44:3930–3935
30. Pollack MS, Heagney SD, Livingston PO, Fogh J (1981) HLA-A,B,C and DR alloantigen expression of forty-six cultured human tumor cell lines. J Natl Cancer Inst 66:1003–1012
31. Carrel S, de Tribolet N, Gross N (1982) expression of HLA-DR and common acute lymphoblastic leukemia antigens on glioma cells. Eur J Immunol 12:354–357
32. Daar AS, Fabre JW (1983) The membrane antigens of human colorectal cancer cells: demonstration with monoclonal antibodies of heterogeneity within and between tumors and anomalous expression of HLA-DR. Eur J Cancer Clin Oncol 19:209–220
33. Shackelford DA, Strominger JL (1983) Analysis of the oligosaccharides on the HLA-DR and DC1 B cell antigens. J Immunol 130:274
34. Tosi R, Tanigaki N, Centis D, Ferrara GB, Pressman D (1978) Immunological dissection of human Ia molecules. J Exp Med 148:1592–1611
35. Corte G, Damiani G, Calabi F, Fabbi M, Bargellesi A (1981) Analysis of HLA-DR polymorphism by two-dimensional peptide mapping. Proc Natl Acad Sci USA 78:534–558
36. Accolla RS, Gross N, Carrel S, Corte G (1981) Distinct forms of both α and β subunits are present in the human Ia molecular pool. Proc Natl Acad Sci USA 78:4549–4551
37. Accolla RS (1983) Analysis of the structural heterogeneity and polymorphism of human Ia antigens. J Exp Med 159:378–393
38. Wake CT, Long EO, Strubin M, Gross N, Accolla RS, Carrel S, Mach B (1982) Isolation of c-DNA clones encoding HLA-DR chains. Proc Natl Acad Sci USA 79:6979–6983
39. Alexander S, Hubbard SC, Strominger JL (1984) HLA-DR antigens of autologous melanoma and B lymphoblastoid cell lines: differences in glycosylation but not protein structure. J Immunol 133:315–320
40. Cillo C, Mach JP, Schreyer M, Carrel S (1984) Antigenic heterogeneity of clones and subclones from human melanoma cell lines demonstrated by a panel of monoclonal antibodies and flow microfluorometry analysis. Int J Cancer 34:11–20
41. Fidler IJ (1978) Tumor heterogeneity and the biology of cancer invasion and metastasis. Cancer Res 38:2651–2660
42. Fidler IJ, Hart IR (1982) Biological diversity in metastatic neoplasms: origins and implication. Science 217:998–1003
43. Woodruff MFA (1983) Cellular heterogeneity in tumors. Br J Cancer 47:589–594
44. Nicolson GL (1984) Cell surface molecules and tumor metastasis. Exp Cell Research 150:3–22
45. Lindahl P, Leary P, Gresser I (1972) Enhancement by interferon of the expression of surface antigens on murine leukemia L1210 cells. Proc Natl Acad Sci USA 69:721–723
46. Heron I, Hokland M, Berg K (1978) Enhanced expression of B2-microglobulin and HLA antigens on human lymphoid cells by interferon. Proc Natl Acad Sci USA 75:6215–6219
47. Fellous M, Kamoun M, Gresser I, Bono R (1979) Enhanced expression of HLA antigens and beta 2 microglobulin on interferon-treated human lymphoid cells. Eur J Immunol 9:446–449
48. Kelley VE, Fiers W, Strom TB (1984) Cloned human interferon-γ but not interferon-α or β induces expression of HLA-DR determinants by fetal monocytes and myeloid leukemic cell lines. J Immunol 132:240–245
49. Imai K, Ng AK, Glassy MC, Ferrone S (1981) Differential effect of interferon on the expression of tumor-associated antigens and histocompatibility antigens on human melanoma cells: relationship to susceptibility to immune lysis mediated by monoclonal antibodies. J Immunol 127:505–508
50. Liao SK, Kurong PC, Khosravi M, Dent PB (1982) Enhanced expression of melanoma-associated antigens and B2-microglobulin on cultured human melanoma cells by interferons. J Natl Cancer Inst 68:19–25

51. Basham TY, Merigan TC (1983) Recombinant interferon-γ increases HLA-DR synthesis and expression. J Immunol 130:1492–1494
52. Ziegler A, Uchaneka-Ziegler B, Rosenfelder G, Braun DG, Wernet P (1981) Heterogeneity of established human hematopoietic cell lines: surface antigens detected by monoclonal antibodies and glycosphingolipid patterns. In: Leukemia markers. Knapp, Düsseldorf, pp 317–320
53. Carrel S, Schmidt-Kessen A, Giuffrè L (1985) Recombinant interferon-γ can induce the expression of HLA-DR and -DC on DR-negative melanoma cells and enhance the expression of HLA-ABC and tumor associated antigens. Eur J Immunol 15:118–123
54. Houghton AN, Thomson TM, Gross D, Oettgen HF, Old LJ (1984) Surface antigens of melanomas and melanocytes. Specificity of induction of Ia antigens by human γ-interferon. J Exp Med 160:255–269
55. Nakamura M, Mauser T, Pearson GPN, Daley MJ, Geffer ML (1984) Effect of IFN-γ on the immune response in vivo and on gene expression in vitro. Nature 307:381–382
56. Rosa F, Hatat D, Abadie A, Wallach D, Revel M, Fellous M (1983) Differential regulation of HLA-DR mRNAs and cell surface antigens by interferon. EMBO J 2:1585–1589
57. Reitz MS, Mann DL, Eiden M, Trainor CD, Clarke MF (1984) DNA methylation and expression of HLA-DR. Mol Cell Biol 4:890–897
58. Pollack MS (1981) The detection of weak allogeneic stimulation by DR-positive cell lines. Transplant Proc 13:1947–1951
59. Du Pont Guerry IV D, Zehngebot LM, Mitchel KF, Zmijewski CM, Lask EJ (1984) HLA-DR histocompatibility leukocyte antigens permit cultured human melanoma cells from early but not advanced disease to stimulate autologous lymphocytes. J Clin Invest 73:267–271
60. Zehngebot LM, Alexander MA, Guerry IV D, Cines DB, Mitchell K, Herlyn M (1983) Functional consequence of variation in melanoma antigen expression. Cancer Immunol Immunother 16:30–34
61. Fossati G, Taramelli D, Balsari A, Bogdanovich G, Andreola S, Parmiani G (1984) Primary but not metastatic human melanomas expressing DR antigens stimulate autologous lymphocytes. Int J Cancer 33:591–597
62. Knuth A, Danowski B, Oettgen HF, Old LJ (1984) T-cell-mediated cytotoxicity against autologous malignant melanoma: analysis with interleukin-2-dependent T-cell cultures. Proc Natl Acad Sci USA 81:3511–3515
63. de Vries JE, Spits H (1984) Cloned human cytotoxic T lymphocyte (CTL) lines reactive with autologous melanoma cells. I. In vitro generation, isolation, and analysis to phenotype and specificity. J Immunol 132:510–519
64. Accolla R S(1983) Human B cell variants immunoselected against a single Ia antigen subset have lost expression of several Ia antigen subsets. J Exp Med 157:1053–1058

Class II HLA Antigens in Benign and Malignant Lesions of Melanocytic Origin *

D. J. Ruiter, S. G. van Duinen, M. Tsujisaki, and S. Ferrone

Table of Contents

Introduction

Following the unexpected detection of immunologically functional class II HLA antigens on melanoma cells in long-term culture [1, 2], several investigators have analyzed the expression of these antigens by surgically removed benign and malignant lesions of melanocytic origin [3–6]. These studies have been facilitated by the availability of monoclonal antibodies (MoAbs) which have contributed to the application of immunohistochemical techniques.

Detection of class II HLA antigens in melanoma has both theoretical relevance and practical implications. Characterization of class II HLA antigens expressed by melanoma cells can contribute to our understanding of the role of immunologic factors in the biology and in the clinical course of melanoma. Furthermore, detection of class II HLA antigens in melanoma may have practical implications, since these antigens have been suggested to be a useful marker to discriminate between benign and malignant lesions of melanocytic origin and to provide useful information for the prognosis of the disease. The aim of this chapter is threefold:

1. To describe the MoAbs and the methodology used by the various investigators to analyze the expression of class II HLA antigens in surgically removed lesions of melanocytic origin
2. To review the information available in the literature about the distribution
3. To discuss the biological and clinical significance of these findings

* This work was supported by NIH grants A121384 and CA38469, by a grant from the Cancer Research Institute, New York, NY, USA, and by the Netherlands Foundation for the Fight against Cancer

Anti-Class II HLA MoAbs and Immunohistochemical Techniques

A number of MoAbs have been utilized to characterize class II HLA antigens in melanoma [7–20]. For most of the antibodies used, it is not known whether the corresponding determinants are restricted to HLA-DR, DQ, or DP antigens or are shared by the gene products of the various loci of the HLA-D region. In view of the differential distribution in normal and malignant tissues of HLA-DR, DQ, and DP antigens (P. G. Natali, personal communication) one should exercise caution when comparing results obtained with different antibodies. Most of the anti-class II HLA antibodies tested during a recent workshop recognize determinants shared by HLA-DR and DP antigens, a few are restricted to HLA-DR or DQ antigens [18, 19]. Only one antibody, MoAb VIC-Y, recognizes the γ-chain of class II HLA antigens, which is detectable only in cytoplasm [20]. Limited information is available about the specificity of the other antibodies on tissue sections [14, 21]. The majority of the antibodies used react only with frozen tissues: only a limited number (i.e., MoAbs 3.87, SG520, and CR3.43) react with formalin-fixed paraffin-embedded tissues [13, 14].

Immunohistochemical analysis of normal tissues, and especially of melanocytic lesions, requires special conditions. An immunoenzyme technique is preferred to immunofluorescence, because better information about the morphology is obtained, especially if nuclear counterstaining is performed [4]. In order to avoid confusion with melanin pigment, the use of 3-amino-ethylcarbazole is advocated, giving a red staining product [4]. For the detection of small amounts of antigen, amplification techniques or alternatively the avidin-biotin technique can be used [22]. In sections of normal skin, Langerhans cells and sweat duct epithelium can be used as an internal control [23]. Staining of endothelial cells is too variable to be useful for this purpose.

Distribution of Class II HLA Antigens in Melanocytic Lesions

Class II HLA antigens have not been detected either in normal melanocytes in tissue sections or in cultured melanocytes [3–5, 15, 24–26]. However, melanocytes acquire class II HLA antigens following in vitro incubation with recombinant immune interferon (IFN-γ) [27]. Three lines of evidence indicate that HLA-DR antigens are more susceptible to induction by IFN-γ than HLA-DQ antigens: (a) the percentage of melanocytes which acquire HLA-DQ antigens is lower than that acquiring HLA-DR antigens; (b) the appearance of HLA-DQ antigens is delayed as compared to HLA-DR antigens; (c) the dose of IFN-γ required to induce the expression of the latter is lower than for the former. These results are at variance with those of Mach [27], who reported a coordinate regulation of HLA-DR, DQ, and DP genes by IFN-γ. This discrepancy can be reconciled by postulating that both transcriptional and posttranscriptional events play a role in the IFN-γ-induced enhancement of the cell surface expression of class II HLA antigens. Melanocytes from various donors differ in their sensitivity to IFN-γ. The effects of IFN-γ are dose- and time-dependent. Representative examples are shown in Fig. 1. It is noteworthy that class II HLA antigens are not detected in a subpopulation of melanocytes treated with IFN-γ. Whether this subpopulation represents melanocytes with a level of class II HLA antigens below the sensitivity

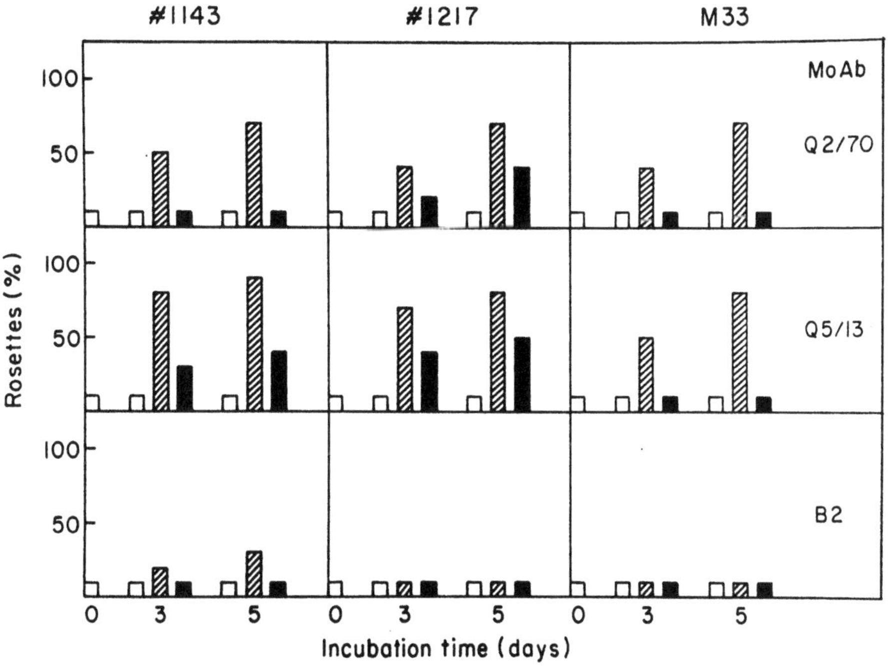

Fig. 1. Reactivity in the mixed hemadsorption assay of control (□) and IFN-γ treated melanocytes from three donors with the anti-HLA-DR MoAb Q2/70, with the anti-HLA-DR + DQ DP MoAb Q5/13, and with the anti-HLA-DQ MoAb B2.
Melanocytes were incubated with IFN-γ [Final concentration 500 U/ml (■) or 1000 U/ml (■)]. The mixed hemadsorption was performed as described by Metzgar and Oleinick [69]

of the assay used, cells which do not express receptors for IFN-γ, or cells at a stage of differentiation unable to express class II HLA antigens is not known at present. The appearance of class II HLA antigens on melanocytes is reversible, since melanocytes which have acquired class II HLA antigens following incubation with IFN-γ lose these antigens following incubation with IFN-γ free medium [28]. The molecular profile of class II HLA antigens synthesized by melanocytes in the presence of IFN-γ is similar to that of B lymphoid cell-derived class II HLA antigens. The effect of IFN-γ is not specific for melanocytes, since a similar phenomenon has been described for a variety of cell types, including endothelial cells, dermal fibroblasts, keratinocytes, fetal monocytes, normal and leukemic myeloid cells, and a variety of tumor cell lines of nonlymphoid origin [27, 29–35]. The effect of IFN-γ on melanocytes is not restricted to class II HLA antigens, since it also induces a melanoma-associated antigen with the apparent molecular weight of 100 K.

With the exception of one report [36], there appears to be general agreement about the absence of class II HLA antigens in common nevocellular nevi. However, in nevocellular nevi with congenital characteristics scattered class II HLA positive dendritic cells may be found amidst negative nevocellular nevus cells [26]. The nature of these cells is not known; they are not stained by the majority of MoAbs to melanoma-associated antigens tested or by MoAb OKT6 [26], which is a marker for Langerhans cells [37]. In two halo nevi we have observed focal class II HLA-positive nevus cell nests, especially those invaded by T lymphocytes

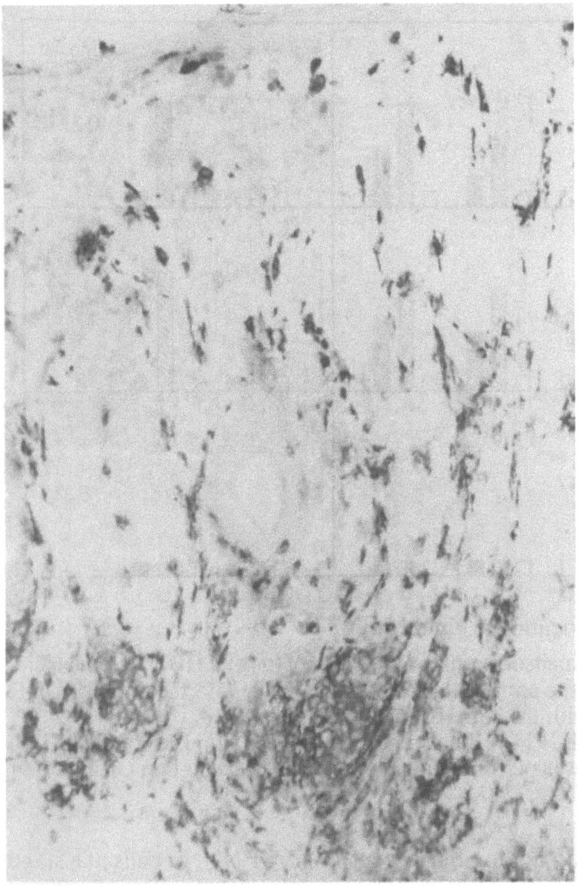

Fig. 2. Primary cutaneous melanoma showing focal staining with the MoAb Q2/70 of HLA-DR antigens at the lower margin of the tumor. Frozen section, two-step immunoperoxidase procedure with nuclear counterstaining. × 160

[38]. One of the positive lesions showed marked atypia of nevocellular cells and was therefore considered as a dysplastic nevus with marked regression resulting in the clinical appearance of halo nevus. Focal staining for class II HLA antigens is reported in few dysplastic nevi [5, 6, 26, 39]. It was striking in our series that the two positive lesions showed marked nevocellular atypia [39]. With the exception of one study [25], focal staining for class II HLA antigens is reported in about 35% of primary cutaneous melanoma lesions (Fig. 2), and diffuse staining in about 10%. Remarkably, Bröcker et al. [13] found an increased proportion of melanoma cells stained by anti-class II HLA MoAbs in tumors with a Breslow thickness of 1.5 mm or more. The highest percentage of class II HLA-positive primary melanoma lesions was found in the group of melanomas invading the reticular dermis (Clark level IV). The mononuclear cell infiltrate within the primary melanoma lesions was more often marked in class II HLA-positive than in class II HLA-negative melanomas.

In large series of melanoma metastases the majority of lesions studied show expression of class II HLA antigens. Based on our own experience, about 35% of the lesions show staining sporadically, 55% locally, and 10% diffusely [40]. Staining tends to be in the peripheral zones of the tumors and perivascular (Fig. 3).

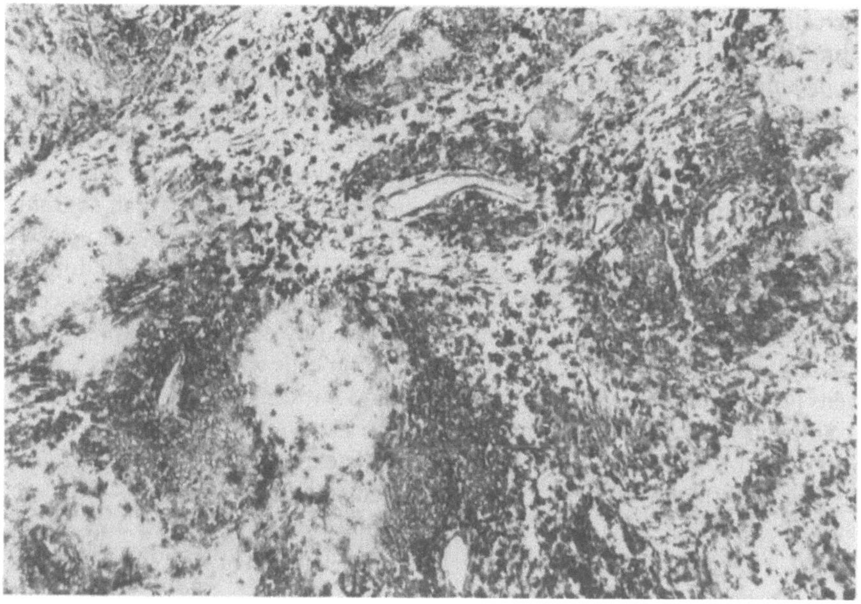

Fig. 3. Melanoma metastasis showing perivascular staining for HLA-DR antigens using the MoAb Q2/70. Frozen section, two-step immunoperoxidase procedure with nuclear counterstaining. ×160

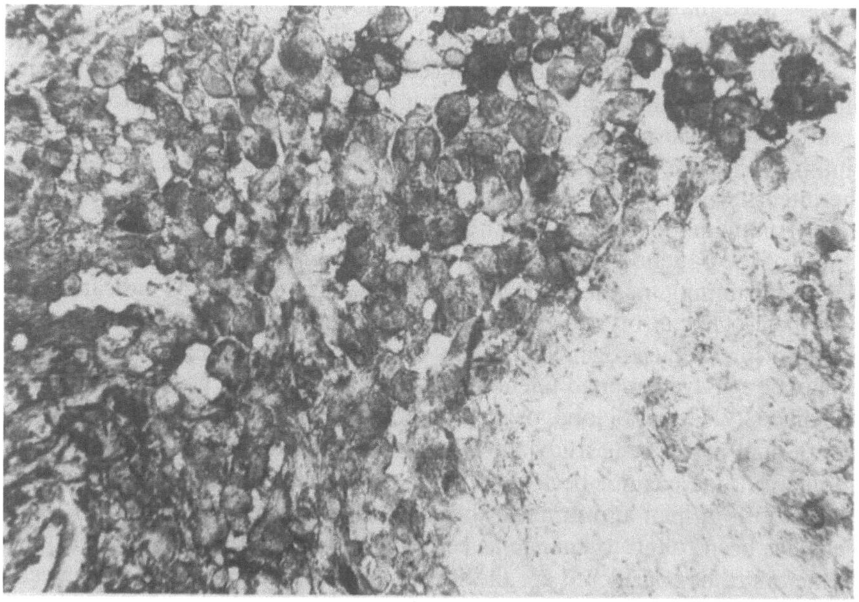

Fig. 4. Melanoma cells showing both diffuse intracellular and peripheral staining for class II HLA antigens using the MoAb Q2/70. Note the sharp demarcation towards the area with negative tumor cells. Frozen section, two-step immunoperoxidase procedure with nuclear counterstaining. ×400

The cellular distribution of class II HLA antigens in melanoma cells is both membrane-bound and cytoplasmic as illustrated in Fig. 4. The discrimination between melanoma cells stained and other non-neoplastic cells in the tumor stroma, such as macrophages and dendritic cells, may be difficult, even in counterstained sections. In our own experience, the percentage of melanoma cells expressing class II HLA antigens is mostly lower, occasionally equal to, that of those expressing class I HLA antigens [26, 40]. Thus far we have found no lesion which contains more melanoma cells stained by anti-class II HLA MoAbs than by anti-class I HLA MoAbs. Furthermore, analysis of individual melanoma cells with double-labeling immunofluorescence and double-labeling immunoelectron microscopy has shown that class II HLA antigens are expressed by cells which express class I HLA antigens and are rarely, if at all, detected on cells which lack class I HLA antigens [41]. We have identified three expression patterns of class II and class I HLA antigens in melanoma lesions [40]:

Pattern A: More than 50% of melanoma cells express class I HLA antigens (high expression) and 50% or less express class II HLA antigens (low expression)

Pattern B: Low expression of class I HLA and low expression of class II HLA

Pattern C: High expression of class I HLA and high expression of class II HLA.

As indicated earlier, the theoretically possible pattern D has not been observed. Pattern A was found in about 40% of melanoma metastases, pattern B in 50%, and pattern C in 10% [40]. HLA antigen expression patterns B or C were found in a significant ($p < 0.01$) number of melanoma metastases containing 50% or less tumor cells stained by the MoAb M2-2-4 [40], which recognizes a melanoma-associated antigen that is largely present on melanocytic lesions [42].

Like other types of tumor-associated antigens [11, 17], class II HLA antigens have a variable expression on melanoma cells. This heterogeneity occurs among lesions isolated from different patients, among autologous lesions removed from different anatomic sites from one patient [43], and especially among cells within a lesion [44, 45]. The level of expression of class II HLA antigens, as measured by the intensity of staining, does not appear to correlate with the presence of melanin. It remains to be seen whether the anatomic site of the lesion and the treatment of the patient have an influence on the degree of staining. However, if the degree of staining for HLA antigens is expressed in patterns as indicated earlier [40], heterogeneity of these staining patterns among various autologous lesions is limited. The heterogeneity is likely to reflect several mechanisms. Among them may be cell-cycle-related phenomena, polyclonal origin, generation of phenotype diversity within a clone, or spontaneous hybridization and chromosome loss. Although in a recent study the expression of class II HLA antigens on a melanoma cell line has not been found to be cell-cycle-dependent [45], in other cell types, both in man and in mice, the cell surface expression of class II HLA antigens has been found to change as cells move through the growth cycle [46]. Other factors to be considered are the stage of differentiation of melanoma cells and the neoplastic evolution of tumor cells to more aggressive variants (i.e., tumor progression) [47].

There is limited information about the expression of HLA-DR, DQ, and DP antigens in primary and metastatic melanoma lesions. In a recent study in our laboratory, analysis of four primary melanoma lesions and seven metastatic lesions with MoAbs specific for the gene products of the three loci of the HLA-D region has shown that in surgically removed lesions, as in melanoma cells in long-term culture [48], HLA-DR antigens are expressed more frequently than HLA-DQ antigens. HLA-DP antigens have an intermediate frequency. Five melanoma lesions were found to express the phenotype HLA-DR-positive, HLA-DQ-negative, HLA-DP-positive; and one HLA-DR-positive, HLA-DQ-negative, HLA-DP-negative. The phenotype HLA-DR-negative, HLA-DQ-negative, HLA-DP-positive was not detected in any lesion.

Biological and Clinical Implications

The information in the literature we have reviewed clearly indicates that malignant transformation of melanocytes may be associated with the appearance of class II HLA antigens. The frequency of the phenomenon ranges from 10% to 100% of the melanoma lesions tested. This variability is likely to reflect a number of factors. Among them are the nature of the lesion, (e.g., tumor thickness, tumor cell type), tumor heterogeneity, sampling of lesions, differences in sensitivity of the assays used, and the difficulties in discriminating tumor cells from other stained cells in tissue sections [26]. Although in our own experience the staining patterns of melanocytic lesions with a number of MoAbs to distinct monomorphic determinants of class II HLA antigens selected for reactivity on normal skin have been superimposable [26], the role of the specificity of the antibodies cannot be excluded because of the differential expression of HLA-DR, DQ, and DP antigens in melanoma lesions.

Several mechanisms may be suggested for the expression of class II HLA antigens in melanoma. This phenomenon may reflect the derepression of genes coding for class II HLA antigens in malignant cells, as documented for embryonal enzymes and antigens in tumor cells [49]. Alternatively, the appearance of class II HLA antigens may reflect the expression of these antigens at the particular stage of differentiation within the melanocytic lineage [50], as occurs on cells of the myeloid lineage [51]. Finally, the induction of class II HLA antigens in melanocytes by IFN-γ suggests a similar mechanism for the expression of class II HLA antigens by melanoma cells [27]. Whatever the mechanism, it should be noted that the association between appearance of class II HLA antigens and malignant transformation of cells is not restricted to melanoma, but occurs in a variety of cell lineages [52]. However, the phenomenon is markedly more frequent in melanoma than in other types of malignancies. This may be related to the presence of an often dense adjacent mononuclear infiltrate, that has been shown to consist mainly of T (both helper/inducer and cytotoxic/suppressor) lymphocytes [4, 25, 53]. Two studies have investigated the functional properties of class II HLA antigens synthesized by melanoma cells by determining their ability to induce the proliferation of allogeneic and autologous T cells [54, 55]. Both studies have shown that melanoma cells from primary lesions which express class II HLA antigens can induce the proliferation of both autologous and allogeneic T lymphocytes. On the other hand, class II HLA antigen-bearing melanoma cells from metastatic lesions can stimulate allogeneic T cells, but do not stimulate autologous T cells. The authors have concluded that expression of class II HLA antigens by melanoma cells is necessary, but not sufficient, to induce proliferation of autologous T cells in in vitro cultures [54, 55]. The role of HLA-DR, DQ, and DP antigens in the stimulation of T cells by melanoma cells is not known, since the antibodies used to analyze the expression of class II HLA antigens have not been characterized in their reactivity with the gene products of the HLA-D region. Limited information is available about the mechanism(s) underlying the differential stimulatory activity of melanoma cells from primary and metastatic lesions. Recently, Taramelli et al. [56] have reported that melanoma cells from metastatic lesions display a suppressive effect on responding lymphocytes, but do not absorb or inactivate interleukin-2. An alternative mechanism suggested by the differential expression of HLA-DR and DQ antigens in melanoma lesions and by the reported role of the latter antigens in autologous mixed lymphocyte reactions [57] is the lack of expression of HLA-DQ antigens by the melanoma cells isolated from the metastatic lesions tested. Limited information is available about the ability of class II HLA antigen-bearing melanoma cells to present soluble antigens to antigen-reactive T cells [48]. Results obtained with other types of tumor cells which express class II HLA antigens [58, 59] suggest that melanoma cells may be able to present antigens. In view of the effect of class II HLA antigens on the immunogenicity of leukemia-associated antigens [60] and of the reduced immunogenicity in xenogeneic combinations of human melanoma-associated antigens expressed by cells which lack class II HLA antigens [61], it will be of interest to determine whether class II HLA antigens influence the immunogenicity of human melanoma-associated antigens in autologous combinations.

No comparison has been published between the phenotypes of class II HLA antigens synthesized by melanoma cells and by autologous B lymphoid cells. This lack of information probably reflects the lack of MoAbs to class II HLA allospecificities and the difficulties in analyzing surgically removed tissues with conventional anti-HLA alloantisera. Although analysis of the HLA phenotype of a limited number of melanoma cell lines in long-term culture has not identified any genetically unorthodox HLA-D coded allospecificity [52], it will be of interest to compare the HLA phenotype of surgically removed melanoma lesions with that of autologous normal tissues, since changes in the HLA phenotype have been described in cells which have undergone malignant transformation [62].

Because of the differential distribution in benign and malignant lesions of melanocyte origin, it has been suggested that class II HLA antigens may be a useful marker in the differential diagnosis of melanocytic lesions. However, class II HLA antigens have been found locally in few dysplastic nevi with marked atypia [26]. Moreover, from a practical viewpoint, the low number of melanocytic cells stained by anti-class II HLA MoAbs in most primary cutaneous melanomas reduces the usefulness of class II HLA antigens for diagnostic purposes [26].

The quantitation of class II HLA antigens in melanoma lesions may provide some useful information for prognosis, since quantitative variation in class II HLA antigen expression plays a central role in immune regulation [63], and progression of malignancy appears to be associated with an increase in the number of melanoma cells expressing these antigens [13, 26]. Thus Bröcker et al. [13] reported an increased expression of class II HLA antigens in primary lesions with a Breslow thickness higher than 1.5 mm and in those which gave rise to early metastases. We have found a higher percentage of melanoma cells stained by anti-class II HLA MoAbs in metastases than in primary lesions [26]. Furthermore, we have found a relationship between the level of expression of class II HLA antigens in metastases and the survival of patients with melanoma metastases [40]. Specifically, a significantly shorter survival has been found when metastases express a high or a low level of both class II and class I HLA antigens than when a low expression of class II HLA antigens is associated with a high level of class I HLA antigens [40]. The significance of this finding is strengthened by the lack of correlation between expression of HLA antigens in melanoma lesions and other known prognostic parameters, i.e. number of metastases, tumor thickness, and ulceration of primary cutaneous melanoma [64]. No simple explanation can be offered to account for the association between increase in the expression of class II HLA antigens and progression in malignancy. Expression of class II HLA antigens by melanoma cells may reflect an arrest in their differentiation which results in an increase in their malignancy. Alternatively, expression of class II HLA antigens by melanoma cells may influence their interaction with the host immune system by generating suppressor T cells and/or by inducing the formation of antibodies which protect tumor cells from immune attack. Finally, class II HLA antigens may mediate cell-cell interactions, leading to the production of factors which promote tumor growth.

Conclusions

Only a few years have passed since the unexpected appearance of class II HLA antigens on melanoma cells was first described. However, a relatively large amount of knowledge has already accumulated. This information contributes to the characterization of the regulatory mechanism(s) which control the expression of class II HLA antigens and of their functional properties. Furthermore, if additional studies with large numbers of patients confirm the prognostic significance of the level of class II HLA antigens in melanoma lesions, then quantitation of these antigens is likely to become a routine procedure in surgical pathology. These approaches will be greatly facilitated by the development of anti-class II HLA MoAbs which react with paraffin-embedded tissues.

Several questions remain to be answered for a complete characterization of the biological profile, functional properties, and clinical relevance of class II HLA antigens synthesized by melanoma cells. Some of these questions, relating to the serological polymorphism, functional properties and clinical significance of class II HLA antigens in melanoma, have been discussed above. We will conclude this chapter by discussing some questions that are of great interest to us and some of the technical problems an investigator faces when studying class II HLA antigens in surgically removed lesions of melanocyte origin.

The gene products of the three loci of the HLA-D region appear to have a differential distribution in melanoma lesions, but how does the class II HLA phenotype correlate with the metastasizing properties of melanoma cells and with the clinical course of the disease? Are the class II HLA allospecificities all genetically appropriate? If inappropriate allospecificities are expressed by melanoma cells, are they immunogenic in the host? Does immunity to these antigens influence the clinical course of the disease? HLA-DR antigens synthesized by two melanoma cell lines have been found to differ from those synthesized by autologous B lymphoid cells in their carbohydrate composition [65, 66], but does this reflect a general phenomenon, and does it occur also with HLA-DQ and DP antigens? Do these abnormalities play any role in the interaction of melanoma cells with other cells, since carbohydrates on class II HLA antigens may mediate carbohydrate-specific recognition, as described in a number of mammalian systems [67]?. Do changes in the glycosylation of class II HLA antigens affect their antigenic profile, since we have shown that carbohydrates may influence the antigenic profile of class I HLA antigens [68]? How do the functional properties of class II HLA antigens synthesized by melanoma cells compare with those of class II HLA antigens synthesized by immune cells? Can melanoma cells in lesions not stained by anti-class II HLA MoAbs be induced to express these antigens? Are melanoma cells from primary lesions and from metastases from various anatomic sites equally susceptible to modulation in the expression of class II HLA antigens by modulators such as interferons?

Can the testing of melanoma lesions for class II HLA antigens provide any information which cannot be obtained with conventional histopathological techniques? Is the appearance of class II histocompatibility antigens in melanoma restricted to the human species or does this also occur in other animal species? The latter information is not only interesting from a phylogenetic view point, but will also aid in the selection of animal models for experiments which cannot be performed in man for ethical reasons.

A major factor in the analysis of class II HLA antigens in surgically removed melanoma lesions has been the availability of MoAbs, which have greatly facilitated the application of immunohistochemical techniques. However, the lack of reactivity of most of the available antibodies with paraffin-embedded tissues as opposed to cryostat sections has hampered the extensive application of this approach and has been an obstacle to retrospective studies utilizing the collections of tissues available in most departments of pathology.

References

1. Winchester RJ, Wang CY, Gibofsky A, Kunkel HG, Lloyd KO, Old LJ (1978) Expression of class II HLA on cultured human malignant melanoma cell lines. Proc Natl Acad Sci USA 75:6235–6239
2. Wilson BS, Indiveri F, Pellegrino MA, Ferrone S (1979) DR (Ia-like) antigens on human melanoma cells. Serological detection and immunochemical characterisation. J Exp Med 148:658–668
3. Natali PG, Cordiali Fei P, Cavaliere R, Di Filippo F, Quaranta V, Pellegrino MG, Ferrone S (1981) Class II HLA on freshly explanted human malignant melanoma. Detection with MoAb and correlation with clinical parameters. Clin Immunol Immunopathol 19:250–259
4. Ruiter DJ, Bhan AK, Harrist TJ, Sober AJ, Mihm MC Jr (1982) Major histocompatibility antigens and mononuclear inflammatory infiltrate in benign nevomelanocytic proliferations and malignant melanoma. J Immunol 129:2808–2815
5. Thompson JJ, Herlyn MF, Elder DE, Clark WH, Steplewski Z, Koprowski H (1982) Use of MoAb in detection of melanoma-associated antigens in intact human tumors. Am J Pathol 107:357–361
6. Thompson JJ, Herlyn MF, Elder DE, Clark WH, Steplewski Z, Koprowski H (1982) Expression of DR antigens in freshly frozen human tumors. Hybridoma 1:161–168
7. Ng AK, Pellegrino MA, Imai K, Ferrone S (1981) HLA-A,B antigens, class II HLA, and tumor associated antigens on prostate carcinoma cell lines: serologic and immunochemical analysis with MoAb. J Immunol 127:443–447

8. Quaranta V, Pellegrino MA, Ferrone S (1981) Serological and immunochemical characterization of the specificity of four MoAb to distinct determinants expressed on subpopulations of human class II HLA. J Immunol 125:548–665
9. Reinherz EL, Kung PC, Pesando JM, Ritz J, Goldstein G, Schlossman SF (1979) Ia determinants on human T cell subsets defined by monoclonal antibodies: activation stimuli required for expression. J Exp Med 150:1472–1480
10. Lloyd KO, Ng J, Dippold WG (1981) Analysis of the biosynthesis of HLA-DR glycoproteins in human malignant melanoma cell lines. J Immunol 126:2408–2417
11. Koprowski H, Steplewski Z, Herlyn D, Herlyn M (1978) Study of antibodies against human melanoma produced by somatic cell hybrids. Proc Natl Acad Sci USA 75:3405–3410
12. Acolla RS, Gross N, Carrel S, Corte G (1981) Distinct forms of both α and β subunits are present in the human Ia molecular pool. Proc Natl Acad Sci USA 78:4549–4551
13. Bröcker EB, Suter L, Sorg C (1984) HLA-DR antigen expression in primary melanomas of the skin. J Invest Dermatol 82:244–247
14. Ghosh AK, Gatter KC, Mason DY (1984) Immunocytochemical characterization of monoclonal anti-HLA-DR antibodies. Dis Markers 2:223–233
15. Epenetos AA, Bobrow LG, Adams TE, Collins CM, Isaacson PG, Bodmer WF (1985) A monoclonal antibody that detects HLA-D region antigen in routinely fixed, wax embedded sections of normal and neoplastic lymphoid tissues. J Clin Pathol 38:12–17
16. Adams TE, Bodmer JG, Bodmer WF (1983) Production and characterization of monoclonal antibodies recognizing the α-chain subunits of human Ia alloantigens. Immunology 50:613–614
17. Wilson BS, Herzig A, Lloyd RV (1984) Immunoperoxidase staining for Ia-like antigens in paraffin-embedded tissues from human melanoma and lung carcinoma. Am J Pathol 115:102–116
18. Workshop on monoclonal antibodies to human MHC class II antigens (1984). Dis Markers 2:363–369
19. Crumpton MJ, Bodmer JG, Bodmer WF, Heyes JM, Lindsay J, Rudd CE (1984) Biochemistry of class II antigens: workshop report. In: Albert ED, Baur MP, Mayr WR (eds) Histocompatibility testing 1984. Springer, Berlin Heidelberg New York Tokyo, pp 29–37
20. Quaranta V, Majdic O, Sintl G, Liszka K, Hönigsmann H, Knapp W (1984) A human Ia cytoplastic determinant located on multiple forms of invariant chain (γ, γ2, γ3). J Immunol 132:1900–1905
21. Natali PG, Segatto O, Ferrone S, Tosi R, Corte G (1984) Differential tissue distribution and ontogeny of DC-1 and HLA-DR antigens. Immunogenetics 19:109–115
22. Polak J, Van Noorden S (1983) Immunocytochemistry. Wright, Bristol
23. Harrist TJ, Ruiter DJ, Bhan AK, Mihm MC Jr (1983) The distribution of major histocompatibility antigens in normal skin. Br J Dermatol 109:623–633
24. Natali PG, Giacomini P, Russo C, Steinbach G, Fenoglio C, Ferrone S (1983) Antigenic profile of human melanoma cells. Analysis with monoclonal antibodies to histocompatibility antigens and to melanoma-associated antigens. J Cutan Pathol 10:225–237
25. Poppema S, Bröcker EB, De Ley L, Terbrack D, Visscher T, Ter Haar A, Macher E, Thé HT, Sorg C (1983) In situ analysis of the mononuclear infiltrate in primary malignant melanoma of the skin. Clin Exp Immunol 51:77–82
26. Ruiter DJ, Bergman W, Welvaart K, Scheffer E, Van Vloten WA, Russo C, Ferrone S (1984) Immunohistochemical analysis of malignant melanomas and nevocellular nevi with monoclonal antibodies to distinct monomorphic determinants of HLA antigens. Cancer Res 44:3930–3935
27. Kindt TJ, Mach B, Sogn JA, Robinson MA, Kulaga H, Möller E, Carlsson B, Wallin J, Bach FH (1984) Editorial review: identical or distinct functional roles for products of the HLA-DR, DC, and SB loci. Scand J Immunol 20:471–492
28. Houghton AN, Thomson TM, Gross D, Oettgen HF, Old LJ (1984) Surface antigens of melanoma and melanocytes. Specificity of induction of Ia antigens by human γ-interferon. J Exp Med 160:255–269
29. Pober JS, Gimbrone MA Jr (1982) Expression of Ia-like antigens by human vascular endothelial cells is inducible in vitro: demonstration by monoclonal antibody binding and immunoprecipitation. Proc Natl Acad Sci USA 79:6641–6645

30. Pober JS, Gimbrone MA Jr, Cotran RS, Reiss CS, Burakoff SJ, Fiers W, Ault KA (1983) Ia expression by vascular endothelium is inducible by activated T cells and by human γ-interferon. J Exp Med 157:1339–1346
31. Collins T, Korman AJ, Wake CT, Boss JM, Kappes DJ, Fiers W, Ault KA, Gimbrone MA Jr, Strominger JL, Pober JS (1984) Immune interferon activates multiple class II major histocompatibility complex genes and the associated invariant chain gene in human endothelial cells and dermal fibroblasts. Proc Natl Acad Sci USA 81:4917–4921
32. Basham TY, Nickoloff BJ, Merigan TC, Morhenn VB (1984) Recombinant gamma interferon induces HLA-DR expression on cultured human keratinocytes. J Invest Dermatol 83:88–93
33. Schwartz R, Momburg G, Moldenhauer G, Dörken B, Schirrmacher V (1985) Induction of HLA class-II antigen expression on human carcinoma cell lines by IFN-gamma. Int J Cancer 35:245–252
34. Koefler HP, Ranyard J, Yelton L, Billing R, Bohman R (1984) γ-Interferon induces expression of the HLA-D antigens on normal and leukemic human myeloid cells. Proc Natl Acad Sci USA 81:4080–4084; Cancer 35:245–252
35. Kelley VE, Fiers W, Strom TB (1984) Cloned human interferon-γ, but not interferon -β or -α, induces expression of HLA-DR determinants by fetal monocytes and myeloid leukaemic cell lines. J Immunol 132:240–245
36. Holzmann B, Johnson JP, Kandewitz P, Braun-Falco O, Riethmüller G (1984) Differential expression of antigens 15.75 and p3.58 on primary melanoma and benign nevi. Behring Inst Mitt 74:24–26
37. Murphy GF, Bhan AK, Sato S, Harrist TJ, Mihm MC Jr (1981) Characterisation of Langerhans cells by the use of monoclonal antibodies. Lab Invest 45:465–472
38. Bergman W, Willemze R, de Graaff-Reitsma C, Ruiter DJ (1985) Analysis of major histocompatibility antigens and the mononuclear cell infiltrate in halo nevi. J Invest Dermatol 85:25–29
39. Ruiter DJ, Bergman W, Steylen PN, Scheffer E (1984) Histopathological aspects of dysplastic nevi. In: Ruiter DS, Welvaart K, Ferrone S (eds) Cutaneous melanoma and precursor lesions. Nijhoff, The Hague, The Netherlands, pp 239–248
40. Van Duinen SG, Ruiter DJ, Bröcker EB, Sorg C, Welvaart K, Ferrone S (1984) Association of low level of HLA-A,B,C antigens on high level of Ia antigens in metastatic melanoma with a high grade of malignancy. J Invest Dermatol 82:558
41. Van Duinen SG, Ruiter DJ, Ferrone S (submitted) Expression of class II MHC antigens on freshly obtained melanoma cells in restricted mainly to cells which also express class I MHC antigens
42. Suter L, Bröcker EB, Brüggen J, Ruiter DJ, Sorg C (1983) Heterogeneity of primary and metastatic human malignant melanoma as detected with monoclonal antibodies in cryostat sections. Cancer Immunol Immunother 16:53–58
43. Albino AP, Lloyd KO, Houghton AN, Oettgen HF, Old LJ (1981) Heterogeneity in surface antigen and glycoprotein expression of cell lines derived from different melanoma cells of the same patient. J Exp Med 154:1764–1778
44. Natali PG, Cavaliere R, Bigotti A, Nicotra MR, Russo C, Ng AK, Giacomini P, Ferrone S (1983) Antigenic heterogeneity of surgically removed primary and autologous metastatic human melanoma. J Immunol 130:1462–1466
45. Burchiel SW, Martin JC, Imai K, Ferrone S, Warner NL (1982) Heterogeneity of HLA-A,B, Ia-like, and melanoma-associated antigen expression by human melanoma cell lines analyzed with monoclonal antibodies and flow cytometry. Cancer Res 42:4110–4115
46. Sarkar S, Glassy MC, Ferrone S, Jones OW (1980) Cell cycle and the differential expression of HLA-A,B and HLA-DR antigens on human B lymphoid cells. Proc Natl Acad Sci USA 77:7297–7301
47. Fidler IJ, Hart IR (1982) Biological diversity in metastatic neoplasms: origins and implications. Science 197:893–897
48. Pollack MS, Chin-Louid J, Moshief RD (1984) Functional characteristics and differential expression of class II DR, DS, and SB antigens on human melanoma cell lines. Human Immunol 9:75–82
49. Sell S (1978) Cancer markers: diagnostic and developmental significance. In: Waters H (ed) Handbook of cancer immunology, vol 3. Garland STPM, New York

50. Houghton AN, Eisinger M, Albino AP, Cairncross JG, Old LJ (1982) Surface antigens of melanocytes and melanomas. Markers of melanocyte differentiation and melanoma subsets. J Exp Med 156:1755–1766
51. Fitchen JH, Foon KA, Cline MH (1981) The antigenic characteristics of hematopoietic stem cells. N Engl J Med 305:17–25
52. Pellegrino MA, Natali PG, Ng AK, Imai K, Russo C, Bigotti A, Wolf P, Ferrone S (1982) Unorthodox expression of Ia-like antigens on human tumor cells of nonlymphoid origin: immunological properties, structural profile, significance and clinical relevance. In: Nakamura RM, Dito WR, Tucker ES (eds) Immunological analysis: recent progress in diagnostic laboratory immunology. Masson, New York, pp 159–173
53. Kornstein MJ, Brooks JSJ, Elder DE (1983) Immunoperoxidase localisation of lymphocyte subsets in the host response to melanoma and nevi. Cancer Res 43:2749–2754
54. Fossati G, Taramelli D, Dalsari A, Bogdanovich G, Andreola S, Parmiani G (1984) Primary but not metastatic human melanomas expressing DR antigens stimulate autologous lymphocytes. Int J Cancer 33:591–597
55. Guerry IV DP, Alexander MA, Herlyn MD, Zehngebot LM, Mitchell KF, Zmijewski CM, Lusk EJ (1984) HLA-DR histocompatibility leukocyte antigens permit cultured human melanoma cells from early but not advanced disease to stimulate autologous lymphocytes. J Clin Invest 73:267–271
56. Taramelli D, Fossati G, Balsari A, Marolda R, Parmiani G (1984) The inhibition of lymphocyte stimulation by autologous human metastatic melanoma cells correlates with the expression of HLA-DR antigens on the tumor cells. Int J Cancer 34:797–806
57. Gonwa TA, Picker LJ, Raff HV, Goyert SM, Silver J, Stobo JD (1983) Antigen-presenting capabilities of human monocytes correlates with their expression of HLA-DS, an Ia determinant distinct from HLA-DR. J Immunol 130:706–711
58. McKean DJ, Infante AJ, Nilson A, Kimoto M, Fathman CG, Walker E, Warner N (1981) Major histocompatibility complex-restricted antigen presentation to antigen-reactive T cells by B lymphocyte tumor cells. J Exp Med 154:1419–1431
59. Glimchez LH, Kim KJ, Green I, Paul WE (1982) Ia antigen-bearing B cell tumor lines can present protein antigen and alloantigen in a major histocompatibility complex-restricted fashion to antigen-reactive T cells. J Exp Med 155:445–459
60. Guy K, Van Heyningen V, Ziegler A, Steel MC (1984) Disparity in HLA-DC antigen expression on chronic lymphocytic leucaemia cells. Dis Markers 2:287–293
61. Faille A, Turmel P, Charron DJ (1984) Differential expression of HLA-DR and HLA-DC/DS molecules in a patient with hairy cell leukaemia: restoration of HLA-DC/DS expression by (12-0-tetradeconyl phorbol-13-acetate), 5-azacytidine, and sodium butyrate. Blood 64:33–38
62. Pellegrino MA, Ferrone S, Brautbar C, Hayflick L (1976) Changes in HLA antigen profiles on SV40 transformed human fibroblasts. Exp Cell Res 97:340
63. Janeway CA Jr, Bottomly K, Babich J, Conrad P, Conzen S, Jones B, Kaye J, Katz M, McVay L, Murphy DB, Tite J (1984) Quantitative variation in Ia antigen expression plays a central role in immune regulation. Immunol Today 5:99–105
64. Van Duinen SG (1984) Pathobiologic and diagnostic aspects of human cutaneous melanoma. Thesis, Leiden; Kanters, Alblasserdam, Netherlands
65. Wilson BS, Imai K, Natali PG, Kay NE, Cavaliere R, Pellegrino MA, Ferrone S (1982) Immunochemical analysis of the antigenic profile of human melanoma cells with monoclonal antibodies. In: Reisfeld RA, Ferrone S (eds) Melanoma antigens and antibodies. Plenum, New York, pp 401–433
66. Alexander S, Hubbard SC, Strominger JL (1984) HLA-DR antigens of autologous melanoma and B lymphoblastoid cell lines: Differences in glycosylation but not protein structure. J Immunol 133:315–320
67. Ashewell G, Morell AG (1977) Carbohydrates on class II major histocompatibility complex antigens may mediate carbohydrate-specific recognition. Trends Biochem Sci 2:76
68. Wilson BS, Glassy MC, Quaranta V, Ng AK, Ferrone S (1981) Effect of tunicamycin on the assembly and antigenicity of HLA antigens: analysis with monoclonal antibodies. Scand J Immunol 14:201–205
69. Metzgar RS, Oleinick SR (1968) The study of normal and malignant cell antigens by mixed agglutination. Cancer Res 28:1366–1371

Molecular Genetics

Molecular Polymorphism of Human Immune-Response-Genes

J. I. Bell and H. O. McDevitt

Table of Contents

Introduction

The observations that in mice the humoral response to a specific antigenic challenge is in some instances genetically controlled [49], and that the genetic loci responsible for this modulation of the murine immune response map to the class II region within the major histocompatibility complex (MHC) [7], have led to the conclusion that the I region in mice and the D region in man encode at least some of the immune-response (Ir) genes. Understanding the structure and polymorphism of the genes within these regions has therefore become an important priority among those studying the genetic basis of the immune response. The original observations on the function of Ir genes have been substantially broadened, so that these genes are now acknowledged to govern the response to a wide variety of antigenic challenges and to control both humoral and cell-mediated immune responses [72]. In man, there is now evidence that these genes function in a similar manner to regulate immune responsiveness [67, 68] and map to the class II region of the MHC. The products of this region are highly polymorphic, and it is likely that these polymorphisms are responsible for the variability observed between individuals in immune responsiveness. An understanding of structural differences between alleles of the class II loci is an important step toward understanding the molecular basis of immune responsiveness. An additional by-product of such studies may be to reveal how the genes of the class II region have acquired and maintained such extensive amounts of polymorphism.

The products of the class II loci of the MHC in the mouse and in man show strong structural similarities [31]. They are expressed under normal circumstances on the surface of B cells, antigen-presenting cells, and activated T cells. Aberrant expression may be observed on vascular endothelium, thyroid epithelium, or biliary epithelium in association with active autoimmune disease or transplant rejection [4, 22]. Each class II molecule is a heterodimer, consisting of an α or heavy chain (34000 kb) and a β or light chain (29000 kb) [31]. Both chains have two extracellular domains, a transmembrane region and a cytoplasmic domain. The membrane proximal domain of both α and β chains have disulfide bonds and both show some homology to immunoglobulin [80]. The membrane distal domain of the β chain but not the α chain has a disulfide loop.

Five sets of molecules have been mapped to this region in the mouse by genetic and serologic analysis [60]. Of these, I-A and I-E have been defined at a molecular level by cloning studies [75], while the other subregion products, from I-J, I-C, and I-B, have been more difficult to clearly identify. They may be the products of other recently defined loci ($E\beta_2$, $E\beta_3$, $A\beta_2$, or $A\beta_3$) [15], or may represent the result of effects of genes outside the MHC [24].

In man, several subregions within the MHC have been identified by cellular typing and serology. Two sets of products, DQ and DR, have been identified by cellular typing, antisera, and monoclonal antibodies, while a further subregion (DP) has been identified with primed lymphocyte typing [71]. More loci have been defined by recent molecular studies. Again, all these regions maintain high levels of polymorphism. Although our understanding of precisely how Ir genes function is currently vague, an appreciation of the nature of this structural polymorphism may help reveal their role in the immune response. In this chapter, we will review the new insights into the structural basis of human class II polymorphisms provided by restriction fragment length polymorphism studies and nucleic acid sequence of alleles, and will discuss how these polymorphisms may relate to the function of Ir genes.

Organization of the Human Class II Region

Cloning studies have identified many more class II loci than have previously been acknowledged. Three subregions have been identified; DR, DQ, and DP (see Fig. 1). The DP subregion has been mapped centromeric to the DR and DQ subregions [71], and consists thus far of two α and two β chains [82]. The α chains and β chains are ordered alternately and the α genes are both oriented in the opposite direction to the β chains, implying a duplication event during the evolution of the subregion. There is evidence available to suggest that in at least some haplotypes, $DP_{\alpha 2}$ and $DP_{\beta 2}$ are not expressed [30, 70]. A $DP_{\alpha 2}$ sequence has revealed two 1-bp mutations and subsequent translational frame shifts, an abnormal first domain splice function, and a premature stop codon on the cytoplasmic tail [70]. The first of these alterations is most likely to inactivate the gene. Similarly, the $DP_{\beta 2}$ locus has been shown to have a single-base deletion and translational frame shift in the $\beta 2$ domain, producing three new stop codons [30]. The DQ subregion is thought to contain two α and two β chain genes. Of these, DQ_α and DQ_β are

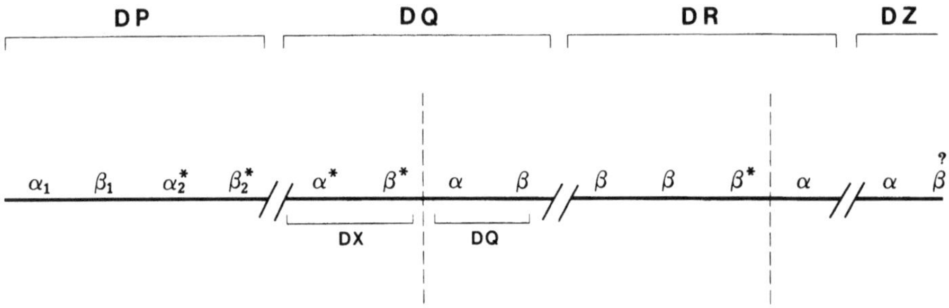

Fig. 1. The organization of the human class II region of the MHC. The *stars* indicate loci not currently known to be expressed. The *vertical lines* outline the region where RFLP is known to be extensive. The exact locations of DZ_α, DZ_β (DO_β), and DR_α are uncertain

known to be expressed, while DX_α has never been identified except as a genomic clone [2] and on Southern blotting studies [74]. DX_β has similarly been identified only on Southern blots, suggesting that both DX α and β chains are expressed either at low levels or not at all.

The DR subregion contains one α chain and at least three β chains in some haplotypes. One β chain is a pseudogene in the DR4 haplotype [41], as it has numerous deviant splice junction signals, two premature stop codons due to point mutations, and a translational frame shift resulting from a 2-bp insertion in codon 183 [41]. At least two other DR_β chains are expressed. We have identified by sequence analysis two distinct cDNA DR_β clones from a lymphoblastoid cell line homozygous by consanguinity for DR3 (unpublished observations). No other DR_β cDNA clones have been identified after partial sequence analysis of 20 further clones. Only one DR_α chain has been identified [42]; it is expressed and nonpolymorphic.

One additional set of loci has been identified and mapped to the human class II region. DZ_α was initially described by Spielman et al. [74], and a genomic DZ_α gene has now been completely sequenced [82]. There is some evidence that this locus may be expressed as cDNA clones, as sequences very similar to those predicted by the genomic DZ_α clones have been obtained [26]. Northern blots with the DZ_α probe have also demonstrated very low levels of expression in some cDNA lines [82]. An additional β chain, DO_β, has also recently been cloned and may prove to be the β chain associated with DZ_α [78]. It has sequence homology to both DQ_β and DR_β. As cDNA clones have been identified for this locus, it may prove to be expressed in lymphoblastoid lines.

The organization of the human class II region includes, therefore, at least six α chains, four of which appear to be expressed, and eight β chains, five of which have been shown to be expressed. It is likely, however, that different haplotypes will possess different numbers of loci and different numbers of expressed products. This is true in other multigene families, such as the α globins, where different haplotypes with two, three, or four α globin genes have been identified [81].

Comparison with the mouse I region indicates that for the β chains the number of loci are comparable (six in mouse, eight in man), while for the α chains there are many fewer in the mouse (two compared to six in man), although this discrepancy may be resolved when cosmid clones are screened with α chain probes at low stringencies.

Class II Polymorphism

Cellular, Serological, and Biochemical Analysis

As previously suggested, the polymorphism in immune response to particular stimuli is paralleled by extensive polymorphism among the genes encoding the Ir gene products in the class II region of the MHC. The original identification and mapping of these genes depended largely on mixed lymphocyte reactivity resulting from these polymorphisms [3], and similarly, serological definition of DR types was based on their polymorphic determinants [84]. Cellular typing and serology have been largely responsible for the understanding we have of the extent of variability between haplotypes in populations. The currently acknowledged serological and cellular types have recently been reviewed [62]. In addition to the polymorphisms defined in these ways, monoclonal antibodies have permitted their analysis in two other ways, with two-dimensional gel electrophoresis [61] and with selective N-terminal amino acid sequencing [17]. Subgroups of DR specificities have been clearly defined using two-dimensional gels [19, 61] on the basis of their electrophoretic mobility. This has confirmed that the polymorphism among human populations is likely to be significantly more extensive than that defined serologically. Similarly, monoclonal antibodies have been used to purify distinct β chains from different lymphoblastoid cell lines, and these have been submitted to protein sequencing of their N-termini [17]. These studies have indicated a distinct pattern of tyrosine residues for DR_β chains from the haplotypes DR1–DR7 with the exception of DR2 and DR4, which were identical [17]. Similarly, the pattern of tyrosines in DQ_α and DQ_β chains identified at least three different DQ_α alleles and six distinct DQ_β alleles.

These techniques have all led to an understanding of the amount of allelic polymorphism present among class II region alleles. However, two other techniques are now available to provide additional, more precise information. The first of these is restriction fragment length polymorphism (RFLP), which may permit analysis of the extent of polymorphism at or near individual class II loci with a sensitivity greater than that previously attained. The second is nucleic acid sequencing, which has for the first time permitted evaluation of the exact nature of the polymorphisms and their sites in the molecule.

Restriction Fragment Length Polymorphism

The use of Southern blotting and labeled DNA probes to identify bands of differing sizes that reflect polymorphic restriction endonuclease recognition sites had been proven to be an effective means of identifying structural genetic polymorphisms in other gene families such as β globin before it was utilized to study the MHC. By chance alone, the majority of polymorphic restriction sites do not lie within the coding region of genes, but instead are most commonly found in noncoding regions (flanking sequences, untranslated regions, or introns). The polymorphisms may be linked, however, to coding region polymorphisms and hence can be used as linkage markers for different coding region products. The utility of this linkage was first demonstrated by Kan and Dozy [29], in their studies of the *Hpa*I polymorphism associated with the sickle mutation in the β globin gene. These observations were extended to the β thalassemias using a range of polymorphisms throughout the β globin cluster [63]. The availability of class II region probes has made it feasible to use this technology to define molecular polymorphisms at different loci and study them easily in populations. It was hoped that RFLPs would enable a molecular dissection of polymorphism at individual loci and would allow a molecular assessment of polymorphisms that was more sensitive than that already observed with serology and cellular typing. To date, many of these hopes have been realized.

Class II RFLP's Reflect Coding Region Polymorphisms

Evidence that class II RFLPs would be useful in reflecting changes in coding region sequences has been easily obtained. When DNA from homozygous cell lines is examined and a DR_β probe [5] is used for hybridization, the patterns of bands obtained are distinct for each of the haplotypes DR1–DR7 (Fig. 2) (Bell et al., unpublished observation) [64]. When multiple representatives of individual haplotypes are then studied, the basic patterns of bands are consistent for any haplo-

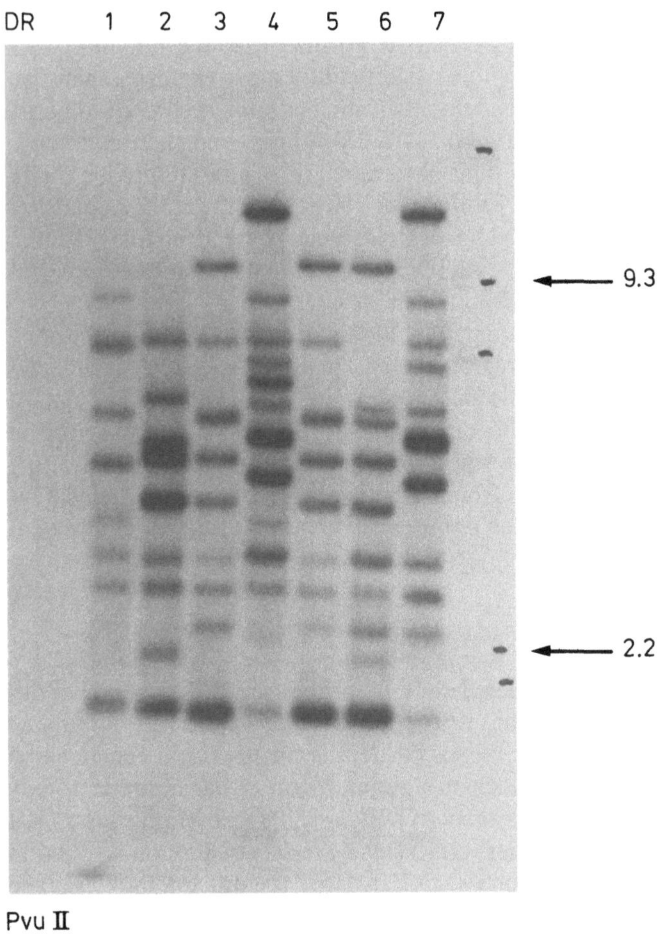

Fig. 2. A Southern blot of consanguineous homozygous cell lines of DR types 1–7, digested with the enzyme *Pvu*II and probed wit a full-length DR_β cDNA probe. This demonstrates the distinct patterns between DR types. Marker sizes based on λ cut with *Hind*III and given in kb

type [6]. The implication from these observations is that the RFLPs are linked to the structural coding region polymorphisms that have been defined serologically as DR1–DR7. This linkage has been similarly found with a DR_α probe [76] and a DQ_α probe [74].

RFLPs Subdivide Serologically Defined Haplotypes

To be useful as a means of improving our ability to detect new polymorphisms in populations, RFLPs must be used to do more than simply identify already defined serological polymorphisms. They have, in part, achieved this goal as it has been possible to subdivide single DR haplotypes using an appropriate restriction enzyme and probe. For example, the DR3 haplotype can be divided into two subtypes using the *Bgl*II enzyme and a DR_β probe (Fig. 3) [6]. A fundamental question relating to these subdivisions is whether they indicate real coding region polymorphisms beyond those defined serologically. There is some evidence that they do. For example, in DR2-homozygous cell lines, one subdivision seen with the DQ_β probe identifies the cell line Akiba (DR2/Dw12) as being distinct from several DR2/Dw2 lines (Fig. 4) [6]. This indicates that this subdivision reflects a coding region polymorphism. Less RFLP is seen between Akiba and other DR2 lines using a DR-subregion-specific probe (unpublished observation). Interestingly, sequence comparison of the Akiba haplotype has indicated that it differs greatly from the PGF (DR2/Dw2) sequence at the DQ_β locus, as suggested by the RFLPs (T. Sazazuki, personal communication).

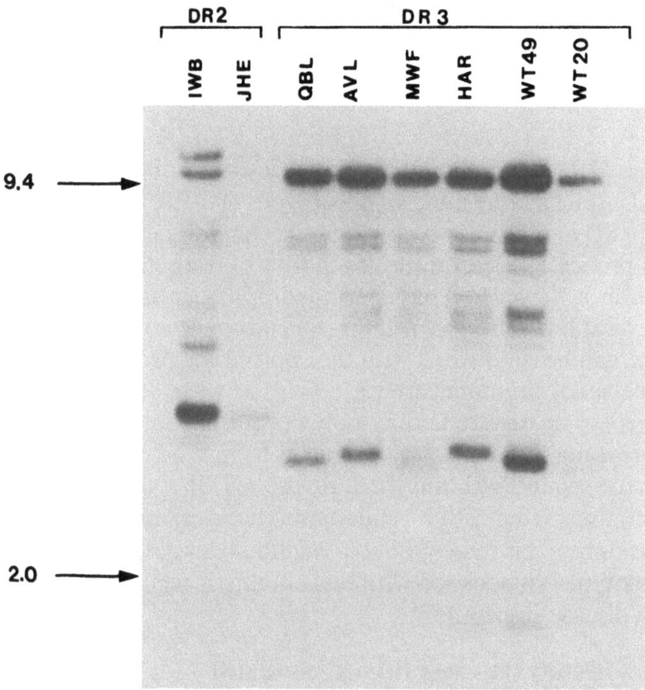

Fig. 3. A Southern blot of homozygous cell lines of DR types one and three cut with the enzyme *Bgl*II and probed with a full-length DR_β cDNA probe. The DR3 pattern is broken into three subtypes RFLP [6]

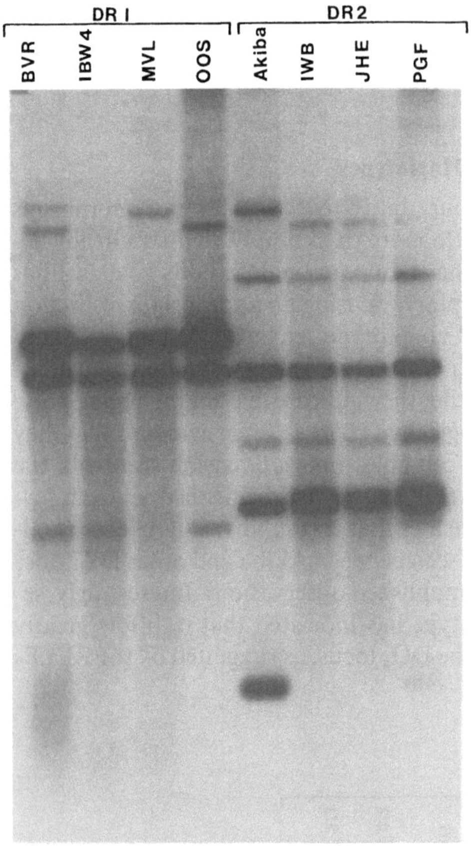

Fig. 4. A Southern blot of DNA from consanguineous homozygous typing cells digested with *BglII* and probed with a DQ_β probe. Lanes 1–4 are DR1 cell lines, lanes 5–8 are DR2 cell lines. The polymorphism between Akiba (DR2/Dw12) and the other DR2/Dw2 lines is clearly shown

Overall, the haplotypes DR1, 3, 5, and 6 are relatively easily subdivided (unpublished observation). Despite a large number of subtypes of DR4, defined with two-dimensional gels [20, 61] and cellular typing [65], this haplotype is not easily subdivided with β chain probes. With appropriate choices of restriction enzymes and subregion-specific probes, however, it has been possible to identify restriction fragments specific for several Dw subtypes of DR4 (D. Hardy, personal communication). Similarly, DR2 can be subdivided with the appropriate probes and enzymes (B. Morley-Lee, personal communication).

RFLPs are likely to reflect linkage to coding polymorphisms not yet defined by cellular or serological typing. Evidence for this comes from the subdivision of DR3 using the restriction enzyme *BglII* and the DR_α probe [77]. One DR3 subtype thus defined is highly associated with juvenile-onset diabetes, much more so than the DR3 haplotype alone. This indicates, at a functional level, that the subdivision of the DR3 haplotype is associated with real coding or regulatory polymorphisms important in disease susceptibility.

Subregion-Specific Probes Identify the Class II Loci Associated with Some RFLPs

The band patterns obtained on Southern blots using a full-length cDNA DR_β chain probe (Fig. 2) are complex even when only one haplotype is studied and

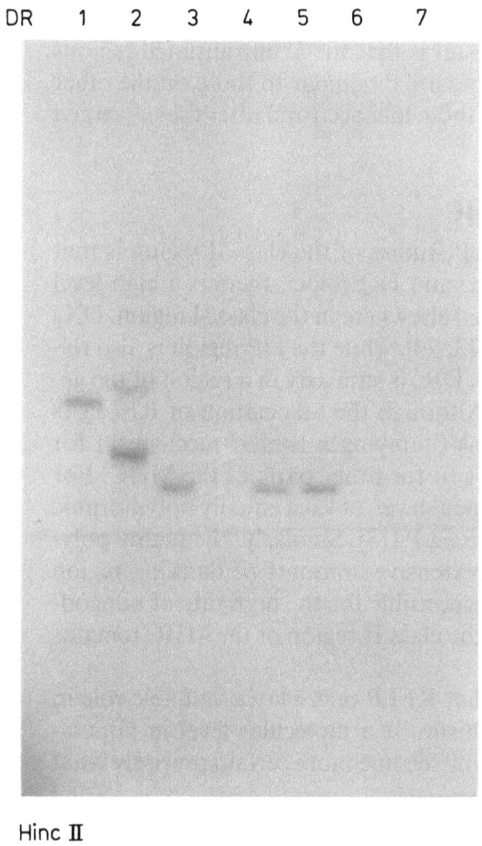

Fig. 5. Pattern of bands obtained on a Southern blot of homozygous lines of DR types 1–7 digested with *Hinc*II and probed with a 3′ untranslated region DR_β probe. The band pattern is greatly simplified compared to that seen with the whole DR_β chain probe (see Figs. 2 and 3). The bands for the DR4 and DR7 lines are not visible at this stringency (hybridized at 42 °C in 50% formamide and washed at 65 °C in 0.1 × SSC)

high stringency conditions are used. This is the result of extensive cross-hybridization between homologous members of this gene family. Although such bands patterns have the advantage of identifying polymorphisms throughout the whole haplotype, and hence might be useful in looking for RFLPs associated with autoimmune diseases, it is also important to know which subregion and locus the polymorphisms are associated with. This can be achieved by using subregion-specific probes. Analysis of sequences from clones representing DR, DQ, and DP β chains has indicated that the 3′ untranslated regions of these clones are unique and could be used to identify bands from individual subregions. We have used a 3′ untranslated region from the DR1 β chain [5] as a subregion-specific probe. The pattern observed using this probe is greatly simplified over that seen with the whole probe (Fig. 5). At high stringency, a DQ_β probe which includes only the first and second domains also produces subregion-specific patterns, with two or three major bands per haplotype (Fig. 4). Utilizing these probes obviously limits the amount of polymorphism one might see around a particular locus. However the benefits of interpreting a relatively simplified pattern, particularly in heterozygotes, are significant.

One interesting finding obtained with our DR-subregion probe is that at very high stringency, it does not hybridize to any bands in DNA from DR4 or DR7 haplotypes (Fig. 5). This observation implies that the 3′ untranslated regions of these DR_β chains differ significantly from those of other haplotypes. This homology would allow hybridization at lower stringency, which is what is observed with our probe. A further implication of this result is that the 3′ untranslated regions of all DR_β loci on DR4 and DR7 haplotypes are dissimilar to those on the other haplotypes, suggesting that duplication of these loci occurred after they diverged as distinct haplotypes.

RFLPs Vary in Frequency Through the MHC

One of the striking conclusions from RFLP studies of the class II region is that for the sequences around the DR β, DQ α, and DQ β loci, there is a high level of RFLP. This is in contrast to that observed elsewhere in the class II region. DX_β and DX_α are associated with little RFLP [73, 74], while the DP region is also relatively devoid of such polymorphisms [82]. DR_α is similarly in a region of the genome where RFLPs are infrequent [77]. Although the association of RFLPs is with the most polymorphic coding regions (implying a similar mechanism for their mutations), such comparisons do not fit for other parts of the MHC. For example, class I loci, which are, at a serological level, at least equally polymorphic to class II loci, have much less associated RFLP [13]. Similarly, the highly polymorphic C4 loci are not associated with extensive amounts of flanking region polymorphism [10]. What mechanism is responsible for the high rate of noncoding region polymorphism in the middle of the class II region of the MHC remains to be determined.

Current evidence indicates, therefore, that RFLP may play a valuable role in further defining and clarifying polymorphisms at a molecular level in populations. As more data becomes available, it will become more certain precisely what that role will be.

Nucleic Acid Sequencing of Class II Alleles

The final analysis of class II allelic polymorphisms will depend upon the availability of amino acid sequences. Although one laboratory has successfully generated several full-length protein sequences [18, 34, 87], most sequence data has been derived from nucleic acid sequencing of genomic or cDNA clones. This has now provided a sizeable amount of information on both the molecular details of allelic polymorphisms and their location in the protein.

α Chains

Studies of allelic polymorphism in the mouse have revealed that E_α is relatively invariant [46, 52, 58], while the A_α chains show much more variability. The variation in A_α molecules is largely clustered in residues 11–15, 53–59, and 69–77 in the membrane distal domain [8].

In man, the DR_α chain has been sequenced by six independent groups [33, 36, 42, 76, 87]. Only one amino acid polymorphism has been described [42]. This lack of polymorphism in the coding region of this gene is shared by its flanking regions as there have been few associated restriction enzyme site polymorphisms identified [76]. DQ_α has proved to be more polymorphic. The variability among alleles at this locus is largely limited to one variable region stretching from residues 29–56 [1, 2, 18, 69]. One clone, pIIα-5, has a single residue deleted at position 56 and evidence of alternative splicing in the 3′ UT region [69].

Restriction fragment patterns associated with DQ_α are polymorphic and reflect the DR haplotype they are associated with. DX_α has never been demonstrated to be expressed. Sequence has been obtained for a single genomic clone [2]. Little RFLP is associated with it.

Four DP_α allelic sequences are available [2, 70, 83]. There is little polymorphism associated with these alleles, although some productive base-pair alterations are distributed throughout the coding sequence. This pattern of polymorphism is atypical for class II loci in that it is slight and not clustered. RFLPs are also rare adjacent to this locus [73]. The second DP_α locus is most probably not expressed (see above).

The DZ_α locus has not been evaluated for allelic polymorphism. No polymorphic restriction sites have been identified adjacent to the gene [83].

β Chains

In the mouse, substantial amounts of allelic sequencing has been performed on E_β and A_β alleles. Among A_β alleles, variable regions are evident in the membrane distal domain in residues 8–17, 60–66, and 85–89 [12, 40, 45]. Several haplotypes have two codons deleted in the last of these variable regions (P. Estess, personal communication). Five E_β alleles have been sequences [55, 57, 58, 66]. Again, the variability is confined to the membrane distal domain and is clustered in residues 1–13, 24–35, and 68–75.

This complex allotypy, with multiple clustered amino acid variations in the membrane distal domain, is also seen among human *β* chain alleles. Sequences of DR *β* chain alleles, when compared, reveal three regions of variability in residues 9–13, 26–32, and 70–74 (Fig. 6) [5, 21, 34, 44]. These show remarkable similarity in position to those variable regions of E_β alleles. The DR_β alleles expressed are derived from at least two distinct loci, and the products of these loci are as similar to each other as they are to allelic products of the same locus, even in their 3′ untranslated regions (unpublished observations).

The DQ_β sequences for three different alleles have been published [5, 9, 37, 40, 69]. Two of these sequences have been sequenced by two independent groups. Variability is prominent in residues 53–58, 66–77, and 84–90. One major region of variability in A_β alleles, in residues 6–12, is absent among DQ_β alleles. As previously described, DR_β and DQ_β loci are surrounded by multiple polymorphic restriction sites.

The DP_β sequences of three alleles have been compared [30]. Again, the first domain includes most of the variable positions, which are clustered in residues 8–9, 56–69, and 84–87 [30].

The molecular basis of class II allelic polymorphisms in mouse and man are remarkably similar. In both, the A_α or DQ_α chains are variable, while the other *α* chains are much less so. The *β* chains all show the same pattern of variability, with discrete regions of hypervariability restricted to the membrane distal domains. The polymorphisms themselves are complex and are surrounded by strong conserved regions. Although it is not certain, it appears likely that these regions of polymorphisms may be critical regions in the molecule that determine its ability to effectively present antigen and act as a modulator of immune response.

```
          1                                                                                  21
2918.4    Gly Asp Thr Arg Pro Arg Phe Leu Trp Gln Leu Lys Phe Glu Cys His Phe Phe Asn Gly Thr
DRb1      --- --- --- --- --- --- --- --- Glu Leu --- --- Ser --- --- --- --- --- --- --- ---
pII-b-3   --- --- --- --- --- --- --- --- Glu Tyr Ser Thr Ser --- --- --- --- --- --- --- ---
pII-b-4   --- --- --- --- --- --- --- --- Glu Glu Val --- --- --- --- --- --- --- --- --- ---
DR2/2     --- --- --- --- --- --- --- --- --- --- Pro --- Arg --- --- --- --- --- --- --- ---

          22                                                                                 42
2918.4    Glu Arg Val Arg Leu Leu Glu Arg Cys Ile Tyr Asn Gln Glu Glu Ser Val Arg Phe Asp Ser
DRb1      --- --- --- --- Phe --- --- --- His Phe His --- --- --- --- Tyr Ala --- --- --- ---
pII-b-3   --- --- --- --- Tyr --- Asp --- Tyr Phe His --- --- --- --- Asn --- --- --- --- ---
pII-b-4   --- --- --- --- --- --- --- --- Arg Val His --- --- --- --- Tyr Ala --- Tyr --- ---
DR2/2     --- --- --- --- Phe --- Asp --- Tyr Phe --- --- --- --- --- --- --- --- --- --- ---

          43                                                                                 63
2918.4    Asp Val Gly Glu Tyr Arg Ala Val Glu Glu Leu Gly Arg Pro Asp Ala Glu Tyr Trp Asn Ser
DRb1      --- --- --- --- --- --- --- --- Arg --- --- --- --- --- --- --- --- --- --- --- ---
pII-b-3   --- --- --- --- Phe --- --- --- Thr --- --- --- --- --- --- --- --- --- --- --- ---
pII-b-4   --- --- --- --- --- --- --- --- Thr --- --- --- --- --- --- --- --- --- --- --- ---
DR2/2     --- --- --- --- Phe --- --- --- Thr --- --- --- --- --- --- --- --- --- --- --- ---

          64                                                                                 84
2918.4    Gln Lys Asp Leu Leu Glu Gln Arg Arg Ala Ala Val Asp Thr Tyr Cys Arg His Asn Tyr Gly
DRb1      --- --- --- --- --- --- --- Lys --- Gly Gln --- --- Asn --- --- --- --- --- --- ---
pII-b-3   --- --- --- --- --- --- --- Lys --- Gly Arg --- --- Asn --- --- --- --- --- --- ---
pII-b-4   --- --- --- --- --- --- Arg --- --- --- --- --- --- --- --- --- --- --- --- --- ---
DR2/2     --- --- --- Ile --- --- --- Ala --- --- --- --- --- --- --- --- --- --- --- --- ---

          85                                                                                 105
2918.4    Val Gly Glu Ser Phe Thr Val Gln Arg Arg Val Glu Pro Lys Val Thr Val Tyr Pro Ser Lys
DRb1      --- Val --- --- --- --- --- --- --- --- --- His --- Gln --- --- --- --- --- Ala ---
pII-b-3   --- Val --- --- --- --- --- --- --- --- --- His --- --- --- --- --- --- --- --- ---
pII-b-4   --- --- --- --- --- --- --- --- --- --- --- Gln --- --- --- --- --- --- --- --- ---
DR2/2     --- Val --- --- --- --- --- --- --- --- --- Gln --- --- --- --- --- --- --- --- ---

          106                                                                                126
2918.4    Thr Gln Pro Leu Gln His His Asn Leu Leu Val Cys Ser Val Ser Gly Phe Tyr Pro Gly Ser
DRb1      --- --- --- --- --- --- --- --- --- --- --- --- --- --- --- --- --- --- --- --- ---
pII-b-3   --- --- --- --- --- --- --- --- --- --- --- --- --- --- --- --- --- --- --- --- ---
pII-b-4   --- --- --- --- --- --- --- --- --- --- --- --- --- --- Asn --- --- --- --- --- ---
DR2/2     --- --- --- --- --- --- --- --- --- --- --- --- --- --- --- --- --- --- --- --- ---

          127                                                                                147
2918.4    Ile Glu Val Arg Trp Phe Arg Asn Gly Gln Glu Glu Lys Ala Gly Val Val Ser Thr Gly Leu
DRb1      --- --- --- --- --- --- --- --- --- --- --- --- --- --- --- --- --- --- --- --- ---
pII-b-3   --- --- --- --- --- --- --- --- --- --- --- --- --- Thr --- --- --- --- --- --- ---
pII-b-4   --- --- --- --- --- --- --- --- --- --- --- --- --- Thr --- --- --- --- --- --- ---
DR2/2     --- --- --- --- --- --- Leu --- --- --- --- --- --- --- --- Gly --- --- --- --- ---

          148                                                                                168
2918.4    Ile Gln Asn Gly Asp Trp Thr Phe Gln Thr Leu Val Met Leu Glu Thr Val Pro Arg Ser Gly
DRb1      --- --- --- --- --- --- --- --- --- --- --- --- --- --- --- --- Phe --- --- --- ---
pII-b-3   --- His --- --- --- --- --- --- --- --- --- --- --- --- --- --- --- --- --- --- ---
pII-b-4   --- --- --- --- --- --- --- --- --- --- --- --- --- --- --- --- --- --- --- --- ---
DR2/2     --- --- Asp --- --- --- --- --- --- --- --- --- --- --- --- --- --- --- --- --- ---

          169                                                                                189
2918.4    Glu Val Tyr Thr Cys Gln Val Glu His Pro Ser Val Thr Ser Pro Leu Thr Val Glu Trp Arg
DRb1       --- --- --- --- --- --- --- --- --- --- --- --- --- --- --- --- --- --- --- --- Ser
pII-b-3   --- --- --- --- --- --- --- --- --- --- --- --- --- --- --- --- --- --- --- --- ---
pII-b-4   --- --- --- --- --- --- --- --- --- --- --- --- Met --- --- --- --- --- --- --- ---
DR2/2     --- --- --- --- --- --- --- --- --- --- --- --- --- --- --- --- --- --- --- --- ---

          190                                                                                210
2918.4    Ala Arg Ser Glu Ser Ala Gln Ser Lys Met Leu Ser Gly Val Gly Gly Phe Val Leu Gly Leu
DRb1      --- --- --- --- --- --- --- --- --- --- --- --- --- --- --- --- --- --- --- --- ---
pII-b-3   --- --- --- --- --- --- --- --- --- --- --- --- --- --- --- --- --- --- --- --- ---
pII-b-4   --- --- --- --- --- --- --- --- --- --- --- --- --- --- --- --- --- --- --- --- ---
DR2/2     --- --- --- --- --- --- --- --- ---

          211                                                                                230
2918.4    Leu Leu Phe Leu Gly Ala Gly Leu Phe Ile Tyr Phe Arg Asn Gln Lys Gly His Ser Gly Leu
DRb1      --- --- --- --- --- --- --- --- --- --- --- --- --- --- --- --- --- --- --- --- ---
pII-b-3   --- --- --- --- --- --- --- --- --- --- --- --- --- --- --- --- --- --- --- --- ---
pII-b-4   --- --- --- --- --- --- --- --- --- --- --- --- --- --- --- --- --- --- --- --- ---

          231                     237
2918.4    Gln Pro Thr Gly Phe Leu Ser
DRb1      --- --- --- --- --- --- ---
pII-b-3     --- --- Arg --- --- --- ---
pII-b-4   Pro --- --- --- --- --- ---
```

Fig. 6. A comparison of the amino acid sequence obtained for five different DR_{β} chains. 2918.4 is a DR1 β chain [5], $DR_{\beta 1}$ was obtained from a DR4,6 library [44], and pII-β-3 and pII-β-4 were obtained from a DR3,6 library [21]. The DR2/2 protein sequence was obtained from a DR2-homozygous cell line [34]. The regions of variability in the first domain are clearly shown

Generation of Ir Gene Polymorphism

The available data on Ir gene polymorphism can be applied to several important questions. The first question is how the variability that has been documented arose. The second is whether other mechanisms might exist beyond alterations in the structural genes to generate even more polymorphism than is already apparent.

Generation of Polymorphism at a Genomic Level

Two mechanisms have been proposed as the generators of class II diversity, gene conversion and point mutation. There is strong evidence in the mouse for gene conversion leading to diversity among both class I and class II loci. The bml mutant has been suggested to be the result of a gene conversion from the Q10 gene to the mutant K^b gene [53, 85]. In the I region, the bm12 mutant was identified as having a mutant A^b_β allele [23, 43, 59] which altered responsiveness to some I-A-restricted antigens. The nucleic acid sequence of the A^{bm12}_β gene differs from the parental A^b_β gene by three nucleotides [50]. This region of the molecule is identical over 44 nucleic acid residues to that found in the E^b_β allele [57, 86], and it is hence likely that it was transferred by a gene conversion event from E^b_β to A^b_β to produce A^{bm12}_β. This event documents that gene conversion is a likely generator of diversity in the class II region and that the variable regions exchanged are important in regulating immune responsiveness.

As pointed out by Benoist et al. [8], however, it is unlikely that the variability seen amongst class II alleles can all be explained by gene conversion. There is a much less extensive reservoir of loci to be drawn upon for gene conversion events in the class II region than in the class I region. An additional mechanism for generating polymorphism might be point mutation followed by marked selection in favor of variability in some regions of the molecule.

Although mutation rates (based on the frequency of silent substitutions) are identical in the first and second domains [21], the second domain has been shown to have a lower rate of replacement substitution than the first domain, suggesting that the difference in replacement rate between the first and second domains could be accounted for by selection against replacement in the second domain rather than selection for replacement in the first domain [21]. This analysis considers the first domain as being homogeneous, however, which it is clearly not. Replacement in conserved portions of the first domain may be strongly selected against (as in the second domain), but when averaged with variable regions where selection is in favor of replacement, the first domain appears to have a replacement rate no greater than that predicted by substitution rate alone. A further indication that selection has been acting to promote change in first domain variable regions is the impressive ratio of productive to nonproductive changes in the first domain of A_α (4.9 vs 0.33) and E_β (8.3 vs 2.2) [8, 54]. These ratios provide clear evidence for selection in favor of variability in selected regions of the membrane distal domain.

Other Potential Mechanisms of Polymorphism

There are several mechanisms that may operate to increase the level of fundamental polymorphism beyond that encoded in the genome. The first of these mechanisms is alternative splicing. This has been documented to occur at the 3′ untranslated regions of DQ_α genes [69] and in the cytoplasmic tail of DP_β genes [30]. These alternative splicing events do not affect the part of the molecule interacting with antigen. However, among class I genes, alternative splicing has been documented to have an effect on the polymorphism of extracellular domains [35, 79]. The splice acceptor site involved in this event is conserved between class I genes and class II β chains, potentially allowing a similar event to lead to functionally important class II polymorphism.

An additional mechanism for generating diversity among class II products involves transassociation of α and β chains from two different haplotypes. This has been well documented in the mouse [27], and has recently been confirmed to occur in man [11, 17]. Perhaps more significant might be associations between α and β chains of different subregions. Although such associations were sought and never found in the mouse using two-dimensional gels, recent transfection experiments suggest that they may be possible [16], and may have been overlooked in the past because their products are normally found at very low levels.

Regulatory polymorphisms may potentially be important in producing heterogeneity beyond that provided by structural genes. Both tissue-specific regulation of expression and the regulation of levels of expression may prove to be important in varying immune responsiveness. In mice, absence of I-E expression is found in the haplotypes b, s, f, and q [28]. This is thought in some strains to be due to a deletion of the promoter and first exon [47] of E_α, while other strains (f and q) produce an apparently aberrant E_α in mRNA [47]. Twenty percent of wild mice do not express I-E [14], some because of the $E_{\alpha\theta}$ promoter deletion, but others potentially because of more subtle alterations in regulatory sequences. A variation in expression resulting from these polymorphisms could be important functionally, but their identification might initially be difficult. RFLPs may be important signposts to their presence, as they will demonstrate linkage to regulatory polymorphisms as well as to polymorphisms in structural genes.

All these mechanisms have the potential to increase the total level of polymorphism present in these molecules much beyond that defined by genomic sequences.

Ir Gene Function and Its Relation to Class II Polymorphism

The accumulating body of information on the molecular basis of class II allelic polymorphism allows several conclusions to be made as to the role of these polymorphisms in determing Ir gene function. In mice, the case for identity between Ir gene products, Ia antigens, and class II products is now very strong. In man, there has been more difficulty in establishing the presence of Ir genes, because of the need to work with outbred heterozygous populations. It has now been clearly established, however, that Ir genes exist in man and most probably map to the class II region of the human MHC [67]. This was first observed with streptococcal cell wall antigens and has since been documented for the antigen responsible for cedar pollen allergy [68]. By analogy with the mouse, it appears likely that the polymorphism in responsiveness in man may relate to variability in the class II alleles. Because of the clustered nature of the human class II polymorphisms, and because of their association with the membrane distal domain, it has been suggested that on folding, the variable regions converge to form the antigen binding site [8]. This would permit polymorphism to have a direct effect on the functional aspects of the Ir genes in determining what antigenic determinants could be bound by a particular class II molecule. Another model would suggest that polymorphisms affect tertiary protein structure by distant effects on conformation, so that an antigen binding site might alter due to changes in amino acid sequence that have an impact on overall structure but are not directly related to the antigen binding site. These possibilities may not be resolved until the three-dimensional structure of these molecules is resolved by crystallography.

That these polymorphic regions are central to the function of Ir genes is clearly shown by the bm12 mutant [51]. This mutation involves a putative gene conversion event from E_β^b to A_α, leading to the A_β^{bm12} allele (see above). The function of these A_β alleles changes in association with this gene conversion event, in that the A_β^{bm12} exhibits differential responsiveness to I-A-restricted antigens [25, 43, 59]. This situation not only reveals that gene conversion events may be responsible for class II variability, it also demonstrates that the variable regions of these alleles are important derterminants in T cell recognition and that they determine ultimately whether an immune response can be raised. Based on this observation, they are the central structural elements determining the genetic variability in immune response.

A complete understanding of the range of structural polymorphisms in class II molecules and of the variations in response to particular antigenic challenges in main remain challenges for the future. Our current state of understanding would strongly suggest that these functional and structural polymorphisms are closely associated and that a better understanding of the structural components will contribute greatly to a clear picture of the manner in which Ir genes function, and the manner in which class II genotype influences susceptibility to a wide variety of autoimmune diseases.

References

1. Auffray C, Korman AJ, Roux-Dosseto M, Bono R, Strominger JL (1982) cDNA clone for the heavy chain of the human B cell alloantigen DC1: strong sequence homology to the HLA-DR heavy chain. Proc Natl Acad Sci USA 79:6337
2. Auffray C, Lillie JW, Arnot D, Grossberger D, Kappes D, Strominger JL (1984) Isotypic and allotypic variation of human class II histocompatibility antigen α-chain genes. Nature 308:327
3. Bach FH, Amos DB (1967) Hu-1 major histocompatibility locus in man. Science 156:1506
4. Barclay AN, Mason AW (1983) Graft rejection and Ia antigens. Paradox resolved? Nature 303:382
5. Bell JI, Estess P, St. John T, Saiki R, Watling DL, Ehrlich HA, McDevitt HO (1985) DNA sequence and characterization of human class II major histocompatibility complex β chains. Proc Natl Acad Sci USA 82:3405–3409
6. Bell JI, McMurray AJ, Denney DW, Watling DL, Foster LS, McDevitt HO (1985) Restriction fragment length polymorphisms among thirty consanguineous homozygous cell lines. (to be published)
7. Benacerraf B, McDevitt HO (1972) Histocompatibility-linked immune response genes. Science 175:273
8. Benoist CO, Mathis DJ, Kanter MR, Williams VE, McDevitt HO (1983) Regions of allelic hypervariability in the murine A_α immune response gene. Cell 34:169

9. Boss JM, Strominger JL (1984) Cloning and sequence analysis of the human major histocompatibility complex gene DC-3β. Proc Natl Acad Sci USA 81:5199
10. Carroll MC, Campbell RD, Bentley DR, Porter RR (1984) A molecular map of the human major histocompatibility complex class III region linking cmplement genes C4, C2, and factor B. Nature 307:237
11. Charron DJ, Lotteau V, Turmel P. (1984) Hybrid HLAA-DC antigens provide molecular evidence for gene trans-complementation. Nature 312:157
12. Choi E, McIntyre L, Germain RN, Seidman JG (1983) Murine I-A_β chain polymorphism: nucleotide sequences of three allelic I-A_β genes. Science 221:283
13. Coppin HL, Denney DW Jr, Weissman SM, McDevitt HO (1985) HLA-B locus polymorphism: studies with a specific hybridization probe. Proc Natl Acad Sci USA (in press)
14. Dembic Z, Singer PA, Klein J (1984) E^o: a history of a mutation. EMBO J 3:1647
15. Devlin JJ, Wake CT, Allen H, Widera G, Mellor AL, Fahrner K, Weiss EH, Flavell RA (1984) The major histocompatibility complex of the C57BL/10 mouse: gene organization and function. In: Cantor H, Chess L, Sercarz E (eds) Regulation of the immune system. Liss, New York (UCLA symposia on molecular and cellular biology)
16. Germain RN, Lechler RI, Norcross MA, Bentley DM, Margulies DH (1985) Advances in gene technology: molecular biology of the immune system. In: Streilein JW, Ahman F, Black S, Blomberg B, Voellmy RW (eds) Cambridge University Press, Cambridge
17. Giles RC, DeMars R, Chang CC, Capra JD (1985) Allelic polymorphism and transassociation of molecules encoded by the HLA-DQ subregion. Proc Natl Acad Sci USA 82:1776
18. Gotz H, Kratzin H, Thinnes FP, Yang CY, Kruse T, Pauly E, Kolbel S, Egbert G, Wernet P, Hilschmann N (1983) Amino acid sequence comparison between DR and DC subclass antigens derived from a lymphoblastoid B cell line homozygous at the HLA loci. Hoppe-Seylers Z Physiol Chem 364:749
19. Goyert SM, Silver J (1983) Further characterization of HLA-DS molecules: implications for studies assessing the role of human Ia molecules in ell interactions and disease susceptibility. Proc Natl Acad Sci USA 80:5719
20. Groner JP, Watson AJ, Bach FH (1983) Dw/LD-Related molecular polymorphism of DR4 β-chains. J Exp Med 157:1687
21. Gustafsson K, Wiman L, Emmoth E, Larhammar D, Bohme J, Hyldig-Nielsen JJ, Ronne H, Peterson PA, Rask L (1984) Mutations and selection in the generation of class II histocompatibility antigen polymorphism. EMBO J 3:1655
22. Hanafusa T, Chiovato L, Doniach D (1983) Aberrant expression of HLA-DR antigen on thyrocytes in Grave's disease: relevance for autoimmunity. Lancet II:1111
23. Hansen TH, Melvold RW, Arn JS, Sachs DH (1980) Evidence for mutation in an I-A gene. Nature 285:340
24. Hayes CE, Klyczed KK, Krum DP, Whitcomb RM, Hullett DA, Cantor H (1984) Chromosome 4 Tt gene controls murine T cell surface I-J expression. Science 223:559
25. Hockman PS, Huber BT (1984) A class II gene conversion event defines an antigen-specific Ir gene epitope. J Exp Med 160:1925
26. Inoko H, Ando A, Kimura M, Ogala S, Tsuju K (1984) Isolation and characterization of the cDNA clones and the genomic clones of the HLA class II antigen heavy chains. In: Albert E, Baur MP, Mayr WR (eds) Histocompatibility testing 1984. Springer, Berlin Heidelberg New York Tokyo, pp 559–564
27. Jones PP, Murphy DB, McDevitt HO (1978) Two-gene control of the expression of a murine Ia antigen. J Exp Med 148:925
28. Jones P, Murphy D, McDevitt HO (1981) Variable synthesis and expression of DC_α and A_e (E_β) polypeptide chains in mice of different H-2 haplotypes. Immunogenetics 12:321
29. Kan YW, Dozy AM (1978) Polymorphism of DNA sequence adjacent to human β-globin structural gene: relationship to sickle mutation. Proc Natl Acad Sci USA 75:5631
30. Kappes DJ, Arnot D, Okada K, Strominger JL (1984) Structure and polymorphism of the HLA class II SB light chain genes. EMBO J 3:2985
31. Kaufman JE, Auffray C, Korman AJ, Shackelford DA, Strominger S (1984) The class II molecules of the human and murine major histocompatibility complex. Cell 36:1
32. Klein J, Figueroa F (1981) Polymorphism of the mouse H-2 loci. Immunol Rev 60:23

33. Korman AJ, Auffray C, Schamboeck A, Strominger JL (1982) The amino acid sequence and gene organization of the heavy chain of the HLA-DR antigen: homology to immunoglobulins. Proc Natl Acad Sci USA 79:6013
34. Kratzin H, Yang C, Gotz H, Pauley E, Korbel S, Egert G, Thinnes FP, Wernet P, Altevogt P, Hilschmann M (1981) Primarstruktur menschlicher Histokompatibilitatsantigene der Klasse II. Hoppe-Seylers Z Physiol Chem 362:1665
35. Lalanne J-L, Cochet M, Kummer AM, Gachelin G, Kourilsky P (1983) Different exon-intron organization at the 5' part of a mouse class I gene is used to generate a novel H-2K^d-related mRNA. Proc Natl Acad Sci USA 80:7461
36. Larhammar D, Gustafsson K, Claesson L, Bill P, Wiman K, Schenning L, Sundelin J, Widmark E, Peterson PA, Rask L (1982) Alpha chain of HLA-DR transplantation antigens is a member of the same protein superfamily as the immunoglobulins. Cell 30:153
37. Larhammar D, Schenning L, Gustafsson K, Wiman K, Claesson L, Rask L, Peterson P (1982) Complete amino acid sequence of an HLA-DR antigen-like β chain as predicted from the nucleotide sequenced similarities with immunoglobulins and HLA-A, -B, and -C antigens. Proc Natl Acad Sci USA 79:3687
38. Larhammar D, Anderson G, Bill P, Bohme J, Claesson J, Denaro M, Emmoth E, Gustafsson K, Hammerling U, Heldin E, Hyldig-Nielson JJ, Und P, Schenning L, Servenius B, Widmark E, Rask L, Peterson P (1983) Molecular analysis of human class II transplantation antigens and their genes. Hum Immunol 8:95
39. Larhammar D, Hyldig-Nielsen JJ, Servenius B, Andersson G, Rask L, Peterson PA (1983) Exon-intron organization and complete nucleotide sequence of a human major histocompatibility antigen DCβ gene. Proc Natl Acad Sci USA 80:7313
40. Larhammar D, Hammerling G, Denaro M, Lund T, Flavell RA, Rask L, Peterson P (1984) Structure of the murine immune response I-A_β gene and an adjacent β-chain second domain exon. Cell 34:179
41. Larhammar D, Servenius B, Rask L, Peterson PA (1985) Characterization of an HLA DR_β pseudogene. Proc Natl Acad Sci USA 82:1475
42. Lee J, Trowsdale J, Travers PJ, Carey J, Grosveld F, Jenkins J, Bodmer W (1982) Sequence of an HLA-DR α-chain cDNA clone and intron-exon organization of the corresponding gene. Nature 299:750
43. Lin CCS, Rosenthal AS, Passmore HC, Hanson TH (1981) Selective loss of antigen-specific Ir gene function in IA mutant B6.C-H.2^{bm12} is an antigen presenting cell defect. Proc Natl Acad Sci USA 78:6406
44. Long EO, Wake CT, Gorski J, Mach B (1983) Complete sequence of an HLA-DR β-chain deduced from a cDNA clone and identification of multiple non-allelic DR β chain genes. EMBO J 2:289
45. Malissen M, Hunkapiller T, Hood L (1983) Nucleotide sequence of a light chain gene of the mouse I-A subregion. Aβ^d. Science 221:750
46. Mathis DJ, Benoist CO, Williams VE II, Kantor MR, McDevitt HO (1983) The murine E_α immune response gene. Cell 32:745
47. Mathis DJ, Benoist CO, Williams VE II, Kanter M, McDevitt HO (1983) Several mechanisms can account for defective DC_α gene expression in different mouse haplotypes. Proc Natl Acad Sci USA 80:273
48. Matis LA, Jones PP, Murphy DB, Hedrick SM, Lerner EA, Janeway CA Jr, McNicholas JM, Schwartz RH (1982) Immune response gene function correlates with the expression of an Ia antigen. II. A quantitative deficiency in $A_{e:E}\alpha$ complex expression causes a corresponding defect in antigen-presenting cell function. J Exp Med 155:508
49. McDevitt HO, Chinitz A (1969) Genetic control of the antibody response: relationship between immune response and histocompatibility (H-2) type. Science 163:1207
50. McIntyre K, Seidman J (1984) Nucleotide sequence of mutant I-A_β^{bm12} gene is evidence for genetic exchange between mouse immune response genes. Nature 308:551
51. McKenzie IFC, Morgan GM, Sndrin MS, Michaelides MM, Melvold RW, Kohn HI (1979) B6.C-H-2^{bm12}, a new H-2 mutation in the I region in the mouse. J Exp Med 150:1323
52. McNicholas J, Steinmetz M, Hunkapillar T, Jones P, Hood L (1982) DNA sequence of the gene encoding the E_α Ia polypeptide of the Balb/c mouse. Science 218:1229
53. Mellor AL, Weiss EH, Ramachandran K, Flavell RA (1984) A potential donor gene for the bm1 gene conversion event in the C57BL mouse. Nature 306:792

54. Mengle-Gaw L (1984) Sequence analysis of allelic I-E_β immune response genes. PhD thesis, Stanford University
55. Mengle-Gaw L, McDevitt HO (1983) Isolation and characterization of a cDNA clone for the murine I-E_β polypeptide chain. Proc Natl Acad Sci USA 80:7621
56. Mengle-Gaw L, McDevitt HO (1984) Allelic variation in mouse Ia chain genes in regulation of the immune system. In: Sercarz E, Cantor H, Chess L (eds) Regulation of the immune system. Liss, New York (ULCA symposia on molecular and cellular biology, new series, vol 18)
57. Mengle-Gaw L, Connor S, McDevitt HO, Fathman CG (1984) Gene conversion between murine class II major histocompatibility complex loci. Functional and molecular evidence from the BM12 mutant. J Exp Med 160:1184
58. Mengle-Gaw L, McDevitt HO, Benoist C, Mathis D (1985) Class II MHC α-L chain association: clues from the u-haplotype. Proc Natl Acad Sci USA (in press)
59. Michaelides M, Sandrin M, Morgan G, McKenzie IFC, Ashman R, Melvoid RW (1981) Ir gene function in an I-A subregion mutant B6.C-H-2^{bm12}. J Exp Med 153:464
60. Murphy DB (1981) Genetic fine structure of the H-2 gene complex. In: Dorf ME (ed) The role of the major histocompatibility complex in immunobiology. Garland, New York
61. Nepom BS, Nepom GT, Mickelson E, Antonelli P, Hansen JA (1983) Electrophoretic analysis of human HLA-DR antigens from HLA-DR homozygous cell lines. Correlation between β chain diversity and HLA-D. Proc Natl Acad Sci USA 80:6962
62. Nomenclature for factors of the HLA system (1984) Tissue Antigens 24:73
63. Orkin SH, Kazazian HH Jr, Antonarakis SE, Goff SC, Boehm CD, Sexton JP, Waber PG, Giardina PJV (1982) Linkage of β-thalassaemia mutations and β-globin gene polymorphisms with DNA polymorphisms in human β-globin gene cluster. Nature 296:627
64. Owerbach D, Lernmark A, Rask L, Peterson P, Platz P, Svejgaard A (1983) Detection of HLA-D/DR-related DNA polymorphism in DLA-D homozygous typing cells. Proc Natl Acad Sci USA 80:3758
65. Reinsmoen NL, Bach FH (1982) Five HLA-D clusters associated with HLA-DR4. Hum Immunol 4:249
66. Saito H, Maki R, Clayton LK, Tonegawa S (1983) Complete primary structures of the E_β chain and its gene of the mouse major histocompatibility complex. Proc Natl Acad Sci USA 80:5520
67. Sasazuki T, Kaneoka H, Nishimura Y et al. (1980) An HLA-linked immune suppression gene in man. J Exp Med 152:297S
68. Sasazuki T, Nishimura Y, Muto M, Ohat N (1983) HLA linked genes controlling immune response and disease susceptibility. Immunol Rev 70:51
69. Schenning L, Larhammar D, Bill P, Wiman K, Johnson AK, Rask L, Peterson PA (1984) Both α and β chains of HLA-DC class II histocompatibility antigens display extensive polymorphism in their amino-terminal domains. EMBO J 3:447
70. Servenius B, Gustafsson K, Widmark E, Emmoth E, Andersson G, Larhammar D, Rask L, Peterson PA (1984) Molecular map of the human HLA-SB (HLA-DP) region and sequence of an SB_α (DP_α) pseudogene. EMBO J 3:3209
71. Shaw S, Kavathas P, Pollack MS, Charmot D, Mawas C (1981) Family studies define a new histocompatibility locus, SB, between HLA-DR and GLO. Nature 293:745
72. Shreffler DC, David CS (1975) The H-2 major histocompatibility complex and the I immune response region: genetic variation, function, and organization. Adv Immunol 20:125
73. So AKL, Trowsdale J, Bodmer JG, Bodmer WF (1984) DNA polymorphism of HLA-DR_β and HLA-DP_β genes. In: Albert ED, Baur MP, Mayr WR (eds) Histocompatibility testing 1984. Springer, Berlin Heidelberg New York Tokyo, pp 565–568
74. Spielman R, Lee JS, Bodmer WF, Bodmer J, Trowsdale J (1984) Six HLA-D_α chain genes on human chromosome 6: polymorphisms and associations of DC_α-related sequences with DR types. Proc Natl Acad Sci USA 81:3461
75. Steinmetz M, Minard K, Horvath S, McNicholas T, Frelinger J, Wake C, Long E, Mach B, Hood L (1982) A molecular map of the immune response region from the major histocompatibility complex of the mouse. Nature 300:35

76. Stetler D, Das H, Nunberg JH, Saiki R, Sheng-Dong R, Mullis KB, Weissman SM, Erlich HA (1982) Isolation of a cDNA clone for the human HLA-DR antigen α chain by using a synthetic oligonucleotide as a hybridization probe. Proc Nat Acad Sci USA 79:5966
77. Stetler D, Grumet C, Erlich HA (1985) Polymorphic restriction endonuclease sites linked to the HLA-DR_α chain gene: localization and use as genetic markers in insulin-dependent diabetes mellitus. Proc Natl Acad Sci USA (in press)
78. Tonnelle C, DeMars R, Long EO (1985) A gene encoding an MHC class II beta chain distinct from DR, DQ, and DR beta chains is expressed in a human B cell line. Proceedings of American Societies for Experimental Biology, 69th annual meeting, abstracts of papers. Fed Proc 44(3)
79. Transky TC, Lalanne JL, Kourilsky P (1984) Alternative splicing in the 5′ moiety of the H-$2K^d$ gene transcript. EMBO J 3:2383
80. Travers P, Blundell TL, Sternberg MJE, Bodmer WF (1984) Structural and evolutionary analysis of HLA-D-region products. Nature 310:235
81. Trent JJ, Wainscoat J, Weatherall DJ (1981) A new triplicated α-globin gene arrangement in man. Br J Haematol 49:149
82. Trowsdale J, Lee JS, Kelly A, Carson S, Austin P, Travers P (1984) A linkage map of two HLA-SB alpha and beta genes: an intron in one of the SB beta genes contains a processed pseudogene. Cell 38:241
83. Trowsdale J, Young JAT, Kelly AP, Austin PJ, Carson S, Meunier H, So A, Ehrlich HA, Spielman RS, Bodmer J, Bodmer WF (1985) Structure, sequence, and polymorphism in the HLA-D region. Immunol Rev (in press)
84. Van Leeuwen A, Schit HRE, Van Rood JJ (1973) Typing for MLC (LD): II. The selection of nonstimulator cells by MLC inhibition tests using DS-identical stimulator cells (MISIS) and fluorescence antibody studies. Transplant Proc 5:1539
85. Weiss E, Golden L, Zakut R, Mellor A, Fahrner K, Juist S, Flavell RA (1983) The DNA sequence of the H-$2k^b$ gene: evidence for gene conversion as a mechanism for the generation of polymorphism in histocompatibility antigens. EMBO J 2:453
86. Widera G, Flavell RA (1984) Nucleotide sequence of the murine I-E^b_β immune response gene: evidence for gene conversion events in class II genes of the major histocompatibility complex. EMBO J 3:1221
87. Yang C, Kratzin H, Gotz H, Thinnes FP, Kruse T, Egert G, Pauly E, Kolbel S, Wernet P, Hilschmann N (1982) Mitteilung: Aminosäuresequenz der N-terminalen 179 Reste der α-Kette des HLA-DW2/DR2-alloantigens. Hoppe-Seylers Z Physiol Chem 363:671

Molecular Genetics as a Tool in Clinical Transplantation *

E. Möller, J. Wallin, and B. Carlsson

Table of Contents

HLA Typing in Transplantation: Historical Comments

After the discovery of the HLA region in the mid 1960s and the observation that kidney grafts exchanged between HLA-identical sibs had excellent survival, national, and international graft exchange programs were initiated all over the world to optimize patients' changes of getting HLA-"matched" grafts. These collaborative efforts began in the last years of the 1960s, before the definition of HLA-C, D, or DR. Those scientists who had used the MLC reaction to select donor-recipient pairs for living related kidney allografts were not surprised when it was shown later that HLA-A,B matching did not seem to have a major influence on necro-kidney graft survival, since by this time Yunis and Amos [40] had already described that MLC activation was induced by antigens encoded by an HLA-linked locus not identical to A or B.

These findings spurred the efforts to define products of this locus, which would later be referred to as HLA-D. The designation HLA-C had been reserved for serologically defined antigens encoded by a locus between A and B [28].

Jörgensen et al. [14], Dupont et al. [9], and Mempel et al. [20] introduced the technique of typing for HLA-D antigens using homozygous typing cells (HTCs). During the 1975 International Histocompatibility Workshop in Aarhus, several

* The experiments cited herein were supported by grants from STU (Swedish Board of Technical Development) and the Swedish Medical Research Council

HLA-D products were defined with this technique, and many alleles of the new locus were found to occur in strong linkage disequilibrium with HLA-B genes [18]. Thus, the lymphocyte-defined (LD) determinant(s) in linkage disequilibrium with B7 was called LD-7a (Dw2), and with B8, LD-8a (Dw3). Results from many centers had already indicated that a low MLC reactivity of donor cells against recipient stimulator cells in vitro was correlated with superior graft survival, which led to the intense efforts in trying to find means of defining these LD determinants with serological reagents [7, 26]. MHC restriction had been described in 1974 [41], and some investigators commented that one might not be able to find antibodies which would recognize alloantigenic determinants in a fashion that correlated completely with specific T cell recognition [21]. However, during the 1977 workshop in Oxford, many different laboratories had defined antibodies, mostly from multiparous women with reactivity patterns that corresponded relatively well with HLA-D types in panel cells [4]. The determinants defined by serological reagents were therefore referred to as HLA-D-related (DR). Relatively good reagents were found that defined Dw1, 2, and 3, and were referred to as DR1, 2, and 3. However, the sera that reacted with cells that had been typed as Dw4 also reacted with a fraction of cells that were not Dw4, i.e., DR4 was broader than Dw4. Readers who would like to know the details of the development and the most recent information on recognition of "D" specificities with antisera are referred to the chapter by Schreuder and van Leeuwen in this volume (Alloantisera Against Human Class II Antigens).

What is HLA-D?

Let us discuss the problem of HLA-D in the light of the more recently gained knowledge that there are at least three loci that encode class II antigens in the HLA region, now referred to as DP, DQ, and DR. The first definition of DP by Shaw et al. [30] and by Termijtelen et al. [33] demonstrated products of this locus as strong stimulators of a secondary MLR in the PLT assay. These data would indicate that DP antigens would not induce a strong MLR, and the conclusion could be drawn that DP compatibility is of little importance in transplantation, since a low MLC reactivity of donor cells against recipient cells is associated with good kidney graft survival. But there is good reason to believe that HLA-D, which stimulates strong primary MLR, consists of a combination of products of at least both the DQ and the DR locus. In fact, it is impossible to presently tell if products of one locus are of greater importance than products of the other for initiation of MLC responses [23].

The definition of HLA-D originates from the use of HTCs. Anybody who has carried out HTC typing knows that it is difficult to define a "typing" response. Ryder et al. [27] introduced the stabilized relative response (RR) for a statistical analysis of these reactivities. Good typing cells were those that gave a clear biphasic response pattern when tested against a panel of responder cells. However, most cells did not induce this clear response pattern, but gave a substantial proportion of cells with a relative response in the "gray area" between the two phases. These responder cells often ended up in the gray area when retested. In addition, two identical typing cells should ideally give a straight line correlation when compared on the same responder panel.

Most of the HTCs were selected from family studies where haploidentical responder cells gave a low response. However, these cells, which were often known to be DR-homozygous, did not necessarily have to be DQ- or DP-homozygous. Since little or no linkage disequilibrium exists between DP on the one side and DQ/DR on the other, most of the commonly used HTCs were probably not DP-homozygous. Alternatively, the good typing reagents were also DP-identical, but those cells that did not give clear biphasic response patterns were DP-heterozygous. It should be remembered that most HTCs used were not consanguineous.

Today, the D region encompasses DQ and DP in addition to DR, and the highest degree of relative responsiveness that is compatible with a D region match still has to be established. Our conclusion would be that MLC responses observed with mixtures of cells from HLA-identical sibs are the only acceptable figures for a complete HLA-D match.

What is HLA-DR?

DR is only one of the three class II loci of the HLA-D region. Historically, those determinants which could be recognized by B cell-reactive sera, mostly from multiparous women, and which on panel cells reacted in a way that correlated to D-typing, were named DR. But if one accepts that the D-region contains DP, DQ, and DR genes, what is the identity of the antigens conventionally called DR? The assay most commonly used for DR typing is microcytotoxicity. Cytotoxic reactions are dependent on a high concentration of cell surface antigens to ensure adequate complement fixation [22]. There would be no problem with DR typing were DR antigens the only ones adequately expressed on peripheral blood monocytes and B lymphocytes; however, DQ antigens are also expressed on B cells and at least on a subset of blood monocytes [25]. The relative expression of DP on mononuclear cells in the blood is not yet known. Perhaps DP has a lower surface representation than DQ or DR, making it impossible to find serological reagents that define individual DP specificities.

Most sera from multiparous women contain mixtures of antibodies against A, B, C, and D region encoded antigens. By absorption, the content of class I antibodies is eliminated. We believe that most of these sera contain mixtures of antibodies against DR, DQ, and perhaps also DP. Most of these sera are weak and often have to be used undiluted to give good cytotoxicity. This implies that if sera with a high correlation coefficient to HLA-D typed panel cells have been selected, the best typing sera should contain an optimal mixture of DR and DQ (and possibly DP) antibodies. The old description of positive cytotoxicity only after adding two nonrelated antibodies reacting with different determinants on the same cell is again relevant [22]. Have we fooled ourselves into believing that one could define serological reagents that reacted with products of a putative single locus, and instead ended up with "good" DR typing reagents which contain optimal mixtures of antibodies reacting with determinants from different loci? One could say that the extreme difficulty of finding good DR typing reagents argues in favor of this idea, and that we have for a long time discarded sera that would indeed define products of individual loci, since it was not believed that other reaction patterns were relevant.

We shall here argue that the current definition of DR could be partly erroneous, and be based on artificial antibody mixtures in "good" typing sera. One has to consider that both DR and DQ molecules are expressed on class II positive blood lymphoid cells and monocytes. A further complication comes from recent findings by Böhme et al. [5], who have shown that a varying number of DR β chain genes exist in haplotypes with different DR types. The data show that in DRw8 positive haplotypes only a single β chain gene exists in the DR locus, whereas in DR4- or DR7-positive haplotypes as many as four DR β chain genes are present (J. Böhme, personal communication). The first problem arises from the fact that more than one DR-containing molecule is expressed from a single haplotype. DNA sequence data have shown that at least one of the DR4-associated β chain genes is a pseudogene [19], and other data indicate that as many as three distinct β chain sequences can be obtained from cDNA of a DR4-positive cell line (D. Larhammar and F. Bach, personal communication). The DQ locus contains a constant number of two α and β genes per haplotype [5]. Biochemical evidence from Karr et al. [16, 17] shows that possibly two distinct DQ molecules can be expressed, one of which contains the DQ-allospecific serological determinants. Data from DNA sequence studies do not argue against the evidence that both DQ α and β genes could be functional. For DP, finally, there is evidence for two α and β genes, but also that only one of each can be expressed and the other pair is nonfunctional [15, 29, 36].

In the following we shall present our data on studies of HLA-D region genes using cDNA probes specific for DR, DQ, and DP α and β genes. Our conclusion will be that certain DR "specificities" are formed by combinations of class II antigens. At the end of the chapter we shall discuss the implications of this idea for the use of DR typing in clinical transplantation.

DR β Gene Polymorphism Detected with cDNA Probes

In collaboration with the Department of Cell Research, Uppsala University, we have studied different cells that have been well defined using HTCs and serological reagents included in the Ninth International Histocompatibility Workshop for restriction fragment length polymorphism (RFLP) that can be detected after DNA-DNA hybridization using cDNA probes.

It has already been shown by Wake et al. [37] and by Andersson et al. [2] and reported by different groups in the proceedings of the Ninth Workshop [1] that cDNA probes can be used to "type" cells. This means that after digestion of genomic DNA with different restriction enzymes, DNA size separation on agarose gels and transfer onto nitrocellulose filters according to Southern [31], p32-labeled full-length cDNA probes will hybridize with DNA of different sizes to form a pattern that is detected using autoradiography. Thus, Andersson et al. [2] found that DNA-DNA hybridizations with cDNA probes on material from cells from unrelated but HLA-Dw/DR-identical homozygous individuals will give rise to identical RFLPs. Since most endonucleases will cut the genomic DNA in intronic parts, these findings indicate that there is a conserved allele-specific nucleotide sequence.

A consistent finding in our study of a large panel of DR-heterozygous cells has been the rather limited heterogeneity that exists between different DR alleles using this method of resolution [6, 38]. Only cells that are DR1, 2, or 4 have specific bands that do not exist in other phenotypes.

These findings could indicate that the degree of polymorphism that can be detected with this method is too small and that allele specific variations in exonic parts of the DNA are not detected with the present methods. However, for the present discussion we shall argue that the specificity of our detection system is adequate. In addition, DR3, 5, w6, and w8 form a group regarding the distribution of restriction fragments. The DR β cDNA patterns of DRw8 are included in those of cells with DR5, which in turn is completely included in that of DR3. DRw6 seems to be divided into two groups in our material; one group is completely identical to DR3 and the other group lacks a 11-kb *Pvu*II band, which we have found to be strongly associated with the serological determinant DRw52. Most of these experiments, which have in part been reported elsewhere [6, 24, 38], have been performed with genomic DNA digested with *Bam*HI and *Pvu*II. We have recently tried to resolve the possible allelic differences between DR3- and DRw6-positive cells by digestions with *Kpn*I, *Pst*I, *Eco*RV, and *Hin*dIII without finding further polymorphism. Recently, however, Hyldig-Nielsen (personal communication) reported that DR3 could be distinguished from DRw6 using the endonuclease *Taq*I. It needs to be shown that this difference is not detecting the allelic variation that we associate with DRw52.

Recent data from many different kinds of experiments clearly indicate that the DRw52 and w53 specificities are present on distinct DR β chains from those that carry the conventional DR epitopes. Tosi et al. [35] first reported that at least three loci encoded class II MHC antigens, referred to as DR, BR, and DC. DC is now known to correspond to DQ, and BR is identical to the DRw52 and w53 specificities. Hurley et al. [12, 13] published evidence to show that DRw52 and DR5 could be present on separate DR β chains, or possibly in certain instances also on the same chain.

As mentioned above, Böhme et al. [5] have clearly established that the number of DR β genes varies in different haplotypes. Cells from individuals who are DRw8 carry only one DR β gene/haplotype, whereas cells from individuals who are DR1 have two, and most other phenotypes are associated with three distinct β genes.

The elucidation of RFLPs from a large panel of Dw/DR-homozygous and -heterozygous cells have shown that certain DR types are more closely related than others [5]. Thus, as mentioned above, clearly distinct patterns exist for DR1, 2, and 4. DR7-positive cells give rise to band patterns that are closely related to those of DR4. DR4 cells have a *Pvu*II band of 5.8 kb that is absent in DR7-positive cells, but otherwise the combination of DR β bands are extremely similar. Furthermore, the RFLP pattern of DRw8 cells is less complex than the pattern from cells of other haplotypes, which is to be expected since the DRw8 haplotype only contains a single DR β gene. Böhme et al. [5] have used this information to deduce a phylogenetic tree for evolution of DR polymorphism, where a primordial gene for DR β chains first differentiated DR7 and 4 from the rest of the alleles, and the other branch threw off the variants that gave rise to DR1 and 2. The main branch contains the DRw8 allele, before the gene duplication occurred which lead to the 3, 5, w6 variants.

DQ Gene Polymorphism Detected with cDNA Probes for α and β Chains

The interpretation of bands detected with cDNA β chain probes can be difficult. This is partly due to the fact that irrespective of carefully chosen stringency conditions, a certain degree of cross-hybridization between genes of different class II loci is hard to avoid. Therefore, it is important to know the band patterns that are obtained with probes for the different β chains in order to identify bands which are the result of cross-hybridization with genes of other class II loci.

In the DQ molecule both α and β chains vary [8]. We have used both types of probes to study allelic variation of DQ RFLPs. When testing a large number of heterozygous panel cells, the close linkage disquilibrium between DR and DQ becomes immediately obvious. Groups of HLA-DR-identical cells from unrelated individuals, which often give identical RFLPs with the DR β chain probe, also demonstrate striking similarities of their DQ β patterns. This is demonstrated in

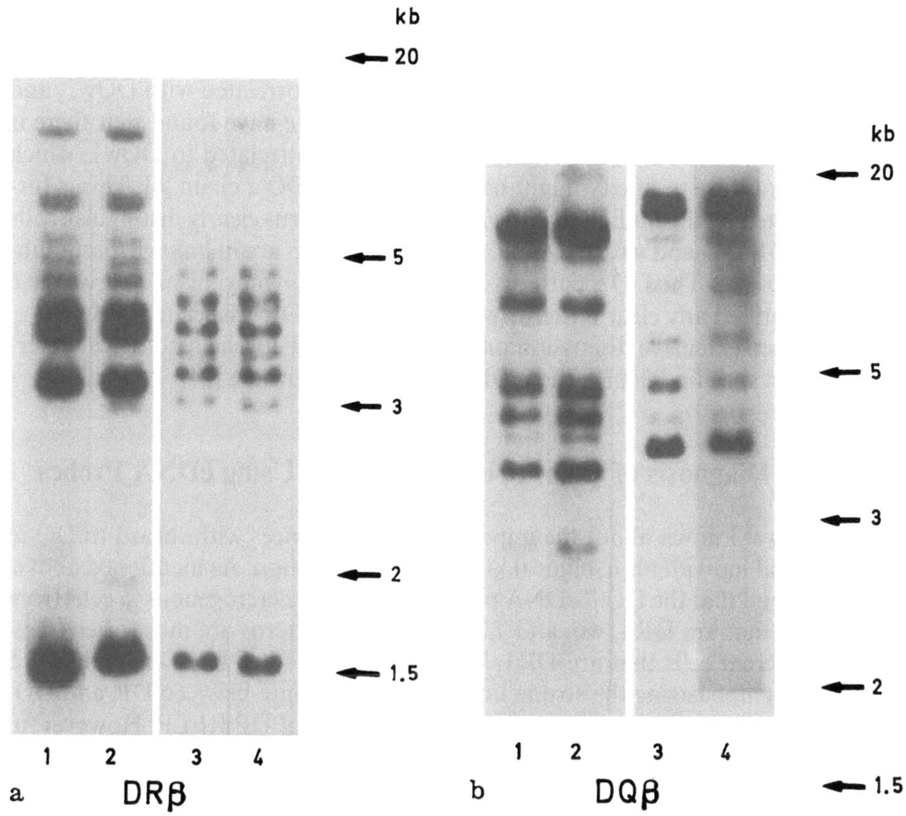

Fig. 1. a Southern blots after DNA digestion with *Pvu*II and hybridization with a full-length DR β cDNA probe. Lanes 1 and 2 contain material from two unrelated individuals both typed as DR2,5, and lanes 3 and 4 are from two individuals typed DR3,4. **b** Southern blots from the same four individuals after DNA digestion with *Bam*HI and hybridization with a full-length DQ β chain probe. The figure demonstrates the close linkage disequilibrium between DR and DQ, since identical DQ patterns are found with DR identical cells. However, the polymorphism is quite extensive for the DQ β patterns, and cells with the DR phenotypes 4,w6, and 7 are associated with at least two distinct DQ β patterns

Fig. 1, where groups of cells from two DR2,5 typed unrelated individuals and two DR3,4 individuals are tested with both DR and DQ β probes.

Böhme et al. [5] and we have earlier correlated the genotypic polymorphism of DQ in DR-identical cells. Thus, there is a pattern of DQ RFLP which occurs in cells from DR1-positive individuals and is usually not present in cells from other individuals, again emphasizing the close linkage disequilibrium between DR and DQ. The degree of DQ polymorphism in this assay is at least as marked as that of DR, and thus by far exceeds the hitherto defined serological DQ polymorphism. Concordant data have indicated the presence of specific DQ genotypic patterns associated with particular DR types. There is one prominent DQ pattern associated with DR2 which is different from that of DR1. In other cells the DQ patterns can vary more. Thus, two distinct DQ genotypes are associated with DR4 in our panel of cells, and at least two exist also for DRw6 and DR7. We have speculated that these DQ subgroups within a single DR specificity are associated with distinct Dw splits of the same DR specificity [24]. These DQ subgroups have not yet been characterized and correlated to Dw typing using HTCs.

Studies using the DQ α chain probe have given results that have been difficult to interpret directly. Spielman et al. [32] demonstrated that using the DQ α probe, the RFLPs could be statistically associated with certain earlier defined serological specificities. Thus, they found a group of bands that correlated with DQw1, and yet other patterns correlating with DRw52 and 53. We have found that there is a 4.5-kb band after *Pvu*II digestion which is closely correlated to DQw1, which indicates that this specificity might be present on the DQ α chain [6]. This is further supported by the finding that the DQ β chain patterns clearly distinguish cells which are DR1, 2, and w6, those DR specificities which are in linkage disequilibrium with DQw1. The DQ α patterns show a limited polymorphism, and we have not yet identified any clear patterns which are closely DR-associated.

For a more extensive discussion on the association between serological determinants and specific RFLPs, the reader is referred elsewhere [24].

Aid in the Diagnosis of Class II Incompatibility Using cDNA Probes

Little is as yet known about the importance of differences with regard to DQ in DR-identical individuals in clinical kidney transplantation. As mentioned above, we have found that the DQ β cDNA probe patterns are heterogenous in cells from individuals that are DR4, w6, and 7, whereas DQ patterns are most often identical in different cells that are DR1. The same is true for DR2, DR3, and DR5 cells, again emphasizing the strong linkage disequilibrium between DR and DQ.

cDNA probes are now also available for the study of DP RFLP. However, in our assays we have not yet identified patterns that correlate with DP determinations using specific PLT cloids. The DP typing of our panel cells has been carried out by Nancy Reinsmoen in Minneapolis. Similar data were recently reported by Hyldig-Nielsen et al. (personal communication). The reason for this finding is not yet known, but there are several possibilities. One is that digestion of DNA with the endonucleases used in the studies so far has not been adequate to detect existing polymorphism. This is believed to be less probable, since little variation exists in genomic DNA sequences when DNAs encoding DP α and β chains are compared (see Peterson et al., and Rask, Genes and Antigens of the HLA-D Region, in this volume). There are two different DP α and β genes, and yet another alternative would be that available sequence data are derived from a set of less variable DP chains. Again, this is hard to reconcile with the idea that extensive cross-hybridization is to be expected from different α and β genes encoded by the same locus. Therefore, the observed DP specificities detected in the PLT assay have not been possible to detect with the molecular approach using cDNA probes. It is likely that future development in this area will resolve this important question.

We have speculated that DP incompatibility might be of major importance in bone marrow transplantation. A high proportion of transplanted patients suffer from severe graft-vs-host disease (GVHD). In most centers performing bone marrow transplantations, HLA-identical sibs are specifically selected as donors, and it is rare that HLA-incompatible donors are accepted. DP was discovered by Shaw et al. [30] in combinations of HLA-A, B, C, DR-identical cells from unrelated individuals that would result in a low primary MLC response, but gave a strong stimulation in the PLT assay. Already these findings demonstrated that DP alleles are not in close linkage disequilibrium with DR.

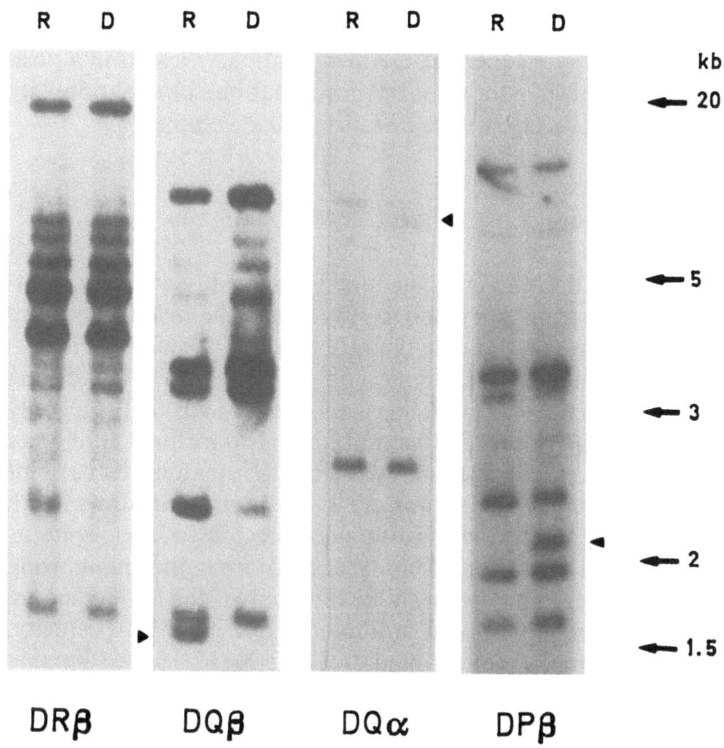

Fig. 2. DNA from two HLA-A, B, C, DR-identical sibs, donor and recipient for bone marrow transplantation, was tested with full-length probes for DR β, DQ α and β, and DP β chains. No polymorphism is detected with the DR β probe, but clearly distinct patterns are revealed with DQ α and β as well as with the DP β probes. Differences are indicated with *arrows*. These RFLPs support the notion that the two sibs are DR-identical but DQ- and DP-incompatible due to a recombination in a maternal haplotype. Since the mother is DR7-homozygous, the recombination is not informative as to the location of the DQ locus with regard to DR and DP

In light of the high recombination frequency between DR and DP, estimated at a genetic distance of 3.3 cM by Termijtelen et al. [34], we set out to study our sib combinations selected for bone marrow transplantation after HLA-D, B, C, DR serological determinations, combined with a negative MLC test (cutoff point $\leq 8\%$ RR).

In 37 combinations tested so far, only one instance was found where cells from serologically identical sibs gave a positive PLT. This combination also gave a mutual MLC response of 30%–40%, in spite of DR identity. DNA-DNA hybridization with DR β, DQ α and β, and DP β probes revealed identical DR β patterns but clear difference both in DQ (α and β) and in DP β RFLPs (Fig. 2). Therefore, the two sibs were most probably DQ- and DP-incompatible, due to a recombination that had occurred in a maternal haplotype. The mother turned out to be DR7- homozygous, but heterozygous for DQw2 and 3 when tested with reagents of the Ninth Workshop. It was impossible to establish whether the recombination occurred between B and DR or between DR and DQ. The clinical course was complicated, and the patient died of a GVHD. This is extremely rare in HLA-identical sib donor-recipient pairs in our patient material, and *we conclude that DQ and/or DP incompatibility is important in bone marrow transplantation.* We have not yet identified any cell combinations that give a completely negative MLC response but a clearly positive PLT response as indicative of a DP incompatibility, and we tentatively conclude that DP incompatibility results in a positive MLC, although it is lower than for most DR-incompatible combinations (see Sanchez-Perez and Shaw, HLA-DP: Current Status, in this volume).

Use of Monoclonal Antibodies to Define Class II Antigens

We have presented the view that the DR type that is assigned to a cell is a combination of class II determinants which could in certain cases be encoded by more than one class II locus. In order to resolve the problem of dissection of the different class II antigens, their relative distribution on different tissues, and during the differentiation of cells, it is imperative to have reliable reagents that react only with products of one locus and not with other molecules. Monoclonal antibodies are the perfect tools for these studies. Before discussing these matters, let us point out that a monoclonal antibody, by definition, reacts in a homogeneous way with the immunizing antigen and is often believed to recognize only a single epitope. The antibodies are often selected for strong reactivity with the immunizing antigen. The specificity of this reaction would be high only if the antibodies are of low affinity. High-affinity monoclonal antibodies have a lower specificity, since cross-reactivity with similar determinants will increase with the binding strength, and therefore might turn out to be useless for biochemical characterization of class II antigens, since there is a high degree of homology between antigens of the different loci.

The repertoire of the B cell population is complete, and therefore antibodies will exist that react with all configurations possible. The total number of possible determinants has been calculated to be 10^{17} (A. Coutinho, personal communication). It has also been agreed that there are only 10^{6}–10^{7} immunocompetent B cell clones at any one time in a given individual (mouse!). Therefore, if the reactivity patterns and the degeneracy of antibodies are similar for all specificities, each monoclonal could be able to physiologically interact with at least 10^{11} different determinants. Therefore it will be important to carefully characterize the specificity of monoclonal antibodies used for typing purposes or for the purification of class II antigens. It is interesting to point out that the first cDNA encoding a class II β chain was produced from mRNA of a cell which could direct the in vitro synthesis of β chains that reacted with a rabbit anti-DR β chain serum. When the cDNA was sequenced, it turned out to specify an I-A like β chain, now known as DQ [39].

Elsewhere in this volume is a summary of available class II monoclonal antibodies available for typing (Colombani and Lepage, Monoclonal Antibodies Against Human HLA Class II Antigens). From our tentative scheme of the HLA-D region and its products, one would expect that allospecific monoclonal antibodies specific for DR1 and 2 would be identified. However, the group of DR4 and 7 would be hard to dissect, just like the group of DR3, 5, 6, and w8 antigens. One might expect that a DRw8 monoclonal antibody would recognize also DR5, 6, and 3, and in addition, that no *DR-specific* antibody would be able to clearly distinguish DR3 from DR6.

What Are the Dw Splits of DR?

From the chapter by Schreuder and van Leeuwen in this volume (Alloantisera Against Human Class II Antigens), the reader can get comprehensive information about the various splits that have been defined with both sera and HTCs of the conventional DR specificities. We have speculated that many of these splits emanate from different DQ associations with DR. There is also the possibility of splits within a single DR specificity, if more than one DR molecule can be expressed and D-heterogeneity is associated with an epitope on one DR β chain. Yet another complexity arises from the fact that the number of DR β genes expressed might differ within the groups of cells carrying a single DR "specificity". To exemplify this idea for the Dw4, w10, w13, w14, and w15 splits associated with DR4, the D differences might be due either to distinct combinations of polymorphic DR β chains expressed on the cell surface, or to the combination of distinct DR and DQ antigens (see [3]).

Class II Compatibility in Clinical Transplantation

There are several points that need to be clarified before any conclusions can be drawn as to the relative importance of products of distinct class II loci in transplantation:

1. Tissue distribution of DR, DQ, and DP antigens. Not all cells that are expressing or can be induced to express class II antigens necessarily express equal amounts of specificities of different loci. Nunez et al. [25] have shown that the tissue distribution of DQ antigens varies on subsets of monocytes, and other reports have described differences in expression of distinct class II antigens on differentiating B cells [11]. As long as it is not known whether DP antigens are expressed at all in cells which could be immunogenic in the kidney, no conclusions

can be reached as to the relative importance of DP matching for kidney graft survival.

2. The level or variability of the DQ α and β genes probably exceeds that which can be recognized with serological or cellular reagents today. As we have discussed, the differences between haplotypes that can be distinguished with DNA-DNA hybridization are not necessarily biologically relevant. However, not only data from studies using various DNA probes, but also biochemical evidence, suggest that the polymorphism of DQ molecules exceeds that recognized serologically (for references see [10]). We have also implied that certain of the Dw splits of well-established DR specificities are associated with DQ incompatibilities, demonstrating the importance of DQ for initiation of MLC responses and the importance of these antigens in immune reactions.

Very little is as yet known about the expression of alloantigenic determinants on DP molecules, since these determinants cannot be typed with antisera. This difficulty might be related to the density of DP-antigenic determinants on peripheral blood lymphocytes, which influences the reactivity of DP-containing cells with cytotoxic antibodies. Other assays might turn out to be more appropriate for the definition of DP.

3. The studies partly reported here have shown that certain DR specificities seem to be more closely related phylogenetically than others. One such group is formed by DR4 and 7, another by DR3, 5, w6, and w8.

If it is correct that DRw8 cells only express a single DR molecule which greatly resembles or is identical to molecules present in individuals who are DR3, 5, or w6, the presence of DRw8 should not be considered as a DR incompatibility in individuals who are DR3, 5, or w6, but only in individuals who are DR1, 2, 4, or 7. Therefore, one might have to reconsider the importance of DR matching in transplantation in these terms. We would argue that some so-called DR mismatches are no mismatches, whereas others which seem to be ideal matches might contain relevant mismatches for products of closely linked loci. Relevant to this discussion are, for example, donor-recipient pairs who share DR4, since at least two different DQ genotypes associate with DR4, and a DQ mismatch could create the incompatibility necessary for induction of graft rejection.

Finally, we cannot leave this discussion without pointing out that most grafts are transplanted into class II-incompatible recipients, but results are excellent with modern and appropriate immunosuppressive treatment irrespective of the degree of matching.

Acknowledgments. Skilful technical assistance was provided by Brith Otterud and Birgitta Hagström. We thank Jan Böhme, Lars Rask, and Per Peterson, Dept. of Cell Research, Wallenberg Laboratory, Uppsala University for fruitful collaboration and the continuous supply of DNA probes used in this study.

References

1. Albert ED, Baur MP, Mayr WR (eds) (1984) Histocompatibility testing 1984. Springer, Berlin Heidelberg New York Tokyo
2. Andersson M, Böhme J, Andersson G, Möller E, Thorsby E, Rask L, Peterson PA (1984) Genomic hybridization with class II transplantation antigen cDNA probes as a complementary technique in tissue typing. Hum Immunol 11:57

3. Bach FH (1985) The HLA class II genes and products. The HLA-D region. Immunol Today 6:89
4. Bodmer WF, Batchelor JR, Bodmer JG, Festenstein H, Morris PJ (eds) (1977) Histocompatibility testing 1977. Munksgaard, Copenhagen
5. Böhme J, Andersson M, Hammerling U, Andersson G, Möller E, Peterson PA, Rask L (1985) HLA DR β genes vary in number between different DR specificities, whereas the number of DQ β genes is constant. J Immunol 135:2149
6. Carlsson B, Böhme J, Lundgren G, Möller E, Peterson PA, Rask L, Ringdén O, Wallin J (1985) HLA class II genes studied with genomic hybridization in kidney and bonemarrow transplantation donor-recipient pairs. Transplant Proc 17:952
7. Cochrum KC, Perkins HA, Payne RO, Kountz SL, Belzer FO (1973) The correlation of MLC with graft survival. Transplant Proc 5:391
8. Corte G, Calabi F, Damiani A, Bargellisi A, Tosi R, Sorréntino R (1981) Human Ia molecules carrying DC 1 determinants differ in both a and b-subunits from Ia molecules carrying DR determinants. Nature 292:357
9. Dupont B, Jersild C, Hansen GS, Nielsen LS, Thomsen M, Svejgaard A (1973) Typing for MLC determinants by means of LD-homozygous and LD-heterozygous test cells. Transplant Proc 5:1543
10. Giles RC, Capra JD (1985) Structure, function, and genetics of human class II molecules. Adv Immunol 37:1
11. Heyningen van V, Guy K, Newman R, Steele CM (1982) Human MHC class II molecules as differentiation markers. Immunogenetics 16:459
12. Hurley CK, Nunez G, Winchester R, Finn OJ, Levy R, Capra JD (1982) The human HLA-DR antigens are encoded by multiple β-chain loci. J Immunol 129:2103
13. Hurley CK, Giles RC, Nunez G, DeMars R, Nadler L, Winchester R, Stastny P, Capra JD (1984) Molecular localization of human class II MT2 and MT3 determinants. J Exp Med 160:472
14. Jörgensen R, Lamm LU, Kissmeyer-Nielsen F (1973) Mixed lymphocyte culture with inbred individuals. An approach to MLC typing. Tissue Antigen 3:323
15. Kappes DJ, Arnot D, Okada K, Strominger JL (1984) Structure and polymorphism of the HLA class II light chain genes. EMBO J 3:2985
16. Karr RW, Kannapell CC, Zangara RJ, Goyert SM, Silver J, Schwartz BD (1983) An HLA-DR5 homozygous cell line express two DS (Ia-like) molecules. J Exp Med 158:1374
17. Karr RW, Alber C, Goyert SM, Silver J, Duquesnoy RJ (1984) The complexity of HLA-DS molecules: A homozygous cell line expresses multiple HLA-DS alfa chains. J Exp Med 159:1512
18. Kissmeyer-Nielsen F (ed) (1975) Histocompatibility testing 1975. Munksgaard, Copenhagen
19. Larhammar D, Servenius G, Rask L, Peterson PA (1985) Characterization of an HLA-DR pseudogene. Proc Natl Acad Sci USA 82:1475
20. Mempel W, Grosse-Wilde H, Barumann P, Netzel B, Steinbauer-Rosenthal I, Scholz S, Berrams J, Albert ED (1973) Population genetics of the MLC response: typing for MLC determinants using homozygous and heterozygous reference cells. Transplant Proc 5:1529
21. Möller E (1974) Specificity of hapten-reactive T and B mouse lymphocytes. Affinity and avidity of T and B cell receptors and anti-hapten antibodies as a factor of dose and time after immunization. Scand J Immunol 3:339
22. Möller E, Möller G (1962) Quantitative studies of the sensitivity of normal and neoplastic mouse cells to the cytotoxic action of iso-antibodies. J Exp Med 115:527
23. Möller E, Carlsson B, Wallin J (1984) Distinct or overlapping functions of human class II genes. Scand J Immunol 20:403
24. Möller E, Carlsson B, Wallin J (1985) Implication of structural class II gene polymorphism for the concept of serologic specificities. Immunol Rev 85:107
25. Nunez G, Giles RC, Ball EJ, Hurley CK, Capra JD, Stastny P (1984) Expression of HLA-DR, MB, MT, and SB antigens on human mononuclear cells: Identification of two phenotypically distinct monocyte populations. J Immunol 133:1300
26. Ringdén O, Berg B (1977) Correlation between magnitude of MLC and kidney graft survival in intra-familial transplantation. Tissue Antigens 10:364

27. Ryder LP, Thomsen M, Platz P, Svejgaard A (1975) Data reduction in LD typing. In: Kissmeyer-Nielsen F (ed) Histocompatibility testing 1975. Munksgaard, Copenhagen, p 557
28. Sandberg L, Thorsby E, Kissmeyer-Nielsen F, Lindholm A (1970) Evidence of a third sublocus within the HL-A chromosomal region. In: Terasaki P (ed) Histocompatibility testing 1970. Munksgaard, Copenhagen, p 165
29. Servenius B, Gustafsson K, Widmark E, Emmoth E, Anderson G, Larhammar D, Rask L, Peterson PA (1984) Molecular map of the human HLA-SB (HLA-DP) region, and sequence of an SBα (DPα) pseudogene. EMBO J 3:3209
30. Shaw S, Johnson AH, Shearer GM (1980) Evidence for a new segregant series of B-cell antigens that are encoded in the HLA-D region and that stimulate secondary allogeneic proliferative and cytotoxic responses. J Exp Med 152:565
31. Southern EM (1975) Detection of specific sequences among DNA fragments separated by gel electrophoresis. J Mol Biol 98:503
32. Spielman RS, Lee J, Bodmer WF, Bodmer JG, Trowsdale J (1984) Six HLA-D region alpha-chain genes on human chromosome 6: polymorphisms and associations of DC alpha-related sequences with DR types. Proc Natl Acad Sci USA 81:3461
33. Termijtelen A, Bradley BA, van Rood JJ (1980) A new determinant defined by PLT, coded for in the HLA region and apparently independent of the HLA-D and DR loci. Tissue Antigens 15:267
34. Termijtelen A, Khan PM, Shaw S, van Rood JJ (1983) Mapping SB in relation to HLA and GLO1 using cells from first-cousin marriage offspring. Immunogenetics 18:503
35. Tosi R, Vismara D, Tanigaki R, Ferrara GB, Cicimarra F, Buffolano W, Follo D, Auricchio S (1983) Evidence that celiac disease is primarily associated with a DC locus allelic specificity. Clin Immunol Immunopathol 28:395
36. Trowsdale J, Kelly A, Lee J, Carson S, Austin P, Travers P (1984) Linkage map of two HLA-SB α and two HLA-SB β-related genes: an intron in one of the SB α genes contains a processed pseudogene. Cell 38:241
37. Wake C, Long E, Mach B (1982) Allelic polymorphism and complexity of the genes for HLA-DR beta gene. Direct analysis by DNA-DNA hybridization. Nature 300:372
38. Wallin J, Böhme J, Carlsson B, Möller E, Peterson PA, Rask L (1984) HLA class II polymorphism: restriction fragment patterns correlated to Ninth Workshop serology and function. In: Albert ED, Baur MP, Mayr WR (eds) Histocompatibility testing 1984. Springer, Berlin Heidelberg New York Tokyo, pp 572–576
39. Wiman K, Larhammar D, Claesson L, Gustafsson K, Schenning L, Bill P, Böhme J, Denaro M, Dobberstein B, Hammerling U, Kvist S, Servenius B, Sundelin J, Peterson PA, Rask L (1982) Isolation and identification of a cDNA clone corresponding to an HLA-DR antigen beta chain. Proc Natl Acad Sci USA 79:1703
40. Yunis EJ, Amos DB (1971) Three closely linked genetic systems relevant to transplantation. Proc Natl Acad Sci USA 68:3031
41. Zinkernagel RM, Doherty PC (1974) Restriction of in vitro T cell-mediated cytotoxicity in lymphocytic choriomeningitis within a syngeneic or semiallogeneic system. Nature 248:701

Biological Implications

The Role of Human Class II Molecules in Activation of T4 Lymphocytes *

E. Qvigstad, Ø. Bruserud, and E. Thorsby

Table of Contents

Introduction

While B lymphocytes can bind antigen directly, T lymphocytes recognize antigen only when presented together with major histocompatibility complex (MHC)-encoded class I or II molecules in the membrane of antigen-presenting cells (APC). This is called MHC restriction and was first shown in animal studies (see [5, 25] for references). The parts of the MHC molecule which are co-recognized together with antigen are often called restriction elements.

Human T lymphocytes may be divided into several different subsets. On the basis of reactivity with some monoclonal antibodies, two major subsets can be identified: the OKT4 or Leu3-positive subset, T4, and the OKT8 or Leu2-positive subset, T8. T4 lymphocytes co-recognize antigenic epitopes together with restriction elements on HLA class II molecules in the APC membranes, while T8 lymphocytes use parts on class I molecules as restriction elements (see [32] for references).

* Work supported by grants from the Norwegian Cancer Society, The Norwegian Diabetes Society, and the University of Oslo

The fine specificity of restriction, i.e., which parts of the HLA molecule provide the restriction element, is less well known. This review will first summarize some of our own studies on the nature of the restricting elements on HLA class II molecules.

The MHC molecules wich restrict T cells also participate in the regulation of the responsiveness to given antigens. Immune response (Ir) genes which control the degree and type of T cell responses have for many years been known to be present in the MHC chromosomal complex [6, 22]. More recently, it has become clear that the MHC class I and II molecules are the products of these Ir genes [17, 41]. How the restricting MHC molecules regulate the T cell responses to given antigens is, however, less clear. The determinant selection hypothesis suggests that by virtue of their allotypic variations, some MHC class I or II molecules may not be able to associate with a given antigen or antigenic epitope and are hence unable to present it to the T lymphocytes in an immunogenic form [4, 34]. Thus, low responsiveness might be due to insufficient antigen presentation to T cells. In contrast, the clonal deletion model maintains that nonresponsiveness is not determined on the antigen-presenting level, but is due to lack of specific T lymphocytes able to recognize an antigen in the context of a given MHC restriction element [16, 38]. This model is also called the "hole in the T cell repertoire" model. A third view holds that unresponsiveness is due to generation of suppressor T cells to given combinations of antigen plus MHC restriction elements. Possibly all three mechanisms may operate, depending upon antigen, mode of immunization, etc.

The second part of this review describes some of our own studies on the possible immunoregulatory effect of HLA class II molecules on T cell responses to viral antigens.

HLA Class II Molecules

The molecular biology of HLA class II molecules is treated elsewhere in this volume (P. A. Peterson and L. Rask, J. Silver and S. M. Goyert, T. Collins et al., H. Kratzin et al., R. Sorrentino and G. Corte, M. Sanchez-Perez and S. Shaw, J. I. Bell and H. O. McDevitt). A schematic outline of HLA class I and II molecules is given in Fig. 1. The class II molecules are encoded for in the HLA-D region of the HLA complex. The region codes for three main sets of molecules: DP(SB), DQ(DC), and DR. On the DR molecules both determinants activating allogeneic B cells, designated DR (DR1-DRw14), as well as determinants inducing T cell proliferation, designated D (Dw1-Dw19), are known. In the DR subregion there are at least three β gene loci, one of which contains a pseudogene. Genes of one of the other DR β loci, DRβ_1, determine allelic variants of the DR β chains responsible for the DR1-DRw14 determinants. Genes of the other DR β locus, DR β_2, may code for another set of allelic chains responsible for the serological determinants DRw52 and DRw53 (formerly called MT2 and MT3). The DQ and DP regions encode for the DQw1-3 and DPw1-6 specificities respectively [8].

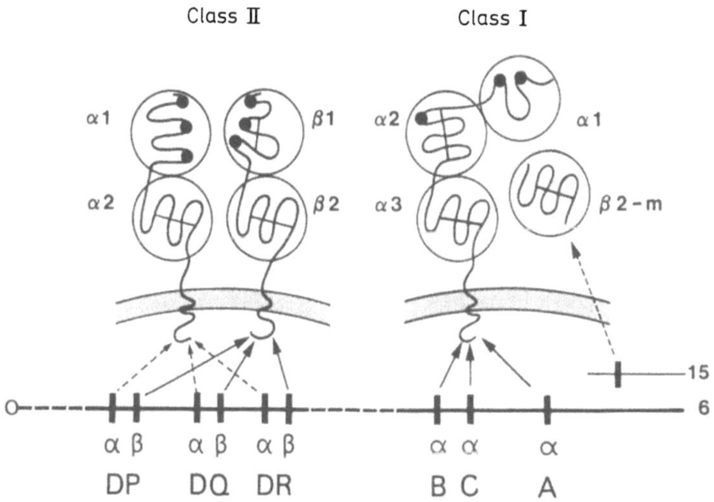

Fig. 1. The HLA class I and II molecules. Three different class II molecules are known (DR, DQ, and DP), and each consists of one α and one β polypeptide chain encoded by loci in the class II region on chromosome No. 6. Both the class II α and β chains have two extracellular domains (α_1 and α_2, β_1 and β_2), one transmembrane portion, and a shorter cytoplasmatic portion. The allelic variations are mainly localized in the first domains, especially the first domain of DRβ, DQα, and DQβ. Most variations are centered around different clusters of residues in the first domains, as illustrated by *black dots* in the figure. The HLA class I α chain loci (A, B, and C) are also shown

HLA Class II Molecules as Restriction Elements

The involvement of HLA class II molecules in T cell activation has been shown in many in vitro studies. The first involved crude T cells from in vivo sensitized donors, which were restimulated in vitro with the relevant antigen, for example purified protein derivative (PPD), together with autologous or allogeneic APC. Antigen-specific proliferative T cell responses required that the APC used shared both, or at least one, of the HLA-DR determinants with the T cell donor. Using T cell suspensions enriched for antigen-specific T cell blasts [19], evidence was also obtained that some T cells might be restricted by elements other than those present on the HLA-DR molecules [42]. Sharing of HLA class I molecules played no role.

Restriction Elements Used by Antigen-Specific Cloned T Cells

A more refined method to study the fine specificity of restriction, i.e., which parts of the MHC molecules constitute the restriction elements, was introduced when cloning of proliferative human T lymphocytes became possible [20, 21, 40]. We have mainly been working with proliferative T lymphocyte clones (TLC) specific for *Chlamydia trachomatis*, and a brief outline of the cloning procedure will first be given [28].

Peripheral blood mononuclear (PBM) cells in serum-supplemented medium are stimulated with antigen (i.e., *C. trachomatis*) for 6 days. T cell blasts are then separated from nonresponding small T cells on Percoll density gradients [19]. The blast-enriched suspension is diluted in serum-supplemented medium containing interleukin-2 (IL-2) (conditioned medium), so that an average of one blast is plated in every third well of a Terasaki microtest tray. Feeder cells are added together with antigen in optimal concentration. After incubation for 7 days, growing TLC are transferred to 96-well flat-bottomed trays and expanded, new feeder cells and antigen being added weekly. They are then screened using autologous APC as well as APC from allogeneic donors, with or without antigen. All tested clones are antigen-specific and do not respond to allogeneic APC without antigen, as previously reported [28]. The TLC used in the studies to be reported here are all T4.

Restriction by Elements on DR Molecules

When studying the class II restriction of *Chlamydia*-specific proliferative TLC, we observed that most of the TLC were restricted by one or the other DR determinant of the T cell donor [27]. Typical examples of HLA-DR restriction of four TLC from the cell donor BS are shown in Table 1. The individual BS has the HLA profile: HLA-A3; B7,15; DR1,4; DRw53, DPw4. All the TLC were restimulated by antigen together with autologous APC (first line in Table 1). Two TLC (BS1 and BS5) responded to the antigen only when allogeneic APC expressing DR4 were used. Two other TLC (BS11 and BS24) were usually only restimulated in the presence of antigen and allogeneic APC expressing DR1. However, the TLC BS11 was not always able to respond to antigen in conjunction with APC expressing DR1 (first allogeneic donor in Table 1).

Taken together, the results indicate that the TLC illustrated in Table 1 all use restriction elements on DR molecules, but also that the two clones BS11 and BS24 may use different restriction epitopes, both being present on DR1 molecules. No significant preferential restriction by any DR molecules could be seen, i.e., a similar number of DR1 and DR4 restricted TLC was found.

Table 1. HLA-DR restriction of chlamydial TLC

APC[b]	DR	Ag[c]	TLC[a]			
			BS1	BS5	BS11	BS24
Autologous	1.4	+	2352	3895	4081	7587
		−	163	246	183	354
Allogeneic	1.4	+	2070	2910	298	4842
Allogeneic	1.2	+	174	322	5507	8405
Allogeneic	1.3	+	173	176	5397	11472
Allogeneic	1.7	+	153	349	6009	7795
Allogeneic	4.2	+	2089	2416	153	165
Allogeneic	4.5	+	4325	3379	252	595
Allogeneic	4.6	+	3434	6183	834	221
Allogeneic	2.5	+	209	268	626	391
Allogeneic	3.8	+	371	350	769	191

Results expressed as mean cpm (SEM usually $<10\%$ of mean) · cpm in allogeneic combinations without antigen comparable with autologous antigen-free controls

[a] Ten thousand cells in each case

[b] Ten thousand non-T cells irradiated with 20 Gy

[c] Final chlamydial antigen concentration in wells: 2×10^6 IFU/ml

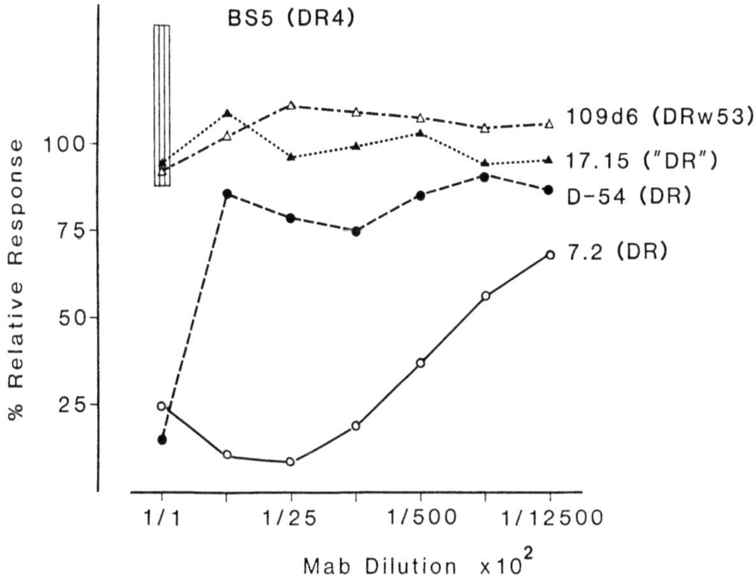

Fig. 2. Effect of different MoAb on the proliferative response of a DR4-restricted TLC (BS5), using antigen-pulsed monocytes as APC. The base value (in normal serum) from which the % relative response was calculated is 4522 cpm. Final dilution of MoAb in the wells is shown on the abscissa, and the designations and class II molecules which the MoAb recognize are also indicated. The *vertical striped column* shows the combined results using different HLA class I, -DQ- or -DP-reactive MoAb which were not blocking the response

To further study whether the restricting elements for these TLC are present on DR molecules, inhibition experiments with monoclonal antibodies (MoAb) against HLA molecules were carried out. The TLC were restimulated with autologous APC plus antigen in the presence or absence of different dilutions of MoAb in culture medium. One typical experiment, showing the effects of MoAb on the proliferative responses of a DR4-restricted TLC from donor BS, is illustrated in Fig. 2. We observe that only MoAb reactive with DR determinants (7.2 and D-54) were able to inhibit the proliferative responses. In our experiments, MoAb reactive with DQ or DP molecules or HLA class I molecules had no inhibitory activity on the DR-restricted TLC.

Restriction Elements on DR4-Expressing Molecules

The studies reported above show that DR molecules may provide restricting elements for T4 cells, but not which parts of the DR molecules are most important in this respect. To try to provide some answers to this question, we investigated TLC from a donor (GR) with HLA profile HLA-A19; B15,40; DR4,4; DRw53; DPw2. These TLC were restimulated with antigen (*C. trachomatis*) plus APC from some but not all donors carrying DR4, as reported elsewhere [27]. In the mixed lymphocyte culture (MLC) experiments we could demonstrate that those DR4-positive individuals who were able to provide the "correct" restricting element carried other T cell-activating determinants than those DR4-positive individuals whose APC were not able to restimulate the TLC. This would be in accordance with previous reports that several different HLA-D clusters may be as-

Table 2. HLA-DR4 subtype restriction of chlamydial TLC

APC	DR	Dw	Ag	TLC	
				GR14	GR15
Autologous	4.4	Dw14	+	11623	4069
			–	569	139
Allogeneic	4.0	Dw14	+	8497	3882
Allogeneic	3.4	Dw14	+	9969	3451
Allogeneic	4.0	Dw14	+	15151	4901
Allogeneic	4.6	Dw4	+	208	173
Allogeneic	4.7	Dw4	+	193	159
Allogeneic	3.4	Dw4	+	149	131
Allogeneic	4.8	Dw4, Dw14	+	11763	4093
Allogeneic	4.6	Dw4, KT2	+	224	141
Allogeneic	4.4	KT2	+	167	111
Allogeneic	4.4	KT2	+	172	231
Allogeneic	4.8	Dw13	+	383	281
Allogeneic	1.4	Dw13	+	195	149

See notes to Table 1

sociated with HLA-DR4 [2, 24, 33]. The relationship between the restriction elements for these TLC and some of the DR4-associated D determinants (i.e., Dw4, Dw10, Dw13, Dw14, Dw15, and KT2) was then studied in more detail with *Chlamydia*-specific TLC from donor GR.

TLC from GR were tested with non-T cells as APC from 20 allogeneic nonrelated DR4-positive individuals expressing different DR4-associated D determinants. Some representative results are given in Table 2. It can be seen that autologous APC together with antigen induced strong responses of both clones. In addition, allogeneic APC expressing Dw14 were all able to restimulate the TLC together with *Chlamydia* antigen. In contrast, APC expressing other DR4-associated D types (Dw4, Dw13, and KT2) were not able to restimulate the TLC together with antigen. The restriction elements for these TLC seem therefore to be closely associated with Dw14, and less closely with DR4. We conclude that in this case there exists a very close relationship between an alloactivating T cell determinant and parts of the DR molecule responsible for the restriction elements [31].

Restriction by Elements on DRw53 Molecules

During our studies we found that some TLC from donor BS were restimulated with antigen and most APC expressing DR4 or DR7. The true clonal nature of these TLC was ascertained in subcloning experiments.

Since the DRw53 specificity is strongly associated with both DR4 and DR7, we investigated whether parts of the DRw53 molecule might provide the restricting elements for these clones. A panel of donors were typed for DRw53, using the Ninth Histocompatibility Workshop antisera, and then used as APC donors in our experiments. Some results are given in Table 3. As can be seen, and has been reported in more detail elsewhere [27], the restriction pattern of TLC BS4 and BS37 closely follows the expression of DRw53 in the APC used for antigen restimulation, with a few exceptions (see below).

Table 3. Probable HLA-DRw53 restriction of chlamydial TLC

APC	DR	Alloantisera typing[a]			Ag	TLC	
		9w734	9w743	9w735		BS4	BS37
Autologous	1.4	0	0	2	+	3083	4341
					−	159	141
Allogeneic	2.7	3	3	3	+	3088	2900
Allogeneic	5.7	4	4	4	+	2986	3832
Allogeneic	1.7	3	3	3	+	3243	3746
Allogeneic	4.6	2	0	2	+	3597	2506
Allogeneic	4.8	2	1	3	+	4450	2346
Allogeneic	7.8	3	3	4	+	118	152
Allogeneic	7.0	3	3	3	+	230	312
Allogeneic	3.8	0	0	1	+	250	360
Allogeneic	2.0	0	0	1	+	188	228
Allogeneic	3.8	0	0	2	+	114	120
Allogeneic	2.5	0	0	0	+	247	198
Allogeneic	6.0	0	0	0	+	242	232
Allogeneic	1.3	2	0	2	+	264	362
Allogeneic	1.2	0	0	0	+	236	310
Allogeneic	2.4	2	1	3	+	1781	2342
Allogeneic	7.8	4	4	4	+	3944	7852
Allogeneic	4.5	2	0	3	+	3863	3522
Allogeneic	2.7	4	4	4	+	2758	2254

See notes to Table 1

[a] Alloantisera typing with Ninth International Histocompatibility Workshop (9w) sera. No reactivity above background is indicated by 0, while 4 means >80% killing

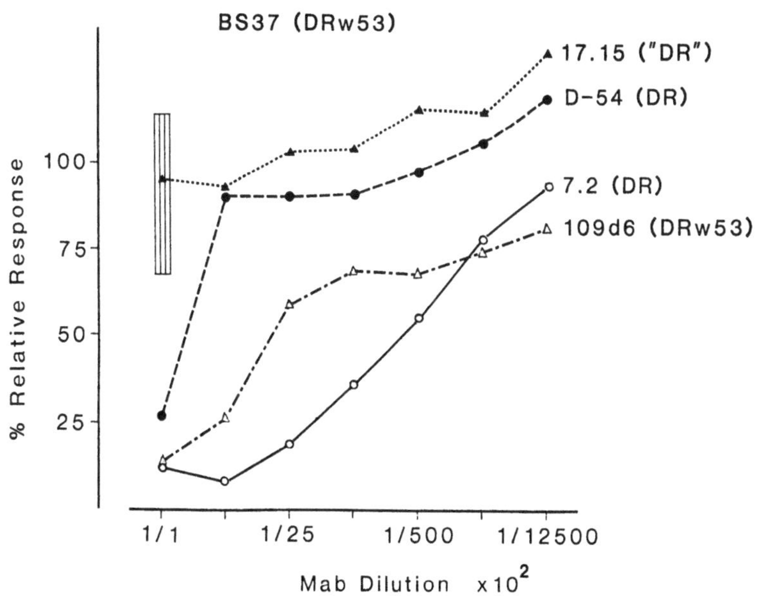

Fig. 3. Effect of MoAb on the proliferative response of a DRw53-restricted TLC. The base value for the TLC is 6816 cpm. See legend to Fig. 2 for further explanation

TLC BS4 and BS37 were then tested in blocking studies with various MoAb. MoAb 109d6, which detects a determinant closely associated but not identical to DRw53 [43], selectively inhibited the DRw53-restricted TLC without any effect on the other DR-restricted TLC, as illustrated in Figs. 2 and 3 [29].

On the other hand, APC from a few donors apparently expressing the DRw53 specificity (allogeneic donors 6 and 7 in Table 3), were not able to restimulate an antigen-specific response of these TLC. In order to study this on the genomic level, we used a DNA probe which hybridizes with genes for the DR β chains, and determined the restriction fragment length polymorphisms (RFLP) of the panel of APC donors. We found complete concordance between the presence of a 9.3-kb band in the *Hind*III digest of DNA from these APC donors and the ability of the APC to provide the "correct" restriction element, i.e., to restimulate an antigen-specific response [26]. The precise structural basis of the restriction element for TLC BS4 and BS37 must await further biochemical and molecular genetic studies. Taken together, however, our results indicate that the restriction element is closely associated with but not identical to the serologically defined DRw53 specificity, and can presently only be detected at the genomic level.

Restriction by Elements on DP Molecules

Chlamydia-specific TLC may also use parts of the DP molecules as restriction elements (Table 4) [30]. One TLC generated from donor BS (BS110) did not follow any of the DR specificities of donor BS in its restriction specificity. Instead, it closely followed the DPw4 specificity of a panel of APC donors, established with cloned alloreactive DPw4-specific T cells. One exception was observed; APC from one donor expressing DPw2 (and DR1) was also able to restimulate the TLC together with *Chlamydia* antigen. Thus, while the T cell-alloactivating determinants and those restricting the T cell responses to soluble antigens are often closely associated (see above), they may not always be completely identical.

It follows that *Chlamydia*-specific T lymphocytes may be restricted by elements on both DR and DP molecules, while we have never found evidence of elements

Table 4. HLA-DP restriction of chlamydial TLC

APC	DR	DP	Ag	TLC BS110
Autologous	1.4	4.0	+	10354
			−	394
Allogeneic	1.6	2.3	+	222
Allogeneic	1.0	3.0	+	174
Allogeneic	3.4	2.0	+	240
Allogeneic	4.8	2.0	+	126
Allogeneic	4.6	2.0	+	190
Allogeneic	2.5	4.0	+	4138
Allogeneic	2.5	4.0	+	7146
Allogeneic	2.3	4.0	+	11426
Allogeneic	3.8	3.4	+	3020
Allogeneic	3.8	4.0	+	4492
Allogeneic	1.0	2.0	+	7042

See notes to Table 1

on DQ molecules restricting the response. Others, however, have reported on DQ-restricted T cell lines [3, 18].

Virus antigen-specific TLC have also been reported to use parts of the DP molecules as restriction elements [14].

Immunoregulation of T Lymphocyte Responses by HLA Class II Molecules

Evidence of an immunoregulatory function of various DR molecules has been shown for the T lymphocyte response to both gluten antigens [39] and *Mycobacterium leprae* antigens [13]. An HLA-linked control of the T lymphocyte responses to streptococcal cell wall antigens, schistosomal antigens, and cedar pollen antigens has also been shown [37]. Scott et al. [39] found a lower frequency of HLA-DR3- and DR7-restricted gluten-specific T lymphocytes than gluten-specific T lymphocytes restricted by elements on other DR molecules. Since HLA-DR3 and DR7 are both associated with celiac disease, this DR-associated hyporesponsiveness may be important for development of the disease.

To study whether the T lymphocyte responses to certain viruses were similarly controlled by HLA class II molecules, we studied the responses to mumps, Coxsackie B4, and varicella-zoster viral antigens. We selected these viruses because they have all been suspected to play a role in the development of Type 1 diabetes mellitus. The frequencies of HLA-DR3 and -DR4 are markedly increased among Type 1 diabetics, whereas there is a decrease in the frequency of HLA-DR2, which is therefore postulated to have a protective effect [11].

HLA-DR-Restricted T Lymphocyte Responsiveness to Mumps Virus

In preliminary studies we compared the T lymphocyte responsiveness to mumps viral antigens in DR3- and DR4-positive healthy individuals. The in vitro responses were found to be significantly higher in DR4-positive individuals than in DR3-positive individuals, thus indicating a different regulatory function of these two DR determinants [10]. That DR molecules were implicated as restriction elements was shown in inhibition studies using MoAb specific for different HLA class II molecules. A majority of the mumps-reactive T lymphocytes, in the presence of antigen and APC were strongly inhibited by MoAb against the DR molecules, and less inhibited by MoAb against DQ and DP molecules [12].

We then used a limiting dilution assay to estimate the frequencies of mumps-specific antigen-reactive T lymphocytes (ARTL) restricted by different DR-associated restriction elements. This method has been described in detail elsewhere [11], and is schematically outlined in Fig. 4. Briefly, antigen-stimulated cultures were incubated for 6 days and the ARTL blasts then recovered by Percoll separation. The T blasts were further enriched by culture in the presence of IL-2 (step 1), and then investigated using the limiting dilution assay (step 2).

A typical experiment is shown in Fig. 5. Various numbers of enriched mumps-specific T blasts from a DR3,4 heterozygote Type 1 diabetic patient were cultured together with mumps antigen and APC sharing either DR3 or DR4 of the T blast donor. As can be seen, the number of positive cultures decreased more rapidly when DR3-expressing APC were used than with DR4-expressing APC. In this ex-

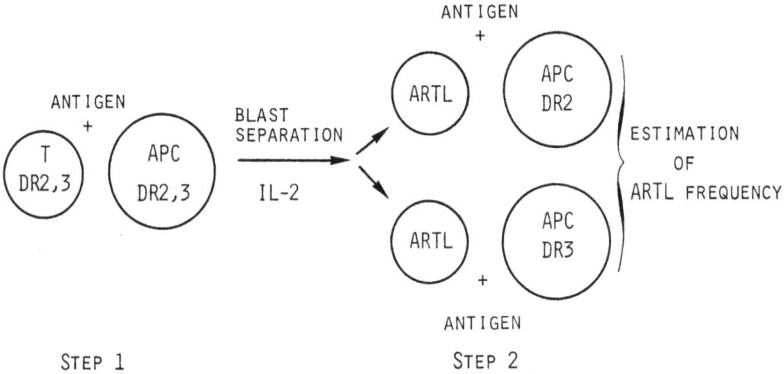

Fig. 4. The methods used to estimate the frequencies of T lymphocytes restricted by DR-associated restriction elements. In step 1, T lymphocytes (DR2,3) and autologous APC were cultured with antigen for 7 days, and the antigen-specific blasts then recovered by Percoll density gradient separation. The blasts were further enriched by culture in the presence of IL-2 for 6 days. The enriched blasts were then tested in the limiting dilution assay (step 2). Various numbers of enriched T blasts were restimulated together with antigen and a fixed number of allogeneic APC (5000/well). The T blasts were tested in parallel, using APC from two different donors, each sharing one DR determinant, either DR2 or DR3, with the T lymphocyte donor. ^{3}H-thymidine incorporation was assayed after 3 days

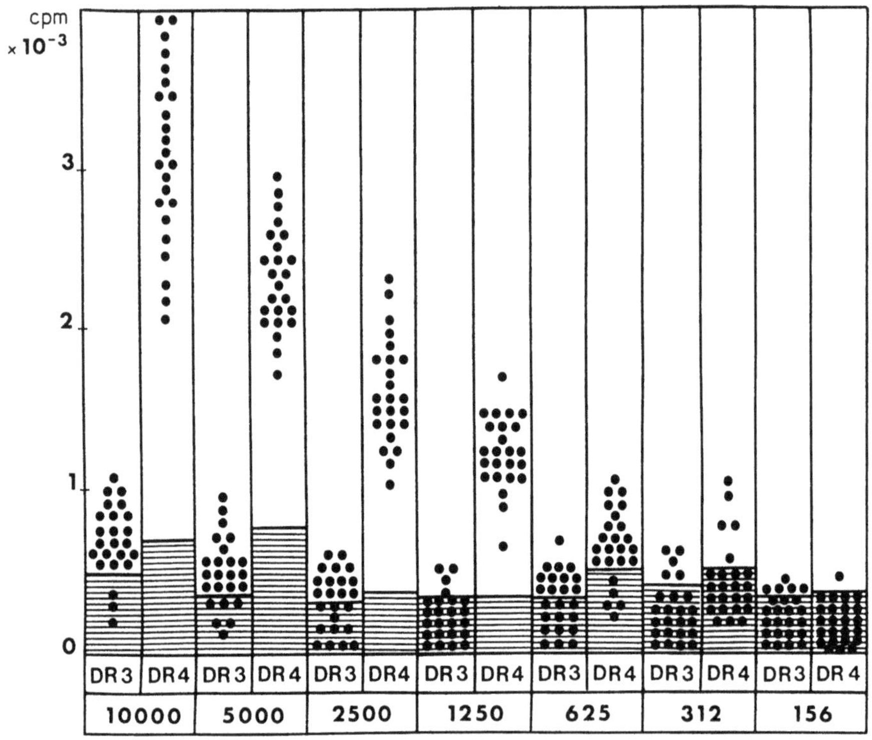

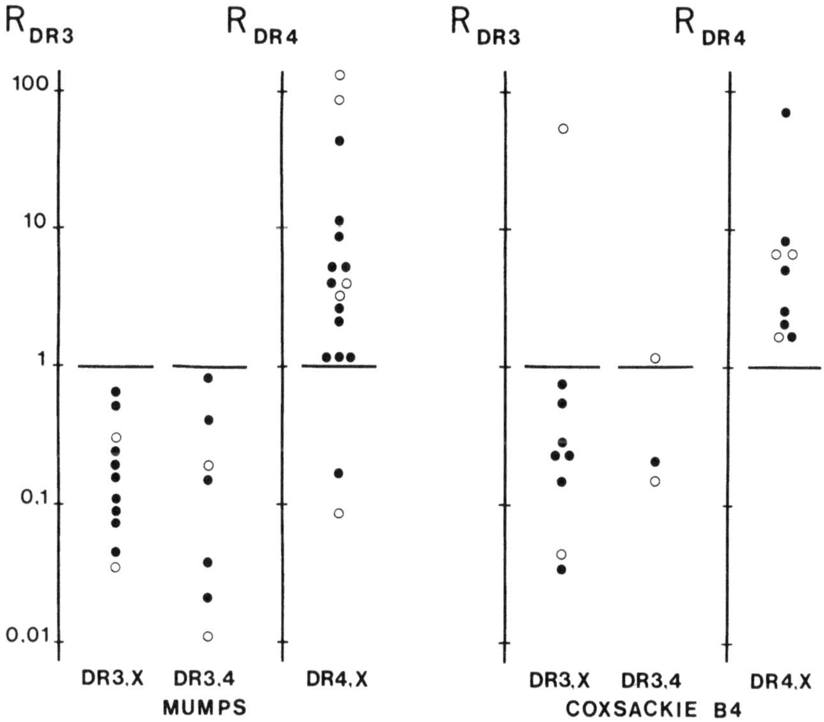

Fig. 6. The relative frequency of T blasts responding to mumps and Coxsackie B4 in healthy individuals (●) and Type 1 diabetic patients (○) expressing DR3, DR4, or both (*X* being any DR determinant other than DR3 or DR4). The relative frequency of ARTL (*R*) was defined as follows:

$$R_{DR3} = \frac{\text{frequency of DR3-restricted ARTL}}{\text{frequency of ARTL restricted by the other DR determinant}}$$

The R_{DR4} was calculated correspondingly

periment the frequency of DR4-restricted ARTL was estimated to be 1:525, whereas the frequency of DR3-restricted ARTL was 1:3630.

The overall results are shown in Fig. 6. A decreased frequency of DR3-restricted ARTL ($R_{DR3} < 1$) to mumps was found for all the 18 healthy individuals and the four diabetics investigated, whereas an increased frequency of DR4-restricted ARTL ($R_{DR4} > 1$) was found in the major proportion of DR4-positive in-

Fig. 5. Enriched mumps-specific T lymphocyte blasts were prepared from a DR3,4 heterozygote Type 1 diabetic patient. Different numbers of blasts were restimulated with antigen and APC sharing either DR3 or DR4 with the T lymphocyte donor. At the *bottom* of the figure is indicated the number of T blasts/well and the DR determinant shared in the restimulation. Each *dot* represents the response (cpm) of incorporated ^{3}H-thymidine in a single culture. Those antigen-stimulated cultures were scored as positive (i.e., assumed to contain at least one ARTL) in which the response exceeded mean cpm + 3 SD of the 12 corresponding antigen-free controls (*shaded area*). The distribution of the ARTL was assumed to be of the Poisson type. Accordingly, the ARTL frequency was calculated as the inverse number of T blasts giving 37% negative cultures. In this particular experiment, the frequency of DR3-restricted ARTL was calculated to be 1:3630, the frequency of DR4-restricted ARTL 1:525 (details in [11])

Table 5. The frequency of ARTL to mumps and Coxsackie B4 in healthy DR2,3 and DR2,4 heterozygotes

Donor	HLA-DR		Antigen	
	T cell	APC	Mumps	Coxsackie B4
TS	2.3	2 (6)	1:16238	1: 5248
		3 (6)	<1:30000	<1:10000
AH	2.3	2 (7)		1: 3236
		3 (8)		<1:10000
RH	2.3	2 (4)	1: 1230	1: 1288
		3 (8)	1:19498	<1:10000
RW	2.3	2 (4)	1: 3313	1: 537
		3 (8)	1:15488	1: 707
GS	2.4	2 (6)	<1:10000	1:16982
		(3) 4	1: 4467	1: 7762
EH	2.4	2 (3)	1: 1288	
		4 (7)	1: 312	
∅B	2.4	2 (6)	1: 1000	
		(1) 4	1: 625	

dividuals tested. There seemed to be no difference between healthy individuals and Type 1 diabetics in this respect. No particular high or low frequency of ARTL was seen when DR2 restricted the response (Table 5).

HLA-DR-Restricted T Lymphocyte Responses to Coxsackie B4 Virus

Very similar findings were made when Coxsackie B4 instead was used as antigen. Judging from inhibition studies, a majority of Coxsackie-B4-reactive T lymphocytes seemed to be restricted by epitopes on the DR molecules [12]. Furthermore, when frequencies of Coxsackie-B4-specific ARTL were estimated using the limiting dilution assay, a decreased frequency of DR3-restricted ARTL was found for a majority of DR3-positives tested, whereas the majority of the DR4-positives showed an increased frequency of DR4-restricted ARTL (Fig. 6). There seemed to be no difference between healthy individuals and diabetics.

As can be seen from Table 5, again the frequency of DR2-restricted ARTL was greater than that of DR3-restricted ARTL and lower than that of DR4-restricted ARTL.

For both the mumps and the Coxsackie B4 virus investigations, varicella-zoster and PPD responses were also tested. However, no differences in ARTL frequencies were found, whether DR2, DR3, or DR4 restricted the responses [12].

Comments

In this review we have summarized some of our data on the involvement of HLA class II molecules in antigen activation of human T4 cells. Activation requires corecognition of an antigenic epitope in conjunction with a restriction element present on class II molecules in the APC membrane. DR and DP class II molecules appear to be able to express restricting elements, of which a given T cell is only able to "use" one. Using *C. trachomatis* as antigen, we were not able to show any DQ-restricted TLC.

How T cells recognize antigen in the context of HLA molecules is not fully known. Recent data suggest that the T cell receptor is made up of two chains (α and β) linked by an interchain S-S bridge [35, 36]. This would favor participation of both subunits in the formation of a single combining site, which would be more compatible with a "single recognition site" model for the T cell receptor, i.e., joint recognition of antigen and MHC products. The T3 molecules seem to be very closely related to the receptor in the cell membrane [9], while the T4 and T8 molecules may be important in facilitating cell-cell interactions, possibly by providing an additional affinity ligand binding [7]. This is schematically illustrated in Fig. 7, where it is assumed that the T cell receptor (T_R) recognizes antigen together with variable parts of the HLA molecules, while the T4 (or T8) molecules recognize more constant parts of the HLA molecules [32].

One explanation of the fine specificity of restriction is that the same variable parts which are immunogenic in allogeneic combinations are constituting the restriction elements. Data presented here indicate that the restricting elements may often not be identical to the parts of the class II molecules which induce alloantibody production, although overlapping may occur. Closer associations have been found between the restricting elements and those parts of the class II molecules which induce proliferation of allogeneic T cells (the "D determinants"), but in some cases the restricting element could only be detected at the genomic level. More studies are needed using class II molecules which are better biochemically characterized, as well as cells transfected with class II molecules [1, 23]. Available data indicate, however, that several different restriction elements may be expressed by each type of class II molecule.

The restriction elements which are co-recognized may be dependent upon the antigen, i.e., the restriction and antigen specificity are closely associated [15]. Whether function (i.e., helper, cytotoxicity, suppression) is also associated with different restriction molecules or elements remains to be clarified. If it turns out that function and restriction are closely associated, then different functional T cell subsets might selectively be activated by virtue of the restriction elements, for example by the use of MoAb blocking the response involving irrelevant restriction molecules.

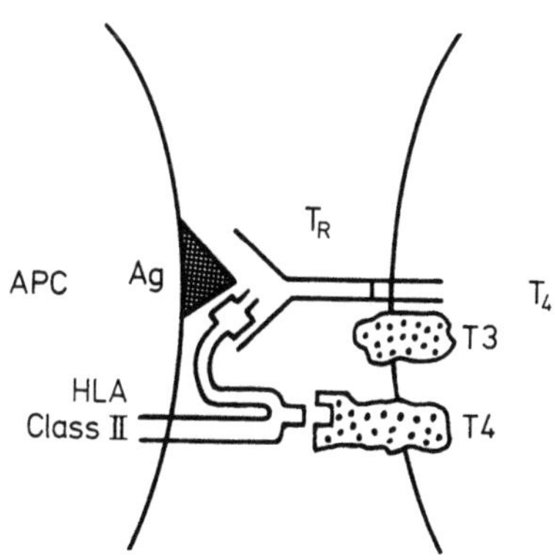

Fig. 7. A highly schematic illustration of T-APC interaction. The T cell receptor (T_T) is assumed to recognize a complex of antigen and variable parts of the HLA molecule in the APC membrane. T4-positive cells recognize antigen together with variable parts of HLA class II molecules, while the T4 molecule provides an additional ligand binding to constant parts of HLA class II molecules (see also [32])

The second part reviews some of our studies on the immunoregulatory function of the restricting class II HLA molecules in antigen-specific T lymphocyte activation. In HLA-DR heterozygote healthy individuals and Type 1 diabetics we found an apparently different immunoregulatory function of HLA-DR3 and HLA-DR4 on the proliferative T lymphocyte response to mumps and Coxsackie B4 virus. The frequency of ARTL to these viruses was found to be lower when elements on DR3 were restricting the response and higher when elements on DR4 were restricting the response, compared to the ARTL frequencies when other DR molecules provided the restricting elements. More studies are needed to ascertain the mechanisms behind these differences, i.e., whether they are due to different numbers of preexisting responding T cells or whether activation of suppressor T cells in vitro is influencing the results. The important point is that the elements on the class II molecules which are co-recognized together with antigen, influence the type and degree of T cell responsiveness.

Whether our results may provide an explanation for the development of Type 1 diabetes mellitus is at present conjectural, and needs further studies. A causal role of viruses in Type 1 diabetes has been suspected, but has not been proven. Viral infections might cause β cell damage directly or might initiate an autoimmune process against the pancreatic β cells. A DR3-associated hyporesponsiveness to mumps and Coxsackie B4 might then act synergistically with other factors, as discussed elsewhere [12]. Also, since T lymphocytes consist of several functional subsets, the decreased frequency of DR3-restricted ARTL to mumps and Coxsackie B4 might involve a functional subset other than those responsible for the increased frequency of DR4-restricted ARTL. Thus, it remains to be seen which functional subpopulation is responsible for this increased frequency.

In conclusion, our studies demonstrate that (1) human T4 cells recognize antigens together with restriction elements present on class II molecules (DR, DQ, or DP); (2) these restriction elements are often not completely identical to the parts of the molecules known to induce alloantibody production or activation of allogeneic T cells, and some of them may be detectable at the genomic level; and (3) the restriction elements have an antigen-specific immunoregulatory function on T cell responses, which may provide an explanation for some of the associations between HLA determinants and diseases.

References

1. Austin P, Trowsdale J, Rudd C, Bodmer W, Feldmann M, Lamb J (1985) Functional expression of HLA-DP genes transfected into mouse fibroblasts. Nature 313:61–64
2. Bach FH, Watson AJ (1983) Dw/LD associated molecular polymorphism of DR4 β-chains: intramolecular localization of polymorphic sites. J Immunol 131:1622–1625
3. Ball EJ, Myers L, Stastny P (1984) Inhibition of antigen-specific T-cell lines by monoclonal antibodies. Dis Markers 2:327–336
4. Benacerraf B (1978) A hypothesis to relate the specificity of T-lymphocytes and the activity of I region-specific Ir genes in macrophages and B lymphocytes. J Immunol 120:1809–1812
5. Benacerraf B (1981) Role of MHC gene products in immune regulation. Science 212:1229–1238
6. Benacerraf B, McDevitt HO (1972) Histocompatibility-linked immune response genes. A new class of genes that controls the formation of specific immune responses has been identified. Science 175:273–279

7. Bensussan A, Meuer SC, Schlossmann SF, Reinherz EL (1984) Delineation of an immunoregulatory amplifier population recognizing autologous Ia molecules. Analysis with human T cell clones. J Exp Med 159:559–576
8. Bodmer WF (1984) The HLA system, 1984. In: Albert ED, Baur MP, Mayr WR (eds) Histocompatibility testing 1984. Springer, Berlin Heidelberg New York Tokyo, pp 11–22
9. Borst J, Coligan JE, Oettgen H, Pessano S, Malin R, Terhorst C (1984) The δ- and ε-chains of the human T3/T-cell receptor complex are distinct polypeptides. Nature 312:455–458
10. Bruserud Ø, Thorsby E (1985a) T lymphocyte responses to Coxsackie B4, mumps and varicella-zoster. Influence of HLA-DR restriction elements. Tissue Antigens 26:41–50
11. Bruserud Ø, Thorsby E (1985b) HLA-DR3 and DR4 control T lymphocyte responses to mumps and Coxsackie B4 virus. Studies on patients with Type 1 diabetes mellitus and healthy subjects. Diabetologia 28:420–426
12. Bruserud Ø, Stenersen M, Thorsby E (1985) HLA-association in insulin-dependent diabetes mellitus: hypo- and hyperresponsiveness to mumps and Coxsackie B4 are associated with HLA-DR3 and DR4 respectively. Tissue Antigens 26:179–192
13. DeVries RRP, Van Eden W, Ottenhoff THM (1985) HLA-class II immune response genes and products in leprosy. Prog Allergy 36:95–113
14. Eckels DD, Lake P, Lamb JR, Johnson AH, Shaw S, Woody JN, Hartzman RJ (1983) SB-restricted presentation of influenza and herpes simplex virus antigens to human T-lymphocyte clones. Nature 301:716–718
15. Eckels DD, Sell TW, Bronson SR, Johnson AH, Hartzman RJ, Lamb JR (1984) Human helper T-cell clones that recognize different influenza hemagglutinin determinants are restricted by different HLA-D region epitopes. Immunogenetics 19:409–423
16. Ischii N, Klein J, Nagy ZA (1983) Different repertoires of mouse T cells for bovine insulin presented by syngeneic and allogeneic cells. Eur J Immunol 13:658–662
17. Klein J (1984) What causes immunological nonresponsiveness? Immunol Rev 81:177–202
18. Krensky AM, Clayberger C, Greenstein JL, Crimmins M, Burakoff SJ (1983) A DC-specific cytolytic T lymphocyte line is OKT8^{+}. J Immunol 131:2777–2780
19. Kurnick JT, Altevogt P, Lindblom J, Sjøberg O, Danneus A, Wigzell H (1980) Long-term maintenance of HLA-D restricted T cells specific for soluble antigens. Scand J Immunol 11:131–136
20. Kurnick JT, Hayward AR, Altevogt P (1981) Helper and suppressor-inducer activity of human T cells and their cloned progeny maintained in long-term culture. J Immunol 126:1307–1311
21. Lamb JR, Eckels DD, Lake P, Johnson AH, Hartzman RJ, Woody JN (1982) Antigen-specific human T lymphocyte clones: induction, antigen specificity and MHC restriction of influenza virus-immune clones. J Immunol 128:233–238
22. McDevitt HO, Chinitz A (1969) Genetic control of the antibody response: relationship between immune response and histocompatibility (H-2) type. Science 163:1207–1208
23. Moen T, de Preval C, Rabourdin-Combe C, Mach B, Gaudernack G, Bondevik E, Thorsby E (1985) Mouse L cells expressing human HLA-DR antigens after transfection with class II genes do not stimulate human T lymphocytes. In: Albert ED, Baur MP, Mayr WR (eds) Histocompatibility testing, 1984. Springer, Berlin Heidelberg New York Tokyo, pp 595–598
24. Nepom BS, Nepom GT, Mickelson E, Antonelli P, Hansen JA (1983) Electrophoretic analysis of human HLA-DR antigens from HLA-DR4 homozygous cell lines: correlation between β-chain diversity and HLA-D. Proc Natl Acad Sci USA 80:6962–6966
25. Paul WE, Benacerraf B (1977) Functional specificity of thymus-dependent lymphocytes. Science 195:1293–1300
26. Paulsen G, Qvigstad E, Gaudernack G, Rask L, Winchester R, Thorsby E (1985) Identification, at the genomic level, of an HLA-DR restriction element for cloned antigen-specific T4 cells. J Exp Med 161:1569–1574
27. Qvigstad E, Thorsby E (1983) Class-II HLA restriction of antigen-specific human T-lymphocyte clones. Evidence of restriction elements on both DR and MT molecules. Scand J Immunol 18:299–306

28. Qvigstad E, Digranes S, Thorsby E (1983) Antigen-specific proliferative human T-lymphocyte clones with specificity for *Chlamydia trachomatis*. Scand J Immunol 18:291–297
29. Qvigstad E, Gaudernack G, Thorsby E (1984a) Antigen-specific T cell clones restricted by DR, DRw53 (MT), or DP (SB) class II HLA molecules. Inhibition studies with monoclonal HLA-specific antibodies. Hum Immunol 11:207–217
30. Qvigstad E, Moen T, Thorsby E (1984b) T-cell clones with similar antigen specificity may be restricted by DR, MT(DC), or SB class II HLA molecules. Immunogenetics 19:455–460
31. Qvigstad E, Thorsby E, Reinsmoen NL, Bach FH (1984c) Close association between the Dw14 (LD40) subtype of HLA-DR4 and a restriction element for antigen-specific T-cell clones. Immunogenetics 20:583–588
32. Reinherz EL, Acuto O, Fabbi M, Bensussan A, Milanese C, Royer HD, Meuer SC, Schlossman SF (1984) Clonotypic surface structure of human T lymphocytes: functional and biochemical analysis of the antigen-receptor complex. Immunol Rev 81:95–129
33. Reinsmoen NL, Bach FH (1982) Five HLA-D clusters associated with HLA-DR4. Hum Immunol 4:249–258
34. Rosenthal AS (1978) Determinant selection and macrophage function in genetic control of the immune response. Immunol Rev 40:136–152
35. Saito H, Kranz DM, Takagaki Y, Hayday AC, Eisen HN, Tonegawa S (1984a) Complete primary structure of a heterodimeric T-cell receptor deduced from cDNA sequences. Nature 309:757–762
36. Saito H, Kranz DM, Takegaki Y, Hayday AC, Eisen HN, Tonegawa S (1984b) A third rearranged and expressed gene in a clone of cytotoxic T lymphocytes. Nature 312:36–40
37. Sasazuki T, Nishimura Y, Muto M, Ohta N (1983) HLA-linked genes controlling immune response and disease susceptibility. Immunol Rev 70:51–75
38. Schwartz RH (1978) A clonal deletion model for Ir gene control of the immune response. Scand J Immunol 7:3–10
39. Scott H, Hirschberg H, Thorsby E (1983) HLA-DR3 and -DR7 restricted T cell hyporesponsiveness to gluten antigens: a clue to the aetiology of coeliac disease. Scand J Immunol 18:163–168
40. Sredni B, Volkman D, Schwartz RH, Fauci AS (1981) Antigen-specific human T cell clones: Development of clones requiring HLA-DR compatible presenting cells for stimulation in the presence of antigen. Proc Natl Acad Sci USA 78:1858–1862
41. Thorsby E (1978) Biological function of HLA. Tissue Antigens 11:321–329
42. Thorsby E, Berle E, Nousiainen H (1982) HLA-D region molecules restrict proliferative T cell responses to antigen. Immunol Rev 66:39–56
43. Toguchi T, Burmester G, Nunez-Rolden A, Gregersen P, Seremetis S, Lee S, Szer I, Hurley C, Winchester R (1984) Evidence for the separate molecular expression of four distinct polymorphic Ia epitopes on cells of DR4 homozygous individuals. Hum Immunol 10:69–81

Class II HLA Antigens in Autoimmune and Immune-Mediated Diseases

M. Jeannet

Table of Contents

Introduction

The observation that susceptibility to virus-induced leukemia is controlled in mice by the major histocompatibility complex (MHC) [114a] stimulated a search for a similar relationship between the HLA system, the MHC of man, and malignant human diseases. Later on, after McDevitt and Benacerraf [122] had shown that MHC-linked immune-response genes in mice control a variety of regulatory interactions of the immune system, attempts were made in man to establish the role of the HLA system in the pathogenesis of various autoimmune diseases. During the past 12 years many associations between HLA determinants and diseases have been found, in general weaker for the class I and stronger for the class II antigens. Exceptions which will not be discussed in this review are the strong association discovered between HLA-B27 and ankylosing spondylitis, and the weaker associatins established with two disorders with no relation to autoimmunity, A3 and hemochromatosis and B47 and congenital adrenal hyperplasia.

There are two different types of relationships between the HLA system and diseases. One of these is *association,* which is sought by means of population studies in which the frequencies of HLA alleles in unrelated patients are compared with those of healthy controls. The other, *genetic linkage,* is recognized by family studies showing that affected relatives share HLA haplotypes more often than expected according to genetic laws. The genes of hemochromatosis and congenital adrenal hypoplasia, the two nonautoimmune diseases mentioned above, as well as the gene of cerebellar ataxia, are tightly linked with the HLA genes and have been recognized as definitively located in the HLA region.

Population studies have shown DR3 to be significantly associated with several autoimmune diseases, but often B8, CW7, and A1 also have an increased frequency, because of the well-established linkage disequilibrium between these alleles. Recently described HLA determinants, such as those coded by the DQ and DP loci, have not yet been extensively studied in immune-mediated diseases, and new associations will most probably be described in the near future.

Disease heterogeneity may hamper the search for associations between disease and HLA antigens and may explain the weakness of some of the associations found, as well as the controversial results obtained in some studies. On the other hand, in several instances, clinical heterogeneity has been revealed or confirmed by the finding of different HLA associations in different forms of the disorder. Well-known examples are the various forms of juvenile rheumatoid arthritis, insulin-dependent and non-insulin-dependent diabetes, and the two clinical forms of myasthenia gravis.

Another aspect of HLA and disease associations which will often be mentioned in this review is the fact that different associations are frequently observed for the same disorder in different ethnic groups. This is of course explained by the wide variations of the frequencies of HLA antigens observed in different populations. In contrast, certain associations, as DR4 in rheumatoid arthritis, are found in many different ethnic groups, and this has of course interesting implications for the pathogenesis of the disease.

Another frequently observed phenomenon is the stronger specific HLA and disease association seen in a population with a higher frequency of a particular antigen than in a population with a lower frequency of the same antigen. This phenomenon has been observed, for example, in Behçet's disease, where the strongest associations with B5 have been observed in populations with a high B5 frequency, such as Japanese and Jews. In contrast, the incidences of several autoimmune diseases strongly associated with the A1, B8, DR3 haplotype in Caucasoids, are very low in the Japanese population, in which this haplotype is lacking [41].

From the great number of studies carried out on the association of HLA class II antigens and diseases during the past 10 years, we have made a selective review, deliberately omitting those with weak associations not confirmed by other independent studies.

Association Between HLA and Autoimmune Diseases

Rheumatic Diseases

Systemic Lupus Erythematosus

Genetic factors play an important predisposing role in the expression of human systemic lupus erythematosus (SLE), although there is also a strong influence of sex hormones [152]. Monozygotic twins have a 70% disease concordance, and the lack of concordance in the remaining 30% could be due to incomplete penetrance or the effect of environmental factors [27]. Although the disease shows a considerable clinical heterogeneity, many reports have shown associations with B8 and DR3, two determinants which are in linkage disequilibrium in Caucasians [26, 34, 154, 165]. It is worth mentioning that both DR2 and DR3, and also DQW1, were found to have an increased frequency in American and English patients [26, 154, 155, 170], whereas in continental Europe, an association with DR3 only was found [34, 165]. In contrast, several studies found similar frequencies of all DR antigens in SLE patients compared with normal controls [16, 19]. Whereas in blacks with SLE, an association was also found with DR3 and DR2 [2, 102], in Japanese no particular association was observed with DR antigens [104]. It has been suggested that there is a relationship between HLA-DR2 and DR3 and the severity of the disease, particular organ involvement, or the level of circulating autoantibodies [1, 19, 43, 78, 154]. However, this has not been confirmed by others [26, 170]. A distinct subset of lupus, with characteristic skin lesions, has a higher association with HLA-DR3 than observed in the classical form of SLE [178]. The association between SLE and DR2 found in many patients is of interest in view of the association described between the haplotype A10, B18, DR2 and deficiency of the second component of complement (C2) [69] and the increased frequency of an allele of C2 among SLE patients [74]. More recently an increased frequency of null alleles at the C4 loci, which are in linkage disequilibrium with DR3, has been found in SLE [43, 93]. Several components of the complement sequence (C2, C4, and factor B) are coded by genes located in the HLA region. Moreover, subjects with complement component deficiencies have an unusual propensity for development of lupus-like syndromes and other autoimmune diseases [99, 110]. The HLA-DR association with SLE may represent linkage disequilibrium with a defective complement gene or an abnormal immune-response gene leading to abnormal immune responses, such as the defective Fc receptor functions and impaired ability to clear immune complexes described by Lawley et al. [111] not only in patients, but also in normal subjects with DR3. Batchelor et al. [16], in a study of 26 patients with hydralazine-induced SLE, found an association with DR4, but this finding has not been confirmed [28].

In families with multiple cases of lupus, the HLA haplotypes do not segregate consistently with the disease [1, 10, 115, 169]. This suggests that a genetically determined disorder of immune regulation not linked to the HLA complex is a factor predisposing to autoimmune phenomena in these families. However, the increased frequency of HLA-DR antigens in patients and the finding by Schur and Carpenter [169] that parents of SLE patients share HLA haplotypes more often than expected suggest that HLA-linked genes also operate in the expression of SLE. It appears therefore likely that SLE is a multigenic disorder. Genetic studies in mice also strongly suggest that multiple genes are responsible for the development of the murine lupus-like disease, although no strong association with the MHC has been found [152].

Rheumatoid Arthritis

Rheumatoid arthritis (RA) is a chronic inflammatory disorder characterized, like SLE, by clinical heterogeneity, and by the absence of a specific biological marker. Although no association of RA with HLA-A and B antigens has been demonstrated, there is a significant association with HLA-DR4, not only in Caucasians [179], but also in blacks [2, 180], in Mexicans [76], in Japanese [129], and in Chippewa Indians [83], but not in Yokima Indians [205]. Two specificities, DRW53 and DQW3, which are in linkage disequilibrium with DR4, also usually have an increased frequency in RA, whereas DR2 is often decreased. An increase of DR1, but not of DR4, has been reported in Asian Indian patients [133], but also in Jewish patients [166] and in Swiss patients with low rheumatoid factor titers [185]. Recently, a significantly increased frequency of a new HLA-DR determinant, MC1, strongly associated with DR1 and DR4, was found in adult RA patients [55]. In these patients MC1 was more strongly associated with the disease than DR4 and DR1, suggesting that MC1 may be a more useful RA marker. Dawkins et al. [43] and Christiansen et al. [35] have shown that RA is associated with particular supratypes (haplotypes) which involve alleles at multiple loci between HLA-B and DR. One supratype which is rare in the normal population has also been found in insulin-dependent diabetes, suggesting some relationship between the two diseases. In contrast to a number of other MHC-associated diseases, there is no evidence of increased HLA haplotype sharing between affected siblings [35]. Moreover, identical twins show a low concordance.

In several studies, the frequency of DR4 appeared to have a relationship with the severity of the disease [181, 211], but this is somewhat controversial. In our own study [185] DR4 was associated with the titer of the rheumatoid factor and with the amount of circulating immune complexes. In fact, the frequency of DR4 in rheumatoid-factor-negative patients is identical to that in controls [54, 95, 180]. In contrast, conflicting results have been published concerning the correlation between DR4 and either cellular or humoral immunity to human type II collagen [56, 105, 176, 177, 210].

Several reports have described an association between HLA-DR3 and the development of toxic responses to gold and D-penicillamine in the treatment of RA [13, 17, 177, 197, 209]. In these studies, proteinuria, rash leukopenia, or thrombocytopenia were found in 50%–90% of the gold-treated patients who were DR3-positive; however, HLA typing only has a limited prognostic value, since many patients exhibiting toxic reactions are not DR3-positive. Finally, the B8 DR3 phenotype was found associated with clinical rheumatoid vasculitis in one study [40], although another study failed to report such an increase in DR3 frequency [171].

Juvenile Chronic Arthritis

Both clinical and genetic heterogeneity have hampered the search for an association with HLA in juvenile chronic arthritis (JCA). Different subtypes based on different onset symptoms have different HLA antigen distributions, and the studies performed so far are often conflicting. The frequency of the DR4 antigen seems to be significantly increased in the small subset of patients having a disease similar to adult RA, with polyarthritis and rheumatoid factor [66, 181]. This association between DR4 and rheumatoid factor production in both RA and JCA suggests that the DR4 gene may act as an immune-response gene for autoantibody production against self IgG [66]. In fact, Nepom et al. [131] have observed a surprisingly homogeneous structure of the HLA-DR4 molecule in patients with seropositive JCA, suggesting also that this determinant may be the product of a disease-susceptibility immune-response gene. The pauciarticular onset type of JCA and the polyarticular onset type without production of rheumatoid factor are both associated with the DR5 and the DR8 antigens [7, 66, 75, 181, 182]. The majority of males with pauciarticular late childhood onset disease are B27-positive, and many develop ankylosing spondylitis. The Still's type of JCA, characterized by onset with high peaks of fever, seems to show an increased frequency of DR2 [181].

Behçet's Disease

Behçet's disease is a chronic multisystemic disorder of unknown origin with arthritis, recurrent iritis, and oral and genital ulcers. Although its strong association with HLA-B5 has been confirmed in several ethnic groups, an increased frequency of the class II antigen DRW52 has recently been shown in Japanese patients [138].

Sjögren's Syndrome

HLA typing studies have documented differences between primary Sjögren's, an autoimmune exocrinopathy associated with B8, DR3 and DRW52, and the secondary form of the disease, associated with RA and the DR4 antigen [36, 89, 127, 149]. In a recent study [206], the DRW52 (MT2) specificity was found more strongly associated with primary Sjögren's syndrome than DR3, both in whites and in blacks. Moreover, this specificity was also significantly increased when the disease was secondary to RA or SLE. In contrast, the presence of anti-Ro (SS-A) and anti-La (SS-B) antibodies was more closely associated with the DR3 and also the DR2 antigens. The study of several families having one or more members with primary Sjögren's syndrome, and various other autoimmune diseases and autoantibodies, has suggested the interaction of HLA-linked, but also non-HLA-linked genes [156].

Progressive Systemic Sclerosis

Somewhat divergent results have been reported concerning possible HLA associations in progressive systemic sclerosis (scleroderma) (PSS), an autoimmune disease of unknown etiology. Whereas in Canadian patients an increased frequency of DR5 was observed [73], in Dutch patients a strong association with B8 and DR3 was found [103]; both DR5 and DR3 are raised in English patients [110]. Moreover, among the Dutch patients, those possessing the B8/DR3 antigens had a strongly depressed cellular response, suggesting an association of the haplotype B8, DR3 with impaired cellular immunity. In the CREST syndrome, a limited form of PSS, an increased prevalence of DR3 has also been observed [72].

Dermatomyositis

An association between HLA-DR3 and juvenile dermatomyositis has been observed in whites and Latin Americans [67]; DR3 was also found increased in polymyositis, but not in dermatomyositis, in another study [90].

Idiopathic Pulmonary Fibrosis

Although idiopathic pulmonary fibrosis (IPF) is not a rheumatic disease, rheumatologic problems are not infrequent in patients with IPF. Moreover, IPF may be a clinical feature of several rheumatic autoimmune diseases, such as SLE and PSS. The circulating T lymphocytes of patients with IPF appear to be sensitized to type I collagen. It is therefore of interest that an association of IPF with HLA-DR2 has recently been observed [114].

Diseases of Blood Vessels

Systemic Vasculitis

Few studies of the class II HLA antigens' distribution in systemic vasculitis have so far been accomplished. A significant increase in the frequency of HLA-DR2 was found in patients with Wegener's granulomatosis, but not in those with polyarteritis nodosa or Churg-Strauss vasculitis [59].

Polymyalgia Rheumatica and Giant Cell Arteritis

Several reports have described an increased frequency of HLA-DR4 in patients with polymyalgia rheumatica and giant cell arteritis [8, 14, 32]. Another study confirmed the association with DR4, but also demonstrated a significant increase in the prevalence of HLA-DR3 in these two diseases [116].

Takayasu's Disease

In Takayasu's disease (aortic arch syndrome), a rare inflammatory disease involving large arteries, strong association has been observed with DR4 and MB3 in North Americans [199]. In the Japanese population, DR2 and DQW1 (MB1) have been found significantly increased [126], but this observation has not been confirmed in another study [135]. However, the two studies agree on the increased frequency of a class I antigen BW52.

Buerger's Disease

In Buerger's disease (thromboangiitis obliterans) a disorder with a high prevalence in some ethnic groups, an increased frequency of DR2 and DR3, as well as very low frequency of B12, has been observed in Caucasoids [47]. However, the possible implication of the HLA system in the susceptibility to this disorder awaits confirmation.

Endocrine Gland and Metabolic Disorders

Grave's Disease

Grave's disease is considered to be an autoimmune disorder, perhaps linked with a deficiency in antigen-specific suppressor T lymphocytes. This defect seems to be genetically linked, since there is a relatively high rate of concordance in identical twins and a strong association with B8, DR3, and DRW52 in Caucasians [18, 62], and with DR5 and DRW53 in Japanese [163]. The severity of the disease may also be genetically related, since patients with DR3 are more likely to relapse than those without it [123]. It has recently been shown that thyroid cells spontaneously express HLA-DR in vivo in autoimmune thyroid disease, in contrast to normal thyroid cells [80]. This abnormal expression of HLA-DR seems to be one of the earliest manifestations of the disease; the thyroid epithelial cells become functional antigen-presenting cells, allowing helper T lymphocytes to recognize thyroid autoantigens and therefore initiating the whole process of autoimmunization. Viral infections, by eliciting the local production of interferon, might be responsible for this abnormal expression of DR.

Hashimoto's Disease

An association between HLA-DR5 and Hashimoto's thyroiditis with goiter has been observed [63, 190, 203], whereas atrophic autoimmune thyroiditis is associated with DR3 [125] suggesting that hypertrophic and atrophic thyroiditis are two different disease entities and not different stages of the same disease.

Idiopathic Addison's Disease

Idiopathic Addison's disease is associated with DW3 and DR3, also when it occurs together with autoimmune thyroid disease or diabetes mellitus [64, 188]. However, it is not DR3-associated when occurring with hypoparathyroidism and chronic mucocutaneous candidiasis (type I polyglandular autoimmunity).

Premature Ovarian Failure

HLA-DR3 was also found significantly increased in a subgroup of the syndrome of isolated premature gonadal failure, suggesting its possible autoimmune origin [201].

Insulin-Dependent Diabetes Mellitus

The familial nature of insulin-dependent diabetes mellitus (IDDM) is well known, but the mode of inheritance remains obscure. Most probably, viruses (Coxsackie B4 and B5, mumps, rubella, CMV), contribute to the pathogenesis. There is also evidence of autoimmunity (islet-cell antibodies, infiltration of pancreatic islets by lymphocytes and macrophages). There is a high concordance (30%–50%) of the disorder in identical twins, and over half the affected siblings share both parental HLA haplotypes in kindreds with a high prevalence of the disease [184]. Early studies established that non-insulin-dependent diabetes is not associated with HLA and that IDDM is associated with HLA-B8 and B15 [132, 174]. Later, a stronger association was observed with the D/DR region (DR3/DW3 and DR4/DW4) [15, 46, 183, 188]. DR2/DW2 seem to confer a protective effect. As with most other disease-associated antigens, individuals homozygous for either of these antigens appear to have the same relative risk as individuals possessing only a single dose of the antigen, i.e. no gene dose effect is observed. However, DR3 and DR4 have an additive effect, as observed by the higher frequency of IDDM in DR3/DR4 individuals. Among the five HLA-D specificities associated with DR4, the frequency of DW4 was found highly significantly increased in IDDM [12]. Analysis of cross-overs between HLA-DR and GLO in IDDM patients has allowed the mapping of the putative susceptibility genes towards the HLA-DR locus [160]. Moreover, no significant association has been found between alleles of the DP (SB) locus and IDDM, suggesting again that the susceptibility genes are tightly linked with HLA-DR [44].

The frequency of DR4 may be increased in patients with an earlier age of onset of the disease [183, 208]. DR4 is increased in all ethnic groups, while the increase of DR3 is observed mainly in Caucasoids [20, 184]. Among Japanese, IDDM is associated with DR4, DRW9, and DRW53 (MT3) [20, 163]. The excess of DR3/DR4-heterozygous patients in Caucasoids strongly suggests the existence of two different HLA-linked susceptibility genes, one associated with DR3 and the other with DR4. Moreover, the associations of IDDM and certain complement allotypes, as well as the increased frequency of several different "extended" haplotypes or supratypes, provides evidence for further genetic heterogeneity [20, 158]. A low-insulin antibody response seem strongly associated with a particular B8-DR3 supratype, while thyrogastric autoantibodies are more closely associated with supratypes containing a null allele of the C4A locus [121]. Genetic heterogeneity is also suggested by the finding that the A1, B8, DR3 haplotype is more involved in the persistence of islet-cell antibodies than in their initiation [50]. In a recent study of the suppressor T cell function of patients with IDDM, there was a trend for a higher proportion of HLA-DR3-positive diabetics than DR3-negative patients to have abnormal immunoregulation [96]. These observations suggest that in IDDM, as in other autoimmune diseases, the HLA system determines abnormalities in immunoregulation which contribute to disease susceptibility; however, other genetic systems almost certainly also play an important role. For the future, the use of DNA probes for HLA region genes should identify the HLA-related genes responsible for susceptibility to IDDM [139, 140].

Polyglandular Autoimmune Syndromes

IDDM occurs frequently in patients with Schmidt's syndrome, a rare condition characterized by polyglandular failure of probable autoimmune origin. In patients with IDDM and Grave's disease, atrophic thyroiditis or Addison's disease, the incidence of B8 and DR3 is greater than for each disorder alone [193]. Patients with IDDM and Hashimoto's disease, in contrast, are predominantly B8, DRW3-negative.

Disorders of the Blood

Pernicious Anaemia

Pernicious anemia belongs to the group of organ-specific autoimmune diseases, but there is evidence for genetic heterogeneity and complexHLA associations. In one report an increased frequency of DW2 and of DW5 was demonstrated [189]. The presence of intrinsic factor antibody was associated with DW2 but not with DW5. Pernicious anemia may be linked with Hashimoto's disease, since they are both associated with DR5, and since thyroid autoantibodies are frequently found in both disorders. Another report has shown an association with DR2 and DR4 in the form of pernicious anemia which is not associated with an endocrine disorder, and with DR3 and DR4 in patients with coexisting endocrine disease [194]. The association with DR2 has been confirmed in the Dutch population [195].

Idiopathic Thrombocytopenic Purpura

Although acute idiopathic thrombocytopenic purpura (ITP) has features characteristic of autoimmune diseases, e.g., high levels of platelet-associated immunoglobulin, there is no evidence that it occurs preferentially in persons with genetically determined abnormalities of the immune system. Chronic ITP, in contrast, is often associated with other immunologically mediated diseases, such as SLE, autoimmune hemolytic anemia, thyroiditis, or myastenia gravis. Serological abnormalities, such as antinuclear antibodies, antithyroid antibodies, and a positive Coomb's test, are frequent in patients with ITP. However, no clear association with class I or class II HLA antigens has been so far established in ITP. The moderately increased frequency of DR2 observed in Ashkenazy Jews by Karpatkin et al. [106], has not been seen in Caucasoids [87]. In a kindred with chronic ITP in monozygotic twin girls and in an older sister, high-titer antinuclear antibodies found in the sisters, their parents, and other members of the family appeared to be linked to the HLA complex [108]. However, in other kindreds there was no linkage. As in other autoimmune diseases, it appears that several genes besides HLA may determine the immunological abnormalities in ITP.

Leukemias

In mice, an immunological mechanism is involved in the defense against virus-induced malignancies. Studies showing a close relationship between the H-2 system and virus-induced leukemias stimulated the search for associations between HLA antigens and the various forms of leukemia in man. However, despite numerous studies, especially involving acute lymphoblastic leukemia (ALL) [82, 97], a role for the HLA system in human leukemia has only recently been established [200, 204, 207]. In 55 families in which one of the children developed ALL, a highly significant increase in shared HLA-DR antigens was observed between the father and the mother [207]. Moreover, the number of homozygotes among the patients was twice the expected value in families where the parents shared an HLA-B and an HLA-DR antigen. These findings strongly suggest that a recessive gene associated with the HLA system is involved in the susceptibility to childhood ALL. Similar findings have been made in acute myeloid leukemia (Carpentier and Jeannet, unpublished). In chronic lymphocytic leukemia and to a lesser degree in hairy cell leukemia, increased frequencies of DR5, DRW52 (MT2), and DQw3 (MB3) have been observed [207]. These findings suggest that the primary association of disease susceptibility is with the non-DR class II determinants.

Aplastic Anemia

Early studies showed an increased frequency of HLA-A2 in aplastic anemia [3, 41 a]. Recently Chapuis et al. (unpublished) observed an overrepresentation of HLA-B5, B7, and DR2 in genotyped patients with aplastic anemia. In addition, the parents of affected children, as in ALL, showed increased compatibility at the DR locus, suggesting that recessive genes linked to HLA-DR could confer a particular susceptibility to this disorder. A cell-mediated immunological mechanism has recently been proposed for aplastic anemia; the observed association with DR2 is therefore of interest, since this determinant is implicated in other immune-mediated diseases such as SLE, Goodpasture syndrome, multiple sclerosis, etc.

Hodgkin's Disease

As for acute leukemia, conflicting results have been reported during the past years concerning a possible association of Hodgkin's disease with HLA. The preliminary observation of an excess of HLA-identical pairs in affected siblings and of shared haplotypes among first cousin pairs, suggesting the possible existence of a disease susceptibility gene in the HLA region [91], did not reach the level of statistical significance in a more recent international study [92]; further studies are therefore necessary to establish the possibility of a genetic linkage between HLA and susceptibility to Hodgkin's disease.

Diseases of the Gastrointestinal Tract and Liver

Celiac Disease

Celiac disease, a disease of the mucosa of the small intestine, is caused by gluten sensitivity. Ten to fifteen percent of first-degree relatives have the disorder, and about 70% of identical twins are concordant for the disease. The association between celiac disease and HLA was among the first to be discovered [61]. B8, DR3, DR7 have been successively found increased in this disorder, with a particularly increased risk for DR3/DR7 heterozygotes [21, 45, 168]. All patients lacking DR3 and DR7 seem to possess DR4. Moreover, B7 and DR2 may be associated with a protective gene.

In pairs of affected siblings, there is a moderate excess of sib-pairs sharing two HLA haplotypes, which confirms the linkage with HLA and suggests the existence of more than one HLA-linked gene [168]. Evidence has recently been presented that the concomitant increased frequency of DR3 and DR7 is secondary to the stronger association with DQW2 (DC3), itself in linkage disequilibrium with both DR3 and DR7 in the population [192]. The disease susceptibility gene coded in the HLA region may govern an abnormal immune reaction to a gluten fraction. In fact, Qvigstad et al. [151] have recently shown that there exists a gluten-specific hyporesponsiveness of T helper cells in conjunction with DR3 and DR7.

Ulcerative Colitis

Although the etiology of ulcerative colitis is still obscure, evidence implicating immunological mechanisms has been presented. Two reports have shown an increased frequency of DR2, one in Japanese and the other in Sicilian patients [11, 33]. However, other investigators found associations with different antigens, and further work is needed to firmly establish an HLA association in this disorder.

Chronic Active Hepatitis

Chronic active hepatitis, another disorder with typical autoimmune histological and serological features, is associated with HLA-A1, B8, and DR3 [117]. The association is more evident in female patients with disease onset before age 30 and with positive tests for antinuclear, anti-smooth-muscle, and antimitochondrial autoantibodies [187]. A subgroup of this disorder, which is associated with hepatitis B surface antigen, shows relatively few immunological features and does not appear to be associated with the HLA system.

Primary Biliary Cirrhosis

Primary biliary cirrhosis (PBC), which has clearly autoimmune features, has been found associated with HLA-DR3 [60]. The increased frequency of DR3 in both chronic active hepatitis and PBC, and the fact that some patients present a mixed picture, reinforce the concept that the two disorders have common pathogenic factors. In Japanese, the association is with BW52 and DW12 [163].

Alcoholic Liver Cirrhosis

The frequency of DR2 has been found to be increased in patients with alcoholic cirrhosis [186]. Other studies have shown an increase of B8 and DR3 in this disorder [30, 164]. Although the background to these controversial results remains obscure, they would suggest, if an association with HLA is confirmed, that genetic determinants linked to HLA enhance the rate of development of liver damage in alcoholic patients.

Postschistosomal Liver Cirrhosis

Sasazuki et al. [163] observed that individuals infected with *Schistosoma japonicum* could be divided into high- and low-responder groups by determining their T cell response to the schistosomal antigen in vitro. The low responders had a strong association with the HLA haplotype BW52, DW12, DR2, suggesting the existence of an HLA-linked immune-suppression gene for schistosomal antigen. Most patients with postschistosomal liver cirrhosis were in the high-responder group and had an increased frequency of B44, DEn, and a decreased frequency of BW52, DW12. The high response was associated with a decreased activity of antigen-specific suppressor cells. These studies represent the first clear evidence of the existence of Is gene in man.

Disorders of the Kidney

Goodpasture's Syndrome

Goodpasture's syndrome, a rare disorder, is characterized by the presence of autoantibodies to the glomerular basement membrane, which also react with a similar antigen in the lung, accounting for glomerulonephritis and lung hemorrhage. A strongly increased frequency of HLA-DR2 has been demonstrated in these patients by Rees et al. [153], suggesting that they may have an abnormality of immune responsiveness. Interestingly, MHC-linked susceptibility to the development of autoantibodies to basement membranes has been demonstrated in guinea pigs and in rats [153].

Idiopathic Membranous Nephropathy and Idiopathic Nephrotic Syndrome

Immunological mechanisms are probably involved in idiopathic membranous nephropathy, which has been found to be strongly associated with DR3 and DRW52 (MT2) [70, 107, 128]. In children with idiopathic nephrotic syndrome, a disorder which probably has an immunopathological mechanism, the incidence of DR7 has been found significantly increased [4, 49, 136]. A strong association has recently been found between a rare allele of the C4B locus, C4B*2.9, and primary glomernlonephritis [202]. In these patients the frequencies of the class I and class II antigens are normal.

IgA Nephropathy

IgA nephropathy (Berger's disease) is characterized pathologically by the deposition of IgA in the mesangium. There are strong suggestions that IgA nephropathy may be familial, but no single HLA haplotype was found in all the patients in family studies [101]. In population studies, increased frequencies of BW35, B12, and DR4 have been found [65, 88, 134], but these observations have not been confirmed by other reports [9, 23, 81].

Acute Poststreptococcal Glomerulonephritis

A recent study has shown an increase of DR4 in acute poststreptococcal glomerulonephritis in Venezuela, where it is endemic [112].

Diseases of the Skin

Dermatitis Herpetiformis

Dermatitis herpetiformis, a pruritic vesicular skin disease frequently associated with gluten-sensitive enteropathy, also has a strong association with HLA-B8 and DR3 [119, 175]. Recently, a very strong association has been reported with DQW2 (Te24), suggesting that the susceptibility gene for this disorder is closer to the DQ locus than to the DR locus [144].

Pemphigus Vulgaris

Most Jewish patients with pemphigus, a disorder characterized by circulating antibodies to intercellular cement of the epidermis, possess the HLA-DR4 antigen [143]. However, this association has only been found in Ashkenazy, not in non-Ashkenazy Jews [29]. Recently, a very strong association has been found with DW10, a determinant in strong linkage disequilibrium with DR4 [6].

Herpes Gestationis

In herpes gestationis, a rare blistering skin disease of pregnancy with circulating antibodies which fix C3 to normal basement membrane, an association with DR3 and DR4 has been shown [172]. Moreover, the frequency of HLA alloimmunization, as detected by the presence of lymphocytotoxic antibodies in these women, is very high, with an increased frequency of antibodies directed against B7 and DR2 [181].

Psoriasis

After variable associations of psoriasis with HLA-B13, B17, B37, and BW39, were found in different ethnic groups, the strongest association was shown to be with CW6 and later DR7, in Caucasians, in Japanese, and in non-Ashkenazi Jews [5, 84]. As there is strong linkage disequilibrium between CW6 and DR7, it is difficult to determine which of these two antigens is primarily associated with the disease.

Kaposi's Sarcoma

DR5 has been found associated with both the classical form and the more malignant form of Kaposi's sarcoma, which develops in more than a third of patients with the acquired immunodeficiency syndrome (AIDS) [39, 68, 142]. In contrast, the B8, DR3 haplotype might protect against the malignant manifestations of the primary disease [147].

Mycosis Fungoides

An increase in DR5 has been observed in mycosis fungoides, an uncommon neoplasm of the lymphoreticular system with distinct immunological features [161].

Neurological Diseases

Multiple Sclerosis

In whites from northern Europe, North America, and Australia, multiple sclerosis (MS) is associated with A3 and B7, but more strongly with DW2 and DR2 [98]. No significant association with any antigen was found in Japanese or in Israeli Jews [191]. The DW2/DR2 phenotype seems to be associated with a more rapid progression of the disease, whereas the DW7/DR7 phenotype has been associated with a decreased susceptibility. In some studies, a statistically significant increase in the B8 and DR3 antigens has been observed [48, 118]. It has recently been shown that the frequency of the class II antigen DP4 (SB4) is increased in MS, but this is probably secondary to the primary association between DR2 and MS [124]. Although about 30% of twins are concordant [38], studies of families with multiple cases have failed to consistently show that MS patients within a family share an HLA haplotype, suggesting that susceptibility to MS cannot be due to a single gene closely linked to HLA [38, 57]. Moreover, epidemiological evidence suggests that an environmental agent initiates MS in genetically susceptible individuals, although direct evidence implicating a virus is still lacking.

Myasthenia Gravis

Two forms of myasthenia gravis (MG), a disease of neuromuscular transmission, may exist. One has a high frequency of B8 and DR3 and is characterized by early age at onset, prevalence in females, thymic hyperplasia, a low incidence of antistriational antibodies, but a high titer of antiacetylcholine receptor antibodies. The other form of MG, which has an adult onset, a male predominance, a high incidence of antistriational antibodies, and often a thymoma, shows no association with HLA. The B8, DR3 haplotype seems therefore to protect the patients from the development of a thymoma and antistriational antibodies [42]. In Japanese and in Chinese, MG is associated with DR4 [113]. Approximately 1% of patients with rheumatoid arthritis treated with D-penicillamine develop MG. In this iatrogenic form of MG, an association with DR1 and perhaps also with DR7 has been found [71].

Narcolepsy

The most unexpected HLA-associated disease identified so far is certainly narcolepsy. It also represents the strongest association with a class II antigen observed so far. DR2 and DWQ1 were found to be present in all 137 narcoleptics tissue-typed in the UK, in France, and in Japan [24, 100, 109]. There is no evidence of immunological abnormality in narcolepsy, and the reason for the strong association with DR2 is unknown.

Infectious Disease

Leprosy

Leprosy is the result of the interaction between *Mycobacterium leprae* and the immune system of the host. The majority of infected individuals develop immunity without disease. A minority, however, develop clinical symptoms, ranging from a few self-healing skin lesions with very few bacilli (polar tuberculoid form) to multiple skin lesions with dissemination of massive numbers of bacilli through the body (polar lepromatous form). From tuberculoid to lepromatous leprosy there is a gradual decrease of cellular immunity and an increase in humoral immunity. Evidence was obtained from family studies to indicate that susceptibility to tuberculoid leprosy was HLA-encoded and inherited in a recessive way, and that HLA-DR2 was inherited more often than expected in Indian multicase families [51]. Further studies have shown that DR2 is also increased in Japanese patients, whereas DR3 is very frequent in tuberculoid leprosy and almost absent in the lepromatous form [198]. Moreover, the frequency of DQW1 was found to be increased in several populations of patients with lepromatous leprosy. Family studies have also shown that HLA-linked factors do not confer susceptibility to infection per se, but determine the mode of immune response and therefore the clinical type of leprosy [52]. Recently, an in vitro correlate has been found for the HLA-associated genetic control of leprosy in vivo. HLA-DR3-heterozygous T cells from tuberculoid leprosy patients were cultured with antigen and either HLA-DR3-positive or HLA-DR3-negative homozygous HLA-DR-compatible allogeneic monocytes as antigen-presenting cells. T cell proliferative responses with DR3-positive homozygous monocytes were observed to be lower than with DR3-negative homozygous monocytes [196].

Immunological Abnormalities

IgA Deficiency

A significant association has been found between A1, B8, and DR3 and selective IgA deficiency, which is a rather common immunodeficiency [79, 137]. In another report increased frequencies of the same antigens were found only in patients with total lack of IgA, not in those who had deficiency of only serum IgA [86].

Zw^a-Immunized Mothers

One of the most interesting observations of the past few years in this field is the strong association demonstrated between B8 and DR3 and immunization against the platelet-specific antigen Pl^{A1} in Pl^{A1}-negative mothers giving birth to children with isoimmune neonatal thrombocytopenia [157, 184]. This finding reinforces the increasing body of evidence supporting the notion that the B8, DR3 haplotype which is implicated in most autoimmune disorders, is also associated with immunoregulatory abnormalities in normal individuals.

Allergy

Various studies have provided strong evidence that the IgE level in human is determined by genetic factors not linked to the HLA loci [120]. However, studies conducted in allergic patients undergoing skin testing with various extracts of commonly inhaled allergens demonstrated a significant association between positive tests and the two most frequent haplotypes in Caucasoids, A1, B8, DW3, and A3, B7, DW2 [120]. In addition, the immune response to RA5, a highly purified extract of ragweed, was strongly associated with DW2, whereas IgE responses to Rye I and II, two non-cross-reacting allergens present in ryegrass pollen, were associated with B8 and DW3 [120]. Allergic reactions to pigeon dust in pigeon breeders have also been found to be associated with DR3 [159]. In Japanese, the frequency of DQW3 is significantly increased in patients with asthma [129].

Family studies in allergic patients have failed to provide unequivocal evidence of an HLA-linked immune-response gene control of the response to ragweed or other allergens [22, 25]. Recently, however, in families with allergy to cedar pollen antigen, an HLA-linked immune-suppression gene was demonstrated in the antigen-specific IgE response in vitro [163]. This immune-suppression gene, which is in linkage disequilibrium with DQW3, controlled new responsiveness to cedar pollen antigen through antigen-specific suppressor cells.

It seems likely that the expression of atopic allergy, in close analogy to that of autoimmune diseases, is dependent on both HLA and non-HLA genetic controls as well as various environmental influences.

AIDS

AIDS patients suffering from various opportunistic infections without developing Kaposi's sarcoma have a significantly increased frequency of DR3 [147], whereas this antigen is markedly decreased in patients with AIDS and Kaposi's sarcoma [148]. In contrast, AIDS patients have a normal frequency of DR5, an antigen which is associated with the AIDS-Kaposi syndrome.

Miscellaneous

HLA and Longevity

In mice, the H_2 system has been shown to play a role in life span by inducing an appropriate immune response, or influencing DNA repair capacity. Interestingly, in man the haplotype A1, CW7, B8, DR3 has been found significantly increased in male nonagenarians [150].

Sarcoidosis

Sarcoidosis is a multisystem granulomatous disorder of unknown etiology with both humoral and cellular immunological abnormalities. Recently, a strong association has been shown between B8 and DR3 and the acute-onset form of the disease, with arthritis and bilateral enlargement of the hilar lymph glands [85].

Cancer

Although a number of studies have been devoted to the search for associations between HLA and cancer, no significant and reproducible findings have been reported. However, an increase in DR5 has been reported in renal cell carcinoma [53], and DR3 may be significantly associated with resistance to testicular carcinoma [146] and to basal cell carcinoma [145]. It is therefore possible that the HLA-DR3 haplotype confers resistance to malignancy in general, but this needs confirmation.

Possible Pathogenetic Mechanisms

Two main hypotheses have been proposed to account for the associations observed between HLA and diseases. The first postulates that the HLA determinants as such are involved in the pathogenetic mechanisms, the second implicates HLA-controlled immune-response genes that are associated with HLA through linkage disequilibrium.

Direct Implication of HLA Determinants

HLA antigens may function as cell-surface receptors for viruses, toxins, or hormones. Some evidence has been provided that MHC molecules can function as receptors for certain viruses [94]. Moreover, class I molecules can interact with foreign molecules such as penicillin, gamma endorphins [37], and insulin [173]. The HLA polymorphism may perhaps influence the effectiveness of the receptor for these molecules. This hypothesis could explain associations with diseases in which viral or other microbial agents are implicated. However, it is unlikely to account for many other associations, particularly diseases in which an HLA antigen is present only in half the patients or in which more than one HLA antigen is associated with a single disease.

Immune-Response Genes Linked to HLA

The recognition of HLA antigens is critical for the induction and subsequent activation of immune response. This HLA restriction phenomenon is one of the most convincing argument for the existence of HLA-linked immune-response genes. All recognized steps of the immune response, including antigen presentation by macrophages, help and suppressor phases of the proliferative response, T-B cooperation for antibody production, and the final lytic phase of hapten or virus-modified cell, involve the recognition of HLA determinants by the various immunocytes. T cell recognition of DR molecules together with the specific antigen is also necessary for the release of various lymphokines, such as IL-I, IL-2, and interferon.

The immune network, which is regulated by these cells and their mediators, is therefore under close genetic control by the HLA system. Many studies have provided convincing evidence to support the analogy between the HLA-D region in man and the H-2 I region in mice. The I region in mice is comprised of several loci, of which only two, the I-A and I-E regions, have been shown to code for class II products. In man, only three loci – DR, DQ, DP – have so far been identified in the HLA-D region, but further progress in molecular genetics will certainly unravel the remaining loci in the foreseeable future. It now seems likely that the D region gene products represent themselves the immune-response (Ir) and immune-suppression (Is) gene identified in the mouse. Therefore the Ir and Is genes are implicated in each step of the immune response, leading to important variations in the magnitude of the response in different individuals, according to the inheritance of particular alleles. An abnormal or even a normal Ir gene may lead to an unusually vigorous response to a self antigen under particular circumstances. For instance, the A1, B8, D3 and A3, B7, DR2 haplotypes, which are implicated in several autoimmune diseases and in allergy, have been associated with immunoregulatory abnormalities in normal persons.

As suggested by Marsh et al. [120] these two haplotypes, which are associated with immune hyperresponsiveness, may have conferred a selective advantage for survival in past centuries. This phenomenon would also explain the relatively high frequency of these two haplotypes in the white population. However, possession of the two haplotypes now confers an increased risk of autoimmune and atopic disease.

The most popular explanation for the absence of these two haplotypes in a minority of patients with autoimmune diseases is the hypothesis of the "hitchhiking" gene. The disease-susceptibility gene would not be the class II gene itself, but a closely linked gene "trapped" in a particular haplotype. However, other explanations are possible to account for the weak associations frequently observed.

Autoimmune diseases are clearly multigenic, and other immunogenetic systems have been shown to correlate with certain disorders. Gm, a polymorphic serologic marker on the Fc portion of immunoglobulins, is associated with Graves' disease, myasthenia gravis, IDDM, SLE, Sjögren's syndrome, etc. [141]. When HLA typing and Gm typing are combined, much stronger associations are found. Autoimmune diseases can develop, therefore, only when both classes of genes are inherited together. As suggested by Schoenfeld and Schwartz [167], one set of genes would permit the formation of autoantibodies, whereas the other set would determine the development of organ lesions.

Nonimmunological associations with MHC polymorphism have been reported [58]. Moreover, the involvement of class II antigens in hematopoietic cellular interactions and the regulation of myelopoiesis has recently been recognized [31], but their possible role in hematological and other nonimmunological diseases remains to be investigated. A better understanding of the role of class II antigens in autoimmune disease will probably be achieved by the use of the refined molecular genetic analyses now available [139, 140].

References

1. Ahearn JM, Provost TT, Dorsch CA, Stevens MB, Bias WB, Arnett FC (1982) Interrelationships of HLA-DR, MB, and MT phenotypes, autoantibody expression, and clinical features in systemic lupus erythematosus. Arthritis Rheum 25:1031–1040
2. Alarif LI, Ruppert GB, Wilson R, Barth WF (1983) HLA-DR antigens in Blacks with rheumatoid arthritis and systemic lupus erythematosus. J Rheumatol 10:297–300
3. Albert ED, Thomas ED, Nisperos B, Storb R, Camitta BM, Parkman R (1976) HLA antigens and haplotypes in 200 patients with aplastic anemia. Transplantation 22:528–531
4. Alfiler CC, Roy LP, Doran T, Sheldon A, Bashir H (1980) HLA-DRW7 and steroid-responsive nephrotic syndrome of childhood. Clin Nephrol 14:71–74
5. Amar A, Rubinstein N, Cohen O, Hacham-Zadeh S, Cohen T, Brautbar C (1984) HLA determinants in psoriasis vulgaris in Israel. Tissue Antigens 24:247–249
6. Amar A, Rubinstein N, Hacham-Zadeh S, Cohen O, Cohen T, Brautbar C (1984) Is predisposition to pemphigus vulgaris in Jewish patients mediated by HLA-DW10 and DR4? Tissue Antigens 23:17–22
7. Ansell BM, Albert ED (1984) Juvenile chronic arthritis, pauciarticular type. In: Albert ED, Baur MP, Mayr WR (eds) Histocompatibility testing 1984. Springer, Berlin Heidelberg New York Tokyo, pp 368–374
8. Armstrong RD, Behn A, Myles A, Panayi GS, Welsh KI (1983) Histocompatibility antigens in polymyalgia rheumatica and giant cell arteritis. J Rheumatol 10:659–661
9. Arnaiz-Villena A, Gonzalo A, Mampaso F, Teruel JL, Ortunno J (1981) HLA and IgA nephropathy in Spanish population. Tissue Antigens 17:549–550
10. Arnett FC, Shulman LE (1976) Studies in familial systemic lupus erythematosus. Medicine 55:313–322
11. Asakura H, Tsuchiya M, Aisu S, Watanabe M, Kobayashi K, Hibi T, Ando K, Takata H, Sekugnchi S (1982) Association of the human lymphocyte-DR2 antigen with ulcerative colitis. Gastroenterology 82:413–418
12. Bach FH, Rich SS, Barbosa J, Segall M (1985) Insulin-dependent diabetes-associated HLA-D region encoded determinants. Human Immunol 12:59–64
13. Barger B, Acton RT, Koopman WJ, Alarcon GS (1984) DR antigens and gold toxicity in white rheumatoid arthritis patients. Arthritis Rheum 27:601–605

14. Barrier J, Bignon JD, Soulillou JP, Grolleous J (1981) Increased prevalence of HLA-DR4 in giant cell arteritis. N Engl J Med 305:104–105
15. Batchelor JR, Morris PF (1978) Juvenile onset diabetes. In: Bodmer WF et al. (ed) Histocompatibility testing 1977. Munksgaard, Copenhagen, p 211
16. Batchelor JR, Welsh KI, Mansilla Tinoco R, Dollery CT, Hughes GRV, Bernstein R, Naish PF, Aber GM, Bing RF, Russell GI (1980) Hydralazine induced systemic lupus erythematosus: influence of HLA-DR and sex on susceptibility. Lancet 1:1107–1109
17. Batchelor JR, Dodi IA, Woo P, Panayi GS, Ansell B, Williams PL (1984) A family study of gold-induced nephropathy in patients with rheumatoid arthritis. In: Albert ED, Baur MP, Mayr WR (eds) Histocompatibility testing 1984. Springer, Berlin Heidelberg New York Tokyo, pp 375–378
18. Bech K, Lumholtz B, Nerup J, Thomsen M, Platz P, Ryder LR, Svejgaard A, Siersboek-Nielsen K, Molholm Hansen J, Larsen JH (1977) HLA antigens in Graves' disease. Acta Endocrinol 86:510–516
19. Bell DA, Maddison PJ (1980) Serologic subsets in systemic lupus erythematosus: an examination of autoantibodies in relationship to clinical features of disease and HLA antigens. Arthritis Rheum 23:1268–1273
20. Bertrams J, Baur MP (1984) Insulin-dependent diabetes mellitus. In: Albert ED, Baur MP, Mayr WR (eds) Histocompatibility testing 1984. Springer, Berlin Heidelberg New York Tokyo, pp 348–358
21. Betuel H, Gebuhrer L, Descos L, Bertrand J, Freycon F, Lepetit JC (1980) Coeliac disease and its association with HLA markers. In: Terasaki PI (ed) Histocompatibility testing 1980. UCLA Tissue Typing Laboratory, Los Angeles, p 668
22. Bias WB, Marsh DG (1975) HLA linked antigen E immune response genes: an unproved hypothesis. Science 188:375–377
23. Bignon JD, Houssin A, Soulillou JP, Denis J, Guimbretiere J, Guenel J (1980) HLA antigens and Berger's disease. Tissue Antigens 16:108–111
24. Billiard M, Seignalet J (1985) Extraordinary association between HLA-DR2 and narcolepsy. Lancet 1:227
25. Black PL, Marsh DG, Jarrett E, Delespesse GJ, Bias WB (1976) Family studies of association betwen HLA and specific immune responses to highly purified pollen allergens. Immunogenetics 3:349–368
26. Black CM, Welsh KI, Fielder A, Hughes GR, Batchelor JR (1982) HLA antigens and Bf allotypes in SLE: evidence for the association being with specific haplotypes. Tissue Antigens 19:115–120
27. Block ST, Lockshin MD, Winfield JB, Weksler ME, Imamura M, Winchester RJ, Mollors RC, Christian CL (1976) Immunologic observations on 9 sets of twins either concordant or discordant for SLE. Arthritis Rheum 19:545–554
28. Brand C, Davidson A, Littlejohn G, Ryan P (1984) Hydralazine-induced lupus: no association with HLA-DR4. Lancet 1:462
29. Brautbar C, Moscovitz M, Livshits T, Haim E, Hacham-Zadeh S, Cohen HA, Sharon R, Nelken D, Cohen T (1980) HLA-DRW4 in pemphigus vulgaris patients in Israel. Tissue Antigens 16:238–243
30. Bron B, Kubski D, Widmann JJ, von Fliedner V, Jeannet M (1982) Increased frequency of DR3 antigen in alcoholic hepatitis and cirrhosis. Hepatogastroenterology 29:183–186
31. Broxmeyer HE, Dupont B (1985) A role for class-II major histocompatibility complex antigens in the regulation of myelopoiesis. Prog Allergy 36:303–321
32. Calamia KT, Moore SB, Elveback LR, Hunder GC (1981) HLA-DR locus antigens in polymyalgia rheumatica and giant cell arteritis. J Rheumatol 8:993–955
33. Caruso C, Palmeri P, Oliva L, Orlando A, Cottone M (1985) HLA antigens in ulcerative colitis: a study in the Sicilian population. Tissue Antigens 25:47–49
34. Celada A, Barras C, Benzonana G, Jeannet M (1980) Increased frequency of HLA-DRW3 in systemic lupus erythematosus. Tissue Antigens 15:283–288
35. Christiansen FT, Kelly H, Dawkins RL (1984) Rheumatoid arthritis. In: Albert ED, Baur MP, Mayr WR (eds) Histocompatibility testing 1984. Springer, Berlin Heidelberg New York Tokyo, pp 378–383
36. Chused TM, Kassan SS, Opelz G, Moutsopoulos HM, Terasaki PI (1977) Sjögren's syndrome associated with HLA-DW3. N Engl J Med 296:895–897

37. Claas FHJ, van Rood JJ (1985) The interaction of drugs and endogeneous substances with HLA class-I antigens. Prog Allergy 36:135–150
38. Clerget-Darpoux F, Govaerts A, Feingold N (1984) HLA and susceptibility to multiple sclerosis. Tissue Antigens 24:160–169
39. Contu L, Cerimela D, Pintus A, Cottoni F, Lanasa G (1984) HLA and Kaposi's sarcoma in Sardinia. Tissue Antigens 23:240–245
40. Cunningham TJ, Tait BD, Mathews JD, Muirden KD (1982) Clinical rheumatoid vasculitis associated with the B8 and DR3 phenotype. Rheumatol Int 2:137–139
41. Dausset J, Contu L (1980) The MHC and immune response in man. In: Fougereau M, Dausset J (eds) Immunology 80. Academic, London, p 513 (Progress in immunology, vol 4)
41a. Dausset J, Gluckman E, Lemarchand F, Nunez-Roldan A, Contu L, Hors J (1977) Excès d'HLA-A2 et d'homozygotes HLA-A2 parmi les malades atteints d'aplasie médullaire et maladie de Fanconi. Nouv Rev Fr Hematol (Blood Cells) 18:315–324
42. Dawkins RL (1980) Myasthenia gravis. In: Terasaki PI (ed) Histocompatibility testing (1980) UCLA Tissue Typing Laboratory, Los Angeles, p 662
43. Dawkins RL, Christiansen FT, Kay PH, Garlepp M, McCluskey J, Hollingworth PN, Zilko PJ (1983) Disease associations with complotypes, supratypes, and haplotypes. In: Möller G (ed) Immunological reviews 1983. Munksgaard, Copenhagen, pp 5–22
44. De Jongh BM, Termijtelen A, Bruning GJ, de Vries RRP, van Rood JJ (1984) Relation of insulin-dependent diabetes mellitus (IDD) and the HLA-linked SB system. Tissue Antigens 23:87–93
45. De Marchi M, Carbonara AD (1984) HLA-DR3 and DR7-negative coeliac disease. In: Albert ED, Baur MP, Mayr WR (eds) Histocompatibility testing 1984. Springer, Berlin Heidelberg New York Tokyo, pp 359–362
46. de Moerloose P, Jeannet M, Bailly C, Raffoux C, Pointel JP, Sizonenko P (1978) HLA and DRW antigens in insulin-dependent diabetes. Br Med J 1:823–824
47. de Moerloose P, Jeannet M, Mirimanoff P, Bouvier CA (1979) Evidence for an HLA-linked resistance gene in Buerger's disease. Tissue Antigens 14:169–173
48. de Moerloose P, Jeannet M, Martins-da-Silva B, Werner-Favre C, Rohr J, Gauthier G (1979) Increased frequency of HLA-DRw2 and DRw3 in multiple sclerosis. Tissue antigens 13:357–360
49. de Mouzon-Cambon A, Bouissou F, Dutau G, Barthe P, Parra MT, Serin A, Ohayon E (1981) HLA-DR7 in children with idiopathic nephrotic syndrome. Correlation with atopy. Tissue Antigens 17:518–524
50. Deschamps I, Homberg JC, Janssen F, Lemut H, Vexiau P, Hors J (1984) Islet-cell antibodies (ICA-CFICA) and HLA genotypes in 107 IDD patients and their first-degree relatives. Hum Immunol 10:129–134
51. De Vries RRP, Mehra NK, Vaidya MC, Gupte MD, Meera Khan P, van Rood JJ (1980) HLA-linked control of susceptibility to tuberculoid leprosy and association with HLA-DR types. Tissue Antigens 16:294–304
52. De Vries RRP, Serjeantson SW, Layrisse Z (1984) Leprosy. In: Albert ED, Baur MP, Mayr WR (eds) Histocompatibility testing 1984. Springer, Berlin Heidelberg New York Tokyo, pp 362–367
53. De Wolfe WC, Lage PH, Shepard R, Martin-Alosco S, Yunis EJ (1981) Association of HLA and renal cell carcinoma. Hum Immunol 1:41–44
54. Dobloug JH, Forre D, Thorsby E (1979) HLA-DRW4 and rheumatoid arthritis. Lancet 1:548
55. Duquesnoy RJ, Morrari M, Hackbarth S, Zeevi A (1984) Serological and cellular definition of a new HLA-DR associated determinant, MC1, and its association with rheumatoid arthritis. Hum Immunol 10:165–176
56. Dyer PA, Clague RB, Klouda PT, Firth S, Harris R, Holt PJL (1982) HLA antigens in patients with rheumatoid arthritis and antibodies to native type II collagen. Tissue Antigens 20:394–396
57. Ebers GC, Paty DW, Stiller CR, Nelson RF, Seland TP, Larsen B (1982) HLA typing in multiple sclerosis sibling pairs. Lancet 2:88–90
58. Edidin M (1983) MHC antigens and non-immune functions. Immunol Today 4:269–270

59. Elkon KB, Sutherland DC, Rees AJ, Hughes GRV, Batchelor JR (1983) HLA antigen frequencies in systemic vasculitis: increase in HLA-DR2 in Wegener's granulomatosis. Arthritis Rheum 26:102–105
60. Ercilla G, Parés A, Arriaga F, Bruguera M, Castillo R, Rodés J, Vives J (1979) Primary biliary cirrhosis associated with HLA-DW3. Tissue Antigens 14:449–452
61. Falchuk ZM, Rogentine GN, Strober W (1972) Predominance of histocompatibility antigen HLA-B8 in patients with gluten-sensitive enteropathy. J Clin Invest 51:1602–1606
62. Farid NR, Bear J (1981) The human major histocompatibility complex and endocrine disease. Endocr Rev 2:50–86
63. Farid NR, Sampson L, Noel EP, Barnard JM, Mandeville R, Larsen B, Marshall WH, Carter ND (1979) A study of human leukocyte D locus related antigens in Graves' disease. J Clin Invest 63:108–113
64. Farid NR, Sampson L, Moen H, Barnard JM (1981) Goitrous autoimmune thyroiditis is associated with HLA-DR5. Tissue Antigens 17:265–268
65. Fauchet R, Guegen M, Genetet B, Le Pogamp P, Ramée MP, Chevet D, Simon P (1980) HLA-DR4 antigen and IgA nephropathy (Berger's disease). N Engl J Med 302:1033–1034
66. Førre O, Dobloug JH, Hoyerall HM, Throsby E (1983) HLA antigens in juvenile arthritis. Arthritis Rheum 26:35–38
67. Friedman JM, Packman LM, Maryjowski ML, Radvany RM, Crowe WE, Hanson V, Lerinson JE, Spencer CH (1983) Immunogenetic studies of juvenile dermatomyositis: HLA-DR antigen frequencies. Arthritis Rheum 26:214–216
68. Friedman-Kien AE, Laubenstein LJ, Rubinstein P, Buinovici-Klein E, Marmor M, Stahl R, Spigland I, Soo Kim K, Zolla-Pazner S (1982) Disseminated Kaposi's sarcoma syndrome in young homosexual men. Ann Intern Med 96:693–700
69. Fu SM, Stern R, Kunkel HG, Dupont B, Hansen JA, Day NK, Good RA, Jersild C, Fotino M (1975) Mixed lymphocyte culture determinants and C2 deficiency: LD-7a associated with C2 deficiency in four families. J Exp Med 142:495–506
70. Garavoy MR (1980) Idiopathic membranous glomerulonephritis: an HLA-associated disease. In: Terasaki PI (ed) Histocompatibility testing 1980. ULCA Tissue Typing Laboratory, Los Angeles, p 673
71. Garlepp MJ, Dawkins RL (1984) D-Penicillamine-induced myasthenia gravis. In: Albert ED, Baur MP, Mayr WR (eds) Histocompatibility testing 1984. Springer, Berlin Heidelberg New York Tokyo, pp 384–387
72. Germain BG, Espinoza LR, Bergen LL, Vagesh M, Vasey FB (1981) Increased prevalence of DRW3 in the CREST syndrome. Arthritis Rheum 24:857–859
73. Gladman DD, Keystone EC, Baron M, Lee P, Cane D, Mervert H (1981) Increased frequency of HLA-DR5 in scleroderma. Arthritis Rheum 24:854–856
74. Glass D, Raum D, Gibson D, Stillman JS, Schur PH (1976) Inherited deficiency of the second component of complement. J Clin Invest 58:853–861
75. Glass D, Litvin K, Wallace L, Chlack L, Garovoy M, Carpenter CB, Schur PH (1980) Early-onset pauciarticular juvenile rheumatoid arthritis associated with human leukocyte antigen DRW5, iritis and antinuclear antibody. J Clin Invest 66:426–429
76. Gorodezky C, Lavalle C, Castro-Escobar LE, Miranda-Limon JM, Escobar-Gutierrez A (1981) HLA antigens in Mexican patients with adult rheumatoid arthritis. Arthritis Rheum 24:976–977
77. Grand JT, Husby G, Thorsby E (1983) HLA-DR antigens and gold toxicity. Ann Rheum Dis 42:63–66
78. Griffing WL, Moore S, Luthra MA, McKenna CH, Fathman CG (1980) Associations of antibodies to native DNA with HLA-DRW3: a possible major histocompatibility-linked human immune response gene. J Exp Med 152:319S–325S
79. Hammarström L, Smith CIE (1983) HLA-A, B, C and DR antigens in immunoglobulin A deficiency. Tissue Antigens 21:75–79
80. Hanafusa T, Pujol-Borrell R, Chiovato L, Russell RCG, Doniach D, Bottazzo GF (1983) Aberrant expression of HLA-DR antigen on thyrocytes in Graves' disease: relevance for autoimmunity. Lancet 2:1111–1115
81. Hanly P, Garrett P, Spencer S, O'Dwyer WF (1984) HLA-A, -B, and -DR antigens in IgA nephropathy. Tissue Antigens 23:270–273

82. Harris R, Lawler SD, Oliver RTD (1978) The HLA system in acute leukemia and Hodgkin's disease. Br Med Bull 34:301–304
83. Harvey J, Arnett FC, Bias WB (1981) Heterogeneity of HLA-DR4 in the RA of a Chippewa band. J Rheumatol 8:797–803
84. Hawkins BR, Tiwari JL, Lowe N, Wolfish P, Pollock CA, Cho YW, Terasaki PI (1980) HLA and psoriasis. In: Terasaki PI (ed) Histocompatibility testing 1980. UCLA Tissue Typing Laboratory, Los Angeles, p 711
85. Hedfors E, Lindström F (1983) HLA-B8/DR3 in sarcoidosis. Tissue Antigens 22:200–203
86. Heikkilä M, Koistinen J, Lohman M, Koskimies S (1984) Increased frequency of HLA-A1 and B8 in association with total lack, but not with deficiency of serum IgA. Tissue Antigens 23:280–283
87. Helmerhorst FM, Nijenhuis LE, deLange GG, van den Berg Loonen PM, Jansen MF, van dem Borne AE, Engelfriet CP (1982) HLA antigens in idiopathic thrombocytopenic purpura. Tissue Antigens 20:372–379
88. Hiki Y, Kobayashi Y, Tateno S, Sada M, Kashiwagi N (1983) Strong association of HLA-DR4 with benign IgA nephropathy. Nephron 32:222–226
89. Hinzova E, Ivanyi D, Dula K, Horejs J, Dostal C, Drizhal I (1977) HLA-DW3 in Sjögren's syndrome. Tissue Antigens 9:8–10
90. Hirsch TJ, Enlow RW, Bias WB, Arnett FC (1981) HLA-D related (DR) antigens in various kinds of myositis. Hum Immunol 3:181–186
91. Hors J, Dausset J (1983) HLA and susceptibility to Hodgkin's disease. Immunol Rev 70:167–192
92. Hors J, Bonaiti-Pellie C, d'Agay MF, Rappaport H, Andrieux JM, de Waal LP, de Lauge GG, Feingold N (1984) Hodgkin's disease. In: Albert ED, Baur MP, Mayr WR (eds) Histocompatibility testing 1984. Springer, Berlin Heidelberg New York Tokyo, pp 411–414
93. Hughes GRV, Batchelor JR (1983) Genetics of systemic lupus erythematosus. Br Med J 1:416–417
94. Jacobson S, Biddison WE (1984) Major histocompatibility complex molecules as virus receptors. Immunol Today 5:262–263
95. Jaraquemada D, Pachoula-Papasteriadis C, Festenstein H, Sachs JA, Roitt IM, Corbett M, Ansell B (1979) HLA-D and DR determinants in rheumatoid arthritis. Transplant Proc 11:1306
96. Jaworski MA, Colle E, Guttmann RD (1983) Abnormal immunoregulation in patients with insulin-dependent diabetes mellitus and their healthy first degree relatives. Hum Immunol 7:25–34
97. Jeannet M, Magnin C (1971) HL-A antigens in haematological malignant diseases. Eur J Clin Invest 2:39–42
98. Jersild C, Hansen GS, Svejgaard A (1973) Histocompatibility determinants in multiple sclerosis, with special reference to clinical course. Lancet 2:1221–1225
99. Jersild C, Rubinstein P, Day NK (1976) The HLA system and inherited deficiencies of the complement system. Immunol Rev 32:43–71
100. Juji T, Satake M, Honda Y, Doi Y (1984) HLA antigens in Japanese patients with narcolepsy. Tissue Antigens 24:316–319
101. Julian BA, Quiggins PA, Thompson JS, Woodford SY, Gleason K, Wyatt RF (1985) Familial IgA nephropathy. N Engl J Med 312:202–208
102. Kachru RB, Sequeira W, Mittal KK, Siegel ME, Tedischi M (1984) A significant increase of HLA-DR3 and DR2 in systemic lupus erythematosus among blacks. J Rheumatol 11:417–474
103. Kallenberg CGM, van der Voort-Beelen JM, d'Amaro J, The TH (1981) Increased frequency of B8/DR3 in scleroderma and association of the haplotype with impaired cellular immune response. Clin Exp Immunol 43:478–485
104. Kameda S, Naito S, Tanaky K, Kajiyama K, Kunihiro K, Nishigouri S, Jimi S, Yanase T (1982) HLA antigens of patients with systemic lupus erythematosus in Japan. Tissue Antigens 20:221–222
105. Kammer GM, Trentham DE (1984) HLA-DR4 is not a requisite for autoimmunity to collagen in rheumatoid arthritis. Arthritis Rheum 27:489–494
106. Karpatkin S, Fotino M, Gibofsky A, Winchester RJ (1979) Association of HLA-DRW2 with autoimmune thrombocytopenic purpura. J Clin Invest 63:1085–1088

107. Klouda PT, Manas J, Acheson EJ, Dyer PA, Goldby FS, Harris R, Lawler W, Mallick NP, Williams G (1979) Strong association between idiopathic membranous nephropathy and HLA-DRW3. Lancet 2:770–771
108. Laster AJ, Conley CL, Kickler TS, Dorsch CA, Bias WB (1982) Chronic immune thrombocytopenic purpura in monozygotic twins: genetic factors predisposing to ITP. N Engl J Med 307:1495–1498
109. Laugdon N, Welsh KI, van Daw M, Vaughan RW, Parkes D (1984) Genetic markers in narcolepsy. Lancet 2:1178–1180
110. Laurent MR, Welsh KI (1983) Genetic markers in rheumatological diseases. J Immunogenetics 10:275–291
111. Lawley TJ, Hall RP, Fauci AS, Katz SI, Hamburger MI, Frank MM (1982) Defective Fc-receptor functions associated with the HLA-B8/DR3 haplotype. Studies in patients with dermatitis herpetiformis isolate. Transplant Proc 11:1788–1791
112. Layrisse Z, Rodriguez-Iturbe B, Garcia-Ramirez R, Rodriguez A, Tiwari J (1983) Family studies of the HLA system in acute post-streptococcal glomerulonephritis. Hum Immunol 7:177–185
113. Lee TD, Zhao TM, Bu KJ, Lu CZ, O'Donnell M, Sandler SG (1984) Association of HLA-DR4 with myasthenia gravis in the Chinese. Tissue Antigens 23:127–129
114. Libby DM, Gibofsky A, Fotino M, Waters SJ, Smith JP (1983) Immunogenetic and clinical findings in idiopathic pulmonary fibrosis. Am Rev Respir Dis 127:618–622
114a Lilly F, Boyse EA, Old FJ (1964) Genetic basis of susceptibility to viral leukemogenesis. Lancet 2:1207–1209
115. Lippman SM, Arnett FC, Conley CL, Ness PM, Meyers DA, Bias WB (1982) Genetic factors predisposing to autoimmune diseases. Am J Med 73:827–840
116. Lowenstein MB, Bridgeford PH, Vasey FB, Germain BF, Espinoza LR (1983) Increased frequency of HLA-DR3 and DR4 in polymyalgia rheumatica-giant cell arteritis. Arthritis Rheum 26:925–927
117. Mackay IR, Tait BD (1980) HLA associations with autoimmune-type chronic active hepatitis: identification of B8-DRW3 haplotype by family studies. Gastroenterology 79:95–98
118. Madigand M, Oger JJF, Fauchet R, Sabouraud O, Genetet B (1982) HLA profiles in multiple sclerosis suggest two forms of disease and the existence of protective haplotypes. J Neurol Sci 53:519–529
119. Mann DL, Katz SI, Nelson DL, Abelson LD, Strober W (1976) Specific B-cell antigens associated with gluten-sensitive enteropathy and dermatitis herpetiformis. Lancet 1:110–111
120. Marsh AG, Deborah A, Meyers A, Bias WB (1981) The epidemiology and genetics of atopic allergy. N Engl J Med 305:1551–1559
121. McCann VJ, McCluskey J, Kelly H, Kay PH, Zilko PJ, Christiansen FT, Dawkins RL (1984) Thyrogastric autoimmunity and MHC associated alleles at the C4 locus in patients with type I (insulin-dependent) diabetes. Diabetologia 27 [Suppl]:124–125
122. McDevitt HO, Benacerraf B (1969) Genetic control of specific immune responses. Adv Immunol 11:31
123. McGregor AM, Smith BR, Hall R, Petersen MM, Miller M, Dewar PJ (1980) Prediction of relapse in hyperthyroid Graves' disease. Lancet 1:1101–1103
124. Moen T, Stien R, Bratlie A, Bondevik E (1984) Distribution of HLA-SB antigens in multiple sclerosis. Tissue Antigens 24:126–127
125. Moens H, Farid NR (1978) Hashimoto's thyroiditis is associated with HLA-DRw3. N Engl J Med 299:133–134
126. Moriuchi J, Wakisaka A, Aizawa M, Yasuda K, Yokota A, Tanabe T, Itakura K (1982) HLA-linked susceptibility gene of Takayasu disease. Hum Immunol 4:87–91
127. Moutsopoulos HM, Mann DL, Johnson AH, Chused TM (1979) Genetic differences between primary and secondary sicca syndrome. N Engl J Med 301:761–763
128. Müller GA, Muller C, Liebau G, Kompf J, Ising H, Wernet P (1981) Strong association of idiopathic membranous nephropathy (IMN) with HLA-DR3 and MT-2 without involvement of HLA-B18 and no association to BfF1. Tissue Antigens 17:332–337
129. Nakai Y, Wakisaka A, Aizawa M, Itakura K, Nakai H, Ohashi A (1981) HLA and rheumatoid arthritis in the Japanese. Arthritis Rheum 24:722–725

130. Nakai Y, Kano T, Morinchi J, Wakisaka A, Aizawa M, Tsuneta H, Togashi K, Sakiyama Y, Wagatsuma Y, Matsumoto S (1982) Association between the MB system and asthma in the Japanese. Hum Immunol 4:265–270
131. Nepom BS, Nepom GT, Mickelson E, Shaller JG, Antonelli P, Hansen JA (1984) Specific HLA-DR4-associated histocompatibility molecules characterize patients with seropositive juvenile rheumatoid arthritis. J Clin Invest 74:287–291
132. Nerup J, Platz P, Ortved Anderson O, Christy M, Lyngsoe J, Poulsen JE, Ryder LP, Staub-Nielsen L, Thompson M, Svejgaard A (1974) HLA antigens and diabetes mellitus. Lancet 2:864
133. Nichol FE, Woodrow JC (1981) HLA-DR antigens in Indian patients with rheumatoid arthritis. Lancet 1:220–221
134. Noël H, Descamps B, Jungers P, Bach JF, Busson M, Suer C, Hors J, Dausset J (1978) HLA antigens in three types of glomerulonephritis. Clin Immunol Immunopathol 10:19–23
135. Numano F, Isohisa I, Egami M, Ohta N, Sasazuki T (1983) HLA-DR MT and MB antigens in Takayasu disease. Tissue Antigens 21:208–212
136. Nunez-Roldan A, Villechenous E, Fernandez-Andrade C, Martin-Govantes J (1982) Increased HLA-DR7 and decreased DR2 in steroid responsive nephrotic syndrome. N Engl J Med 306:366–367
137. Oen K, Petty RE, Schroeder ML (1982) Immunoglobulin A deficiency: genetic studies. Tissue Antigens 19:183–188
138. Okuyama T, Kunikane H, Kasahara M, Ohno S, Aizawa M, Conighi C, Perrone S, Mattiuz PL (1984) Behcet's disease. In: Albert ED, Baur MP, Mayr WR (eds) Histocompatibility testing 1984. Springer, Berlin Heidelberg New York Tokyo, pp 397–402
139. Owerbach D, Lernmark A, Platz P, Ryder LP, Rask L, Peterson PA, Ludvigsson J (1983) HLA-D region-chain DNA endonuclease fragments differ between HLA-DR identical healthy and insulin-dependent diabetic individuals. Nature 303:815–817
140. Owerbach D, Hägglöf M, Lernmark A, Holmgren G (1984) Susceptibility to insulin-dependent diabetes defined by restriction enzyme polymorphism of HLA-D region genomic DNA. Diabetes 33:958–965
141. Pandey JP, Fudenberg HH (1984) Immunogenetic markers in autoimmune disease. Ann Intern Med 101:868–869
142. Papasteriadis C, Kaloterakis A, Filiotou A, Economidou J, Nicolis G, Trichopoulos D, Stratigos J (1984) Histocompatibility antigens HLA-A, -B, -DR in Greek patients with Kaposi's sarcoma. Tissue Antigens 24:313–315
143. Park MS, Terasaki PI, Ahmed AR, Tiwari JL (1979) HLA-DRW4 in 91% of Jewish pemphigus vulgaris patients. Lancet 2:441–442
144. Park MS, Terasaki PI, Razzaque Ahmed A, Zone J (1983) The 90% incidence of HLA antigen (Te 24) in dermatitis herpetiformis. Tissue Antigens 22:263–266
145. Pollack MS (1985) Editorial comment on: Prognostic value of HLA in genitourinary tumors. Sagalowsky, chapter author: the possible role of class II HLA markers. In: Catalona WJ, Ratliff TF (eds) Genitourinary cancer 2. Martinus Nijhoff, Higham MA
146. Pollack MS, Vugrin D, Hennessy W, Herr HW, Dupont B, Withmore WF (1982) HLA antigens in patients with germ cell cancer of the testis. Cancer Res 42:2470
147. Pollack MS, Gold J, Metroka CE, Safai B, Dupont B (1984) HLA-A, B, C, and DR antigen frequencies in acquired immunodeficiency syndrome (AIDS) patients with opportunistic infections. Hum Immunol 11:99–103
148. Pollack MS, Falk J, Gazit E, Lawrence D, Safai B, Rubinstein P, Dupont B (1984) Classical and AIDS Kaposi's sarcoma. In: Albert ED, Baur MP, Mayr WR (eds) Histocompatibility testing 1984. Springer, Berlin Heidelberg New York Tokyo, pp 403–406
149. Powell TR, Michalski JP, McCombs CC, Danilovs JA, Terasaki PI, Park MS, Flood T, Boone WB (1980) HLA-BW44 and HLA-DRW4 in male Sjögren's syndrome patients with associated rheumatoid arthritis. Clin Immunol Immunopathol 17:463–468
150. Proust J, Moulias R, Fumeron F, Bekkhoucha F, Busson M, Schmid M, Hors J (1982) HLA and longevity. Tissue Antigens 19:168–173
151. Qvigstad E, Scott H, Thorsby E (1985) HLA class-II restriction of antigen-specific T-cell activation. Prog Allergy 36:73–94

152. Raveché ES (1984) Genetics of human and murine lupus erythematosus. In: Steinberg AD (moderator). Systematic lupus erythematosus: insights from animal models. Ann Intern Med 100:714–727
153. Rees AJ, Peters DK, Compston DAS, Batchelor JR (1978) Strong association between HLA-DRW2 and antibody-mediated Goodpasture's syndrome. Lancet 1:966–968
154. Reinersten JL, Klippel JH, Johnson AH, Steinberg AD, Decker JL, Mann DL (1978) B-lymphocyte alloantigens associated with systemic lupus erythematosus. N Engl J Med 299:515–518
155. Reinersten JL, Klippel JH, Johnson AH, Steinberg AD, Decker JL, Mann DL (1982) Family studies of B lymphocyte alloantigens in systemic lupus erythematosus. J Rheumatol 9:253–262
156. Reveille JD, Wilson RW, Provost TT, Bias WB, Arnett FC (1984) Primary Sjögren's syndrome and other autoimmune disease in families. Ann Intern Med 101:748–756
157. Reznikoff-Eteviant MF, Dangu C, Lobet R (1981) HLA-B8 antigen and anti-PL^{A1} alloimmunization. Tissue Antigens 18:66–68
158. Rich SS, Weitkamp LR, Barbosa J (1984) Genetic heterogeneity of insulin-dependent (type I) diabetes mellitus: evidence from a study of extended haplotypes. Amer J Hum Genet 36:1015–1023
159. Rittner C, Sennekamp J, Mollehaner E, Rösinger N, Niese D, Lüttkenhorst M, Baur MP, Stroehmann I (1983) Pigeon breeder's lung: association with HLA-DR3. Tissue Antigens 21:374–379
160. Rubinstein P, Ginsberg-Fellner F, Falk C (1981) Genetics of type 1 diabetes mellitus: a single recessive predisposition gene mapping between HLA-B and GLO. Am J Hum Genet 33:865–882
161. Safai B, Myskowski PL, Dupont BO, Pollack MS (1983) Association of HLA-DR5 with mycosis fungoides. J Invest Dermatol 80:395–397
162. Sasazuki T, Ohta N, Isohisa I, Numano F, Maezawa H (1979) Association between Takayasu disease and HLA-DHO. Tissue Antigens 14:177–178
163. Sasazuki S, Nishimura Y, Muto M, Ohta N (1983) HLA-linked genes controlling immune response and disease susceptibility. Immunol Rev 70:51–75
164. Saunders JB, Wodak AD, Haines A, Powell-Jackson PR, Portman B, Davis M, Williams R (1982) Accelerated development of alcoholic cirrhosis in patients with HLA-B8. Lancet 1:1381
165. Scherak O, Smolen JS, Mayr WR (1980) HLA-DRW3 and systemic lupus erythematosus. Arthritis Rheum 23:954–957
166. Schiff B, Mizrachi Y, Orgad S, Yaron M, Gazit E (1982) Association of HLA-Aw31 and HLA-DR1 with adult rheumatoid arthritis. Ann Rheum Dis 41:403–404
167. Schoenfeld Y, Schwartz RS (1984) Immunologic and genetic factors in autoimmune diseases. N Engl J Med 311:1019–1029
168. Scholz S, Albert E (1983) HLA and diseases: involvement of more than one HLA-linked determinant of disease susceptibility. Immunol Rev 70:77–88
169. Schur PH, Carpenter CB (1983) Sharing of HLA haplotype by parents of patients with systemic lupus erythematosus. Arthritis Rheum 26:1104–1110
170. Schur PH, Meyer I, Garovoy M, Carpenter CB (1982) Associations between systemic lupus erythematosus and the major histocompatibility complex: clinical and immunological considerations. Clin Immunol Immunopathol 24:263–275
171. Scott DGI, Bacon PA, Tribe CR (1981) Systemic rheumatoid vasculitis. A clinical and laboratory study of 50 cases. Medicine 60:288–297
172. Shornik JK, Stastny P, Gilliam JN (1981)High frequency of histocompatibility antigens HLA-DR3 and DR4 in herpes gestationis. J Clin Invest 68:553–555
173. Simonsen M, Skøodt K, Crone M, Sanderson A, Fujita-Yamaguchi Y, Due C, Rønne E, Linnet K, Olsson L (1985) Compound receptors in the cell membrane: ruminations from the borderland of immunology and physiology. Prog Allergy 36:151–176
174. Singal DP, Blajchman MA (1973) Histocompatibility (HL-A) antigens, lymphocytotoxic antibodies and tissue antibodies in patients with diabetes mellitus. Diabetes 22:429–432
175. Solheim BG, Albrechtsen D, Thorsby E, Thune P (1977) Strong association between and HLA-DW3 associated B cell alloantigen and dermatitis herpetiformis. Tissue Antigens 10:114–118

176. Solinger AM, Stobo JD (1982) Immune response gene control of collagen reactivity in man: collagen unresponsiveness in HLA-DR4 negative responders is due to the presence of T-dependent suppressive influences. J Immunol 129:1916–1920
177. Solinger AM, Bhatnagar R, Stobo JD (1981) Cellular molecular and genetic characteristics of T cell reactivity to collagen in man. Proc Natl Acad Sci USA 78:3877–3881
178. Sontheimer RD, Stastny P, Gilliam HN (1981) Human histocompatibility antigen associations in subacute cutaneous lupus erythematosus. J Clin Invest 67:312–316
179. Stastny P (1978) Association of the B-cell alloantigen DRW4 with rheumatoid arthritis. N Engl J Med 298:869–871
180. Stastny P (1980) Joint report on rheumatoid arthritis. In: Terasaki PI (ed) Histocompatibility testing 1980. UCLA Tissue Typing Laboratory, Los Angeles, pp 681–686
181. Stastny P, Ball EJ, Dry PJ, Nunez G (1983) The human immune response region (HLA-D) and disease susceptibility. Immunol Rev 70:113–153
182. Suciu-Foca N, Godfrey M, Jacobs J, Khan R, Rohowsky C, Foca-Rodi A, Woodward K, Hardy M (1980) Increased frequency of DRW5 in pauciarticular JRA. In: Terasaki PI (ed) Histocompatibility testing 1980. UCLA Tissue Typing Laboratory, Los Angeles, p 953
183. Svejgaard A, Platz P, Ryder LP (1981) Insulin-dependent diabetes mellitus. In: Terasaki PI (ed) Histocompatibility testing 1980. UCLA Tissue Typing Laboratory, Los Angeles, p 638
184. Svejgaard A, Platz P, Ryder LP (1983) HLA and disease 1982 – a survey. Immunol Rev 70:193–218
185. Swiss Federal Commission for the Rheumatic Diseases, subcommission for research (1981) HLA-DR antigens in rheumatoid arthritis. A swiss collaborative study. Rheumatol Int 1:111–113
186. Tait BD, Mackay IR (1982) HLA and alcoholic cirrhosis. Tissue Antigens 19:6–10
187. Tait BD, Mackay IR, Kastelan A, Dausset J, Mayer S, Okochi K (1980) Chronic liver disease including chronic active hepatitis. In: Terasaki PI (ed) Histocompatibility testing 1980. UCLA Tissue Typing Laboratory, Los Angeles, p 657
188. Thomsen M, Platz R, Andersen PO, Christy M, Lyngsoe J, Nerup J, Rasmussen K, Ryder LO, Nielsen LS, Svejgaard A (1975) MLC typing in juvenile diabetes mellitus and idiopathic Addison's disease. Transplant Rev 22:125–147
189. Thomsen M, Jorgensen F, Brundsborg M, Gimsing P, Lanng Nielsen J, Ryder LP, Svejgaard A (1981) Association of pernicious anemia and intrinsic factor antibody with HLA-D. Tissue Antigens 17:97–103
190. Thomsen M, Ryder LP, Bech K, Bliddal H, Feldt-Rasmussen U, Molholm J, Kappergaard E, Nielsen H, Svejgaard A (1983) HLA-D in Hashimoto's thyroiditis. Tissue Antigens 21:173–175
191. Tiwari JL, Morton NE, Lalouel JM, Terasaki PI, Zander H, Hawkins BR, Cho YW (1980) Multiple sclerosis. In: Terasaki PI (ed) Histocompatibility testing 1980. UCLA Tissue Typing Laboratory, Los Angeles, p 687
192. Tosi R, Vismara D, Tanigaki N, Ferrara GB, Ciccimarra F, Buffolano W, Follo D, Aurichio S (1983) Evidence that coeliac disease is primarily associated with a DC locus allelic specificity. Clin Immunol Immunopathol 28:395–404
193. Trence D, Morley JE, Handwerger BS (1984) Polyglandular autoimmune syndromes. Am J Med 77:107–116
194. Ungar B, Mathews JD, Tait BD, Crowling DC (1981) HLA-DR patterns in pernicious anaemia. Br Med J 282:768–770
195. Van den Berg-Loonen EM, Hilterman TCM, Bins M, Nijenhuis LE, Engelfriet P (1982) Increased incidence of HLA-DR2 in patients with pernicious anemia. Tissue Antigens 19:158–160
196. van Eden W, Elferink BG, de Vries RRP, Leiker DL, van Rood JJ (1984) Low T-lymphocyte responsiveness to Mycobacterium leprae antigens in association with HLA-DR3. Clin Exp Immunol 55:140–148
197. van Riel PLCM, Reekers P, van de Putte LBA, Gribnau FWJ (1983) Association of HLA antigens, toxic reactions and therapeutic response to auranofin and aurothioglucose in patients with rheumatoid arthritis. Tissue Antigens 22:194–199
198. van Rood JJ (1984) HLA as a regulator. Ann Rheum Dis 43:665–672

199. Volkman DJ, Mann DL, Fauci AS (1982) Association between Takayasu's arteritis and a B-cell alloantigen in North Americans. N Engl J Med 306:464–465
200. von Fliedner VE, Merica H, Jeannet M, Barras C, Feldges A, Imbach P, Wyss M (1983) Evidence for HLA-linked susceptibility factors in childhood leukemia. Hum Immunol 8:183–193
201. Walfish PG, Gotterman IS, Schewchuk AB, Bain J, Hawe BS, Farid NR (1983) Association of premature ovarian failure with HLA antigens. Tissue Antigens 21:168–169
202. Wank R, Schendel DJ, O'Neill GJ, Riethmüller G, Held E, Feucht HE (1984) Rare variant of complement C4 is seen in high frequency in patients with primary glomerulonephritis. Lancet 1:872–873
203. Weissel M, Hofer R, Zasmeta H, Mayr WR (1980) HLA-DR and Hashimoto's thyroiditis. Tissue Antigens 16:256–257
204. Werner-Favre C, Jeannet M (1979) HLA compatibility in couples with children suffering from acute leukemia or aplastic anemia. Tissue Antigens 13:307–309
205. Willkens RF, Hansen JA, Molmgren JA, Nisperos B, Mickelson EM, Watson MA (1982) HLA antigens in Yakima Indians with rheumatoid arthritis. Arthritis Rheum 25:1435–1439
206. Wilson RW, Provost TT, Bias WB, Alexander EL, Edlow DW, Hochberg MC, Stevens MB, Arnett FC (1984) Sjögren's syndrome. Influence of multiple HLA-D region alloantigens on clinical and serological expression. Arthritis Rheum 27:1245–1253
207. Winchester R, Toguchi T, Szer I, Burmester G, Lo Galbo P, Cuttner J, Capra D, Nunez-Roldan A (1983) Association of susceptibility to certain hematopoietic malignancies with the presence of Ia allodeterminants distinct from the DR series; utility of monoclonal antibody reagents. Immunol Rev 70:155–166
208. Winearls BC, Bodmer JG, Bodmer WF, Bottazo GF, McNally J, Mann JI, Thorogood M, Smith MA, Baum JD (1984) A family study of the association between insulin-dependent diabetes mellitus, autoantibodies and the HLA system. Tissue Antigens 24:234–246
209. Wooley PH, Griffin J, Panayi GS, Batchelor JR, Welsh KI, Gibson TJ (1980) HLA-DR antigens and toxic reaction to sodium aurothiomalate and D-penicillamine in patients with rheumatoid arthritis. N Engl J Med 303:300–302
210. Wooly PH, Luthra HS, O'Duffy JO, Bunch TW, Moore SB, Stuart JM (1984) Anti-type II collagen antibodies in rheumatoid arthritis. Tissue Antigens 23:263–269
211. Young A, Jaraquemada D, Awad J, Festenstein H, Corbett M, Hay FC, Roitt IM (1984) Association of HLA-DR4/DW6 and DR2/DW2 with radiologic changes in a prospective study of patients with rheumatoid arthritis. Arthritis Rheum 27:20–25

The Role of HLA Class II Antigens in Clinical Transplantation

A. Ting

Table of Contents

In this chapter I will discuss the role of matching for the HLA-DR antigens in clinical renal transplantation and the effects of pregraft HLA-DR antibodies on renal allograft outcome.

HLA-DR Matching and Renal Transplantation

Our initial report that HLA-DR matching may be important in improving cadaver graft survival [69] was soon confirmed by others [2, 45, 56]. A DR matching effect has been seen in multicentre studies, where the number of patients analysed is often very large [22, 52, 57], and in single-centre analyses, where the number of patients involved is much smaller [10, 33, 46, 71], although Dyer et al. [25] found no benefit of DR matching in a single-centre study.

Analyses of DR matching are relatively recent compared to those of A,B matching. Nevertheless, there are already a number of reports appearing in the literature suggesting that DR matching may be more effective in some groups of patients than in others. d'Amaro et al. [20] examined the effect of HLA-DR matching in relation to the sex and blood group of the recipient. They found a significant DR matching effect when all male patients were included in the analysis, but the effect was restricted to those males who were blood group A, B or AB (non-O). The difference in 1-year graft survival between the 0- and 2-DR-antigen mismatch groups was 19% in the non-O males and only 5% in the O males. In the female population the results were different: DR matching was less marked, and any effect seen was in the blood group O females. The influence of DR matching may be altered by the DRw6 status of the donor and recipient, as reported by van Rood et al. [77]. In their data the graft survival rate of DRw6-positive kidneys was high (about 75%–80% at 2 years), regardless of the DR match between donor and recipient. Graft survival of DRw6-negative kidneys in DRw6-positive recipients was low (50% at 2 years) regardless of DR matching, and the only patients in which an influence of DR matching could be seen were the DRw6-negative donor–DRw6-negative recipient group.

There is some evidence that DR matching may have a place in living related donor (LRD) transplants where the donor and recipient share one haplotype. In such transplants there will usually be one DR antigen mismatched, but sometimes there may be no DR mismatches. Sutherland et al. [65] found a 92% 1-year graft survival rate in the latter group compared with 82% in the group with one mismatched DR antigen. This difference in survival was not statistically significantly. However, a significant difference was seen between DR matching and the number of recipients who had at least one rejection episode – 24% of those with no DR mismatches and 43% in those with one DR mismatch.

HLA-DR matching appears to be a more effective method for improving cadaver graft survival than A,B matching, and has generated a vast amount of enthusiasm in transplant centres. Perhaps the main reason for this enthusiasm is the limited polymorphism of the alleles, which means that it should be possible to find a DR well-matched kidney for many recipients even with a relatively small recipient pool. In spite of this enthusiasm, a number of important practical questions need to be answered: (1) How important is the quality of the typing? (2) Does the graft survival rate increase as the match grade between donor and recipient increases? (3) Is there an additive effect of DR with A,B matching? (4) Is there an additive effect of DR matching with pregraft blood transfusions? (5) Is DR matching still necessary in patients treated with cyclosporin?

Quality of HLA-DR Typing

There is no doubt that HLA-DR typing is a more difficult procedure to carry out than A,B,C typing, mainly due to the fact that a relatively pure B lymphocyte suspension must be prepared, and this is not always easy, especially from patients with end-stage renal failure. Furthermore, in cadaver donors who have been treated with corticosteroids, DR typing may be virtually impossible from peripheral blood B lymphocytes. Madsen et al. [44] found a reduced expression of DR antigens on peripheral blood B cells after their patients had been treated with corticosteroids. Interestingly, the expression of A,B,C antigens on T lymphocytes was not affected by the same treatment. A reliable DR typing from a cadaver donor can only be obtained from B lymphocytes separated from lymph nodes or from spleen. Even with relatively pure cells, the discrepancy rate for DR typing (different DR types found by two different laboratories) is certainly higher than that for A,B,C typing. This is predominantly due to the poor definition of DRw6. There is no doubt that good quality DR typing is important. Jakobsen et al. [36]

found a 20 times stronger correlation between DR matching and graft survival when the DR type of the donor was repeated until two concordant results were obtained than when the initial DR typing of the donor was used. In the Collaborative Transplant Study (CTS), there was some indication of a better DR matching effect in those grafts typed with the Ninth International Histocompatibility Workshop sera than in those in which only local sera were used for antigen assessment [52].

Degree of HLA-DR Matching Required

From a practical point of view it is relevant to determine whether graft survival increases as the match grade between donor and recipient increases, or if high graft survival can be expected only in the DR-compatible grafts. The data from our centre (Table 1) clearly indicate that grafts with no DR mismatches have a high survival rate which is significantly higher than that for grafts with one or two DR mismatches, and that these latter two groups have similar survival rates. Other single-centre studies have also seen this "all-or-none" effect [10, 33], although a strong "gradation" effect has also been reported [4]. In multicentre studies the data are also at variance. d'Apice et al. [22] conducted a controlled trial where one kidney of a pair was allocated on DR matching and the other on B matching, and the results showed that DR-matched grafts had a better survival rate than those mismatched for either one or two antigens, the latter two groups having similar survival rates. A similar finding was made in the total Scandinavian material of 669 first cadaver grafts [5]. The Eurotransplant analysis of over 4000 first cadaver grafts shows a strong gradation effect [77]. Results from the CTS indicate a gradation effect, with each mismatched antigen decreasing the 1-year graft survival rate by about 8%. There is obviously no agreement on whether DR matching produces an all-or-none effect or a gradation effect, and for the present time a reasonable compromise would be to try to obtain a no-mismatch graft for each recipient, and failing this a graft with one mismatched antigen.

HLA-DR and HLA-A,B Matching

The question of whether DR matching is independent of A,B matching or whether the two are additive is important, and the answer will obviously influence

Table 1. The influence of HLA-DR matching on the survival rate of first cadaver grafts

DR mismatches	Patients	Percent survival (months)			
		12	24	36	60
0	107	79	77	72	64
1	155	70	62	55	47
2	81	68	61	54	51

Actuarial graft survival curves were generated according to the method of Peto et al. [58] and survival rates at specific time points were extracted. The *p* value for a positive trend is 0.0081 the matching policy which is adopted. The data from Eurotransplant show that both DR and A,B matching are important [77]. In an analysis of over 1000 transplants, DR matching did correlate with graft survival: the 2-year survival figures were 73% for grafts with no mismatches, 63% with one mismatch and 57% with two mismatches. However, in the group with no DR mismatches, the 2-year survival rate for grafts which had no, one, two, and three to four A,B mismatches were 82%, 76%, 72%, and 57% respectively. The conclusions drawn by the investigators were that HLA-DR compatibility should be sought, that the donor should be as well matched as possible for HLA-A,B, and that perhaps three or four A,B mismatches in the presence of DR compatibility should not take precedence over DR incompatibility with A,B compatibility. Corry et al. [17] have found that a 1-year graft survival rate of better than 75% could be achieved by matching for two DR antigens regardless of A,B matching, or one DR matching when two or more A,B antigens were also matched.

The CTS data show a near perfect correlation between the number of A,B,DR mismatches and graft survival. Although only 163 of the 5574 transplants had no mismatches, their 1-year survival rate was about 80%, which was over 20% higher than for grafts mismatched for five or six antigens. However, the same success rate could be achieved if only the B and DR antigens were matched, and here of course a much greater proportion of well-matched grafts can be expected. The 414 grafts with no B,DR mismatches had 1 year graft survival of about 80%, whereas in those with four mismatches the survival rate was below 60%. The CTS data show that DR matching is the most important, followed by B and then A matching. A combination of DR and B loci matching appears to provide the maximum advantage. For example, grafts with no DR mismatches have a 1-year graft survival of 70%, which is improved to about 80% when there are also no B mismatches.

Studies from some single centres have shown no A,B matching effect in DR-compatible grafts. Albrechtsen et al. [3] found that the degree of A,B matching did not influence graft survival in DR-compatible grafts, but in the DR-mismatched grafts, A,B matching tended to improve graft survival. This finding has also been made in our own data [74].

Most studies have shown that graft survival can be improved by matching for DR alone, and intuitively one might expect that additional A,B matching would improve graft survival even more. It would be totally impractical to transplant only kidneys with a perfect A,B,DR match. Based on the available data, DR matching may be the most important, followed by B and then A, and perhaps matching policies should be based on this premise.

HLA-DR Matching and Pregraft Blood Transfusions

Graft survival can be improved by both DR matching and pregraft blood transfusions, and although the latter is probably the single most important factor in improving graft survival, one of the risks of transfusions is sensitisation to HLA antigens, which if great may make it difficult to find a crossmatch-negative donor. If the DR matching effect is as good as blood transfusions, then it may provide a method of increasing graft survival without the associated risks of sensitisation seen with multiple blood transfusions. In fact few studies have addressed this problem, since in most centres there are very few, if any, non-transfused patients.

In our own centre, where we have had a relatively large number of non-transfused patients a DR matching effect is seen in both transfused and non-transfused individuals [74]. In the transfused group, those with a DR-compatible kidney had a 1-year graft survival rate of 87%, compared with 73% in those with a mismatched graft ($p=0.02$), and in the non-transfused group the 1-year graft survival in those receiving compatible grafts was 70%, compared with 47% in those receiving incompatible grafts ($p=0.04$). Similar results were obtained by Ayoub and Terasaki [6], but not by d'Apice et al. [22].

The overall data appear to show that DR matching and pregraft blood transfusions exert their effects independently, and one should not be a substitute for the other.

HLA-DR Matching and Cyclosporin

With the introduction of cyclosporin into clinical renal transplantation, and the finding that it is superior to conventional immunosuppressive therapy, the role of HLA matching has been re-examined in patients receiving cyclosporin. At the Tenth International Congress of the Transplantation Society, three groups reported that HLA-DR matching was not necessary in patients treated with cyclosporin [34, 40, 66, 67]. Harris et al. [34] found that in the group of patients treated with azathioprine and prednisolone, those who received a DR-matched kidney had a significantly better graft survival ($p=0.01$) than those who received a one- or two-antigen mismatched graft, the 1-year graft survival rates being 75%, 45%, and 37% respectively. However, in the cyclosporin-treated patients the opposite was seen; the 1-year graft survival rate was 64% for DR-compatible kidneys, 67% for kidneys with one DR mismatch, and 100% for kidneys with two DR mismatches. Taylor et al. [66] found a high graft survival rate in cyclosporin-treated patients irrespective of the degree of DR match of the kidney. One-year survival rates for grafts mismatched for no, one, and two DR antigens were 74%, 78%, and 79% respectively. The Scandinavian multicentre trial was designed to determine whether prospective blood transfusions and DR matching can be omitted in cadaver transplantation in patients treated with cyclosporin [40]. The results showed that a 6-month graft survival of about 75% could be achieved in patients with and without blood transfusions. Furthermore, DR matching had no effect in these patients; the 6-month survival rates for grafts transplanted with no, one, and two DR mismatches were about 77%, 70%, and 82% respectively. Flechner et al. [31] found an 18-month graft survival rate of 92% in one-haplotype disparate LRD transplants with high mixed lymphocyte culture reactivity treated with cyclosporin and prednisolone. Fourteen of the 15 non-transfused and 19 of the 21 transfused patients had successful grafts.

It has been argued by the authors of these publications that if indeed the use of cyclosporin can negate the blood transfusion and DR matching effects, the practical implications are major. Fewer patients would become sensitised as a result of the withdrawal of blood transfusions, the cold ischaemia times would be shortened, since cadaver kidneys would not have to be shipped to other centres, and expensive organ-sharing programmes could be kept to a minimum.

However, not all studies have shown that cyclosporin abrogates the transfusion and HLA-DR matching effects. Cats et al. [14] have analysed data from North America and found that HLA-A,B matching, DR matching and pregraft blood transfusions are effective in increasing the transplant survival rate in patients treated with cyclosporin. In fact the data indicate that these effects are greater in cyclosporin-treated patients than in patients treated with azathioprine and prednisolone, and the authors have suggested that matching and pregraft blood transfusions should be pursued even more vigorously in cyclosporin-treated patients. In the CTS data [52] the group treated with cyclosporin ($n=2198$) had a significantly higher graft survival rate (76% at 1 year) than the 6392 patients without cyclosporin (64% at 1 year). A significant correlation was seen between DR matching and graft outcome in both the cyclosporin-treated and non-cyclosporin-treated patients. The difference between well-matched and poorly-matched grafts in both treatment groups was about 10%. However, poor DR-matched grafts in patients with cyclosporin had a similar survival rate to well DR matched grafts in patients without cyclosporin. HLA-A,B matching also improved graft survival in cyclosporin-treated patients, and a powerful effect was seen with HLA-B and DR matching. Based on these results, Opelz [52] concludes that intelligent combined utilisation of HLA-B,DR matching and cyclosporin treatment may be a key to further improvements in cadaver kidney transplantation.

The results of the effects of HLA matching in patients treated with cyclosporin are only beginning to emerge, and at the present time no definitive conclusions can be drawn from the data. These studies are of course extremely important, for as we have already mentioned, the practical implications of treating all patients with cyclosporin without prior conditioning with blood transfusions and without HLA matching are enormous.

Pregraft HLA-DR Antibodies and Renal Transplantation

It would be impossible to discuss the effects of HLA-DR antibodies on renal allograft outcome without discussing other types of B cell antibodies, since in many cases it is difficult or impossible to determine with certainty that the B cell antibody in the patient's serum is directed at HLA-DR antigens. Therefore, in this section I will discuss first the different types of B cell antibodies which can be detected in the lymphocytotoxic test, and then their relevance to graft outcome.

B Lymphocyte Antibodies Detected by the Cytotoxic Test

Many different specificities of B lymphocyte antibodies can be detected in the cytotoxic test. The data published over the past several years clearly indicate that some specificities are not damaging to renal allograft survival, while others may be damaging. Therefore, it is important to accurately define the type of B cell antibodies present in patients awaiting renal transplantation, for the specificity of the antibody will determine whether or not a transplant can be performed with a B cell-positive crossmatch.

HLA-DR and DQ (Class II) Antibodies

Class II antigens have been found on a number of cells and tissues of the body, although their distribution is less widespread than that of HLA class I antigens. Using a mouse monoclonal antibody to a monomorphic determinant, Daar et al. [19] found class II antigens on epithelial cells in a number of organs and on the capillaries of all organs examined except brain, testis, and placenta. Baldwin et al. [8] found only weak staining of kidney pertibular capillaries with five of the seven human HLA-DR alloantisera examined. Evans et al. [30] used the immunoperoxidase staining technique to test the reactivity of two mouse monoclonal monomorphic class II antibodies and ten human HLA-DR alloantisera detecting DR1, DR3, DR4, and DR7 against sections from eight kidney biopsies. The monoclonal antibodies stained the glomerular, peritubular capillary and venous endothelium, whilst the arterial endothelium was negative. The human alloantisera showed the same pattern of staining as the monoclonal antibodies but the reactions were weaker. The "expected" reactions were seen with all sera, except that a DR1-positive kidney gave negative results with two of the three DR1 sera.

The question which remains unanswered is whether the appropriate HLA-DR antigens is expressed in the kidney cells when it is expressed on the lymphocytes of the same individual, or whether there is variation in the expression of DR antigens in the kidney endothelium. There appears to be little doubt that the class II monomorphic determinant is intensely expressed on all glomerular and peritubular capillaries, but its expression on the endothelium of large vessels may be variable, both within the kidney and between the kidneys of different individuals. On the other hand, the few studies which have looked at the expression of specific HLA-DR antigens using either monoclonal antibodies [8] or human alloantisera [8, 30] have shown variable intensity of staining among the kidneys examined. In some cases a negative reaction was seen when a positive was expected from the HLA typing of the appropriate lymphocytes. This may mean that although the DR antigen is on the lymphocytes, it is not necessarily expressed on the kidney cells.

Interstitial dendritic cells, monocytes and macrophages express class II antigens, although some monocytes appear not to express HLA-DQ antigens [51].

Autoreactive Antibodies

Some renal patients develop B cell antibodies which not only react with normal allogeneic lymphocytes, but also react with their own B cells [59]. Autoantibodies do not react or only react weakly with B lymphocytes from chronic lymphocytic leukaemia (CLL) cells [70] and this property distinguishes them from HLA-DR,DQ antibodies, which do react with CLL cells. In the lymphocytotoxic test, the autoantibody reacts more strongly if the pre-complement incubation step is carried out at 4 °C rather than at 22 °C [53]. The appearance of autoantibodies does not seem to be related to blood transfusions or pregnancies, since they have been found in non-transfused male patients. Furthermore, the antibody is IgM rather than the usual IgG produced after conventional immunisation. The incidence of autoantibodies in dialysis patients has been reported to be as high as 42% [41], although most laboratories find a considerably lower frequency [28] and in some units they are not found at all.

Red Cell Antibodies

Antibodies to some red cell antigens have been detected in the sera of dialysis patients and parous women using the lymphocytotoxic test. Lymphocytotoxic antibodies to blood group A have been described by Jeannet et al. [37]. However, this is a rare occurrence, and in the majority of non-A individuals the anti-A antibody is not lymphocytotoxic. Although these antibodies do occur, they should not be a problem in the crossmatch test, since normally only ABO-compatible kidneys are considered for transplantation. Lymphocytotoxic anti-Lewis antibodies have been described [54], and these react predominantly with B lymphocytes. The Lewis antigen on B lymphocytes is not secreted by the cell, but is adsorbed onto the cell surface from the plasma. Shumak et al. [63] found an auto-anti-I as well as an auto-anti-i which were cytotoxic to the patient's own lymphocytes. A lymphocytotoxic anti-Yk^a was found [16] in a recipient of an HLA identical sibling transplant and this antibody gave a positive B cell crossmatch with the donor. The York system is apparently not an important transplantation antigen, since the transplant showed no evidence of rejection 4 months after operation.

Thus it is apparent that not only the HLA antibodies, but also a large variety of other antibodies with different specificities are reactive in the lymphocytotoxicity test. Furthermore, it would appear that although these non-HLA antibodies can cause a positive lymphocytotoxic crossmatch, they are in themselves not damaging to renal allografts. Therefore, much of the work which now has to be done is to find ways of clearly differentiating the non-damaging from the damaging lymphocytotoxic antibodies so that the significance of a positive crossmatch can be correctly interpreted.

Transplantation with a Positive B Cell Crossmatch

During the mid to late 1970s a number of reports were published showing that successful transplantation could be achieved in the presence of a positive B lymphocyte crossmatch provided the T cell crossmatch was negative [21, 27, 42, 50, 59, 68]. Some authors have even suggested that grafts performed in this situation have a better survival rate than grafts with a negative crossmatch [21]. On the other hand, other reports have indicated that B cell antibodies might be associated with immediate graft failure [1, 9, 13, 24, 47]. Differences in the specificity of B cell antibodies among the patients may provide at least a partial explanation for the observations of the varying effects of B cell antibodies on renal allografts.

Autoreactive Antibodies

There is overwhelming evidence that autoreactive B cell antibodies are not graft damaging, either in cadaver transplants [29, 43, 64, 68, 73] or in LRD transplants

Table 2. Survival rate of first cadaver grafts performed in the presence of a B cell-positive crossmatch due to autoantibodies, non-autoantibodies, and with a negative crossmatch

Type of crossmatch	Patients	Percent survival (months)			
		3	6	12	24
B+, auto+	17	88	88	88	81
B+, auto−	11	46	46	34	34
Negative	100	76	70	65	59

Actuarial graft survival curves were generated according to the method of Peto et al. [58], and survival rates at specific time points were extracted

[49]. Some studies have indicated that autoreactive B cell antibodies may be associated with improved graft survival [29, 72]. Our results of transplantation of first cadaver grafts with a positive B cell crossmatch due to autoantibodies, non-autoantibodies or with a negative crossmatch are shown in Table 2. A high graft survival rate is seen in the autoantibody group (88% at 1 year) which is significantly higher than the survival rate of the non-autoantibody group (34%, $p=0.005$), but not of the negative crossmatch group (65%, $p=0.223$). The negative crossmatch group has a significantly higher actuarial graft survival rate than the B cell-positive non-autoantibody group ($p=0.016$).

HLA-DR Antibodies

The influence of donor-reactive HLA-DR (and/or DQ) antibodies is not clear. Certainly HLA class II molecules are found in kidney tissue such as the peritubular capillaries, glomeruli, some tubular cells, and to a lesser extent on the endothelium of large vessels [19, 32]. Based on this finding, one might expect donor-specific HLA-DR antibodies to be a cause of acute graft failure. There have only been a few reported cases of graft failure in which the recipient has had a pregraft specific DR antibody against the mismatched DR antigen of the donor. For example, Mohanakumar et al. [47] described two cases of second transplants performed with a B cell-positive–T cell-negative crossmatch in which the patients had specific DR antibodies to the mismatched DR antigen of the donor, HLA-DRw6 in one case and HLA-DR2 in the other. Both grafts failed, one at 15 weeks and the other at 5 weeks. Ahern et al. [1] reported two cases of hyperacute rejection in B cell-positive crossmatch transplants. One was in a recipient of an LRD transplant where the only mismatch was DR3. The specificity of the DR3 antibody of the recipient was confirmed by the fact that it could be removed by absorption with a DR3-homozygous cell line. Other cases of early graft failure have been reported with a B cell-positive crossmatch in HLA-A,B-compatible–DR-incompatible grafts where the specificity of the antibody was not clearly defined [9]. Poor graft survival was seen in patients who had a positive B cell crossmatch with sera which demonstrated DR specificity [60]. Indirect evidence that DR antibodies can cause graft rejection comes from studies which have shown that DR antibodies can be eluted from rejected grafts [48].

Some studies have found no deleterious effect of DR antibodies. Jeannet et al. [39] reported successful outcome in 14 of 16 grafts performed across a B cell-positive crossmatch, the majority of which were not due to autoreactive antibodies. The authors claimed that the B cell antibodies were directed at donor HLA-DR, since they were not platelet-absorbable (platelets carry HLA-A,B,C but not HLA-DR,DQ antigens).

Cold Reactive Antibodies

The standard lymphocytotoxic test used for screening sera and for crossmatching is normally carried out with both the pre- and post-complement steps at room temperature (20°–25 °C). Iwaki et al. [35] introduced the cold and warm test by changing the temperature of the pre-complement incubation step to 5 °C and 37 °C respectively; the second incubation step was carried out at room temperature in both tests. Using this method they found that some B cell antibodies reacted at 5 °C only (B cold antibodies), while others reacted at both 5 °C and 37 °C (B warm antibodies). In this initial publication they found that patients with only B cold antibodies had a significantly higher graft survival rate (70% at 6 months) than those patients with B warm antibodies (38%) or no antibodies (47%). In this retrospective study the sera were not crossmatched with the donors' cells, but their presence was determined by screening the sera against random panel cells. However, based on their results the authors postulated that B cold antibodies were enhancing antibodies. Similar results have been found by some [38], but not by others [26, 75]. The B cold antibody is not directed at HLA antigens. There is some evidence that it is an IgM anti-IgM, and may be anti-idiotype [15]. In some cases it may be an autoantibody [53].

Ayoub et al. [7] found that grafts performed across a B cold positive crossmatch had a higher (but not significantly higher) 1-year survival rate (58%) than those due to B warm antibodies (42%) and those with a negative crossmatch (38%). However, patients with strong B warm antibodies (titre $>1:8$) did significantly worse at 6 months (27% graft survival rate) than those with a B cold positive crossmatch. The authors suggested that these high-titred B warm antibodies were directed at HLA-DR antigens, since they were not plåtelet-absorbable. The graft-damaging effects of B warm antibodies has not been confirmed by most laboratories [18, 21, 23, 43, 60], although most studies show that B cold antibodies are not harmful.

Our own data and that of others suggest that (a) B cell autoantibodies can react at both 4 °C and 37 °C, although the reactivity is usually stronger at 4 °C; (b) B cold antibodies are not directed at HLA-DR, but may be autoreactive; (c) a B warm positive crossmatch is not necessarily a contraindication to transplantation, and therefore performing the crossmatch at 37 °C as an additional test is of limited value in eliminating patients who might rapidly reject the graft; and (d) because B cold antibodies are not harmful, such a crossmatch need not be performed. The influence of B cell antibodies on graft outcome probably depends on their specificity rather than their optimal thermal reactivity.

Living Related Donor Transplants

The relevance of donor-specific B cell antibodies in LRD transplants, particularly in patients who have received donor-specific transfusions (DST), is becoming more important with the increasing use of this protocol to improve the survival rate of one-haplotype-mismatched grafts. Salvatierra et al. [61] showed that donor-specific B warm cytotoxic antibodies can develop in some patients. In their first 90 patients treated with DST, 7 (8%) had persistent B warm antibodies while 12 (13%) initially developed B cell antibodies followed by the appearance of T and B cell antibodies. The supposition here was that weak HLA-A,B,C antibodies reacting only with B cells had developed initially, but that with further transfusions these became stronger to react with T and B cells. This latter phenomenon has also been described by Blank et al. [11]. In fact these authors have used this finding to argue that a transplant should not be performed in the presence of a B warm positive crossmatch. However, at the present time the published data do not seem to fully support the argument that a B warm positive crossmatch is a definite contra-indication to transplantation. Salvatierra et al. [62] have reported an unsuccessful transplant with a B warm positive crossmatch. On the other hand, Bow et al. [12] performed successful transplants in two patients with a B warm positive crossmatch in whom the antibody was transient. In one case the B cell antibody disappeared 6 months after the last DST and the patients received a transplant a further 6 months after this date. Vaidya et al. [76] have performed transplants in 16 patients with a B cell-positive crossmatch. Although all grafts were functioning, 10 of the 16 patients (63%) experienced one or more reversible rejection episodes within 3 months of transplantation, compared with an incidence of 37% in patients receiving a transplant with a negative crossmatch.

No attempt was made in any of these studies to characterise the B cell antibodies into HLA-DR, weak HLA-A,B,C or some other specificity, so we have no information as to whether failure or acute rejection episodes in these patients was associated with any one type of antibody. Until more data is available, we have to say that it does appear that successful transplantation can be achieved in the presence of a B cell-positive crossmatch in patients treated with DST. These patients, however, may have a greater risk of acute reversible rejection episodes.

Conclusions

Matching for the HLA-DR antigens can improve renal allograft survival, and its effect may be more pronounced in certain subgroups of patients, such as non-O males. With the recent introduction of cyclosporin and its superiority over conventional immunosuppression, the role of DR matching has to be re-examined in patients treated with cyclosporin. The present data are conflicting, and more studies are needed.

With regard to the role of donor-specific B cell antibodies there is clear evidence that B cell autoantibodies are not harmful, and renal transplantation can certainly proceed if a positive crossmatch is caused by these antibodies. The relevance of non-autoreactive B cell antibodies is far from clear. One reason for this uncertainty is that the specificity of the antibodies is so varied; the antibodies can be directed at HLA-DR antigens or at red cell antigens such as A and Lewis. It has even been suggested that most B cell antibodies found in the sera of dialysis patients are not directed at HLA-DR antigens. To cloud the issue even more, some reactivity with B cells only may be due to weak HLA-A,B antibodies, for it has been shown that B lymphocytes have a greater density of HLA class I antigens than T lymphocytes [55].

In the few studies where a specific DR antibody has been defined and is directed at the mismatched DR antigen of the donor, the grafts have failed, suggesting that DR antibodies may be a cause of graft failure. These reported studies should not be considered as definitive, however, and certainly more work needs to be done in this area. The effect of HLA-DR,DQ antibodies on renal allografts is still questionable. In the reported studies where a well-defined HLA-DR antibody directed at the mismatched DR antigen of the donor was present before transplantation, poor survival was seen. However, in other studies where a B cell-positive crossmatch was thought to be due to HLA-DR antibodies, good graft survival has been reported. The main difficulty in assessing the effect of DR antibodies on graft function is caused by our inability to clearly characterise the specificity of most B cell antibodies. Until reliable methods are available to clearly distinguish DR from non-DR antibodies, the question of the effect of DR antibodies will remain open.

References

1. Ahern AT, Artruc SB, Della Pelle P, Cosimi AB, Russell PS, Colvin RB, Fuller TC (1982) Hyperacute rejection of HLA-AB-identical renal allografts associated with B lymphocyte and endothelial reactive antibodies. Transplantation 33:103–106
2. Albrechtsen D, Flatmark A, Jervell J, Solheim B, Thorsby E (1978) HLA-DR antigen matching in cadaver renal transplantation. Lancet 1:825
3. Albrechtsen D, Moen T, Flatmark A, Halvorsen S, Jakobsen A, Jervell J, Solheim BG, Thorsby E (1981) Influence of HLA-A, B, C, D, and DR matching in renal transplantation. Transplant Proc 13:924–929
4. Albrechtsen D, Bondevik H, Flatmark A, Halvorsen S, Jakobsen A, Jervell J, Moen T, Solheim BG, Sodal G, Thorsby E (1982) HLA matching in first cadaveric renal transplantation in Norway 1969–1981. Transplant Proc 14:182–184
5. Albrechtsen D, Moen T, Thorsby E (1983) HLA matching in clinical transplantation. Transplant Proc 15:1120–1123
6. Ayoub G, Terasaki PI (1982) HLA-DR matching in multicenter, single-typing laboratory data. Transplantation 33:515–517
7. Ayoub G, Park MS, Terasaki PI, Iwaki Y, Opelz G (1980) B cell antibodies and crossmatching. Transplantation 29:227–229
8. Baldwin WM, Claas FHJ, van Es LA, van Rood JJ (1981) Distribution of endothelial-monocyte and HLA antigens on renal vascular endothelium. Transplant Proc 13:103–107
9. Berg B, Moller E (1981) Immediate rejection of a HLA-A,B compatible, HLA-DR incompatible kidney with a positive donor-recipient B-cell crossmatch. Scand J Urol Nephrol [Suppl] 54:36
10. Berg B, Groth CG, Lundgren G, Moller E (1982) The impact of HLA-DR matching on the outcome of cadaver kidney transplantation. Transplant Proc 14:178–181
11. Blank JL, Leo GM, Sollinger HW, Glass NR, Belzer FO (1982) B-warm-positive crossmatch: a contraindication for transplantation in living related transplants undergoing donor-specific transfusion. Transplantation 33:212–213
12. Bow LM, Schweizer RT, Cho S (1984) Successful renal transplantation after transient warm B cell antibody to donor specific transfusions. Transplantation 37:618–619
13. Buckingham JM, Geis WP, Giacchino JL, Popli S, Hano JE, Chejfec G, Jonasson O (1979) B-cell directed antibodies and delayed hyperacute rejection: a case report. J Surg Res 27:268–274
14. Cats S, Terasaki P, Perdue S, Mickey MR (1984) Effect of HLA typing and transfusions on cyclosporine-treated renal-allograft recipients. N Engl J Med 311:675–676
15. Cicciarelli JC, Chia D, Terasaki PI, Barnett EV, Shirahama S (1979) IgM anti-IgM cold lymphocytotoxins to B cells. Transplant Proc 11:1950–1953
16. Connors SM, Myberg SJ, Dodds K, Carpenter CB, Garovoy MR (1979) Successful renal allograft in the presence of York (Yk[a]) and autologous B-cell antibodies. Transplant Proc 11:1944–1946
17. Corry RJ, Schulak JA, Goeken NE, Nghiem DD (1985) The effect of HLA, A, B, and DR matching and blood transfusion in first cadaver kidney transplantation. Transplant Proc 17:756–757
18. Coxe-Gilliland R, Cross DE (1981) Warm B-cell antibodies and DRw matching: their influence on transplant outcome at a single centre. Transplant Proc 13:945–948
19. Daar AS, Fuggle SV, Fabre JW, Ting A, Morris PJ (1984) The detailed distribution of MHC class II antigens in normal human organs. Transplantation 38:293–298
20. d'Amaro J, Hendriks GFJ, Persijn GG, van Rood JJ (1985) Influence of sex and ABO blood group on HLA-A,B, and -DR matching in renal transplantation. Transplant Proc 17:758–760
21. d'Apice AJF, Tait BD (1979) Improved survival and function of renal transplants with positive B cell crossmatches. Transplantation 27:324–328
22. d'Apice AJF, Sheil AGR, Tait BD, Bashir HV (1984) A prospective randomized trial of matching for HLA-A and B versus HLA-DR in renal transplantation. Transplantation 38:37–41
23. Deierhoi MH, Ting A, Morris PJ (1983) Successful renal transplantation despite warm B cell antibodies. Transplantation 36:207–209

24. Dejelo CL, Williams TC (1977) B-cell cross-match in renal transplantation. Lancet 2:241
25. Dyer PA, Johnson RWG, Mallick NP, Harris R (1983) A single center prospective study showing no benefit of HLA-DR matching between cadaver kidney donors and recipients. Transplant Proc 15:137–138
26. Etheredge E, Sicard GA, Anderson CB (1979) Increased detection of leukocytotoxic antibodies by thermal discrimination and their influence on renal allograft survival. Transplantation 27:12–17
27. Ettenger RB, Terasaki PI, Opelz G, Malekzadeh M, Pennisi AJ, Uittenbogaart C, Fine R (1976) Successful renal allografts across a positive cross-match for donor B-lymphocyte alloantigens. Lancet 2:56–58
28. Ettenger RB, Jordan S, Fine RN (1981) Autolymphocytotoxic antibodies in patients on dialysis awaiting renal transplantation. Transplantation 32:248–251
29. Ettenger RB, Jordan SC, Fine RN (1983) Cadaver renal transplant outcome in recipients with autolymphocytotoxic antibodies. Transplantation 35:429–431
30. Evans PR, Trickett LP, Smith JL, MacIver AG, Tate D, Slapak M (1985) Varying expression of major histocompatibility complex antigens on human renal endothelium and epithelium. Br J Exp Pathol 66:79–87
31. Flechner SM, Kerman RH, van Buren C, Kahan BD (1984) Successful transplantation of cyclosporine-treated haploidentical living-related renal recipients without blood transfusions. Transplantation 37:73–76
32. Fuggle SV, Errasti P, Daar AS, Fabre JW, Ting A, Morris PJ (1983) Localisation of MHC (HLA-ABC and DR) antigens in 46 kidneys. Differences in HLA-DR staining of tubules among kidneys. Transplantation 35:385–390
33. Goeken NE, Thompson JS, Corry RJ (1981) A 2-year trial of prospective HLA-DR matching. Effects on renal allograft survival and rate of transplantation. Transplantation 32:522–527
34. Harris KR, Digard NJ, Gosling DC, Gardner B, Campbell MJ, Tate DG, Sharman VL, Slapak M (1985) HLA-DR matching in renal transplant patients on cyclosporine. Transplant Proc 17:42–43
35. Iwaki Y, Terasaki PI, Park MS, Billing R (1978) Enhancement of human kidney allografts by cold B-lymphocyte cytotoxins. Lancet 1:1228–1229
36. Jakobsen BK, Langhoff E, Platz P, Ryder LP, Thaysen JH, Olgaard K, Kristensen JK, Jorgensen HE, Lokkegaard H, Rasmussen F, Sorensen WS, Svejgaard A (1984) The impact of HLA-DR compatibility on cadaver kidney graft survival in a prospective study with special emphasis on the quality of typing. Tissue Antigens 23:94–104
37. Jeannet M, Bodmer JG, Bodmer WF, Schapira M (1973) Lymphocytotoxic sera associated with the ABO and Lewis red cell blood groups. In: Dausset J, Colombani J (eds) Histocompatibility testing 1972. Munksgaard, Copenhagen, pp 493–499
38. Jeannet M, Vassalli P, Hufschmid MF (1980) Enhancement of human kidney allografts by cold B lymphocyte cytotoxins. Transplantation 29:174–175
39. Jeannet M, Benzonana G, Arni I (1981) Donor-specific B and T lymphocyte antibodies and kidney graft survival. Transplantation 31:160–163
40. Klintmalm G, Brynger H, Flatmark A, Frodin L, Husberg B, Thorsby E, Groth CG (1985) The blood transfusion, DR matching, and mixed lymphocyte culture effects are not seen in cyclosporine-treated transplant recipients. Transplant Proc 17:1026–1031
41. Lobo PI (1981) Nature of autolymphocytotoxins present in renal hemodialysis patients. Their possible role in controlling alloantibody formation. Transplantation 32:233–237
42. Lobo PI, Westervelt FB, Rudolf LE (1977) Kidney transplantability across a positive cross-match. Cross-match assays and distribution of B lymphocytes in donor tissues. Lancet 1:925–928
43. Lobo PI, Westervelt FB, Rudolf LE (1978) Kidney transplantation across positive B and T cell crossmatches. Transplantation 26:84–86
44. Madsen M, Kissmeyer-Nielsen F, Rasmussen P, Andersen P (1981) Decreased expression of HLA-DR antigens on peripheral blood B lymphocytes during glucocorticoid treatment. Tissue Antigens 17:195–204
45. Martins-da-Silva B, Vassalli P, Jeannet M (1978) Matching renal grafts. Lancet 1:1047–1048

46. Moen T, Albrechtsen D, Flatmark A, Jakobsen A, Jervell J, Halvorsen S, Solheim BG, Thorsby E (1980) Importance of HLA-DR matching in cadaveric renal transplantation. A prospective one-center study of 17 transplants. N Engl J Med 303:850–854
47. Mohanakumar T, Rhodes C, Mendez-Picon G, Goldman M, Moncure C, Lee H (1981a) Renal allograft rejection associated with presensitization to HLA-DR antigens. Transplantation 31:93–95
48. Mohanakumar T, Waldrep JC, Phibbs M, Mendez-Picon G, Kaplan AM, Lee HM (1981b) Serological characterization of antibodies eluted from chronically rejected human renal allografts. Transplantation 32:61–66
49. Myberg SJ, Connors CM, Carpenter CB, Garovoy MR (1979) Positive crossmatches due to autoantibodies in living-related transplantation. Transplant Proc 11:1954–1957
50. Myburgh JA, Smit JA, Maier G, Shapiro M (1977) B-cell cross-match in renal transplantation. Lancet 2:241–242
51. Neppert J, Nunez G, Stastny P (1984) HLA-A, B, C; -DR; -MB, and SB antigens on unstimulated human endothelial cells. Tissue Antigens 24:40–47
52. Opelz G (1985) Ninth International Histocompatibility Workshop renal transplant study. In: Albert ED, Baur MP, Mayr WR (eds) Histocompatibility testing 1985. Springer, Berlin Heidelberg New York Tokyo, pp 342–347
53. Park MS, Terasaki PI, Bernocco D (1977) Autoantibody against B lymphocytes. Lancet 2:465–467
54. Park MS, Oriol R, Nakata S, Terasaki PI, Ford R, Bernoco D (1979) ABH and Lewis antigens on lymphocytes: screening of pregnant women's sera with the B-cell cytotoxicity test. Transplant Proc 11:1947–1949
55. Pellegrino MA, Belvedere M, Pellegrino AG, Ferrone S (1978) B peripheral lymphocytes express more HLA antigens than T peripheral lymphocytes. Transplantation 25:93–95
56. Persijn GG, Gabb BW, van Leeuwen A, Nagtegal A, Hoogeboom J, van Rood JJ (1978) Matching for HLA antigens of A, B, and DR loci in renal transplantation by Eurotransplant. Lancet 1:1278–1281
57. Persijn GG, van Leeuwen A, Parleviet J, Cohen B, Lansbergen Q, d'Amaro J, van Rood JJ (1981) Two major factors influencing kidney graft survival in Eurotransplant: HLA-DR matching and blood transfusion(s). Transplant Proc 13:150–154
58. Peto R, Pike MC, Armitage P, Breslow NE, Cox DR, Howard SV, Mantel N, McPherson K, Peto J, Smith PG (1977) Design and analysis of randomized clinical trials requiring prolonged observation of each patient. II. Analysis and examples. Br J Cancer 35:1–39
59. Reekers P, Lucassen-Hermans R, Koene RAP, Kunst VAJM (1977) Autolymphocytotoxic antibodies and kidney transplantation. Lancet 1:1063–1064
60. Rhodes CL, Goldman MH, Mendez-Picon G, Lee HM, Mohanakumar T (1984) Multiple specificities of B lymphocyte-reactive antibodies and their significance in renal allograft survival. Transplant Proc 16:1425–1426
61. Salvatierra O, Amend W, Vincenti F, Potter D, Iwaki Y, Opelz G, Terasaki PI, Duca R, Hanes D, Cochrum KC, Hopper S, Feduska NJ (1981a) Pretreatment with donor-specific blood transfusions in related recipients with high MLC. Transplant Proc 13:142–149
62. Salvatierra O, Iwaki Y, Vincenti F, Amend W, Potter D, Opelz G, Terasaki P, Duca R, Hopper S, Feduska N (1981b) Incidence, characteristics, and outcome of recipients sensitized after donor-specific blood transfusions. Transplantation 32:528–531
63. Shumak KH, Rachewich RA, Crookston MC, Crookston JH (1971) Antigens of the Ii system on lymphocytes. Nature 231:148–149
64. Soulillou JP, Bignon JD, Hourmant M, Ythier A, Cozian A, Faye R, Lecogic G, Guenel J (1982) Effect of HLA-A,B, and DR typing, pregraft blood transfusions, and positive anti-B lymphocyte cross-matches on kidney-graft survival – a one center prospective study. Transplant Proc 14:187–190
65. Sutherland DER, Morrow CE, Kaufman D, Fryd DS, Najarian JS, Burke M, Noreen H, Segall M, Bach FH (1983) The effect of mismatching for HLA-DR in recipients of renal allografts sharing one HLA-ABC haplotype with related donors. Transplantation 36:643–647

66. Taylor RJ, Andrews W, Rosenthal JT, Carpenter B, Hakala TR (1984) Influence of DR matching in cadaveric renal transplants performed with cyclosporine. Transplantation 38:616–618
67. Taylor RJ, Andrews W, Rosenthal JT, Carpenter B, Hakala TR (1985) DR matching in cadaveric renal transplantation with cyclosporine. Transplant Proc 17:1194–1196
68. Ting A, Morris PJ (1977) Renal transplantation and B-cell cross-matches with autoantibodies and alloantibodies. Lancet 2:1095–1097
69. Ting A, Morris PJ (1978a) Matching for B-cell antigens of the HLA-DR series in cadaver renal transplantation. Lancet 1:575–577
70. Ting A, Morris PJ (1978b) Reactivity of autolymphocytotoxic antibodies from dialysis patients with lymphocytes from chronic lymphocytic leukemia (CLL) patients. Transplantation 25:31–33
71. Ting A, Morris PJ (1980) Powerful effect of HLA-DR matching on survival of cadaveric renal allografts. Lancet 2:282–285
72. Ting A, Morris PJ (1981) Positive crossmatch transplants – safe or not? Transplant Proc 13:1544–1546
73. Ting A, Morris PJ (1983) Successful transplantation with a positive T and B cell crossmatch due to autoreactive antibodies. Tissue Antigens 21:219–226
74. Ting A, Morris PJ (1984) The influence of HLA-A,B and -DR matching and pregraft blood transfusions on graft and patient survival after renal transplantation in a single centre. Tissue Antigens 24:256–264
75. Ting A, Williams KA, Morris PJ (1980) HLA-DR matching and B-cell crossmatching in renal transplantation. Transplant Proc 12:495–501
76. Vaidya S, Orosz C, Cerilli J, Sommer B, Ferguson R (1984) The clinical significance of donor-specific B cell antibody after donor-specific blood transfusion in renal transplantation. Transplant Proc 16:1447
77. van Rood, Hendriks GFJ, d'Amaro J, Gratama JW, Jager M, van Es A, Persijn GG (1985) HLA matching, patient survival, and immune response genes in renal transplantation. Transplant Proc 17:681–685

Relevance of HLA-D/-DR Matching in a National Kidney Transplant Program

D. Albrechtsen, A. Flatmark, K. J. Berg, T. Moen, and E. Thorsby

Table of Contents

Introduction

The care of patients in terminal renal failure poses great medical and economic challenges. Life-supporting treatment, i.e., dialysis or transplantation, requires expensive personnel and technology. Results are often less than successful, particularly in the elderly and in patients with systemic disease. Since there is a general shortage of organs available for transplantation, patients have to be selected for transplant treatment according to some set of criteria. If few transplants can be performed relative to the number of patients requiring treatment, a rational policy is to select for transplant treatment those patients most likely to have a successful result. High-risk patients are consequently relegated to other, usually inferior treatment modalities. The moral dilemma inherent in this approach is a difficult one for the medical profession, whose prime obligation is to help those in greatest need.

A multitude of factors may influence transplantation results, including age, general health, and immune responsiveness of the recipient, mode of immunosuppressive modulation and treatment, donor organ quality, histocompatibility, operative and postoperative techniques, long-term management, and patient compliance. In evaluating the relevance of any of these factors, the mode of patient selection must be taken into account. In transplant centers which are able to offer kidneys to most patients with terminal renal failure, relatively more high-risk patients receive transplants than in centers which have greater difficulties in meeting need. As a consequence, lower patient and graft survival rates are to be expected in centers of the former type, although overall survival and quality of life in the uremic population as a whole may be considerably improved. Furthermore, factors carrying prognostic significance may be qualitatively and quantitatively different from those observed in centers treating a smaller proportion of the total uremic population. These important consequences of different treatment policies are frequently neglected in reviews of prognostic factors in transplantation, including histocompatibility matching.

In the following we will illustrate the effect of HLA-D/-DR matching in our own material of recipients of kidneys from one HLA haplotype family donors or cadaveric donors, treated in a single center.

Patients and Methods

Incidence of Renal Failure and Transplantation

The Norwegian incidence of chronic terminal renal failure requiring active treatment has increased slowly from 35 to 45 per million, a majority of patients being over 50 years of age. A uniform nationwide policy for the care of these patients, involving renal transplantation at one center and adequate dialysis back-up capacity, has been in operation for several years. By means of an active cadaver organ procurement organization, and also by using family donors, a transplantation rate (first grafts only) of 20–30 per million has been obtained. Presently, approximately 70% of all patients entering chronic renal failure in Norway are actually receiving transplants.

Patients and Transplants

During the period 1978–1984, 742 transplants were performed, including 186 transplants from haploidentical family donors (FD), 368 first transplants from cadaveric donors (CD), and 112 retransplants from cadaveric donors (re-CD). (The remaining 76 patients received grafts from HLA-identical siblings.) The effect of HLA-D/DR matching was studied in these three patient groups. As indicated in Table 1, a majority of the patients were either over 50 years of age (range 5–83 years) or had diabetes or some other systemic disease.

Generally, a family donor was searched for in the following order of preference: (1) HLA-identical; (2) low-MLC-stimulating haploidentical; (3) high-MLC-stimulating haploidentical.

Patients not having a family donor were placed on a waiting list for a cadaver graft. Transplantation was performed only if there was a negative cross-match test against donor cells, mainly detecting T cell antibodies reactive at 37 °C [1], using a recent serum sample. Priority was given to patients having multispecific HLA-A,B,C antibodies, donor-recipient combinations sharing two DR antigens,

Table 1. Patients and transplants prospectively typed for HLA-D/DR (1978–1984)

	Haploidentical family donor ($n=186$)	First cadaveric donor ($n=368$)	Repeat cadaveric donor ($n=112$)
Median age (years)	28	51	43
Age >55 years (%)	8	44	21
Diabetics (%)	17	18	11
Systemic disease (%)[a]	12	7	10
Untransfused (%)	39	31	0
HLA-A,B			
0 mismatches (%)	15	11	16
1–2 mismatches	85	56	63
3–4 mismatches	–	33	21
HLA-DR			
0 mismatches (%)	48	41	36
1 mismatches	52	47	46
2 mismatches	–	12	20
MLC relative response <60 (%)	46	–	–

[a] Collagenosis, systemic lupus erythematosus, amyloidosis, Goodpasture's syndrome, Alport's syndrome, lecithin-cholesterol-acetyltransferase deficiency, Fabry's disease, hemolytic uremic syndrome, Henoch-Schönlein syndrome, oxalosis, cystinosis

clinical urgency, or a long waiting period. Although preference was given to HLA-DR compatible combinations during the period 1978–1982, any match for HLA-A,B, and DR antigens (0–6 mismatches) was accepted, as seen in Table 1.

HLA Typing

Typing for HLA-A,B antigens covering a gene frequency of at least 98% was performed prospectively [2]. Typing for HLA-DR antigens 1–8, covering a gene frequency of approximately 75% in our population, was performed prospectively using peripheral blood non-T cells of recipients and living donors and spleen non-T cells of cadaveric donors as previously described [2, 3]. The HLA-DR type was defined in a rather uniform and conservative manner based mainly on the Seventh International Histocompatibility Workshop criteria and sera [3]. Only detectable HLA-DR antigens were taken into account when determining the HLA-DR match between donor and recipient, thus disregarding potential mismatch for undetected ("blank") antigens. In family transplants, HLA-D matching was performed using one-way mixed lymphocyte culture (MLC) tests, results being expressed as relative response [3]. The haplotype disparity between a family donor and a recipient was based on HLA typing of the whole family.

Immunosuppressive Therapy

In 1978–1982 a conventional *azathioprine + steroid* immunosuppression protocol was used for both FD and CD kidney recipients. Prednisolone 40 mg was given daily for 2 months, then tapered slowly to a low maintenance dose. In 1983–1984 all patients were treated by a *cyclosporin + steroid* protocol, except recipients of HLA-identical sibling transplants, who were still given azathioprine + steroids. FD kidney recipients received cyclosporin (CyA) 15 mg/kg orally for 2 days before transplantation, 10 mg/kg intravenously on days 0 and 1, and 15 mg/kg orally until day 14, and then intake was tapered to a maintenance dose. Prednisolone was tapered from 100 mg to 20 mg by day 8, and further to 10 mg by day 90. CD kidney recipients were started on CyA 15 mg/kg intravenously on day 0, otherwise the same protocol was employed. CyA dosage was generally adjusted to maintain blood levels decreasing from 800 to 200 ng/ml, or lower if toxicity was suspected. During the entire study, rejection episodes were treated with methylprednisolone (boluses of 125–1000 mg to a maximum of 4–6 g).

Other Treatment

All transplants were performed using conventional and standardized techniques. Transfusions (usually leukocyte-depleted) were given for medical reasons only and not to modulate the recipients immunologically, except for donor-specific transfusions given to 29 and five FD kidney recipients in 1981/1982 and 1983 respectively [4]. Approximately one-third of the patients received no blood transfusions prior to transplantation (Table 1).

Analysis of Results

Calculations of graft survival rates included all causes of graft loss, including patients dying with a functioning graft. Transplants were considered successful in patients maintained by dialysis. Statistical significance was evaluated by generalized Wilcoxon (Breslow) tests.

Results

Intraoperatively, no case of hyperacute rejection was observed, all grafts appearently being well vascularized at completion of the operation.

Although a uniform general treatment policy was adhered to, and patient age and disease patterns remained stable during the study period, significantly improved graft survival rates were observed following the change in immunosuppressive regimen to CyA in 1983. Furthermore, while HLA-D/DR matching significantly influenced graft survival in azathioprine-treated recipients, no effect of HLA-DR matching on graft survival has yet been detected in the CyA-treated patients, except possibly for retransplants. The results of the two treatment protocols will therefore be presented separately.

Relevance of HLA-D/DR Matching in Azathioprine-Treated Patients

Haploidentical Family Donor Transplants ($n = 112$)

As illustrated in Fig. 1, there was a trend toward better graft survival in HLA-DR-compatible transplants. One-year graft survival rates were 84% and 76% in matched and mismatched grafts respectively. This was observed irrespective of matching for HLA,A,B antigens (see Table 2).

A similar trend was seen in transplants from haploidentical donors who stimulated their recipients only moderately (relative response <60; Fig. 2). However,

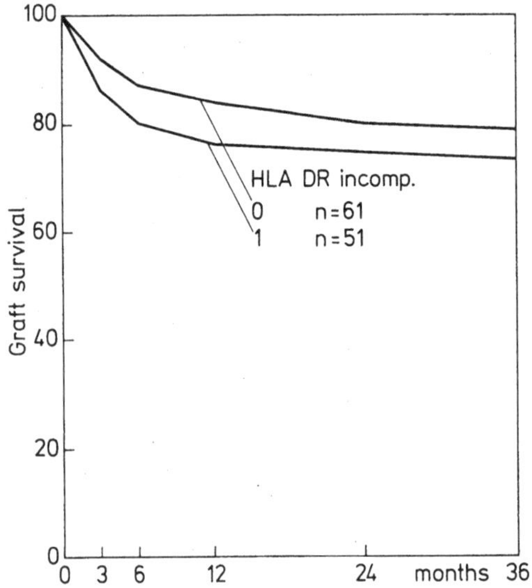

Fig. 1. Influence of HLA-DR matching on graft survival in 112 azathioprine-treated recipients of haploidentical family donor transplants 1978–1982. *0*, HLA-DR incomp. = no detectable mismatched HLA-DR antigen; *1*, HLA-DR incomp. = mismatch for 1 HLA-DR antigen

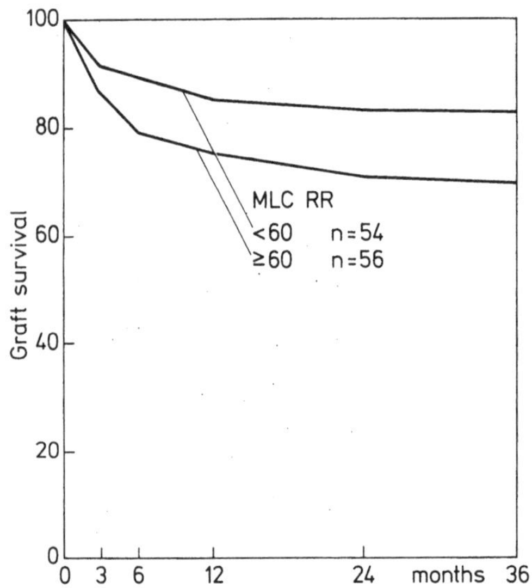

Fig. 2. Graft survival in 110 azathioprine-treated recipients of family donor transplants 1978–1982, stratified according to the degree of MLC response between donor and recipient. *MLC-RR>60,* relative response in MLC > 60% (weak to moderate); *MLC-RR>60,* relative response in MLC > 60% (relatively strong)

Table 2. Graft survival in 112 azathioprine-treated recipients of haploidentical family transplants, stratified according to HLA-A,B and HLA-DR match (1978–1982)

HLA-A,B match	HLA-DR match	*n*	One-year graft survival (%)
0 incompatible	0 incompatible	11	91
	1 incompatible	7	57
1–2 incompatible	0 incompatible	50	82
	1 incompatible	44	71

Table 3. Graft survival in 112 azathioprine-treated recipients of family transplants, stratified according to HLA-D/DR match and pretransplant blood transfusion status (1978–1982)

Pretransplant transfusion	HLA-D/DR match	*n*	One-year graft survival (%)
+	0 DR incompatible	36	86
	1 DR incompatible	31	87
–	0 DR incompatible	25	80
	1 DR incompatible	20	60
+	MLC RR <60[a]	36	89
	MLC RR ≥60	31	84
–	MLC RR <60	18	78
	MLC RR ≥60	25	64

RR, relative response (%)
[a] MLC studies were not performed in two patients

if the pretransplant blood transfusion status of the recipient was taken into account, these trends were only seen in untransfused patients (see Table 3). None of these differences reached statistical significance.

Cadaveric Donor First Transplants (*n*=226)

A significant beneficial influence of matching for HLA-DR antigens was observed, 1-year graft survival rates being 58%, 49%, and 23% in grafts *mismatched* for 0, 1, and 2 antigens respectively, see Fig. 3. The effect persisted for at least 3 years post transplant, and was observed irrespective of matching for HLA-A,B antigens (Table 4).

If patients were stratified according to the number of detectable DR antigens *shared* between the donor and the recipient, a similar picture emerged (Fig. 4). Patients receiving DR-identical grafts (sharing two DR antigens with the donor) had

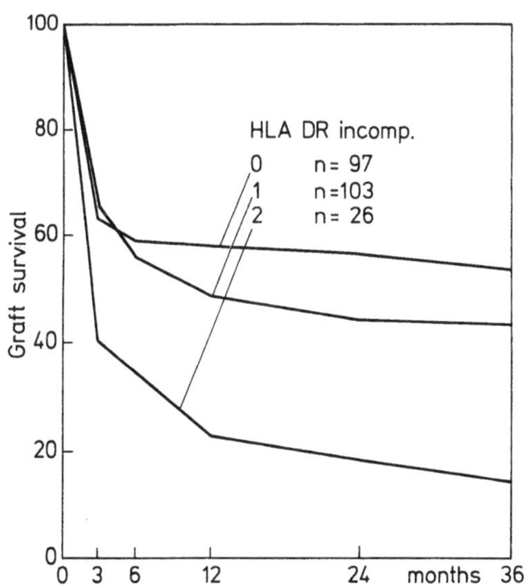

Fig. 3. Graft survival in 226 azathioprine-treated recipients of cadaveric donor first transplants 1978–1982, stratified according to the number of mismatched HLA-DR antigens between the donor and the recipient

Table 4. Graft survival in 226 azathioprine-treated recipients of cadaveric first transplants, stratified according to HLA-A,B and HLA-DR match (1978–1982)

HLA-A,B match	HLA-DR match	*n*	One-year graft survival (%)
0 incompatible	0 incompatible	12	67
	1–2 incompatible	23	52
1–2 incompatible	0 incompatible	59	58
	1–2 incompatible	83	45
3–4 incompatible	0 incompatible	26	54
	1–2 incompatible	23	26

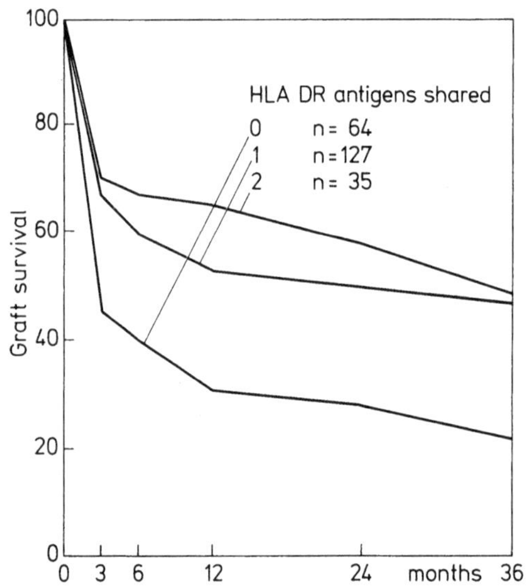

Fig. 4. Graft survival in 226 azathioprine-treated recipients of cadaveric donor first transplants 1978–1982, stratified according to the number of HLA-DR antigens shared between the donor and the recipient

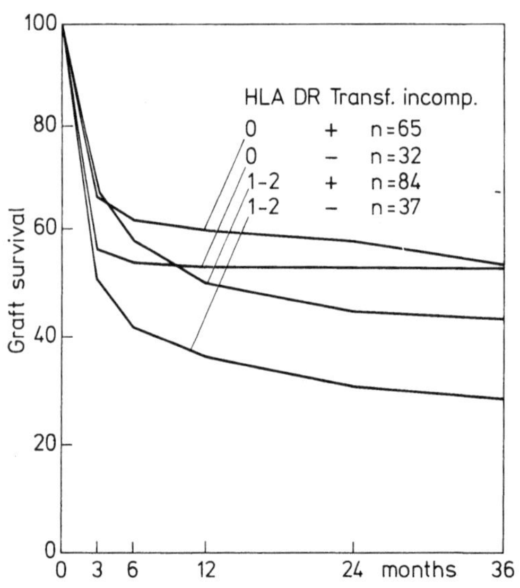

Fig. 5. Graft survival in 226 azathioprine-treated recipients of cadaveric donor first transplants 1978–1982, stratified according to HLA-DR match and pretransplant blood transfusion status

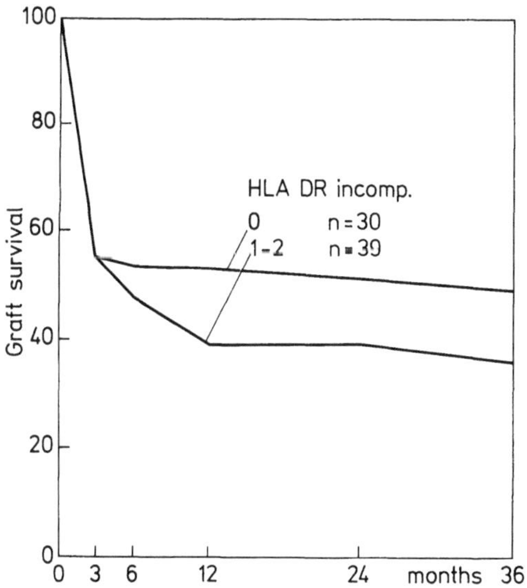

Fig. 6. Influence of HLA-DR matching on graft survival in 69 azathioprine-treated recipients of cadaveric donor retransplants 1978–1982

no better prognosis than patients receiving DR-compatible grafts (no detectable DR mismatch); compare Figs. 3 and 4. Since some of these grafts might be mismatched for DR antigens not detectable due to lack of appropriate reagents, this may indicate a low immunogenecity for these undetected antigens.

As depicted in Fig. 5, the beneficial influence of HLA-DR matching was particularly evident in patients who had not received blood transfusions prior to transplantation.

Cadaveric Donor Retransplants ($n=69$)

Recipients of HLA-DR-compatible cadaveric retransplants also tended to have a better prognosis than those receiving mismatched grafts, although the difference did not reach statistical significance (Fig. 6).

Relevance of HLA-D/DR Matching in Cyclosporin-Treated Patients

Haploidentical Family Donor Transplants ($n=74$)

As indicated in Table 5, CyA treatment greatly improved graft survival in haploidentical transplants, approaching that seen in HLA-identical sibling transplants

Table 5. Graft survival in 74 cyclosporine-treated recipients of haploidentical family transplants, stratified according to HLA-DR match and degree of MLC stimulation between donor and recipient

HLA-DR match	*n*	One-year graft survival (%)
0 DR incompatible	29	96
1 DR incompatible	45	95
MLC RR <60[a]	35	97
MLC RR ≥60	35	93

[a] MLC studies were not performed in four patients

[2]. Following this, no influence of HLA-D/DR matching on graft survival could be observed. Neither HLA-A,B matching nor pretransplant blood transfusion status of the patient influenced the results.

Cadaveric Donor First Transplants ($n=142$)

No effect of HLA-DR matching on *graft survival* was seen among 142 recipients of CD grafts receiving CyA (Table 6). However, a significant effect of HLA-DR matching on the incidence of first *rejection episodes* was observed. In HLA-DR matched transplants ($n=52$), 48% had a rejection episode, compared to 53% and 80% in transplants mismatched for one DR antigen ($n=70$) or two DR antigens ($n=20$) respectively ($p=0.05$).

Table 6. Graft survival in 142 cyclosporine-treated recipients of cadaveric first transplants, stratified according to HLA-DR match

HLA-DR match	n	One-year graft survival (%)
0 DR incompatible	52	71
1 DR incompatible	70	72
2 DR incompatible	20	74

Matching for HLA-A,B antigens and pretransplant transfusion status did not influence graft survival. On the other hand, patients having panel-reactive antibodies (PRA) at the time of transplantation reactive with panel peripheral blood mononuclear cells (PBM) with the KN technique [1], but not reactive against donor PBM, had a graft survival at 1 year of 35% ($n=17$), compared to 79% ($n=125$) among those not having PRA. This difference is statistically significant ($p<0.001$).

Cadaveric Donor Retransplants ($n=43$)

One-year graft survival was 80% in HLA-DR-compatible retransplants ($n=10$), vs 42% in DR-incompatible retransplants ($n=33$) (Table 7).

Table 7. Graft survival in 43 cyclosporine-treated recipients of cadaveric retransplants, stratified according to HLA-DR match

HLA-DR match	n	One-year graft survival (%)
0 DR incompatible	10	80
1–2 incompatible	33	42

Comments

Matching for HLA-D/DR gene products carried considerable prognostic significance in azathioprine-treated recipients of kidney grafts from family and cadaveric donors, particularly in untransfused patients. This is in accordance with results previously published by us [2] and others [5–9]. The introduction of CyA immunosuppression dramatically improved results in the our kidney transplant program, not the least because clinical high-risk patients (age >55 years, diabetes, systemic disease) apparently tolerated treatment far better. At present, no influence of HLA-D/DR matching on graft (and patient) survival can be detected in the CyA material at 1 year post transplant. Similar observations have been reported by others [10–13]. Although rejection episodes occurred significantly more frequently in recipients of poorly DR-matched first transplants, no differences in graft survival at 1 year could be seen. Since the material is relatively small and the observation time short, caution must be exercised in interpreting these data. It may be that other factors, such as graft quality (including ischemia time), age and clinical and immune status of the recipient (as reflected in the presence of PRA), and the dose and mode of CyA administration presently play a more important role in determining graft survival in our material. It is noteworthy that among retransplants, HLA-DR matching seemed to have an effect upon graft survival. The material is small, however, and observation time short. More studies are obviously needed before definite conclusions concerning the influence of HLA-DR matching in CyA-treated recipients of cadaveric donor kidneys can be ade.

Our finding that the presence of PRA at the time of transplantation significantly influenced the results in CyA-treated recipients of CD grafts needs confirmation. As discussed elsewhere [14], such antibodies may also signify cellular presensitization, being more difficult to suppress with CyA. On the other hand, we cannot exclude a deleterious efect of weak donor-reactive antibodies which are not detectable in our cross-match tests against the donor, yet which may act synergistically, with the harmful effects of long ischemia time and CyA toxicity. It is noteworthy that 53% of the first CD grafts to recipients with PRA had primary nonfunction, compared to 20% of the kidneys given to those without PRA at time of transplantation. This is an important topic of current study in our center.

References

1. Kissmeyer-Nielsen F, Kjerbye L (1976) Lymphocytotoxic micro-technique. In: Dausset J et al. (eds) Histocomatibility testing 1967. Munksgaard, Copenhagen, pp 381–383
2. Albrechtsen D, Moen T, Flatmark A, Halvorsen S, Jakobsen A, Jervell J, Solheim BG, Thorsby E (1981) Influence of HLA-A,B,C,D, and DR matching in renal transplantation. Transplant Proc 13:924–929
3. Albrechtsen D, Bratlie A, Nousiainen H, Solheim BG, Thorsby E (1978) Serological typing of HLA-D: predictive value in mixed lymphocyte cultures (MLC). Immunogenetics 6:91–103
4. Leivestad T, Flatmark A, Hirschberg H, Thorsby E (1982) Effect of pretransplant donor-specific transfusions in renal transplantation. Transplant Proc 14:370–373

5. Persijn GG, Gabb BW, van Leeuven A, Nagtegal A, Hoogeboom J, van Rood JJ (1978) Matching for HLA antigens of A, B, and DR loci in renal transplantation by Eurotransplant. Lancet 1:1278–1281
6. Ting A, Morris PJ (1984) The influence of HLA-A,B, and -DR matching and pregraft blood transfusions on graft and patient survival after renal transplantation in a single centre. Tissue Antigens 24:256–264
7. Cochrum KC, Perkins HA, Payne RO, Kountz SL, Belzer LO (1973) The correlation of MLC with graft survival. Transplant Proc 5:391–395
8. Berg B, Groth CG, Lundgren G, Möller E, Ringden O, Wilczek H (1983) Five year experience with DR matching in cadaveric kidney transplantation. Transplant Proc 15:1132–1135
9. Goeken NE, Thompson JS, Corry RJ (1981) A two year trial of prospective HLA-DR matching: effects on renal allograft survival and rate of transplantation. Transplantation 32:522–527
10. European Multicenter Trial Group (1983) Cyclosporine in cadaveric renal transplantation: one-year follow-up of a multicentre trial. Lancet 2:986–989
11. Canadian Multicenter Transplant Study Group (1983) A randomized clinical trial of cyclosporine in cadaveric renal transplantation. N Engl J Med 309:809–815
12. Kahan BD, van Buren CT, Flechner SM, Payne WD, Boileau M, Kerman RH (1983) Cyclosporine immune suppression mitigates immunologic risk factors in renal allotransplantation. Transplant Proc 15:2469–2478
13. Ringden O, Ost L, Klintmalm G, Tillegard A, Fehrman I, Wilczek H, Groth C-G (1983) Improved outcome in renal transplant recipients above 55 years of age treated with cyclosporine and low doses of steroids. Transplant Proc 15:2507–2512
14. Thorsby E (1985) On the antibody cross-match controversies. Transplant Proc 17:1533–1536

The Pig as a Model to Assess the Effect of Class II MHC Antigen Matching on Renal Allograft Survival

M. D. Pescovitz, D. H. Sachs

Table of Contents

Development of the Miniature Swine Transplantation Model at the NIH

Large animals such as dogs [1], monkeys [2], and swine [3] have been valuable models for transplantation biology both because of their size, which permits surgical manipulations similar to those in man, and because they provide an intermediate step between rodents and man in which to reexamine new experimental results. Although most biological principles are conserved among species, fine tuning of the immune system is in some cases different enough to make results in any one species not directly applicable to man. Among the known species differences which could potentially have clinical ramifications for transplants are differences in distribution of class II MHC antigens on vascular endothelium [4] and differences in levels of allogeneic resistance or graft-vs-host disease in the setting of bone marrow transplants [5, 6].

Over the past 12 years, this laboratory has developed a herd of miniature swine for use in studies of transplantation biology [7]. Choice of this species was based on a variety of advantageous characteristics, some of which are as follows:

1. Breeding
   a) gestation period of 112 days
   b) sexual maturity at 6 months

c) estrous cycle of 3 weeks
d) litter size 3–10 animals

2. Size
   a) maximum weight 70–90 kg
   b) weight at puberty 40–60 kg
   c) slower growth rate than domestic swine
3. Inexpensive upkeep: about $1.50 per day per animal (1984)

Foremost among these advantages are the breeding characteristics, which have made genetic manipulations possible in a relatively short time. The entire herd was developed from a single breeding pair selected from widely disparate sources in order to assure disparity at the presumed MHC [7]. Sera obtained following reciprocal immunization of the breeders were absorbed with lymphocytes of each of the progeny in the first litter, and the absorbed sera were used to type lymphocytes of the progeny (Fig. 1). As a result of this analysis, three of the four possible distinct MHC haplotypes were identified and arbitrarily designated *a, c,* and *d.* It is presumed that one of the breeders was either homozygous or did not transmit the *b* haplotype to any of the progeny. By selectively breeding the offspring, three herds homozygous for the MHC, *aa, cc,* and *dd,* were reached by the third generation (Fig. 2). More recently, two recombinant haplotypes *gg* and *ff* have been detected and established (see below). It should be noted that after establishment of MHC-homozygous lines, breeding within lines has been purposely maintained by random, non-brother/sister matings in order to keep background genes diverse. The genetic relationship among these animals therefore simulates the relationships within a human family and provides the possibility to examine transplants between MHC-identical, haplotype-identical, or MHC-mismatched "siblings."

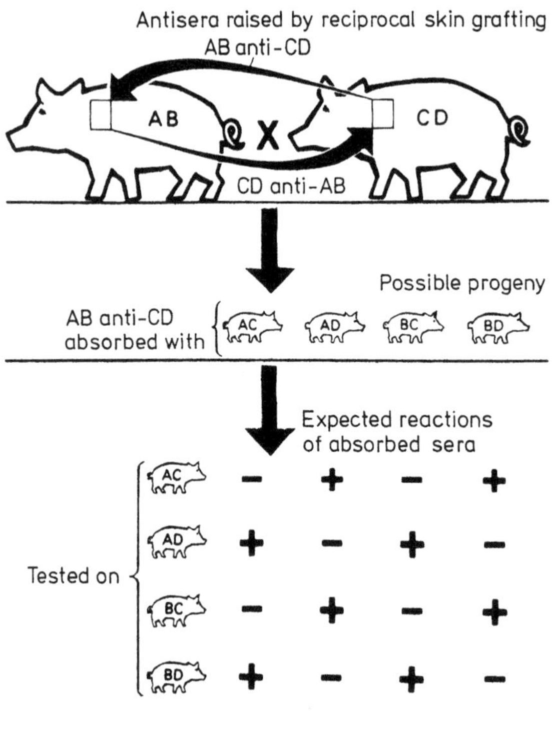

Fig. 1. Method of serological analysis of the first-generation miniature swine. Sera obtained following skin grafting between the parents were adsorbed with lymphocytes of the progeny. These sera were then tested for residual cytotoxic activity on lymphocytes of the progeny in a complement-dependent assay. As a control for adequacy of the absorption, all sera were also tested on the original absorbing animal. The hypothetical results expected from the possible progeny are demonstrated. (Reproduced from [7] by permissionof The Williams and Wilkins Co.)

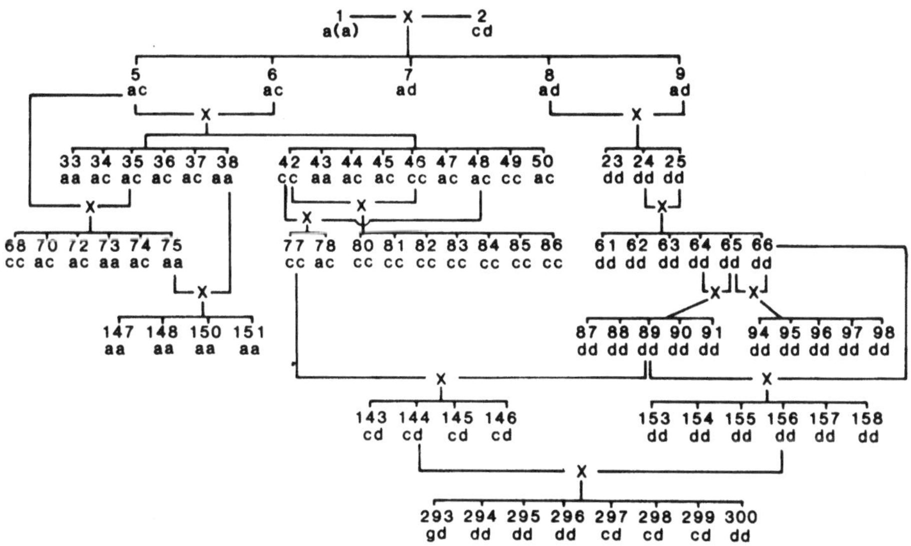

Fig. 2. The pedigree of the miniature swine, showing the segregation of the serologically defined MHC antigens. MHC-homozygous lines were obtained by the third generation. In addition, the first *g* haplotype animal, 293, and its parents, 144 *cd* and 156 *dd*, are shown

The SLA Complex: Biochemistry and Genetics

Swine, like other mammalian species studied to date, have an MHC [8] termed SLA that contains genes encoding for both class I and class II MHC cell surface molecules. The porcine class I MHC products are similar at both the protein and DNA levels to those of other species. They are composed of a 44000-MW heavy chain and a 12000-MW β_2-microglobulin chain [9], both of which have sequence homology to the human and murine analogs. Although there is evidence at the DNA level for six to eight class I genes [10], only two [11] or perhaps three [12] products have been identified on peripheral blood lymphocytes (PBL). The other identified genes possibly include porcine Tla or Qa analogs.

The class II MHC products also consist of two chains – a 32000-MW heavy chain and a 25000-MW light chain [13]. Very little is known about the protein sequence or the molecular biology of the swine class II genes, although, as will be shown below, the homology is sufficient to allow human class II gene probes to cross-hybridize with genomic DNA of the pig. Work from this laboratory with cross-reactive alloantisera [14] and murine anti-IE^k sera [14] and more recently with monoclonal antibodies [15] (J. Lunney, unpublished observation), indicates that at least two class II gene products are expressed on the lymphocyte surface.

Like humans, but unlike mice [16, 17], the porcine class II MHC genes lie outside the cluster of class I MHC genes [12] (Fig. 3). This has been shown definitively by the analysis of two recombinant haplotypes within our herd, the *f* and *g* haplotypes [18, 19]. These haplotypes were found among the progeny of two separate matings of *cd* heterozygotes. Serologically, the original *f* animal typed as a *cc,* but was stimulatory to *cc*-homozygous animals in MLC, while the *g* animal typed as a *cd* but was stimulated by *cc* animals, indicating that the two animals differed by mixed lymphocyte reaction (MLR) determinants for their expected genotypes.

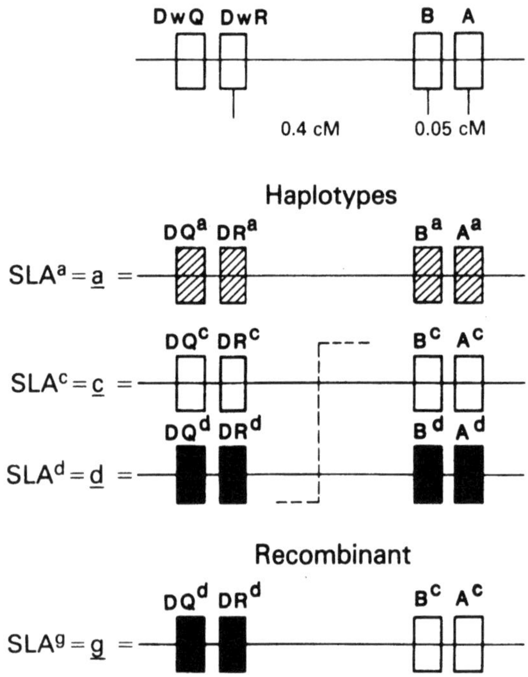

Fig. 3. Schematic representation of the porcine MHC (SLA), demonstrating the class I (A, B) and class II (DR, DQ) antigens. Also shown is the recombination event that led to the MHC-recombinant haplotype *g*

Immunoprecipitation of radiolabeled PBL extracts with alloantisera showed that both recombinants expressed all known class I products of the *c* haplotype and all known class II products of the *d* haplotype [18, 19]. Although the *f* and *g* haplotypes resulted from separate events, they are apparently identical genetically, since they do not stimulate each other in MLR, nor are antibodies produced following reciprocal immunization [19]. Results at the DNA level have confirmed the biochemical and serologic evidence for recombination, confirming the similarity of *f* and *g* in that Southern blot analysis of restriction-enzyme-digested genomic DNA with a human class I cDNA probe disclosed no difference from *cc* (D. H. Sachs, unpublished results), while analysis with a human DRβ cDNA class II probe disclosed no differences from *dd* (Fig. 4). Because of better breeding ability, more animals of the *g* haplotype have generally been available and have therefore been used in most of the renal transplant studies described below.

In both humans [20] and mice [21], the MHC is linked to genes encoding for the class III or complement components – this is also true for swine [22]. Another gene locus linked to the MHC in mice [23], rats [24], and humans [25], but of uncertain immunologic relevance, is the glyoxylase locus, Glo. Recent studies by W. R. Lie indicate that this linkage is conserved in pigs (personal communication). Using progeny of our inbred swine, she found that *aa* animals had high levels of Glo activity, *dd* animals low levels, and in *ad* × *dd*, or *ad* × *ad* backcrosses, high Glo activity correlated the *a* with MHC haplotype.

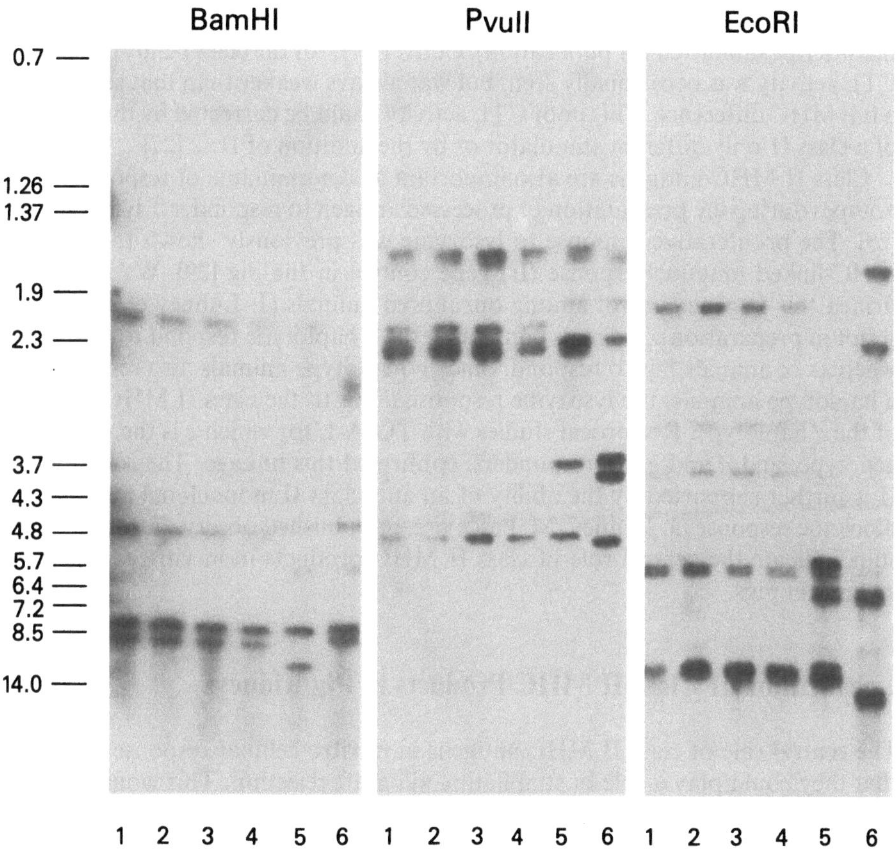

Fig. 4. Southern blot analysis for class II genes of porcine genomic DNA. DNA from PBL was digested with the enzymes *Bam*HI, *Pvu*II, and *Eco*RI as indicated. The probe was a human cDNA DRβ gene from the laboratory of P. Peterson. The haplotypes of the animals are *gg* (lane 1), a newly identified recombinant (lane 2), *ff* (lane 3), *dd* (lane 4), *aa* (lane 5), and *cc* (lane 6). The origin is at the *bottom*

The Role of Porcine Class II MHC Antigens in In Vitro Cellular Responses

In both mouse and human, the class II MHC antigens play an essential role in cellular responses in vitro and in vivo [reviewed in 26]. Using the porcine MHC recombinant haplotype *g*, the role of class I and class II antigens in porcine in vitro immune responses has been studied [27]. In MLR, Thislethwaite et al. found that the majority of the proliferative response was directed toward the class II MHC antigens. He found high levels of proliferation when the MLR was between *gg* and *cc* animals (class II-only difference), but very little proliferation when the stimulation was between *gg* and *dd* (class I-only difference). Despite this high level of proliferation across a class II-only difference, no cytotoxic T lymphocytes (CTL) were detected [27], and this lack of CTL was shown subsequently not to be due to a lack of target antigens on the phytohemagglutinin (PHA)T cell blasts. In the pig, resting as well as stimulated, T cells express class II MHC antigens in levels about 50% that of B cells and roughly equal to macrophages (M. Pescovitz, manuscript submitted for publication). Conversely, for the class I-only difference, CTL activity was occasionally seen, but was always weaker than that seen across a full MHC difference. This poor CTL activity could be corrected by the addition of a class II-only different stimulator or by the addition of IL-2 [27].

Class II MHC antigens are also important as determinants of responder phenotypes during the presentation of processed antigen to responder T lymphocytes [28]. The proliferative response to lysozyme was previously shown to be under MHC-linked immune-response (Ir) gene control in the pig [29]. We have confirmed this Ir gene control among our inbred animals (J. Lunney et al., manuscript in preparation). Animals containing the *d* haplotype respond to lysozyme, whereas *cc* animals fail to respond. Since *g* haplotype animals also respond like *d* haplotype animals, the lysozyme response maps to the class II MHC antigens of the *d* haplotype. Reciprocal studies with TG-A-L for which *c* is the responder genotype, and *d* and *g* nonresponders, confirmed this linkage. The role of class II is further supported by the ability of an anti-class II monoclonal antibody to block the response (J. Lunney, M. Pescovitz, unpublished observation). These results indicate the central role of class II MHC products in in vitro immune responses in pigs.

Localization of Class II MHC Products in Pig Kidneys

The central role of class II MHC antigens in in vitro cellular responses suggests that they could play a role in stimulating allograft rejection. This would require that class II antigens be present on at least some cells in the allograft. In mice [30] and rats [31], expression of class II antigens in the kidney is restricted to the dendritic cells (see Fig. 5a). These cells have been shown to play a major role in rejection both of kidneys [32] and of heart allografts [33]. In human kidneys, class II antigens are also detectable on renal vascular endothelium – one of the first contact regions between lymphoid cells and allograft [34]. Fabre [4] suggested that this difference in anatomy could explain the relative facility with which allografts could be prolonged in rodents. He suggested that a short course of immunosuppression, either pharmacologic or with antidonor antibody (enhancement), would allow the stimulatory donor-type dendritic cells to be replaced with host-type dendritic cells, thereby decreasing the immunogenicity of the graft. This may be analogous to the removal of dendritic cells from tissue by culturing (reviewed in [35]). Fabre [4] also suggested that enhancement may not succeed in humans, because the vascular endothelium, unlike dendritic cells, would not be expected to be replaced and would always bear stimulatory allogeneic class II antigens.

Immunohistologic examination of porcine renal tissue has been carried out in order to examine the pattern of MHC class II antigen distributionin this species [36]. As shown in Fig 5b, large amounts of class II MHC antigens are present on the endothelium of renal arteries and glomeruli, as well as within the interstitial and peritubular areas. It is not clear if the interstitial/peritubular reaction is with capillary endothelium, dendritic cells, or basement membrane. The pig therefore resembles man in regard to the presence of class II MHC antigens on renal endothelial cells, suggesting that it may be a more appropriate model in which to study the effects of class II matching than the mouse or the rat.

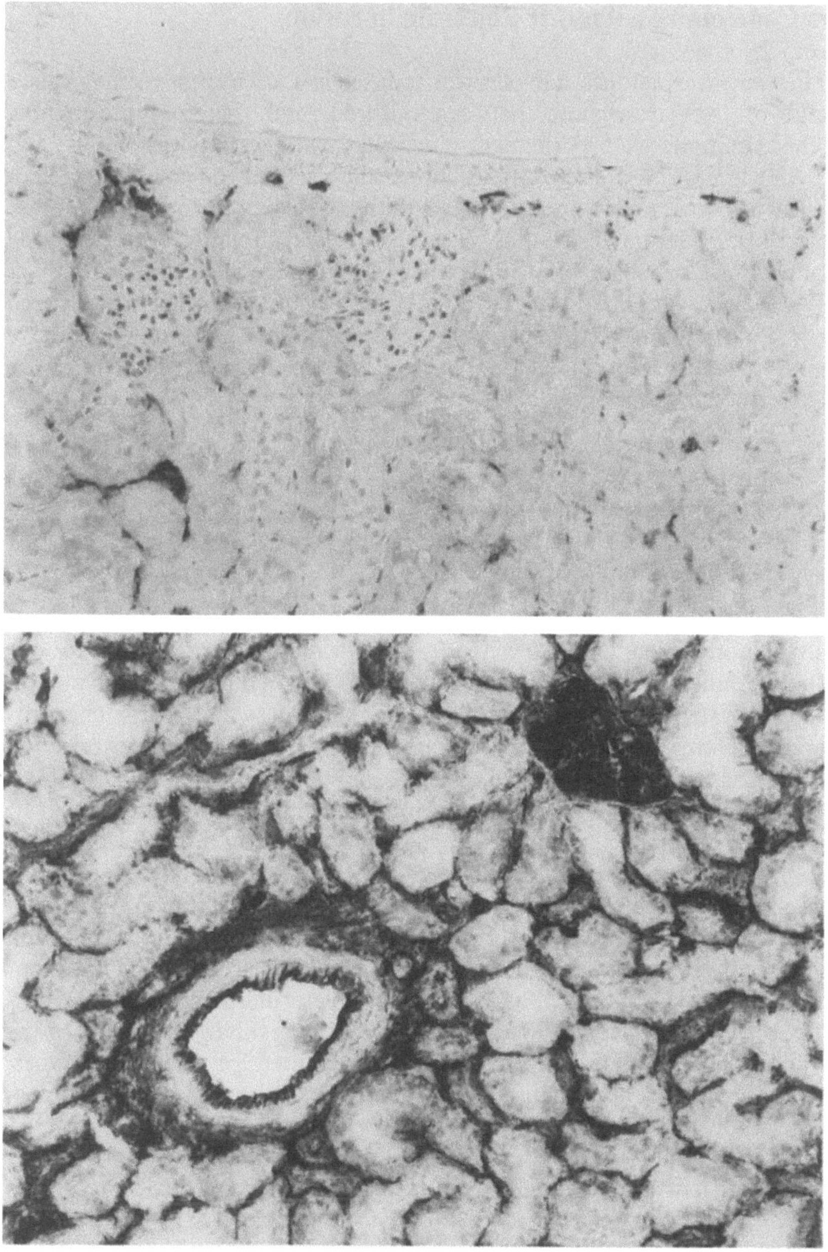

Fig. 5 a, b. The presence of class II MHC antigens on porcine (*dd*) versus mouse (B10.A) kidney. Frozen sections of tissue were stained using an anti-I-E^k monoclonal antibody 40D that also cross-reacts with one of the two class II proteins in pigs and developed with an avidin-biotin-peroxidase reaction. The nuclei were counterstained with cresol green. **a** The mouse kidney (×220) shows only scattered positive cells having the appearance of dendritic cells. The pig kidney **b** (×130) shows intense staining of the vascular endothelium, glomeruli, and peritubular structures. (Reproduced from [36] by permission of The Williams and Wilkins Co.)

Factors Controlling Allograft Rejection in Swine

Interest in liver transplantation in pigs was aroused in 1969 by reports that a large percentage of liver transplants between outbred, and therefore presumably mismatched, animals were permanently accepted without immunosuppression [37]. A major limitation of these studies, however, was that the animals were not genotypically defined with respect to MHC antigens. Using the inbred miniature swine model, the factors controlling rejection of liver allografts were analyzed while controlling for known MHC differences [38]. Under these conditions, liver allograft rejection was found to occur in a similar fashion to other vascularized grafts, e.g., kidney [39], and to depend on the same factors. The factors that have been found to govern allograft survival in swine are summarized in the following list and described in some detail below:

1. Blood group antigens
2. MHC antigens
3. Minor histocompatibility antigens
4. Vascularized vs nonvascularized status of graft
5. Non-MHC linked immune response gene
6. Recipient immune status

Initially, blood groups A and O were identifiable as segregating markers in our herds [40]. Examination of the effect of A-O matching on allograft survival indicated the A-O system to be a histocompatibility system in swine. Mismatching for A-O while matching for MHC resulted in significantly faster skin graft rejection time: 7.66 ± 0.54 days vs 10.75 ± 0.25 days ($p < 0.001$) [40]. In addition, lymphocytotoxic antibodies were detected in four out of six animals following skin graft rejection. These antibodies could be absorbed only with skin donor erythrocytes or nondonor erythrocytes that were matched at the A-O blood group to the donor. Limited results with A-O- and SLA-identical reciprocal skin graft pairs indicated that mismatches at blood groups G, H, and K did not accelerate rejection or induce lymphocytotoxic antibodies [40]. Other blood groups, which are not polymorphic in our herd, may, however, be capable of inducing cytotoxic antibodies or accelerating rejection. Because our chief interest has been study of the MHC, animals of the O blood group (recessive) were bred for transplant studies. The A blood group has been maintained in a subline of the *d* haplotype for possible future studies.

The MHC has been found to exert a major effect on skin [7], liver [38], and renal [39] allograft survival. All allogeneic skin grafts were rejected, but MHC-mismatched grafts were rejected more rapidly: 7.0 ± 0.35 days as compared to 11.8 ± 0.89 days for MHC-matched grafts. This also indicates that non-MHC (i.e., minor histocompatibility) differences lead to allograft rejection.

Both kidney [39] and liver [38] transplants were rejected similarly to skin if mismatched at the MHC. However, vascularized organs behaved differently from skin when MHC-matched, minor-antigen-mismatched. Kirkman et al. [39] reported that all 13 animals of the herd containing the *c* haplotype rejected MHC-matched renal grafts, while two of two *aa* and six of eight *dd* animals permanently accepted such vascularized grafts. Similar results were found for liver grafts [38]. Therefore the three different herds demonstrated different abilities to respond to the mismatched minor histocompatibility antigens when present on vascularized organs, but not when present on skin. A formal backcross analysis was performed to examine the genetics of this survival. When matings were performed between *cd* and *dd*, rejector by nonrejector animals, about half of all progeny (both *cd* and *dd*) accepted MHC-matched allografts [41]. This rejection across minor antigens was therefore shown to be regulated by one, or perhaps two, non-MHC-linked IR genes.

The initial male *g* haplotype animal came from a *cd* parent and the majority of the initial *g* progeny came from matings with *ac* sows. Therefore the non-MHC-linked Ir gene shown to regulate rejection to minor histocompatibility antigens in the MHC-matched setting was most likely also segregating within the *g* herd. This possibility could be of importance in assessing survival of class I-only or class II-only matched grafts using the *g* haplotype, as will be discussed further below. Although best characterized in these inbred swine, results similar to those attributed to this non-MHC-linked Ir gene have been seen in both man [42] and monkey [2, 43]. In addition, MHC-linked genes that regulate allograft survival in rat [44] and man (DR6) [45] have been studied.

An additional factor shown to regulate survival in our swine is the pretransplant immune status. Since these animals receive no pretransplant immunization, serologic cross-matches are, with rare exceptions, negative. If, on the other hand, the animals are immunized by skin grafting, hyperacute or accelerated rejection of the kidney is always seen [46]. This was found despite the absence of detectable antibody in the MHC-matched combinations [46] as determined by complement-mediated lymphocytotoxicity of immune sera or immunofluorescent staining of the rejected donor kidney tissue. However, when MLR or cell-mediated lympholysis (CML) was assayed between recipient and donor, the reactivity, always present following skin grafting, disappeared after the kidney was perfused, only to reappear after the transplant nephrectomy. This pattern suggests that the transplant kidney was absorbing the reactive cells. These results indicate the importance of T cell-mediated responses in this model of hyperacute rejection.

The Effect of Class II MHC Antigen Matching on Renal Allograft Survival

Most single-center studies have found a positive benefit of HLA-DR matching on survival of cadaveric renal allografts [47], although the results of some multicenter studies have been less clear [48]. The true effect of DR matching in man is difficult to assess because of the prevalence of blood transfusions and immunosuppression. In rodents, the effect of class II matching was not consistent [49–51], while large animal models for class II matching have been limited by dependence on rare intra-MHC recombinants among siblings [1], or the use of serologic and mixed lymphocyte reactivity typing as a measure of class II identity [2, 43, 52]. Such large animal models have therefore suffered from an inability to repeat specific combinations of matching and the uncertainty of genotypic class II matching among outbred populations.

The availability of the porcine recombinant haplotype *g* [18, 19] has obviated the problems found in the other large animal models, permitting unlimited repetition of similarly matched combinations, and permitting transplants between animals of known genotype, matching selectively for either class I or class II loci.

Of course, genotypic matching for the MHC is generally not available in man. Results from experimental studies such as these with swine could, however, indicate whether perfect matching for class I or class II antigens would be necessary or beneficial for allograft survival. Therefore a series of transplants was performed between animals of the *g* and *c* haplotypes (class I-matched) and the *g* and *d* haplotypes (class II-matched) [53]. As with all of our transplants, only O blood group animals were used, and other untyped minor histocompatibility differences existed between the animals. All the *dd* animals were of the acceptor phenotype (i.e., they would accept MHC-matched grafts) [41]. Since no in vitro assay is available for the non-MHC-linked Ir gene, all other animals were of unknown Ir gene status, but, as discussed above, a percentage of the recipients were likely to be of rejector phenotype. Recipients underwent bilateral nephrectomy and placement of a left renal allograft according to our standard protocol [53]. Serial posttransplant blood urea nitrogen and creatinine values were obtained to assess renal function. Rejection was defined as death of the animal with uremia and confirmatory gross and microscopic pathology. No exogenous immunosuppression nor blood transfusions were given to avoid confounding the effect of matching.

The overall results [53] are shown in Fig. 6. As discussed above and in confirmation of previous results, the MHC had a powerful effect on allograft survival, such that all fully mismatched grafts were rejected by day 15, while MHC-matched grafts enjoyed longer survival. The division of MHC-matched grafts into those 20% that survived permanently and the remainder that were rejected was similar to that reported previously as the effect of a non-MHC-linked Ir gene [41].

Class I MHC matching alone was first performed using reciprocal transplants between animals of the *ag* and *ac* genotypes to address the question of whether class I matching alone would be sufficient to prolong survival over the fully

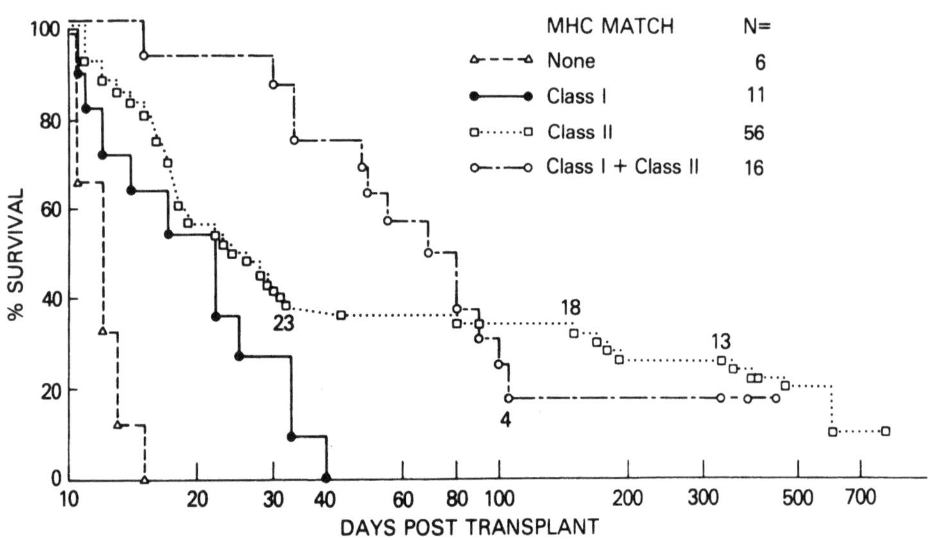

Fig. 6. Overall results of renal allografts in miniature swine. Life table survival curves are shown for each degree of MHC matching. Deaths from all causes after a technically succesful transplant are included. (Reproduced from [53] by copyright permission of The Rockefeller University Press)

mismatched group. These class I matched grafts did in fact have prolonged survival compared to the fully mismatched grafts, but were all eventually rejected (Fig. 6). Although all of the *ac* animals were presumably of the rejector phenotype [41], extrapolating from the class II matched results (see below), about half of the *ag* animals should have been of the acceptor phenotype. To assure that presence of the non-MHC-linked Ir gene did not prevent acceptance, *ag* acceptor animals (i.e., the progeny of animals that had accepted renal allografts) were similarly transplanted and they too rejected *ac* grafts. Acceptor animals of the *ac* genotype are currently being bred to test the reciprocal direction. Therefore, although class I matching does lead to prolonged renal allograft survival over fully mismatched combinations, the class II mismatch appeared sufficient to always cause rejection.

In contrast to class I matching alone, class II matching alone did lead to permanent (>1 year) allograft survival in approximately 30% of animals (Fig. 6). This survival was similar to that of fully MHC-matched animals. The overall survival curve for these animals appears to be bimodal, with 60% of animals rejecting their grafts with a time-course identical to that of class I matched animals (although prolonged over fully mismatched animals), while the remaining 40% showed prolonged or permanent survival. The bimodal nature of the survival can be seen better and at least three factors regulating survival can be identified when the results are analyzed according to specific class II-matched donor-recipient pairs (Fig. 7):

First, mismatched class I antigen gene dose affected length of survival in *dd* recipients of *gg* vs *dg* grafts (groups 6 and 7) and affected the number of permanent survivors in *gg* recipients of *dg* vs *dd* grafts (groups 3 and 4). This antigen-dose effect has been seen in other systems but no satisfactory explanation for it is available [54].

Second, an MHC-linked effect was apparent in that *dd* animals always rejected *dg* grafts, while *gg* animals always accepted *dg* grafts (groups 3 and 6). The decreased survival of the *dd* recipients could have resulted either from a greater response capacity of the *dd* animals than of the *gg* animals, or from a greater antigenicity of class I^c than class I^d. In vitro CML and MLR reactivity is also usually greater in the *d* anti-*c* direction for fully MHC-mismatched animals.

The non-MHC-linked Ir gene previously described for MHC-matched grafts [41] may also have been involved in the *ag*/*ad* reciprocal transplants. In both of these combinations (groups 1 and 5), one-third to one-half of the kidneys survived permanently, while the remainder were rejected by 30 days, a pattern similar to that reported initially for the non-MHC-linked Ir gene in the MHC-matched, minor-antigen-mismatched situation. The *a* and *g* haplotypes were often mated with the *c* haplotype in which this Ir gene segregated. In fact, as discussed above, the original *g* animal was the progeny of a *cd* parent. Therefore, it is likely that the rejector gene was segregating in these *ag* and *ad* animals. Since the presence of the rejector gene causes rejection across minor antigen differences alone, and since minor antigen differences in addition to the class I differences were also present in the class II-matched pairs, it would be expected that the rejector gene would lead to rejection across this greater degree of mismatch as well. The rejector gene from the previous MHC matched studies was apparently dominant. If this same gene functions similarly in the class II-only matched setting, then it would be predicted that all of the progeny of the class II-only matched acceptor by ac-

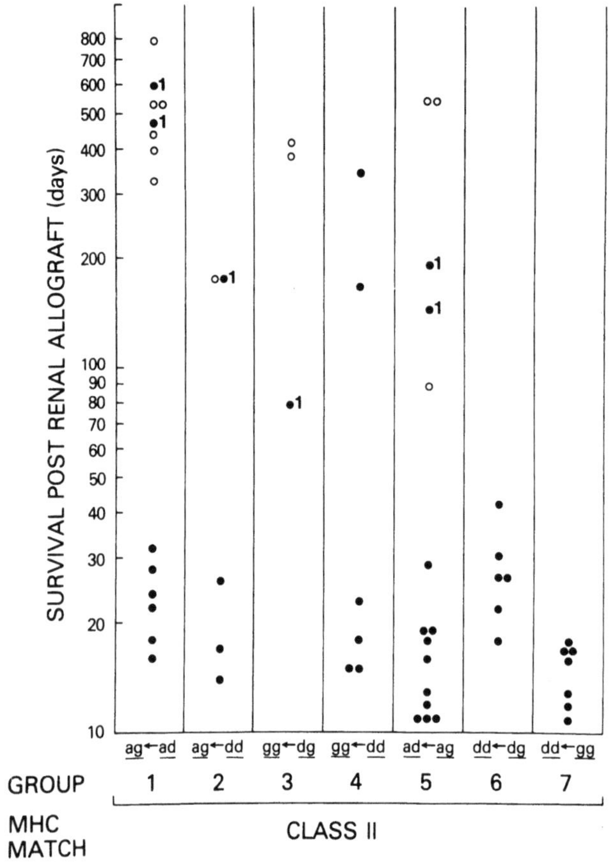

Fig. 7. Analysis of class II-matched renal allograft survival by specific donor-recipient combinations. The recipient MHC type is indicated by the pair of *letters* to the left of each arrow. Animals still alive at the time of analysis (○) and those that died of rejection (●) are indicated. Each circle indicates one animal. A *1* indicates that the animal died from nonrenal causes. (Reproduced from [53] by copyright permission of The Rockefeller University Press)

ceptor breedings should also be acceptors. Such animals are currently being examined to test this hypothesis.

Relevance of the Porcine Model to Human Kidney Transplants

The results reviewed here indicate that class II antigen matching alone leads to prolonged renal allograft survival in pigs. These studies also demonstrate that many other factors contribute to the ultimate result of allograft survival or rejection, including mismatched antigen gene dose, an MHC-linked effect, and a non-MHC-linked Ir gene.

With certain of the swine class II-matched groups, there was a clear advantage in also matching for class I (e.g., *dd* recipients of dg versus *gg* kidney; Fig. 2). In man, the mismatched class I gene dose has been reported to have an inconsistent effect on survival in the presence of DR matching. In cadaver grafts, Ting and

Morris found no greater survival in patients matched for class I as well as class II [55], while Soulillou et al. found an additional increase in survival when also matching for class I [56]. Finally, Watanabe et al. found no difference between one or two HLA-AB-mismatched but DR-identical living related donor transplants (a situation more analogous to the miniature swine model [57]). However, in all these reports, DR matching was phenotypic rather than genotypic, and patients were also given the usual immunosuppression.

In man, the DR6 allele has been reported to be associated with a higher rejection rate [45]. The mechanism behind this is not clear, but it has been suggested that DR6 may function as an Ir gene for MHC antigens. An MHC-linked Ir gene for MHC antigens has also been proposed to explain results of rat skin graft studies [44]. The MHC-linked Ir effect observed in the pig differs from these other systems, however, in that the *gg* and *dd* animals are genotypically identical for class II. Therefore, the gene(s) responsible for the difference in survival must be either class I or closely linked to class I. Isakov recently reported similar results of nonreciprocal survival (i.e., MHC-linked Ir effect) with certain murine thyroid allografts, and suggested that the different survival he had seen resulted from different CTL precursor frequencies [58]. Such studies have not been performed in the pig, and no reports in man have described a similar increase in rejection frequency across specific class I-only differences, although human data would be difficult to analyze in this fashion.

Finally, there is suggestive evidence of other Ir genes in man and monkeys similar to the non-MHC-linked Ir gene seen in the pig. In monkeys that were phenotypically class II-matched, a bimodal survival pattern of renal allografts was found [2, 43], and in man a bimodal pattern of rejection episodes was reported [42]. In both of these systems it would be difficult to prove that the results are due to an Ir gene(s) or to demonstrate non-MHC linkage, since the selective breeding we used to study this phenomenon would be prohibitively time-consuming in monkeys and of course unavailable in man. It might, though, be possible to test recipients prior to transplantation for the presence of such a gene(s). In fact, many studies have been described attempting to predict immune responsiveness prior to transplantation [59]. We are currently examining a variety of non-MHC-linked genetic markers in the pig for possible linkage to the Ir gene.

References

1. Bijnen AB, Westbroek DL, Obertop H, Vriesendorp HM (1979) Genetics of kidney allograft survival in dogs. I. Relevance of subregions of the major histocompatibility complex in recipients without immunosuppressive therapy. Transplantation 28:186–190
2. van Es AA, Balner H (1978) Serologic matching for D locus antigens improves kidney allograft survival in rhesus monkeys. Transplantation 26:187–190
3. Vaiman M, Garnier H, Kunklin A, Hay JM, Parc R, Bacour F, Fagniez PH, Villiers PA, Lecointre J, Bara MF, Nizza P (1972) The SL-A histocompatibility system in the *Sus scrofa* species. Transplantation 14:541–550
4. Fabre JW (1982) Rat kidney allograft model: was it all too good to be true? Transplantation 34:223–225
5. Almaraz R, Ballinger W, Sachs DH, Rosenberg SA (1983) The effect of peripheral lymphoid cells on the incidence of lethal graft versus host disease following allogeneic bone marrow transplantation. J Surg Res 34:133–144

6. Filipovich AH, Ramsay NHC, McGlave P, Quinones R, Winslow C, Heinitz KJ, Arthur D, Kersey JH (1983) Mismatched bone marrow transplantation at the University of Minnesota: use of related donors other than HLA MLC identicle siblings and T cell depletion. In: Gale RP (ed) Recent advances in bone marrow transplantation. Liss, New York, NY, pp 769–783
7. Sachs DH, Leight G, Cone J, Schwarz S, Stuart L, Rosenberg S (1976) Transplantation in miniature swine. I. Fixation of the major histocompatibility complex. Transplantation 22:559–567
8. Vaiman M, Renard C, LaFage P, Ameteau J, Nizza P (1970) Evidence for histocompatibility system in swine (SL-A). Transplantation 10:155–164
9. Metzger JJ, Lunney JK, Sachs DH, Rudikoff S (1982) Transplantation in miniature swine. XII. N-terminal sequences of class I histocompatibility antigens (SLA) and β_2 microglobulin. J Immunol 129:716–721
10. Singer DS, Camerini-Otero RD, Satz ML, Osborne B, Sachs D, Rudikoff S (1982) Characterization of a porcine genomic clone encoding a major histocompatibility antigen: expression in mouse L cells. Proc Natl Acad Sci USA 79:1403–1407
11. Osborne BA, Lunney JK, Pennington L, Sachs DH, Rudikoff S (1983) Twodimensional gel analysis of swine histocompatibility antigens. J Immunol 131:2939–2944
12. Vaiman M, Chardon P, Renard P (1979) Genetic organization of the pig SLA complex. Studies on nine recombinants and biochemical and lysostrip analysis. Immunogenetics 9:353–361
13. Lunney JK, Sachs DH (1978) Transplantation in miniature swine. IV. Chemical characterization of MSLA and Ia-like antigens. J Immunol 120:607–612
14. Lunney JK, Sachs DH (1979) Transplantation in miniature swine. V. Characterization of Ia antigens. J Immunol 122:623–627
15. Lunney JK, Osborne BA, Sharrow SO, Devaux C, Pierres M, Sachs DH (1983) Sharing of Ia antigens between species. IV. Interspecies cross-reactivity of monoclonal antibodies directed against polymorphic mouse Ia determinants. J Immunol 130:2786–2793
16. Steinmetz M, Hood L (1983) Genes of the major histocompatibility complex in mouse and man. Science 222:727–733
17. Steinmetz M (1985) Organization of MHC genes. In: Streilein JW, Ahmad F, Black S, Blomberg B, Voellmy RW (eds) Advances in gene technology: molecular biology of the immune system. Proceedings of the 17th Miami Winter Symposium. ICSU Press, Cambridge, England, pp 23–26
18. Pennington LR; Lunney JK, Sachs DH (1981) Transplantation in miniature swine. VIII. Recombination within the major histocompatibility complex of miniature swine. Transplantation 31:66–71
19. Thistlethwaite JR Jr, Pennington LR, Lunney JK, Sachs DH (1983) Immunologic characterization of MHC recombinant swine: production of SLA class specific antisera and detection of Ia antigens on both B and non-B PBL. Transplantation 35:394–400
20. Porter RR (1985) The complement genes of the HLA complex. In: Streilein JW, Ahmad F, Black S, Blomberg B, Voellmy RW (eds) Advances in gene technology: molecular biology of the immune system. Proceedings of the 17th Miami Winter Symposium. ICSU Press, Cambridge, England, pp 77–80
21. Chaplin DD, Woods DE, Whitehead AS, Goldberger G, Colten HR, Seidman JG (1983) Molecular map of the murine S region. Proc Natl Acad Sci USA 80:6947–6951
22. Vaiman M, Hauptmann G, Mayer S (1978) Influence of the major histocompatibility complex in the pig (SLA) on serum haemolytic complement levels. J Immunogenet 5:59–65
23. Rubinstein P, Vienne K (1982) Genetic control of the quantitative variation of erythrocytic glyoxalase-1 (GLO-1) in mice. Biochem Genet 20:153–162
24. Stolc V, Kunz HW, Gill III TS (1980) The linkage of glyoxylase-1 to the major histocompatibility complex in the rat. J Immunol 125:1167–1170
25. Weitkamp LR (1976) Linkage of GLO with HLA and BF. Effect of population and sex on recombination frequency. Tissue Antigens 7:273–279
26. Shackelford DA, Kaufman JF, Korman AJ, Strominger JL (1982) HLA-DR antigens: Structure, separation of subpopulations, gene cloning and function. Immunol Rev 66:133–187

27. Thistlethwaite JR Jr, Auchincloss H Jr, Pescovitz MD, Sachs DH (1984) Immunologic characterization of MHC recombinant swine: role of class I and II antigens in in vitro immune responses. J Immunogenet 11:9–19
28. Norcross MA, Bentley DM, Margulies DH, Germain R (1984) Membrane Ia expression and antigen-presenting accessory cell function of L cells transfected with class II major histocompatibility complex genes. J Exp Med 160:1316–1337
29. Vaiman M, Metzger JJ, Renard C, Vila JP (1978) Immune response gene(s) controlling the humoral anti-lysozyme response (Ir-lys) linked to the major histocompatibility complex SL-A in the pig. Immunogenetics 7:231–238
30. Benson EM, Colvin RB, Russell PS (1985) Induction of Ia antigens in murine renal transplants. J Immunol 134:7–9
31. Hart DNJ, Fabre JW (1981) Major histocompatibility complex antigens in rat kidney, ureter, and bladder. Transplantation 31:318–325
32. Lechler RI, Batchelor JR (1982) Restoration of immunogenicity to passenger cell-depleted kidney allografts by the addition of donor strain dendritic cells. J Exp Med 155:31–41
33. McKenzie JL, Beard MEJ, Hart DNJ (1984) The effect of donor pretreatment on interstitial dendritic cell content and rat cardiac allograft survival. Transplantation 38:371–376
34. Hart DNJ, Fuggle SV, Williams KA, Fabre JW, Ting A, Morris PJ (1981) Localization of HLA-ABC and DR antigens in human kidney. Transplantation 31:428–433
35. Lafferty K (1980) Immunogenicity of foreign tissues. Transplantation 29:179–182
36. Pescovitz MD, Sachs DH, Lunney JK, Hsu SM (1984) Localization of class II MHC antigens on porcine renal vascular endothelium. Transplantation 37:627–630
37. Calne RY, Sells RA, Pena JR, Davis DR, Millard PR, Hebertson BM, Binns RM, Davies DAL (1969) Induction of immunological tolerance by porcine liver allografts. Nature 223:472–476
38. Flye MW (1980) Immunological assessment of orthotopic liver transplantation in both outbred and MSLA defined inbred miniature swine. Thesis, Duke University, Durham
39. Kirkman RL, Colvin RB, Flye MW, Leight GS, Rosenberg SA, Williams GM, Sachs DH (1979) Transplantation in miniature swine. VI. Factors influencing survival of renal allografts. Transplantation 28:18–23
40. Leight GS, Kirkman R, Rasmusen BA, Rosenberg SA, Sachs DH, Terrill R, Williams GM (1978) Transplantation in miniature swine. III. Effect of MSLA and A-O blood group matching on skin allograft survival. Tissue Antigens 12:65–74
41. Pennington LR, Flye MW, Kirkman RL, Thistlethwaite JR Jr, Williams GM, Sachs DH (1981) Transplantation in miniature swine. X. Evidence for non-SLA-linked immune response gene(s) controlling rejection of SLA-matched kidney allografts. Transplantation 32:315–320
42. Schulak JA, Goeken NE, Nghiem DD, Corry RJ (1982) Effect of DR matching on rejection in first cadaver kidney transplantation. Transplantation 34:382–384
43. Borleffs JCC, Marquet RL, deBy-Aghai Z, van Vreeswijk W, Neuhaus P, Balner H (1982) Kidney transplantation in rhesus monkeys: matching for D/DR antigens, pretransplant blood transfusions, and immunologic monitoring before transplantation. Transplantation 33:285–290
44. Howard JC, Butcher GW (1981) The mechanism of graft rejection and the concept of antigenic strength. Scand J Immunol 14:687–691
45. Hendricks GFJ, Claas FHJ, Persijn GG, Witvliet MD, Baldwin W, van Rood JJ (1983) HLA-DRw6-positive recipients are high responders in renal transplantation. Transplant Proc 14:1136–1138
46. Kirkman RL, Colvin RB, Flye MW, Williams GM, Sachs DH (1979) Transplantation in miniature swine. VII. Evidence for cellular immune mechanisms in hyperacute rejection of renal allografts. Transplantation 28:24–30
47. Berg B, Moller E (1981) The influence of HLA-DR match on the outcome of cadaver renal transplantation in Stockholm during 1977–1980. Tissue Antigens 18:316–328
48. Opelz G, Terasaki PI (1980) International histocompatibility workshop study on renal transplantation. In: Terasaki PI (ed) Histocompatibility testing 1980. UCLA Tissue Typing Laboratory, Los Angeles, pp 592–624
49. Aizawa M (1984) Transplantation immunobiology in the rat. In: Yamamura VY, Tada T (eds) Progress in immunology. Academic, Japan, pp 1439–1448

50. Paris A, Gunther E (1980) Kidney grafting between rats which carry recombinant major histocompatibility haplotypes. Immunogenetics 10:205–209
51. Gallico GG, Butcher GW, Howard JC (1979) The role of subregions of the rat major histocompatibility complex in the rejection and passive enhancement of renal allografts. J Exp Med 149:244–253
52. Borleffs JCC, de By-Aghai Z, Balner H (1981) Variable "predictive value" of matching for MLC nonresponsiveness in rhesus monkeys. Transplant Proc 13:1057–1060
53. Pescovitz MD, Thistlethwaite JR Jr, Auchincloss H Jr, Ildstad ST, Sharp TG, Terrill R, Sachs DH (1984) Effects of class II antigen matching on renal allograft survival in miniature swine. J Exp Med 160:1495–1505
54. Pettirossi O, Sakai A, Kountz SL (1976) Differential survivals of F1 hybrid allografts in parental recipients. Transplantation 21:403–407
55. Ting A, Morris PJ (1984) The influence of HLA-A,B and -DR matching and pregraft blood transfusions on graft and patient survival after renal transplantation in a single centre. Tissue Antigens 24:256–264
56. Soulillou JP, Bignon JD, Houmant M, Ythier A, Cozian A, Faye R, Lecogic G, Guenel J (1982) Effect of HLA-A,B, and DR typing, pregraft blood transfusions, and positive anti-B lymphocyte cross matches on kidney-graft survival – a one-center prospective study. Transplant Proc 14:187–190
57. Watanabe K, Sada M, Uchida H, Endo T, Kashiwagi N (1983) Effects of DR matching and B-cell antibodies on related kidney graft survival. Transplant Proc 15:130–133
58. Isakov N, Bach FH (1984) High frequency of splenic anti-class I cytotoxic T lymphocyte precursors correlates with in vivo rejection of K/D region disparate thyroid and islet grafts in mice. J Immunol 132:50–56
59. Thorsby E, Ettenger R, Garovoy M (1984) Pretransplant immunologic considerations. Transplant Proc 16:1649–1653

Subject Index

MIX
Papier aus verantwortungsvollen Quellen
Paper from responsible sources
FSC® C105338

If you have any concerns about our products,
you can contact us on
ProductSafety@springernature.com

In case Publisher is established outside the EU,
the EU authorized representative is:
Springer Nature Customer Service Center GmbH
Europaplatz 3, 69115 Heidelberg, Germany

Printed by Libri Plureos GmbH
in Hamburg, Germany